Textbook of
Orthopedic Rheumatology

Textbook of
Orthopedic Rheumatology

Under Aegis of Indian Orthopaedic Rheumatology Association

Editor-in-Chief
Manish Khanna
President Emeritus, Indian Orthopaedic Rheumatology Association
Chairperson, Indian Stem Cell Study Group Association
Professor
Department of Orthopedics
Lucknow, Uttar Pradesh, India

Co-Editors
Madhan Jeyaraman
Department of Orthopedics
School of Medical Sciences and Research
Sharda University
Greater Noida, Uttar Pradesh, India

Sathish Muthu
Department of Orthopedics
Government Medical College and Hospital
Dindigul, Tamil Nadu, India

Forewords
Professor GS Kulkarni
Professor M Shantharam Shetty

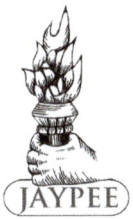

JAYPEE BROTHERS MEDICAL PUBLISHERS
The Health Sciences Publisher
New Delhi | London

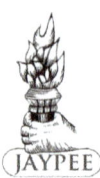 **Jaypee Brothers Medical Publishers (P) Ltd**

Headquarters

Jaypee Brothers Medical Publishers (P) Ltd
EMCA House, 23/23-B
Ansari Road, Daryaganj
New Delhi 110 002, India
Landline: +91-11-23272143, +91-11-23272703
+91-11-23282021, +91-11-23245672
Email: jaypee@jaypeebrothers.com

Corporate Office

Jaypee Brothers Medical Publishers (P) Ltd
4838/24, Ansari Road, Daryaganj
New Delhi 110 002, India
Phone: +91-11-43574357
Fax: +91-11-43574314
Email: jaypee@jaypeebrothers.com

Overseas Office

JP Medical Ltd
83 Victoria Street, London
SW1H 0HW (UK)
Phone: +44 20 3170 8910
Fax: +44 (0)20 3008 6180
Email: info@jpmedpub.com

Website: www.jaypeebrothers.com
Website: www.jaypeedigital.com

© 2022, Jaypee Brothers Medical Publishers

The views and opinions expressed in this book are solely those of the original contributor(s)/author(s) and do not necessarily represent those of editor(s) of the book.

All rights reserved. No part of this publication may be reproduced, stored or transmitted in any form or by any means, electronic, mechanical, photocopying, recording or otherwise, without the prior permission in writing of the publishers.

All brand names and product names used in this book are trade names, service marks, trademarks or registered trademarks of their respective owners. The publisher is not associated with any product or vendor mentioned in this book.

Medical knowledge and practice change constantly. This book is designed to provide accurate, authoritative information about the subject matter in question. However, readers are advised to check the most current information available on procedures included and check information from the manufacturer of each product to be administered, to verify the recommended dose, formula, method and duration of administration, adverse effects and contraindications. It is the responsibility of the practitioner to take all appropriate safety precautions. Neither the publisher nor the author(s)/editor(s) assume any liability for any injury and/or damage to persons or property arising from or related to use of material in this book.

This book is sold on the understanding that the publisher is not engaged in providing professional medical services. If such advice or services are required, the services of a competent medical professional should be sought.

Every effort has been made where necessary to contact holders of copyright to obtain permission to reproduce copyright material. If any have been inadvertently overlooked, the publisher will be pleased to make the necessary arrangements at the first opportunity. The **CD/DVD-ROM** (if any) provided in the sealed envelope with this book is complimentary and free of cost. **Not meant for sale.**

Inquiries for bulk sales may be solicited at: jaypee@jaypeebrothers.com

Textbook of Orthopedic Rheumatology

First Edition: 2022

ISBN: 978-93-5465-187-8

Dedicated to

My parents, teachers, mentors, students and my patients who continue to provide lot of stimulating challenges in our clinical practice.

Contributors

Aarti B Bhattacharya
Professor
Department of Pathology
Hind Institute of Medical Sciences
Lucknow, Uttar Pradesh, India

Abhay Elhence
Professor
Department of Orthopedics
All India Institute of Medical Sciences
Jodhpur, Rajasthan, India

Abhinandan Reddy M
Junior Consultant
Department of Spine Surgery
Indian Spinal Injury Center
New Delhi, India

Ajay SS
Senior Resident
Department of Orthopedics
Sri Devaraj Urs Medical College
Kolar, Karnataka, India

Alok Chandra Agrawal
Professor
Department of Orthopedics
All India Institute of Medical Sciences
Raipur, Chhattisgarh, India

Amrit Kumar Singh
Junior Resident
Department of Orthopedics
School of Medical Sciences and Research
Sharda University
Greater Noida, Uttar Pradesh India

Anil Gowtham Manivannan
Consultant Orthopedic Surgeon
Department of Orthopedics
Arathana Hospital
Pollachi, Tamil Nadu, India

Ankit Kumar Garg
Senior Resident
Department of Orthopedics
All India Institute of Medical Sciences
Raipur, Chhattisgarh, India

Anupam Inamdar
Senior Resident
Department of Orthopedics
All India Institute of Medical Sciences
Raipur, Chhattisgarh, India

Arun Gulati
Senior Resident
Department of Orthopedics
Kalpana Chawla Government Medical College
Karnal, Haryana, India

Arun Kumar Sharma
Associate Professor
Department of Orthopedics
SMS Medical College and Hospital
Jaipur, Rajasthan, India

Arunabh Arora
Junior Resident
Department of Orthopedics
School of Medical Sciences and Research
Sharda University
Greater Noida, Uttar Pradesh India

Arvind Kanchan
Professor
Department of Physiology
Hind Institute of Medical Sciences
Lucknow, Uttar Pradesh, India

Bhaskar Borgohain
Professor
Department of Orthopedics
North Eastern Indira Gandhi Regional Institute of Health and Medical Sciences
Shillong, Meghalaya, India

Bikram Kar
Associate Professor
Department of Orthopedics
All India Institute of Medical Sciences
Raipur, Chhattisgarh, India

Dushyant Chaudhary
Junior Resident
Department of Orthopedics
School of Medical Sciences and Research
Sharda University
Greater Noida, Uttar Pradesh India

Gyaneshwar Tonk
Professor
Department of Orthopedics
LLRM Medical College
Meerut, Uttar Pradesh, India

Harshal Sakale
Associate Professor
Department of Orthopedics
All India Institute of Medical Sciences
Raipur, Chhattisgarh, India

J Mangwani
Consultant Orthopedic Foot and Ankle Surgeon
Department of Orthopedics
University Hospitals of Leicester
Leicester, UK

Jitendra Chowdhary
Consultant
Department of Orthopedics
Orthopedic Centre
Jain Knee and Hip Clinic
Ahmedabad, Gujarat, India

Jitesh K Jain
Consultant Orthopedic and Sports Surgeon
Department of Orthopedics
Rajasthan Hospital
Jaipur, Rajasthan, India

Kashif A Ahmed
Consultant Orthopedic Surgeon
Department of Orthopedics
Rahman Hospital
Guwahati, Assam, India

Krishna Subramanyam
Consultant Orthopedic Surgeon
Department of Orthopedics and Sports Medicine
Yashoda Hospital
Hyderabad, Telangana, India

Kushal Singh
Assistant Professor
Department of Radiodiagnosis
Hind Institute of Medical Sciences
Lucknow, Uttar Pradesh, India

Lalit Kishore
Consultant Orthopedic Surgeon
Department of Orthopedics
Rajeshwar Hospital
Patna, Bihar, India

Contributors

Madhan Jeyaraman
Senior Resident
Department of Orthopedics
School of Medical Sciences and Research
Sharda University
Greater Noida, Uttar Pradesh India

Mahaveer Mali
Senior Resident
Department of Orthopedics
All India Institute of Medical Sciences
Jodhpur, Rajasthan, India

Manish Khanna
President Emeritus
Indian Orthopaedic Rheumatology Association
Chairperson, Indian Stem Cell Study Group Association
Professor
Department of Orthopedics
Lucknow, Uttar Pradesh, India

Manju Agrawal
Assistant Professor
Department of Pharmacology
Pt JNM Medical College
Raipur, Chhattisgarh, India

Md Neshar Ansari
Assistant Professor
Department of Orthopedics
Hind Institute of Medical Sciences
Lucknow, Uttar Pradesh, India

Mukund Madhav Ojha
Senior Resident
Department of Orthopedics
All India Institute of Medical Sciences
Raipur, Chhattisgarh, India

N Nanavati

Naveen Jeyaraman
Senior Resident
Department of Orthopedics
School of Medical Sciences and Research
Sharda University
Greater Noida, Uttar Pradesh India

Neeraj Jain
Consultant Rheumatologist
Department of Rheumatology
Sir Ganga Ram Hospital
New Delhi, India

Omkarnath Gudapati
Professor
Department of Orthopedics
Great Eastern Medical School and Hospital
Ragolu, Andhra Pradesh, India

Prajwal GS
Junior Resident
Department of Orthopedics
JJM Medical College
Davanagere, Karnataka, India

Rahul Ranjan
Assistant Professor
Department of Orthopedics
Darbhanga Medical College
Darbhanga, Bihar, India

Raja TV
Consultant Orthopedic Surgeon
Department of Orthopedics
Visa Medicure
Chennai, Tamil Nadu, India

Rajiv Lakhotia
Professor
Department of Anesthesiology
Hind Institute of Medical Sciences
Lucknow, Uttar Pradesh, India

Rajni Ranjan
Professor
Department of Orthopedics
School of Medical Sciences and Research
Sharda University
Greater Noida, Uttar Pradesh India

Rakesh Kumar
Associate Professor
Department of Orthopedics
School of Medical Sciences and Research
Sharda University
Greater Noida, Uttar Pradesh India

Rashmi Chopra
Orthopedic Consultant Hand and Wrist Surgeon
Department of Orthopedics
Apollo Spectra Hospitals
New Delhi, India

Rashmi Jain
Resident
School of Medical Sciences and Research
Sharda University
Greater Noida, Uttar Pradesh India

Ravi VR
Consultant Orthopedic Surgeon
Department of Orthopedics
Maruti Hospital
Tiruchirappalli, Tamil Nadu India

RB Kalia
Additional Professor
Department of Orthopedics
All Institute of Medical Sciences
Rishikesh, Uttarakhand, India

RC Meena
Professor
Department of Orthopedics
SMS Medical College and Hospital
Jaipur, Rajasthan, India

Sathish Muthu
Assistant Professor
Department of Orthopedics
Government Medical College and Hospital
Dindigul, Tamil Nadu, India

Shashank Tiwari
Consultant Medical Ethics and Clinical Research
Lucknow, Uttar Pradesh, India

Shantanu Lahkar
Consultant Orthopedic Surgeon
Department of Orthopedics
Archana Trauma and Orthopedic Hospital
Dibrugarh, Assam, India

Shilp Verma
Senior Resident
Department of Orthopedics
All India Institute of Medical Sciences
Raipur, Chhattisgarh, India

Shilpa Sharma
Professor
Department of Pediatric Surgery
All India Institute of Medical Sciences
New Delhi, India

Shivakumar Bingi
Consultant Orthopedic Surgeon
Department of Orthopedics
Fortis Hospital
Bengaluru, Karnataka, India

Shivaraj B
Consultant Orthopedic Surgeon
Department of Orthopedics
Fortis Hospital
Bengaluru, Karnataka, India

Shweta Agarwal
Associate Professor
Department of Medicine
Career Institute of Medical Sciences and Hospital
Lucknow, Uttar Pradesh, India

Sribatsa Kumar Mohapatra
Professor
Department of Surgery
Veer Surendra Sai Institute of Medical Sciences and Research
Burla, Odisha, India

SS Jha
Consultant Orthopedic Surgeon
Department of Orthopedics
Harishchandra Orthopaedic
Research Institute
Patna, Bihar, India

Subir Kumar Mukherjee
Consultant Orthopedic Surgeon
Department of Orthopedics
Raipur, Chhattisgarh, India

Sujit Kumar
Senior Resident
Department of Orthopedics
LLRM Medical College
Meerut, Uttar Pradesh, India

Sunil Kumar Gupta
Associate Professor
Department of Dermatology
All India Institute of Medical Sciences
Gorakhpur, Uttar Pradesh, India

THS Bedi
Chief Radiologist
Department of Radiodiagnosis
Bedi Ultrasound Clinic
New Delhi, India

Utkarsh Bansal
Professor
Department of Pediatrics
Hind Institute of Medical Sciences
Lucknow, Uttar Pradesh, India

V Adukia

Venus Khanna
Professor
Department of Pathology
Prasad Institute of Medical Sciences
Lucknow, Uttar Pradesh, India

Vipul Sud
Consultant Plastic Surgeon
Department of Plastic and
Reconstructive Surgery
Batra Hospital and
Medical Research Centre
New Delhi, India

Foreword

I am pleased to write the foreword for this most-needed book on ortho-rheumatology, edited by Manish Khanna. He is a great visionary. It is his idea to start a new branch of orthopedics, "ortho-rheumatology" as a superspecialty in India. He is passionately dedicated to this superspecialty. For the last 25 years he has conducted lectures, conferences and webinars on this topic. This is comparatively a new specialty which has spread over globally. This is a comprehensive book combining the two large branches—medical and orthopedic rheumatology. This book not only covers medical and surgical rheumatology but also related arthropathies, basic sciences and crystal arthritis—a truly comprehensive book. All contributors are authorities in their fields. He has formed, "Indian Stem Sell Study Group Association". In this book, a section is devoted to Regenerative Science in Orthopedic Rheumatology. He is also the Editor-in-Chief of International Journal of Orthopedic Rheumatology.

This book will be of great use not only to general orthopedic surgeons, but also to hand surgeons, foot specialists and spine surgeons as well. I sincerely congratulate Professor Manish Khanna for bringing out this most useful book.

With best wishes.

Professor GS Kulkarni
Director, Postgraduate Institute of Orthopedics, Miraj
Director, Sandhata Medical Research Society
Miraj, Maharashtra, India

Foreword

It is indeed my privilege to script the foreword for this important *Textbook of Orthopedic Rheumatology* edited by Manish Khanna. Rheumatology by itself is a vast specialty involving many specialists requiring a comprehensive care. Orthopedics compiled with rheumatology can play a vital role to put back a crippled patient to fairly normal activity.

This book with various chapters deals with basic sciences to various orthopedic disorders related to rheumatology. There is also a chapter on regenerative medicine and its application in patients with ortho-rheumatological disorders.

Unfortunately, even today with all the biological pursuits, the scientists have achieved, patients with various rheumatological disorders still suffer. I am sure this book with various subsections authored by reputed clinicians and researchers will provide definite guidelines on the management of different orthopedic rheumatological disorders. There is no doubt that this script will not only be a guide to the postgraduates and treating surgeons, but also to the orthopedic fraternity as a whole.

I wish the Editor-in-Chief and all those who have subscribed to this useful book all the very best and may God bless you in all their future endeavors.

With best wishes,

Professor M Shantharam Shetty
Past President, Indian Orthopaedic Association
Pro Chancellor, Nitte University, Mangalore
Chairman, Tejasvini Hospital Group of Institutions
Mangalore, Karnataka, India

Preface

Most often for treating complicated medical ailments there is a common need for involvement of various medical specialists for planning the treatment protocol. Ailments like bone and joint diseases are usually treated by Orthopedists who delve into a more surgical treatment approach. However, the treatment procedure for such patients who have autoimmune diseases and various forms of arthritis is often inclined towards a nonsurgical approach, especially during the initial phase of the disease which is something that is covered under the scope of ortho-rheumatology. While over the years, the patients have either approached rheumatologists first, prior to consulting an orthopedist, and vice versa, the process is often long and tiresome. The similarity between symptoms leads to confusion among patients and sometime delay in the care which results in a progression of the severity. Often times, patients are forced to alternate between two different clinics to merge together one concise plan of treatment. Not to mention, also patients often remain in pain due to the lack of awareness and inability to have access to specialists from two different medical backgrounds to provide them with relief.

The *Textbook of Orthopedic Rheumatology* for orthopedic surgeons aims to lessen this gap and delay in care by bringing forward the awareness and combining two specializations to provide in the needy patients with cutting edge therapies along with a combination of traditionally approached plans. The main aim of this book is to create awareness amongst orthopedic surgeons whilst encouraging broadened research and development.

The book delves into the continuous need for consistency in clinical care. A new wave of emerging high-quality treatment programs for patients who struggle with disease management is set to be the new evolving specialization of orthopedic rheumatology. The integration of orthopedics and rheumatology enables patients to receive the best possible care under one roof for their ailments, thereby minimizing patient effort and ensuring quick and early treatment of progressive ailments.

In addition to covering the technological aspects of this modern medicinal system, this book will target beginning specialists to develop a deeper interest in this combined specialty. The contents of book are prompted by the growing need for understanding, detailed healthcare plans and a full-fledged medical approach to the treatment of ailments that co-exist in a number of orthopedic intervention-beneficial rheumatoid patients.

Manish Khanna

Acknowledgments

I would firstly like to be grateful to the Almighty, who brought the idea to my mind for publishing a textbook on Orthopedic Rheumatology for the orthopedic surgeons. We are further grateful to the tremendous work of the contributors without whom this book would not be possible. I would like to acknowledge the dynamic, stimulating work of our Co-Editors Dr Madhan Jeyaraman and Dr Sathish Muthu who are the real pillars of the various academic work of the *Textbook of Orthopedic Rheumatology*. My heartful thanks to both of these young, dynamic orthopedic surgeons for continuously supporting the project. I would also like to acknowledge the excellent team work for the production of the book by M/s Jaypee Brothers Medical Publishers (P) Ltd, New Delhi, India, especially to Shri Jitendar P Vij (Group Chairman), Mr Ankit Vij (Managing Director), Mr MS Mani (Group President), Ms Chetna Malhotra Vohra (Associate Director—Content Strategy), Ms Pooja Bhandari (Production Head), Ms Saima Rashid (Manager Publishing), Mr Ashish Rajput (Commissioning Editor), and Dr Pratul Roy (Development Editor).

My special thanks to the Medley Company for their support for bringing out this book which was very dear to me for years all together. Last, but certainly not the least we want to acknowledge our Indian patients who are the true backbone for our knowledge. Our patients truly provide all the stimulating challenges to learn in our clinical practice.

Contents

SECTION 1 Basic Sciences in Orthopedic Rheumatology

1. Synovial Joints 3
   Arvind Kanchan

2. Biomechanics of Joints 5
   Subir Kumar Mukherjee, Alok Chandra Agrawal, Mukund Madhav Ojha

3. Pathogenesis of Autoimmune Diseases 13
   Venus Khanna

4. Genetic Basis of Rheumatic Diseases 17
   Aarti B Bhattacharya

SECTION 2 Rheumatoid Arthritis in Orthopedic Rheumatology

5. Introduction of Orthopedic Rheumatology 25
   Manish Khanna

6. Rheumatoid Arthritis: Etiopathogenesis, Clinical Features, and Management 26
   Manish Khanna

7. Ultrasound in Early Inflammatory Arthritis 34
   THS Bedi

8. Recent Advances in the Management of Rheumatoid Arthritis 43
   Neeraj Jain

9. Biological Therapy 47
   Shweta Agarwal

10. Surgical Considerations in Inflammatory Arthritis 54
    Manish Khanna, Rashmi Chopra

11. Challenges in Arthroplasty in Rheumatoid Arthritis 60
    Jitendra Chowdhary

12. Skin Manifestations in Orthorheumatology 63
    Sunil Kumar Gupta

SECTION 3 Spondyloarthropathies in Orthopedic Rheumatology

13. Ankylosing Spondylitis 73
    Manish Khanna, Shantanu Lahkar

14. Surgical Management in Ankylosing Spondylitis 81
    Md Neshar Ansari, Rajiv Lakhotia, Abhinandan Reddy M

15. Other Spondyloarthropathies 91
    Bhaskar Borgohain, Kashif A Ahmed, Shantanu Lahkar

SECTION 4 Crystal-induced Inflammation, Disorders of Cartilage and Bone in Orthopedic Rheumatology

16. Crystal Deposition Disorders 97
    Omkarnath Gudapati

17. Osteoarthritis: Etiology, Pathogenesis, and Management 117
    Venus Khanna, Manju Agrawal, Alok Chandra Agrawal

18.1. Osteoporosis 125
    SS Jha, Lalit Kishore

18.2. Osteomalacia 147
    SS Jha, Rahul Ranjan

18.3. Paget's Disease of Bone 152
    SS Jha, Rahul Ranjan

SECTION 5 Childhood Rheumatic Disease and Tubercular Infection in Orthopedic Rheumatology

19. Juvenile Idiopathic Arthritis 159
    Utkarsh Bansal, Manish Khanna

20. Mycobacterial Infections of Bone and Joints 171
    Gyaneshwar Tonk, Sujit Kumar

SECTION 6 Orthopedic Rheumatological Variants

21. Hand Radiograph: A Marker of Systemic Arthritis and Various Systemic Diseases 187
    Kushal Singh

22. Various Arthritic Joint Disorders 192
    Madhan Jeyaraman, Rakesh Kumar, Anil Gowtham Manivannan

23. Tendinopathies 199
    Madhan Jeyaraman, Naveen Jeyaraman, Ravi VR

24. Periarthritis Shoulder 215
    Krishna Subramanyam

25.1. Myofascial Pain Syndrome 228
    SS Jha, Lalit Kishore

25.2. Fibromyalgia 236
    SS Jha, Lalit Kishore

SECTION 7 Hand and Wrist Involvement in Orthopedic Rheumatology

26. Anatomy of Wrist and Hand 263
    Vipul Sud

27. Approach to Inflammatory Arthritis of Hand 267
    Alok Chandra Agrawal, Mukund Madhav Ojha, Harshal Sakale

28. Arthrodesis and Arthroplasty of the Rheumatoid Wrist and Small Joints of Hand:
    Where do We Stand? 275
    Abhay Elhence, Mahaveer Mali

29. **Pain in Hand: Carpal Tunnel Syndrome, Ulnar Nerve Entrapment at Wrist,
    Kienböck's Disease, and Osteoarthrosis of Carpometacarpal Joint of the Thumb** 279
    RB Kalia

30. **Common Hand Disorders** 292
    Alok Chandra Agrawal, Bikram Kar, Anupam Inamdar

SECTION 8 Foot and Ankle Involvement in Orthopedic Rheumatology

31. **Rheumatoid and Neuropathic Foot** 301
    Alok Chandra Agrawal, Ankit Kumar Garg, Shilp Verma

32. **Diabetic Foot** 310
    RC Meena, Jitesh K Jain, Arun Kumar Sharma

33. **Ankle Osteoarthritis** 316
    J Mangwani, N Nanavati, V Adukia

34. **Hallux Valgus** 325
    Raja TV, Ajay SS, Madhan Jeyaraman

SECTION 9 Regenerative Science in Orthopedic Rheumatology

35. **Introduction to Stem Cells** 335
    Naveen Jeyaraman, Rashmi Jain, Arunabh Arora

36. **Translational Products of Adipose Tissue-derived Mesenchymal Stem Cells:
    Bench to Bedside Applications** 341
    Madhan Jeyaraman, Rajni Ranjan, Amrit Kumar Singh

37. **Ethical Consideration in Stem Cell Research** 348
    Manish Khanna, Shashank Tiwari

38. **Cellular Therapy in Rheumatoid Arthritis** 354
    Sathish Muthu, Madhan Jeyaraman, Manish Khanna

39. **Cytotherapy in Osteoarthritic Knee** 359
    Madhan Jeyaraman, Sathish Muthu, Naveen Jeyaraman

40. **Promising Role of Regenerative Therapy in AVN and Sports Injuries: An Update** 367
    Manish Khanna, Madhan Jeyaraman, Arun Gulati

41. **Regenerative Medicine in Neurological Disorders: Current Understanding** 372
    Shilpa Sharma, Prajwal GS, Shivaraj B

42. **Ulcers and Regenerative Medicine** 381
    Sribatsa Kumar Mohapatra, Dushyant Chaudhary, Shivakumar Bingi

Index 389

Introduction

Most often treating complicated medical ailments leads to an amalgam of medical specialists and treatment plans. The concept of one size fits all does not work in most medical plans. The same has been found in the treatment of rheumatoid and orthopedic conditions.

Certain ailments like bone, joint injuries and diseases, namely, body trauma and osteoarthritis are treated by orthopedists who delve into a more surgical treatment approach. However, the plan of care for patients who have autoimmune conditions and arthritis is often inclined towards a nonsurgical approach and covered under rheumatology.

The question arises then for those patients who need treatment for diseases that require both nonsurgical and surgical efforts. While, over the years, the patients have either approached Rheumatologists first prior to seeing an orthopedist, and vice versa, the process is long and tiresome.

Each specialization deals with separate concerns, for example, orthopedic surgeons deal with joint and musculoskeletal pain and joint replacement surgery. Whilst, patients who suffer from joint pain, stiffness and psoriasis often visit a rheumatologist. The similarity between the symptoms leads to confusion amongst patients and delays in care resulting in the progression of severity.

Often times, patients are forced to go between two different clinics to merge together one concise plan of treatment. Not to mention, patients often remain in pain due to the lack of awareness and inability to have access to specialists from two medical backgrounds to provide relief. Thus, it can be argued that it is essential to understand the dynamics between the two specialists to ensure the timely, most effective treatment.

The Indian Orthopaedic Rheumatology Association (IORA) aims to lessen this gap and delay in care by bringing forward awareness and combining two specializations to provide in need patients with cutting edge therapies with a combination of traditionally approached plans.

Having both specialists under the same hospital structure can also lessen patient effort. Wherein, patients whose joint pain is not amenable with traditional rheumatology efforts, can be referred to an orthopedic surgeon who can further use surgical treatment for the management of the disease.

The gap in communication leads to patients going in circles, sometimes often revisiting different doctors specialized in rheumatology under the impression that the current method of treatment is ineffective, rather than being aware of the orthopedic option.

Here is where the IORA comes into the picture, enabling comprehensive and accelerated care to patients. The main aim of IORA is to create awareness amongst orthopedic surgeons whilst encouraging broadened research and development. The first step is to research into the nuances of this nascent field and create scientific relations on an international and national level.

The limitations the IORA's include lack of infrastructure to provide elaborated care through a multispecialty approach, patient awareness and compliance, expensive biologicals. Patients' environment and lifestyle can also hamper treatment plans. There is also a great need in urban and rural areas for rheumatology specialists.

Despite these limitations, the IORA has surged forward, focusing and encouraging new research coupled with academic advancements in the field of Orthopedic Rheumatology. IORA understands the complexity of uncontrolled rheumatoid arthritis, disease modifying anti-rheumatic drugs (DMARDs), avascular necrosis (AVN) head of femur and osteoarthritis (OA) causing the stress on orthopedic surgical treatment and traditional Rheumatology.

Hence, the IORA has taken up through their peer-reviewed journals the action of providing orthopedic surgeons with insights, knowledge and cutting edge technology awareness. This further enhances and manages rheumatic and orthopedic musculoskeletal disorders. The IORA also provides a platform for newer aspiring researches to provide insight into a diagnostic and clinical guide for treatment through research.

The aim of this book is thus, to foremostly to create awareness, challenge orthopedic and rheumatology specialized to broaden their treatment scope to taking a newer more comprehensible multidimensional approach to the treatment of such diseases.

Basic Sciences in Orthopedic Rheumatology

- **Synovial Joints**
  Arvind Kanchan
- **Biomechanics of Joints**
  Subir Kumar Mukherjee, Alok Chandra Agrawal, Mukund Madhav Ojha
- **Pathogenesis of Autoimmune Diseases**
  Venus Khanna
- **Genetic Basis of Rheumatic Diseases**
  Aarti B Bhattacharya

Synovial Joints

Arvind Kanchan

■ INTRODUCTION

The human skeletal system consists of many joints, where adjacent bones or bone and cartilage articulate with each other to form a connection. Joints are classified based on their mobility as immobile, partially/slightly mobile, or freely mobile joints. The mobility at a particular joint is related to its functional need. Thus, immobile or slightly mobile joints are important for protection of visceral organs, providing stability, and for restricted bodily movements while freely mobile joints can permit as well as tolerate much more widespread movements of the limbs comprising all the synovial joints of body.

■ SYNOVIAL JOINTS

Synovial joint is a fluid-filled cavity which is surrounded by articular cartilages over the bony surfaces, and fibrous articular capsule. The articular capsule also consists of intimal and subintimal membranous lining layers called synovium and subsynovium, respectively. Synovial fluid (SF) spreads over the synovial linings (synovium) and the articular cartilage, as well as ligaments. Synovial joints offer low friction, low wear, and tear resistant mobility between the opposing surfaces of bones **(Fig. 1)**.

Synovium and Subsynovium

Synovium or synovial membrane comprises of a thin sheet of cells that covers the intra-articular surface of the joint capsule. Synovial membrane functions as a selectively-permeable barrier that limits the fluid and molecular movements between SF and blood plasma, hence it contributes to the regulation of SF.

There are two principal types of cells in the synovial membranes (synoviocytes): Type A or macrophage-like synoviocytes (33%) and Type B or fibroblast-like synoviocytes (67%). Type B synoviocytes secrete hyaluronic acid (HA) as well as the constituents of connective tissue matrix like type IV and type VI collagens, laminin, and chondroitin sulfate **(Fig. 2)**.

Subsynovium

Subsynovium layer is situated beneath the synovial membrane. It is a supportive, loose connective tissue layer consisting of blood vessels, nerves, and lymphatics. Adipose and fibrous connective tissues also present in a variable range of proportions. Capillaries present in the superficial region of subsynovium are of both fenestrated and unfenestrated explaining transsynovial fluid passage through capillary fenestra.

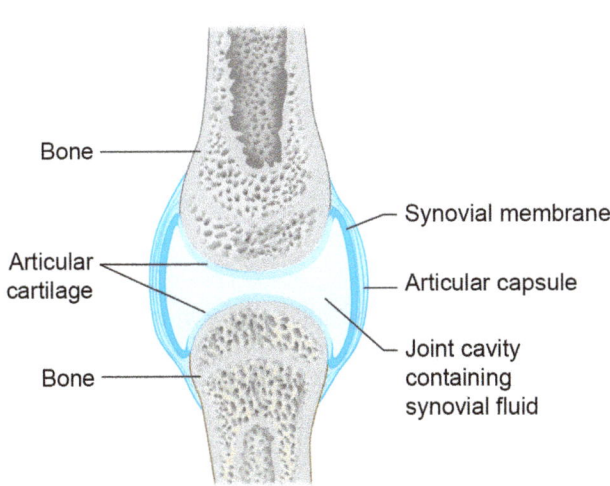

Fig. 1: Synovial joint.

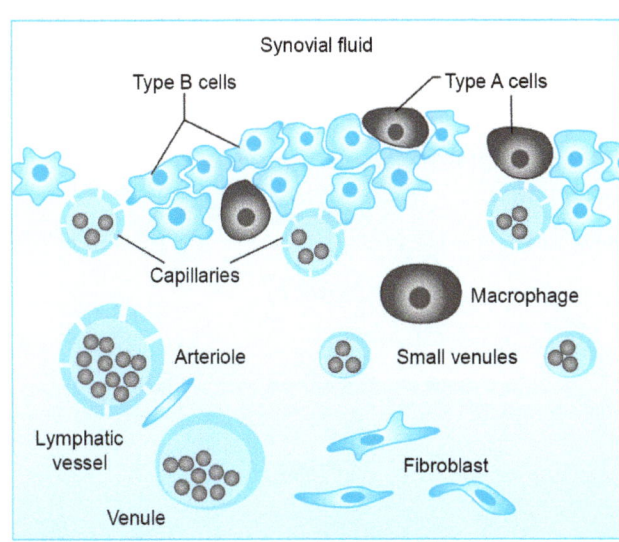

Fig. 2: Synovium and subsynovium.

Cartilage

Articular cartilages are connective tissue over the bone ends responsible for load-bearing, reducing friction, and providing tear and wear resistant surface to facilitate the mobility of joint. It is made up of chondrocytes (cartilage cells) present in a specialized extracellular matrix (ECM). The ECM of articular cartilage consisting of type II collagen and proteoglycan (PG). PG provides the compressive stiffness to the cartilage. The collagenous reticulum provides functional integrity and strength, tensile and shear stiffness to the cartilage. However, the cellular and ECM constituents of cartilage as well as its mechanical properties, vary with its depth from the superficial surface.

■ SYNOVIAL FLUID

Synovial fluid is a non-Newtonian, clear, viscous fluid present inside the joints. It principally functions as a lubricant fluid for the articulating bony surfaces involved in synovial joints, during their whole range of mobility. SF acts as a fluid transport medium for many metabolites and nutrients from circulation to the joint. SF also contains soluble-signaling factors, which mediates effective communication between distinct cell populations in the joint. Thus, SF is required for maintaining the homeostatic mechanisms of joints, owing to the unique properties and functions of its constituents.

Biosynthesis and Composition of Synovial Fluid

Synovial fluid is composed of ultrafiltrate from blood plasma and the molecular substances secreted by synoviocytes (the cells lining the synovium). The synovium behaves as a selectively-permeable membrane that retains and permits only specific molecules, depending on size and density. Higher molecular weight substances in the SF, such as HA and proteoglycan 4 (PRG4), are retained within the synovial cavity and contributing to the lubricant property, while low-molecular-weight substances, such as most of the metabolic byproducts and substrates, cytokines, and growth factors, are returned back to circulation via lymphatics **(Fig. 3)**. Thus, bidirectional transport of molecules across the synovial membrane along with the active secretions from the synoviocytes result in SF, having HA concentration of 1–4 mg/mL and PRG4 concentration of 0.05–0.35 mg/mL during steady state.

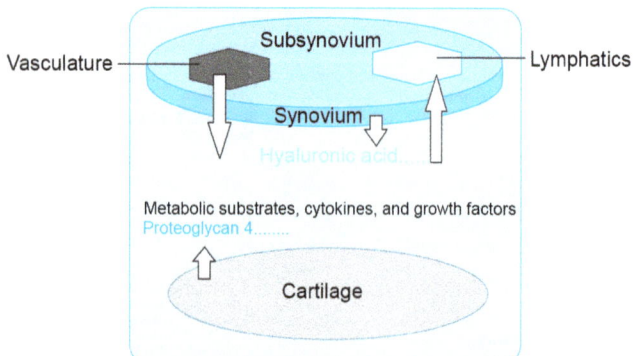

Fig. 3: Biosynthesis and composition of synovial fluid.

Plasma Proteins

The protein constituents of SF is almost comparable to that of blood plasma, though selective permeability of synovial membranes preserves most of larger-sized proteins in the circulation and restrain their passage into the synovial cavity. The protein concentration in SF (25–28 mg/mL) is roughly about one-third of that of plasma. The albumin is most abundant protein macromolecule of SF, followed by transferrin and γ-globulin. Larger proteins, such as β2 macroglobulin, fibrinogen, and α2 macroglobulin, are in low concentration or untraceable in a normal healthy SF.

Lubricating Substances

The principal lubricating substances in the SF are HA and PRG4 (also known as lubricin) and surface-active phospholipids (SAPL). These substances are all ideally placed to contribute to the lubricating function of SF. HA is a nonsulfated glycosaminoglycan made up of repeating polymeric disaccharides D-glucuronic acid and N-acetyl-D-glucosamine. The HA concentration in SF is the major determinant of its viscosity. PRG4/lubricin is a glycoprotein with multiple O-linked β(1-3)Gal-GalNAc oligosaccharides, which mediate the molecule's function as a boundary lubricant. PRG4/lubricin also plays important role in organizing HA and providing SF the ability to dissipate the strain energy. SAPL also possess boundary-lubricating ability of SF at a cartilage–cartilage interface.

Synovial Fluid Rheology

The viscosity and viscoelastic properties of SF strongly correlate with the concentration of HA. Viscoelastic models of SF have demonstrated an elastic-like response from "normal" SF at high frequencies of oscillation. In knee joint, it is estimated that it can be exposed to rates of shear strain up to 10^3 Hz, as well as wide range of variability in frequency. High viscosity at low shear rates and frequencies allows the SF to act as a potential load-bearer. This stabilizes the articular capsule during very small movements at low speeds (e.g., shifts in position). Whereas, at increased shear rates and frequencies (in conditions of extreme joint mobility like during running), the viscosity of SF decreases to very low, leading to the formation of very thin fluid-film that differentiates the cartilage surfaces. Pathological SF exhibits impaired rheological properties.

■ KEY POINTS

- Synovial joints is a fluid-filled cavity which is surrounded by articular cartilage and fibrous articular capsule (synovium and subsynovium).
- Synovial fluid is composed of ultrafiltrate from blood plasma and the molecular substances secreted by synoviocytes.
- Principal lubricating substances in SF are HA and PRG4.

Biomechanics of Joints

Subir Kumar Mukherjee, Alok Chandra Agrawal, Mukund Madhav Ojha

INTRODUCTION

"Nothing happens until something moves."
—**Albert Einstein**

If we look into our surroundings, we will be amazed at the biomechanics involved in the intricate and skilled movements of dancers, musicians, toddlers, and even animals. Needless to say, scholars from aeons ago have devoted themselves in studying movements in animals and humans. Human body may be viewed as a machine comprising different parts that allow movements which occur at different joints formed by the specific parts of body's musculoskeletal system. The very essence of this chapter is to develop a lucid and coherent understanding of clinical useful biomechanical concepts used for elucidating changes in joint functions.

Certain terminologies pertinent to this chapter:
- *Mechanics*—study of forces and their effects.
- *Kinematics*—branch of mechanics that deals with the geometry of the motion of objects, including displacement, velocity, and acceleration, without taking into account the forces that produce the motion.
- *Kinetics*—study of the relationships between the force system acting on a body and changes produced in body motion.
- *Force*—action exerted on a body that causes it to deform or to move.
- *Biomechanics*—study of continuum mechanics (i.e., the study of loads, motion, stress, and strain of solids and fluids) of biological systems and the mechanical effects on the body's movement, size, shape, and structure. It ascends from molecular level to systemic level.
- *Molecular biomechanics*—study of how mechanical forces and deformation affect the conformation, binding/reaction, function, and transport of biomolecules like DNA, RNA, and proteins.
- *Cellular biomechanics*—study of how cells detect mechanical forces or deformations, and transduces them into biological responses, especially for the study of how mechanical forces change cell growth, differentiation, movement, signal transduction, protein secretion and transport, and gene expression and regulation.
- *Tissue biomechanics*—study related to growth and remodeling of tissues as a response to applied mechanical stimuli.

For instance, Julius Wolff in 19th century postulated a law on bone remodeling, famously known as Wolff's law which states that internal architecture of the trabecular and cortical bone in a healthy person or animal will adapt to the loads placed on the bone and it will remodel itself over time to become stronger to resist that type of loading. The reverse also holds true.
- *Systemic biomechanics*—study concerned with highly coordinated mechanical interaction between bones, muscles, ligaments, and joints within musculoskeletal system under control of nervous system.

Why to give emphasis on understanding biomechanics?
There has been constant quest in discovering principles and developing concepts that govern movements. It can be applied for:
- *Performance enhancement*: Biomechanics give a qualitative analysis of the situation thereby aiding sports professionals to adapt techniques needed for effective movements.
- *Designation of sports equipment*: It also helps in modifying and designing equipment keeping in mind the weight distribution, range and time of motion, and shortening or lengthening of equipment.
- Advances in exercise and conditioning programs.

LEVERS

A lever is a rigid bar (bone) that turns about an axis of rotation or fulcrum (joint) when a force (from muscle contraction) is applied against a resistance (weight, gravity, etc.). Levers are used to alter the resulting direction of the applied force. Lever can be categorized on the basis of relationship of fulcrum/arm (A) to force (F) and resistance (R) **(Table 1 and Fig. 1)**.

Section 1: Basic Sciences in Orthopedic Rheumatology

TABLE 1: Classes of lever.

Class I lever	Class II lever	Class III lever (most common)
F-A-R	A-R-F	A-F-R
Resistance and force are always opposite	Resistance and force are in same direction	Resistance and force are in same direction
1. Balanced movements—axis near middle, e.g., erector spinae neck extension 2. Speed and ROM—axis near force, e.g., extension at elbow through triceps contraction 3. Force—axis near resistance	Force—axis near resistance, e.g., plantar flexion through gastrocnemius and soleus contraction	Speed and ROM—axis near force, e.g., flexion of elbow joint through biceps contraction

(A: axis; F: force; R: resistance; ROM: range of motion)

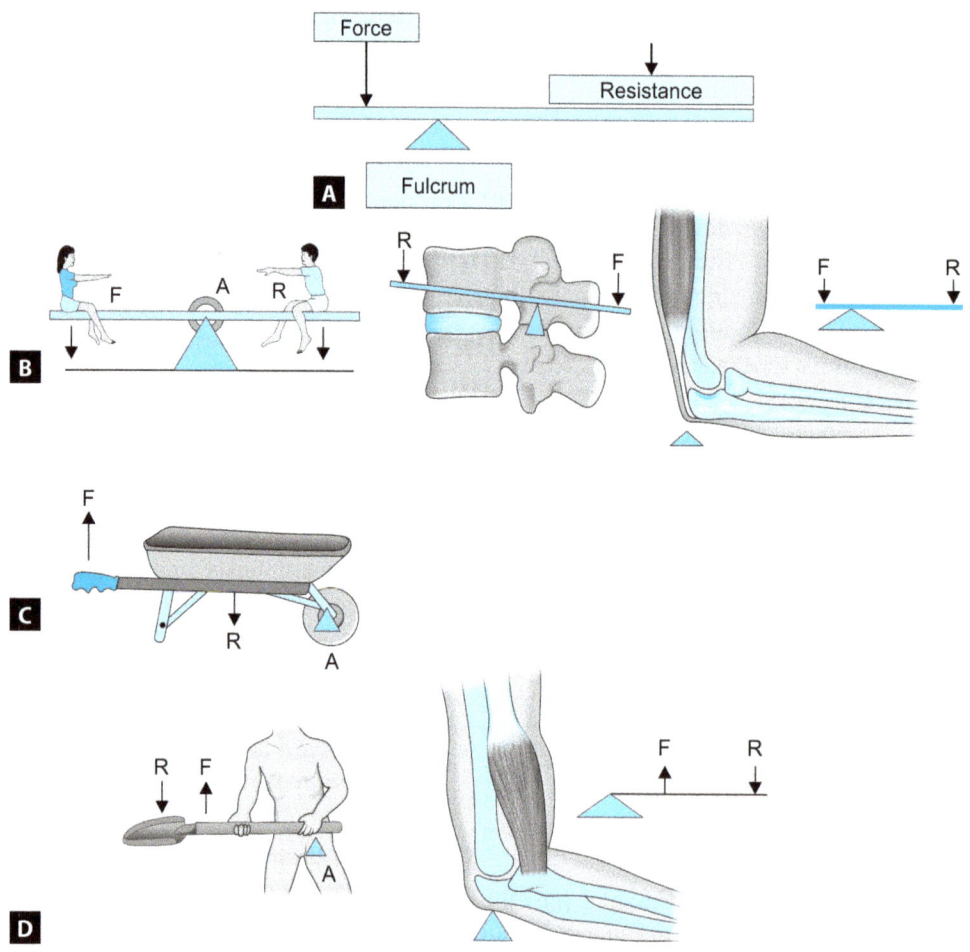

Figs. 1A to D: (A) Lever system showing components; (B) First-class lever system; (C) Second-class lever system; (D) Third-class lever system. [A: axis (fulcrum); F: force; R: resistance]
Source: Chapter 2: Joint anatomy and basic biomechanics. In: Bergmann TF, Peterson DH (Eds). Chiropractic Technique: Principles and Procedures, 3rd edition. Mosby; 2010.

■ BODY PLANES AND AXES OF MOVEMENT

For explaining structural position and movement directions, there should be allocation of body planes with reference to anatomical position. An axis is a line around which movement occurs. Three dimensional coordinate system with X, Y, and Z axes are used in locating the extent of types of movements permissible at each joint like **(Table 2 and Fig. 2)**:

- Rotational—all movements that occur about an axis
- Translational—linear movements along an axis and through a plane
- Curvilinear—translational movements along with rotational movements.

TABLE 2: Body planes with axis and joint movement.

Plane of movement	Axis		Joint movement
Sagittal (extends from anterior to posterior)	Vertical	X (junction of coronal and transverse)	Flexion and extension; lateral to medial and medial to lateral slide*
Coronal (extends from side to side)	Vertical	Z (junction of sagittal and transverse)	Abduction and adduction; anterior to posterior, and posterior to anterior glide*
Transverse (divides into upper and lower)	Horizontal	Y (junction of coronal and sagittal)	Medial and lateral rotation (axial rotation) inferior to superior, and superior to inferior glide* (compression, distraction)

*(slide and glide are used to refer translational movements between joint surfaces.)

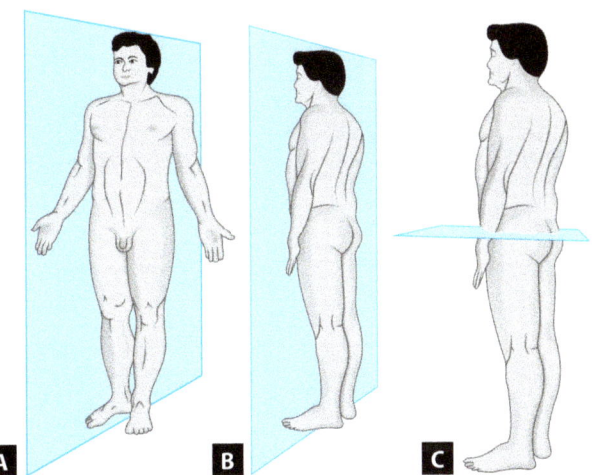

Figs. 2A to C: (A) Midsagittal plane; (B) Coronal plane; (C) Transverse plane.
Source: Chapter 2: Joint anatomy and basic biomechanics. In: Bergmann TF, Peterson DH (Eds). Chiropractic Technique: Principles and Procedures, 3rd edition. Mosby; 2010.

■ JOINT MOTION AND TYPES

Every joint is blessed to exhibit 6° of freedom, three translational and three rotational. The extent of each motion is based on the anatomy of the joint and the plane of the joint surface particularly to spinal joints **(Flowchart 1)**.

■ SYNOVIAL JOINTS

Synovial joints are the most common, highly evolved, and freely movable joints. These are comprised of bony elements, articular cartilage, fibrocartilage, synovial membrane, fibroligamentous joint capsule, and articular joint receptors.

Bony Elements

It is a type of connective tissue with inorganic constituents like salts. Cortical bone is hard outer shell which surrounds cancellous bone thereby providing structural support while cancellous bone is inner part containing marrow and blood vessels for nutrition and also contains trabeculations. It plays crucial role in hematopoiesis. Bone is often considered as storehouse of calcium and phosphorus. It has self-repairing quality with its own tissue. It also has best ability for remodeling, repair, and regeneration.

Articular Cartilage

Speciated, avascular hyaline cartilage covering articulating surfaces of synovial joints thereby relaying loads and minimizing friction. Through zone of calcification, it is adhered to subchondral bone. It has four characteristic histological areas given in **Table 3**.

Articular cartilage derives its nutrition from highly vascularized synovium and intermittent compression and distraction needed for adequate exchange of nutritions and waste products. Possesses limited capacity for cartilage repair hence degeneration of articular cartilage depends on the size and depth of lesion, integrity of surrounding articular surface, age and weight of patient, associated meniscal and ligamentous lesions, and other biomechanical factors.

Fibrocartilage

Mostly found in intervertebral discs, pubis symphysis, etc. It mainly applies "load-unload mechanism" for nutrition and eradication of metabolic wastes. Owing to its higher fiber content, it has pivotal role in bolstering and stabilizing joints with subsequent driving off the compressive force.

Synovial Fluid

An ultrafiltrate derived from blood with supplements from synovium, meant for lubrication, protection, and nutrition of articular cartilage. Earlier, hyaluronic acid (secreted by type B cells) was thought of imparting the viscosity to synovial fluid but now it has been investigated that a glycoprotein named "lubricin" secreted by surface chondrocytes and synovial cells possess the same quality due to its surface active phospholipids.

Joint Lubrication Models

Albeit no model is superior to one other, amalgamation of elastohydrodynamic and boundary lubrication model serves a satisfactory explanation to human synovial joint **(Table 4)**.

■ ARTICULAR NEUROLOGY

Neural innervation of synovial joints is by three or four neuroreceptors, briefly described in **Table 5**.

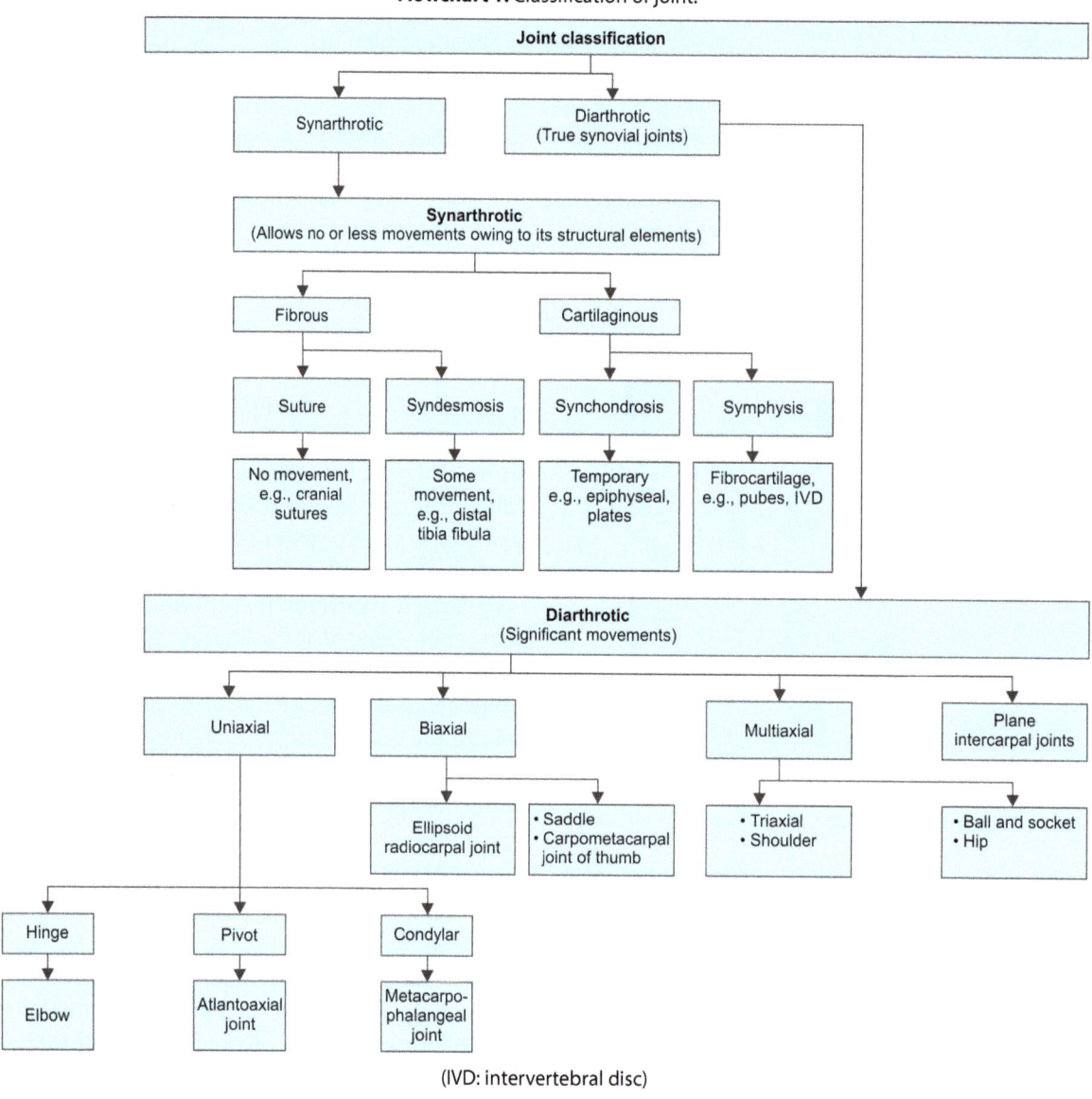

Flowchart 1: Classification of joint.

(IVD: intervertebral disc)

TABLE 3: Zones of articular cartilage.

Gliding zone	Outermost zone with outer superficial layer of random collagen arrangement and inner tangential layer of dense and compact collagen orientation, collateral to joint surface in order to shield deeper elastic cartilage
Transitional zone	Orientational change of fibers from parallel to perpendicular direction
Radial zone	
Zone of calcified cartilage	

TABLE 4: Joint lubrication models.

Hydrodynamic model	Synovial fluid gaps the left out spaces of incongruent joint surfaces and maintains fluid film during movements Advantage—works well with quick movement Disadvantage—inadequate lubrication for slow movements and movements under increased loads
Elastohydrodynamic model	Modified form of previous model. Viscoelastic qualities of articular cartilage minimizes compression stress to lubrication fluid Advantage—explains movements under loading forces Disadvantage—fails to justify lubrication at motion initiation or period of zero velocity during reciprocating movements
Boundary lubrication model	Adsorption of lubricant on joint surface minimizes surface roughness by gap filling and surface coating Advantage—can justify initial movement and zero velocity movements

TABLE 5: Neural innervation of synovial joints.

Receptors	Nature	Location	Function
Type I (low threshold)	Mechanoreceptor	Outer layer of joint capsule	Posture and motion perception
Type II (low threshold)	Mechanoreceptor	Deepest layers of joint capsule	Movement monitoring for reflex actions (completely shut down in immobilized joints)
Type III (slow adapters)	Mechanoreceptor	Intrinsic and extrinsic ligaments of peripheral joints	Monitors motion direction. Braking mechanism against over displacing joint movements
Type IV (very high threshold)	Nociceptor	Fibrous portions of joint capsule, ligaments and synovial folds. (Absent in articular cartilage, synovial linings)	Pain perception (inactive in physiologic joint)

JOINT FUNCTION

The physiologic movements at each joint occurring due to muscular contraction or acting gravity is known as *"osteokinematic movement."* It speaks about the relativity of each joint with each other.

A concatenation of segmental linkage, i.e., connected shoulder girdle, arm, forearm, wrist and hand of upper extremity, is often known as kinematic chain, which can be either closed or open. Fixed distal segment to immovable object while keeping proximal segment free is called closed chain while in open chain, distal segment is free and not connected with fixed object.

Movements occurring at the articulated joint surfaces are known as *arthrokinematic movement*. While evaluating joint motion, it is thus imperative to relate osteokinematic movement to arthrokinematic movement. Various permutations and combinations like roll, spin, and slide occur during relative movements of joint surfaces.

- Roll occurs when points on one bone surface coincides with points on other bone at same interval.
- Spin—rotational movement around mechanical axis. Possible in hip, shoulder, and proximal radius.
- Slide—when single point on moving joint coincides with many points on opposing joint surface.

For normal joint function, joint motion must possess five traits which are joint play, active range of motion, passive range of motion, end feel or play, and paraphysiologic movement. Joint movement beyond the paraphysiologic barrier departs from confinement of anatomic integrity subsequently making an entrance into pathologic zone.

HUMAN MOTION ANALYSIS

It is defined as the systematic study of human motion by careful vigilance, supported by instrumentation for measuring somatic movements, body mechanics, and muscle activity. It is often used to gather quantitative data about the mechanics of the musculoskeletal system during motor performance.

A special branch related to human walking is *"gait analyses."* Eadweard Muybridge is regarded as the "Father of Modern Gait Analysis" attributed to his pioneer work in gait. Carl Pulfrich is widely known as the "Father of Stereophotogrammetry", a technique used to measure 3D landmark coordinates. The quantifiable values to assess human motion analysis are musculoskeletal movements defined by skin markers and measured by motion capture systems and external forces applied by force plates. The 3D trajectories of skin markers derived from stereophotogrammetry, the GRFs (ground reaction forces) and the center of pressure measured via force plates, intersegmental forces, and internal moments at joints of lower limbs are calculated from the solution of equations based on Newton's laws of motion. This process is known as "inverse dynamics analyses."

IMPLEMENTATIONS OF BIOMECHANICS

- Useful diagnostic and investigative tool in research and clinical areas.
- Identification of any deviation from normal movement with simultaneous evaluation of neuromusculoskeletal conditions and treatment planning, e.g., cerebral palsy, osteoarthritis of knee, paraplegia, etc.
- Important role in assistive technology such as prosthetics, orthotics where critical joint motion are precisely evaluated.
- Helps in honing athletic performance, detecting common sports injuries along with posture and movement related problems.

APPLIED BIOMECHANICS

Biomechanics is a continuous evolving branch of science where engineers and doctors work together for the betterment of human disability. Any disarray in the normal kinematics of joints sets off a vicious cycle of disturbed biomechanics which in turn further damages the joint. Principles of biomechanics and human motion analysis are used to study the pathobiomechanics occurring due to various joint pathologies. Purpose of any musculoskeletal surgeries and rehabilitation protocols is to ameliorate the pathobiomechanic processes occurring at joints, bone, or muscles and reinstate the normokinematics so as to work in harmony.

BIOMECHANICS OF FRACTURE FIXATION

In this era where conservative treatment of fracture has shifted to operative procedures, newer techniques and implant designs (dynamic compression plate, locking compression plate, and intramedullary nails) for fracture fixation are available. Biomechanics involved in fracture fixation using these implants persuade the fracture healing. Perren described strain to be the limiting factor for the final outcome of fracture healing **(Table 6)**.

Various parameters like fracture morphology (simple or comminuted), soft tissue status, implant used (plate or nail), implant material (titanium or stainless steel), and mode of implant application affect the final outcome of fracture healing.

Working length of an implant bone construct is the distance between the proximal and distal end points where implant is fixed to the bone across the fracture site. Working length is inversely related to fracture fixation stability. Increasing working length results in decreased fracture stability at far cortex to produce enough micromotion ensuring optimum callus production. This principle is used for secondary fracture healing in comminuted fractures.

BIOMECHANICS OF ARTHROPLASTY

Osteoarthritis is one of the most common causes for disability in the world. It is a disease of the whole joint which includes muscles, tendons, ligaments, synovium, and bone. Altered loading mechanisms, increased mechanical forces, and changed biomechanics in weight-bearing joints are imperative factors responsible for initiation and progression of osteoarthritis. It is most common in weight-bearing joints like hips, knees, and ankle but can also occur in any synovial joint of the body. Biomechanically, knee acting as polycentric joint bears higher shear forces in comparison to hip or ankle joint as it involves sliding, rotating, and rolling motions during movements. Any imbalance between repair mechanisms and destructive forces can sabotage the joint homeostasis resulting in osteoarthritis though congregation of structural reaction of joint tissues to mechanical stimuli is the current cognizance of pathogenesis of osteoarthritis. Joints connected serially act as kinematic chain which allows movement with subsequent stability, congruency, and shock absorption. For optimal load reduction and distribution and painless gliding, alignments, adduction movements, and muscle balancing are principle factors and thus unphysiological loading patterns on one joint may impact the near by joints too. The alignment of lower extremity is known as mechanical axis which is defined as a line drawn from the center of the femoral head to the center of the talus which passes close to the center of the tibial head between the eminentia tibiae, approximately one degree in varus thereby physiologically causing unequal weight distribution of 60–70% on medial compartment and 30–40% on lateral compartment, which is a predisposing factor for medially accentuated tibiofemoral osteoarthritis. The deviation of mechanical axis drastically reduces the load bearing area and amplifying the resultant load to the remaining joint surface. By human motion analysis, gait analysis (a noninvasive, indirect, and most common method) uses video cameras and ground reaction force plates summarize pressure and movements transforming information to external moments relative to internal joint loads. In varus arrangement, the adduction moment (AdM) is a varus torque on the knee joint which is determined by the ground reaction force (GRF—force generated by the foot touching the ground) and by the distance of the GRF vector from the center of the knee joint. At early and late stance phase (heel strike to foot flat and toe off), a valgus moment is present together with maximal compressive forces on lateral knee compartment. During midstance phase, a varus moment occurs to the knee in line with maximum compressive forces on medial knee compartment. Anything which decreases AdM at knee tends to relieve symptoms of osteoarthritis like conservative strategies in form of lateral wedge insole, valgus knee braces, gait modification with toe out gait, weight loss, etc. Joint preserving surgeries can restore normal biomechanics with simultaneous reduction in pain and functional improvement. Young and active patients may get maximum benefit from these surgeries which include correction osteotomy either open or closing wedge, orthobiologics and viscosupplementation, autologous chondrocytes implantations (ACL), transplantation of osteochondral allografts, or mosaicoplasty. In advanced cases where articular cartilage is severely destroyed, total joint replacement is the treatment of choice in which soft tissue balancing plays a key role in deformity correction and restoring the normal alignment.

Biomechanical studies are equally important in understanding hip movements and hip joint reaction forces. The biomechanical principle guide engineers in proper designing of components of hip replacement implants. From various studies conducted in vitro and in vivo have helped in executing therapeutic programs to relieve symptoms thereby delaying the disease progression of

TABLE 6: Strain as the limiting factor.

Strain	Stability at fracture gap	Type of fracture healing
≤2%	Rigid fixation	Primary or direct without callus formation
2–10%	Allows micromotions	Secondary or indirect with callus formation
>10%	Unstable	Leads to nonunion

hip pathology. The biomechanics and biomaterials are important components attributed to the success of total hip arthroplasty in pain alleviation and functional restoration.

BIOMECHANICS OF SPINE AND PRINCIPLE OF DEFORMITY CORRECTION

Any spinal deformity whether acute or chronic commences with instability in at least one motion segment which can be corrected by various methods with its pros and cons. Forces on spine can be divided into component vectors. Instantaneous axis of rotation (IAR) is an axis around which the bending moment applied to a point in space causes rotation or tendency to rotate. It acts as pivot point around which flexion or extension occurs. Loads applied whether acutely or chronically cause deformation in one of two directions involving one or multiple spinal segments.

Principles Considered during Deformity Correction

The load bearing axis must be considered in both sagittal and coronal planes which is shifted ventrally with flexion and dorsally in extension. It is located in ventral region in normal thoracic spine while in dorsal region in normal cervical and lumbar spine. Sagittal balance of the spine should be kept in mind. Central sacral line (CSL) is perpendicular to a line passing through both iliac crests, ascending rostrally in the line with sacral spinous processes. It is often used to assess balance in coronal plane and scoliosis assessment. The length and location of the stabilizing construct are critical. The apical and neutral vertebrae in coronal and sagittal planes must be evaluated. An implant should not be closed at or near an apical vertebra and hence should be long enough to extend to neutral vertebra. Cervicothoracic and thoracolumbar regions are susceptible to deformity if implants are placed to but not beyond these levels. Disc spaces near the junctional zones are usually not parallel to the ground in the standing position thereby applying angular forces to the spine.

BIOMECHANICS OF SHOULDER AND ITS PATHOLOGY

Shoulder joint is the most complex joint of body where four joints (glenohumeral, sternoclavicular, acromioclavicular, and scapulothoracic) with support from muscles, ligament, and capsule work synchronously in balance to attain multidirectional movements at the cost of stability. Humeral head articular surface is about three times that of glenoid cavity and is made stable by static and dynamic stabilizers around the joints. Rotator cuff (supraspinatus, infraspinatus, teres minor, and subscapularis) is a group of muscles which acts as a key dynamic stabilizer to glenohumeral joint stability at rest and during motion. It presses humeral head to glenoid (concavity-compression principle) and helps in overhead arm elevation. Any disruption in balance leads to mechanical dysfunction in form of rotator cuff impingement or glenohumeral instability. Application of the biomechanical concepts of shoulder is helpful in addressing the rehabilitation protocol to these mechanical dysfunctions after musculoskeletal procedures.

BIOMECHANICS OF REHABILITATION BY ORTHOSES AND PROSTHESIS

Group of splints and appliances, which when applied or fixed to a body part to make it work properly, are called as orthoses, whereas prosthesis acts as proxy to the missing part of the body. Understanding biomechanics of normal and pathological gait helps us to prescribe proper orthoses to the patient. Orthoses are basically designed to overcome the abnormal forces acting on body. Biomechanics helps in development of floor reaction orthoses which are used in cerebral palsy patient with crouch gait (severe knee flexion) to improve gait in midstance by preventing forward tibial progression and therefore helping quadriceps muscle in maintaining knee extension.

SUMMARY

This chapter briefly tells about the very importance of biomechanics of joints. Human beings are constantly insulted by different forces on earth. By studying the interrelationship between these forces and human body movements, we can apply biomechanics principles in uplifting the quality of life. Human movements are highly complicated and are governed by sophisticated interaction between nervous and musculoskeletal system. Any insult to, or injury to any single element of this network will lead to undesired consequences in form of disability. Biomechanics principles and human motion analysis help us to study the disease process and planning the treatment.

KEY POINTS

- Understanding biomechanics is essential for planning of treatment, performance enhancement, and improving quality of life.
- Joints may be synarthrotic or diarthrotic.
- Zones of articular cartilage—gliding, transitional, radial, and calcified.
- Joint lubrication models—hydrodynamic, elastohydrodynamic, and boundary lubrication.
- Perren's strain hypothesis >10% strain leads to nonunion.
- Working length is inversely proportional to stability.

FURTHER READING

1. Allard P, Stokes IAF, Blanchi JP. Three-dimensional Analysis of Human Movement. Champaign, IL: Human Kinetics Publishers; 1995.

2. Armfield DR, Stickle RL, Robertson DD, Towers JD, Debski RE. Biomechanical basis of common shoulder problems. Semin Musculoskelet Radiol. 2003;7:5-18.
3. Center for Photogrammetric Training, Ferris State University. History of photogrammetry. Michigan: Ferris State University; 2008.
4. Chapter 2: Joint anatomy and basic biomechanics. In: Bergmann TF, Peterson DH (Eds). Chiropractic Technique: Principles and Procedures, 3rd edition. Mosby; 2010.
5. Chen HL, Lu TW, Wang TM, Huang SC. Biomechanical strategies for successful obstacle crossing with the trailing limb in older adults with medial compartment knee osteoarthritis. J Biomech. 2008;41:753e61.
6. Egloff C, Huegle T, Valderrabano V. Biomechanics and pathomechanisms of osteoarthritis. Swiss Med Wkly. 2012; 142:w13583.
7. Gage JR. Gait analysis for decision-making in cerebral palsy. Bull Hosp Joint Dis Orthop Inst. 1983;43:147e63.
8. Gage JR. Gait Analysis in Cerebral Palsy. London: Mac Keith Press; 1991.
9. Gale LR, Chen Y, Hills BA, Crawford R. Boundary lubrication of joints: characterization of surface-active phospholipids found on retrieved implants. Acta Orthop. 2007;78(3): 309-14.
10. Hak DJ, Toker S, Yi C, Toreson J. The influence of fracture fixation biomechanics on fracture healing. Orthopedics. 2010;33(10):752.
11. Hertling D, Kessler RM. Management of Common Musculoskeletal Disorders: Physical Therapy Principles and Methods, 2nd edition. Philadelphia: JB Lippincott; 1990.
12. Hsu WC, Wang TM, Liu MW, Chang CF, Chen HL, Lu TW. Control of body center of mass motion during level walking and obstacle-crossing in older patients with knee osteoarthritis. J Mech. 2010;26:229e37.
13. Huang SC, Wei IP, Chien HL, Wang TM, Liu YH, Chen HL, et al. Effects of severity of degeneration on gait patterns in patients with medial knee osteoarthritis. Med Eng Phys. 2008;30:997e1003.
14. Jay GD, Torres JR, Rhee DK, Helminen HJ, Hytinnen MM, Cha CJ, et al. Association between friction and wear in diarthrodial joints lacking lubricin. Arthritis Rheum. 2007; 56(11):3662-9.
15. Jay GD, Torres JR, Warman ML, Laderer MC, Breuer KS. The role of lubricin in the mechanical behavior of synovial fluid. Proc Natl Acad Sci U S A. 2007;104(15):6194-9.
16. "Lever of a Human Body" by Alexandra. The Physics Corner; 2014. pp. 1-7.
17. Lin KH, Lu TW, Hsu PP, Yu SM, Liao WS. Postural responses during falling with rapid reach-and-grasp balance reaction in patients with motor complete paraplegia. Spinal Cord. 2008;46:204e9.
18. Lu TW, Chen HL, Wang TM. Obstacle crossing in older adults with medial compartment knee osteoarthritis. Gait Posture. 2007;26:553e9.
19. Lu TW, Wei IP, Liu YH, Wang TM, Hsu WC, Chang CF, et al. Immediate effects of acupuncture on gait patterns in patient with knee osteoarthritis. Chin Med J. 2010;123:165e72.
20. Lucareli PRG, Lima M de O, Lucarelli JG de A, Lima FPS. Changes in joint kinematics in children with cerebral palsy while walking with and without a floor reaction ankle–foot orthosis. Clinics. 2007;62(1):63-8.
21. MacConnail MA, Basmajian JV. Muscles and Movements: A Basis for Human Kinesiology. Baltimore; Williams & Wilkins; 1969.
22. Nordin M, Frankel VH. Basic Biomechanics of the Musculoskeletal System, 2nd edition. Philadelphia: Lippincott Williams & Wilkins; 2001.
23. Robert B. Kinetic Anatomy With Web Resource, 3rd edition. Human Kinetics; 2012.
24. Schlenk RP, Kowalski RJ, Benzel EC. Biomechanics of spinal deformity. Neurosurg Focus. 2003;14(1):1-10.
25. Tung WL, Chu-Fen C. Biomechanics of human movement and its clinical applications. Kaohsiung J Med Sci. 2012; 28(2 Suppl):S13-25.
26. Wang TM, Hsu WC, Chang CF, Hu CC, Lu TW. Effects of knee osteoarthritis on body's center of mass motion in older adults during level walking. Biomed Eng Appl Basis Comm. 2010;22:205e12.
27. Wang TM, Yen HC, Lu TW, Chen HL, Chang CF, Liu YH, et al. Bilateral knee osteoarthritis does not affect inter-joint coordination in older adults with gait deviations during obstacle crossing. J Biomech. 2009;42:2349e56.
28. Wei IP, Hsu WC, Chien HL, Chang CF, Liu YH, Ho TJ, et al. Leg and joint stiffness in patients with bilateral medial knee osteoarthritis during level walking. J Mech. 2009;25:279e87.
29. Weiss C, Rosenberg L, Helfet AJ. An ultrastructural study of normal young adult human articular cartilage. J Bone Joint Surg Am. 1968;50:663.
30. Woo SLY, Adeson WH, Jemmott GF. Measurements of nonhomogeneous directional mechanical properties of articular cartilage in tension. J Biomech. 1976;9:785.
31. Wyke BD. Articular neurology and manipulative therapy. In: Glasgow EF, Twomey LT, Scull ER, Kleynhans AM, Idczak RM (Eds). Aspects of Manipulative Therapy. Edinburgh, UK: Churchill Livingstone; 1985.

Pathogenesis of Autoimmune Diseases

Venus Khanna

INTRODUCTION

Rheumatoid arthritis (RA) is a disorder of autoimmune origin that primarily affects the joints, producing a nonsuppurative, proliferative, and inflammatory synovitis, cartilage, and bony destruction, production of autoantibodies. Rheumatoid factor (RF), anti-citrulline peptidase antibody (ACPA), and systemic involvement leading to cardiovascular, pulmonary, and skeletal complications. Understanding pathogenesis and complications of RA lead to development of new therapies with better outcome. Pathogenesis involves a complex interplay among genetic and environmental factors.

Smoking: Among environmental factors, smoking is most established risk factor. Many studies have confirmed the increased risk of RA in smokers. Risk is more for RF or ACPA positive RA. Studies have shown that risk is increased among persons with susceptibility human leukocyte antigen (HLA) DR4 alleles. Moreover, smoking and HLA-DR4 synergistically increase the risk of RA between 10 and 40 times higher.

Exposure to silica dust: Studies show that incidence of ACPA positive RA is more in miners exposed to silica than in those not exposed. Mechanisms for this are still not established and systemically studied.

Dietary factors: Some studies suggest that red meat may cause increased risk of RA and intake of fruits and oily fish may protect against RA. Mechanisms responsible for the relationship between dietary factors and occurrence of RA have thus far not been investigated systematically.

Lifestyle factors: Risk of RA is more in women than among men. Studies also show inverse relationship between level of education and risk of RA. Adverse life events are also associated with increase risk of RA in animal models. Rodent models show a link between the hypothalamic-pituitary axis and cytokine production. Such neuroimmunological interactions may operate locally or centrally. Studies show increased levels of neurotransmitters in synovitis of RA and peripheral inflammation upregulation cytokines in hypothalamus.

Infectious agents: Epstein-Barr virus (EBV), cytomegalovirus (CMV), proteus species, and their products have long been linked with RA. Underlying mechanisms remain elusive, some form of adjuvant action is postulated. The formation of immune complexes may trigger or induce the RF or result in citrullination of peptidase proteins. Arginine residues are post-translationally converted to citrulline. The marked reaction to these autoantigen suggests that they may be important arthritogenic agents.

Risk of developing RA is more in women than among men. Risk of onset of RA is also associated with adverse life events. Animal models show a link between the hypothalamic-pituitary adrenal axis and cytokine production. The central nervous system is normally involved in immune regulation and homeostatsis, and neuroimmunologic interactions regulate disease development in rodent models of arthritis. Such effects may operate locally (several neurotransmitters are expressed in synovitis in RA) or centrally (cytokines are rapidly up-regulated in the hypothalamus during peripheral inflammation).

The earliest event in RA pathogenesis is activation of the innate immune response, which includes the activation of dendritic cells by exogenous material and autologous antigens. Antigen-presenting cells including dendritic cells, macrophages, and activated B cells, present arthritis-associated antigens to T cells, which then release various cytokines leading to pathogenesis of RA.

ACTIVATION OF THE INNATE IMMUNE SYSTEM

Autoimmune rheumatic disease results from—break in self-tolerance, development of chronic inflammation in one or several organs and ongoing tissue destruction. Break in self-tolerance may result from central tolerance defects. Central tolerance is maintained in thymus in fetal and neonatal period. During this process the T cells that have high affinity for self-antigens are deleted by process of negative selection.

Dendritic cells are the "masterminds" of the immune system that play role in both central and peripheral tolerance.

Dendritic cell precursors are present in bone marrow. They go to peripheral tissues via blood where they capture foreign pathogens and antigens. Then through lymphatic channels they go to the lymphatic organs where they act as key antigen presenting cells responsible for priming of naïve T cells and induce their clonal expansion. During this process dendritic cells undergo maturation, which can be stimulated by various factors like proinflammatory cytokines, tissue factors like hyaluronan fragments, etc.

Mast cells: Along with dendritic cells, mast cells are also seen in synovium of patients with RA. They are usually in excess of tenfold above normal, sometimes described as synovial mastocytosis. Mast cells do not differentiate in the bone marrow; they circulate as committed progenitor cells that deposit in tissues where they complete their differentiation. Granules of mast cells contain natural protease, tryptase, and chymase. Synovial mastocytosis results from increase influx of mast cell progenitors at site of active inflammation. Possible chemoattractants are C5a, LTB4, TGF B, and serotonin. Stem cell factor (SCF) is major regulator of mast cell growth, survival, and differentiation. TNF promotes expression of SCF in synovial fibroblasts resulting in mast cell chemotaxis, maturation, and survival. On activation, mast cells release vasoactive mediators histamine, prostaglandin D2, and leucotrienes, which result in increased vascular permeability leading to edema and fibrin deposition. Mast cells along with other angiogenic factors, may contribute to growth of blood vessels that is seen associated with synovial hyperplasia in RA. Mast cells may activate synovial fibroblasts through TNF and IL-1 to produce matrix metalloproteinase, and prostaglandin E2. Mast cells may facilitate pannus invasion into cartilage and may modulate the functions of chondrocytes.

Macrophages—are cells of mononuclear phagocyte system (MPS). They are naturally present in synovial membrane. Altered differentiation and maturation seen in RA is a result of excess or imbalance of cytokines or growth factors. Both autocrine and paracrine mechanisms get activated and a complex reaction occurs in synovial tissues, influx of preactivated monocytes and their maturation in resident macrophages and interaction with other synovial cells result. Activated macrophages release several proinflammatory cytokines (e.g., MIF, TNF, IL-1, IL-13, IL-15, IL-23, IL-27), nitric oxide, reactive oxygen species, tissue degrading enzymes, acute phase proteins, chemokines, and regulatory molecules like IL-1, IL-10, TGF, TNF-R, etc.

CELLULAR IMMUNITY

T cells: T cells are derived from hematopoietic precursors in bone marrow. Differentiation of these cells occur in thymus where by process of negative selection, autoaggressive T cells are removed and only those T cells remain, which are tolerant toward self antigens. This is by binding of T cell receptor to MHC molecules. Only those thymocytes differentiate into mature lymphocytes that are able to identify self-MHC molecules complexed with foreign antigens. These thymocytes leave the circulation and form peripheral T lymphocytes. In periphery additional mechanisms act to maintain tolerance toward self-structures. On activation T cells perform their function.

T cells are abundant in the synovial fluid in patients with RA but their functional role is not completely understood. In studies, autoreactive T cells against citrullinated self proteins have been identified. Synovium in RA also contain several myeloid cells and dendritic cells that express cytokines and HLA class II molecules that are needed for T cell activation and antigen presentation.

HUMORAL IMMUNITY

B cells are derived from the hematopoietic precursors in the bone marrow. Immature B cells immigrate from the bone marrow into the peripheral blood and then mature in the spleen. Mature B cells undergo germinal center reaction in secondary lymphoid organs. This leads to proliferation of antigen-specific cells. Some B cells respond to specific antigens in T cell-independent manner and this leads to production of IgM antibodies. In patients with RA, IgM-RF, and antibodies against CCP are frequently present in synovial fluid and their presence is an indication of breakdown of immune tolerance. These antibodies can be seen in some patients 6–10 years before the onset of the disease indicating this as the important step in pathogensis.

CYTOKINES

In early RA, IL-4, IL-13, and IL-15 are expressed whereas in chronic disease TNFα and IL-17 have a significant impact. Through complex signal pathways cytokines activate additional cytokines and matrix metalloproteinases (MMPs) involved in tissue degradation. Important cytokines, are IFN-γ from TH-1 cells, activate macrophages and resident synovial cells. IL-17 recruits neutrophils and monocytes. TNF and IL-1 from macrophages stimulate resident synovial cells to secrete proteases that destroy hyaline cartilage, receptor antagonist of NF-κB ligand (RANKL), expressed on activated T cells stimulate bone resorption. Of these cells TNF has been most firmly implicated in the pathogenesis of RA.

Mesenchymal tissue response: The normal synovium contains synovial fibroblasts and macrophages. In RA, synovial fibroblasts contribute to chronic inflammation and joint destruction by direct mechanisms and through interaction with other cells. Fibroblasts get activated by inflammatory as well as through noninflammatory mechanisms like soluble factors, components of extracellular matrix (ECM) and other environmental stimuli like hypoxia and bacterial and viral antigens. Fibroblasts interact with cartilage ECM components through integrin molecules, which are highly expressed on synovial fibroblasts. These molecules also help in fibroblastic proliferation. Other cell surface molecules may be involved in this process. Fibroblasts produce matrix-degrading enzymes mainly MMP and cysteine proteinases (Cathepsins), which lead to resorption of cartilage. Fibroblasts also have a role in neoangiogenesis and accumulation of inflammatory cells, which further release cytokines like TNFα, IL-1, and IFN-γ, which further stimulate fibroblasts.

In RA osteoclastic activity occurs in underlying bone, which allows synovium to penetrate into it and form pannus. Inflammatory cytokines and enzymes released from neutrophils help in degradation of cartilage. Cartilage may also participate in its own degradation as evidences are there for selective damage to type II collagen fibrils in middle and deep layers.

Normally, few osteoblasts and osteoclasts are present at bone surface. In RA there is disbalance between osteoblastic and osteoclastic activity. Osteoclastic activity dominates as seen with increase concentration of macrophage colony stimulating factor (MCSF) and the RANKL, which are required for growth and differentiation of osteoclasts. Osteoblasts are virtually absent in RA indicating minimal repair activity. Few osteoblasts can be seen near endosteal surface close to inflammation site. These are metabolically active and represent bone response to inflammation. TNFα, IL-1, IL-6, and IL-17 also help in osteoclastic growth and differentiation. All these factors lead to rapid bone erosion in RA.

SYSTEMIC CONSEQUENCES

Patients with RA are at increased risk of cardiovascular illness like myocardial infarction, cerebrovascular events, and heart failure. Circulating IL-6, TNF, acute phase reactants, immune complexes, and altered lipid particles increase endothelial activation and render atheromatous plaques unstable.

Rheumatoid arthritis-related dyslipidemia is characterized by low total and high-density lipoproteins (HDL), elevated triglycerides and increase of small, dense low-density lipoprotein (LDL) species. Increased levels of acute phase reactants are an independent cardiovascular risk.

After cardiovascular disease (CVD), the most common systemic manifestation of RA is anemia, which occurs more frequently during the early stage of the disease. In patients with early RA, IL-6 levels are significantly higher than in persons without anemia. Additionally, hemoglobin levels are inversely correlated with IL-6 levels.

Persistent fatigue and high rates of depression are commonly reported in patients with RA. This is caused by upregulation of hypothalamus pituitary axis by various cytokines such as TNFα, IL-1. Thus, depression frequently observed in persons with RA is primarily mediated by the up regulation of cytokines.

Inflammation in RA also affects the brain (fatigue and reduced cognitive function), liver (elevated acute phase response and anemia of chronic disease), exocrine glands (secondary Sjögren's syndrome), muscles (sarcopenia), and bones (osteoporosis). Osteoporosis affects the axial and appendicular skeleton, with only a modest elevation of the acute phase response or subclinical inflammation, and probably occurs before the onset of articular disease.

KEY NOTES

- RA is a chronic inflammatory disease of autoimmune origin primarily affecting joints.
- Environmental factors (smoking, silica exposure), infections (EBV, CMV) also plays a role.
- Earliest event is activation of innate immune response.
- TNFα, IL-6, and IL-1 are the important mediators of cell migration, inflammation, systemic involvement.
- Most common systemic manifestation is CVDs (MI, CVA, etc.)
- IL-6 is raised in patient with anemia in RA.
- TNFα, IL-1 are responsible for HPA dysregulation.

FURTHER READING

1. Bradfield PF, Amft N, Vernon-Wilson E, Exley AE, Parsonage G, Rainger GE, et al. Rheumatoid fibroblast-like synoviocytes overexpress the chemokine stromal cell-derived factor 1 (CXCL12), which supports distinct patterns and rates of CD4+ and CD8+ T cell migration within synovial tissue. Arthritis Rheum. 2003;48:2472-82.
2. Cantaert T, Brouard S, Thurlings RM, Pallier A, Salinas GF, Braud C, et al. Alterations of the synovial T cell repertoire in anti-citrullinated protein antibody-positive rheumatoid arthritis. Arthritis Rheum. 2009;60:1944-56.
3. Choy E. Understanding the dynamics: pathways involved in the pathogenesis of rheumatoid arthritis. Rheumatology. 2012;51(Suppl 5):v3-11.
4. Eijsbouts AM, van den Hoogen FH, Laan RF, Hermus AR, Sweep CG, van de Putte LB. Hypothalamic-pituitary-adrenal axis activity in patients with rheumatoid arthritis. Clin Exp Rheumatol. 2005;23:658-64.
5. Gregersen PK, Silver J, Winchester RJ. The shared epitope hypothesis: an approach to understanding the moleculargenetics of susceptibility to rheumatoid arthritis. Arthritis Rheum. 1987;30:1205-13.
6. Güler-Yüksel M, Allaart CF, Goekoop-Ruiterman YPM, de Vries-Bouwstra JK, van Groenendael JH, Mallée C, et al. Changes in hand and generalised bone mineral density in patients with recent-onset rheumatoid arthritis. Ann Rheum Dis. 2009;68:330-6.
7. Hochberg MC, Johnston SS, John AK. The incidence and prevalence of extra-articular and systemic manifestations in a cohort of newly-diagnosed patients with rheumatoid arthritis between 1999 and 2006. Curr Med Res Opin. 2008; 24:469-80.

8. Holmqvist ME, Wedrén S, Jacobsson LT, Klareskog L, Nyberg F, Rantapää-Dahlqvist S, et al. Rapid increase in myocardial infarction risk following diagnosis of rheumatoid arthritis amongst patients diagnosed between 1995 and 2006. J Intern Med. 2010; 268:578-85.
9. Horvai A. Bone, joints and soft tissue tumors. In: Kumar V, Abbas AK, Aster JC (Eds). Robbins and Cotran The Pathologic Basis of Disease, 9th edition. Philadelphia: Elsevier; 2014. pp. 1209-12.
10. Lebre MC, Jongbloed SL, Tas SW, Smeets TJ, McInnes IB, Tak PP. Rheumatoid arthritis synovium contains two subsets of CD83-DC-LAMP-dendritic cells with distinct cytokine profiles. Am J Pathol. 2008;172:940-50.
11. McInnes IB, Leung BP, Liew FY. Cell-cell interactions in synovitis: Interactions between T lymphocytes and synovial cells. Arthritis Res. 2000;2:374-8.
12. McInnes IB, Schett G. The pathogenesis of rheumatoid arthritis. N Engl J Med. 2011;365:2205-19.
13. Sattar N, McInnes IB. Vascular comorbidity in rheumatoid arthritis: potential mechanisms and solutions. Curr Opin Rheumatol. 2005;17:286-92.
14. Schröder AE, Greiner A, Seyfert C, Berek C. Differentiation of B cells in the nonlymphoid tissue of the synovial membrane of patients with rheumatoid arthritis. Proc Natl Acad Sci USA. 1996;93:221-5.

Genetic Basis of Rheumatic Diseases

Aarti B Bhattacharya

■ INTRODUCTION

Rheumatic diseases include rheumatoid arthritis (RA), Felty's syndrome, Sjögren's syndrome, systemic sclerosis, polymyositis, dermatomyositis, Behçet's disease, spondyloarthropathies including ankylosing spondylitis (AS), reactive arthritis, Reiter's syndrome, psoriatic arthritis, etc.

■ ETIOPATHOGENESIS

The spectrum of rheumatic diseases is wide with conditions of diverse pathology, but most have in common a heritable risk with a common genetic basis, e.g., in RA, systemic lupus erythematosus (SLE) and AS **(Fig. 1)**. Autoimmune mechanisms are involved in the development of rheumatic diseases. The human leukocyte antigen (HLA) locus on chromosome 6 contributes to the risk of almost all autoimmune diseases **(Fig. 2)**. Both genetic and environmental factors play a strong role in its development. Genetic factors have been known to have an influence: some genes can predispose one to a disease while others protect one from a disease. A single major gene has been hypothesized to confer susceptibility for autoimmunity indicating that a postulated autoimmune gene is expressed as an autosomal dominant trait with penetrance of approximately 92% in females and 49% in males. Autoimmune diseases affect roughly 10% of the population in general. The exact cause of autoimmune disease is unknown. It is supposed that variation in the major histocompatibility complex (MHC)

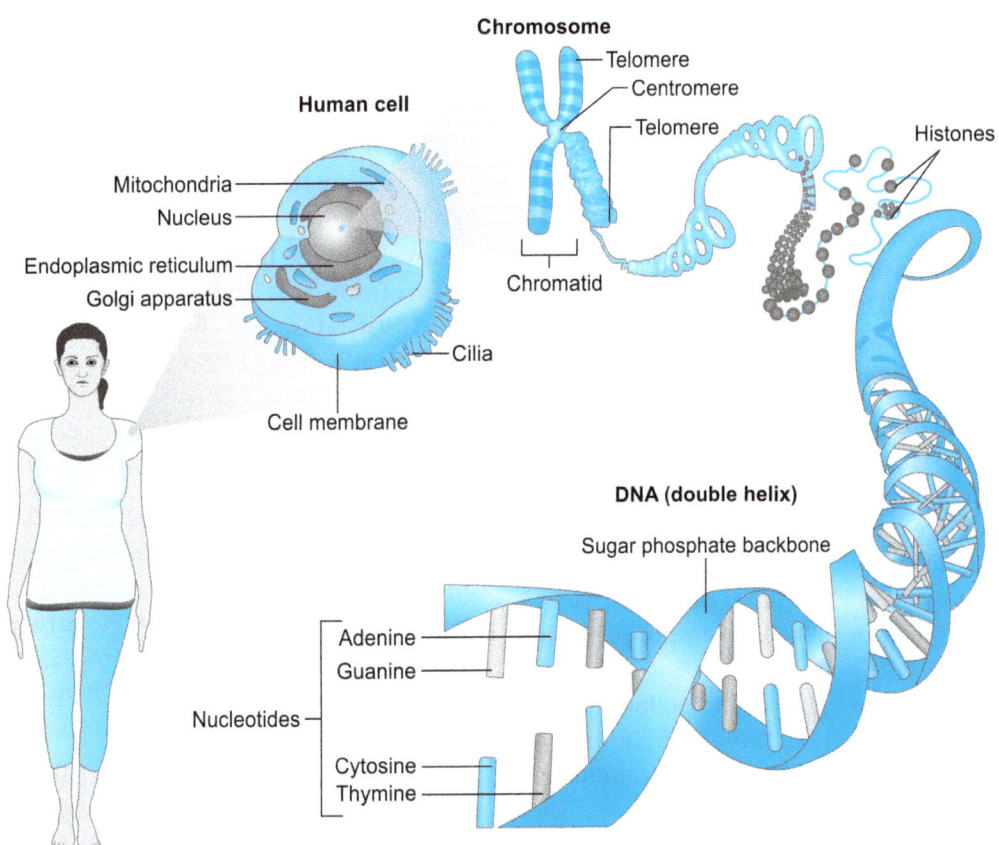

Fig. 1: Basic genetics.

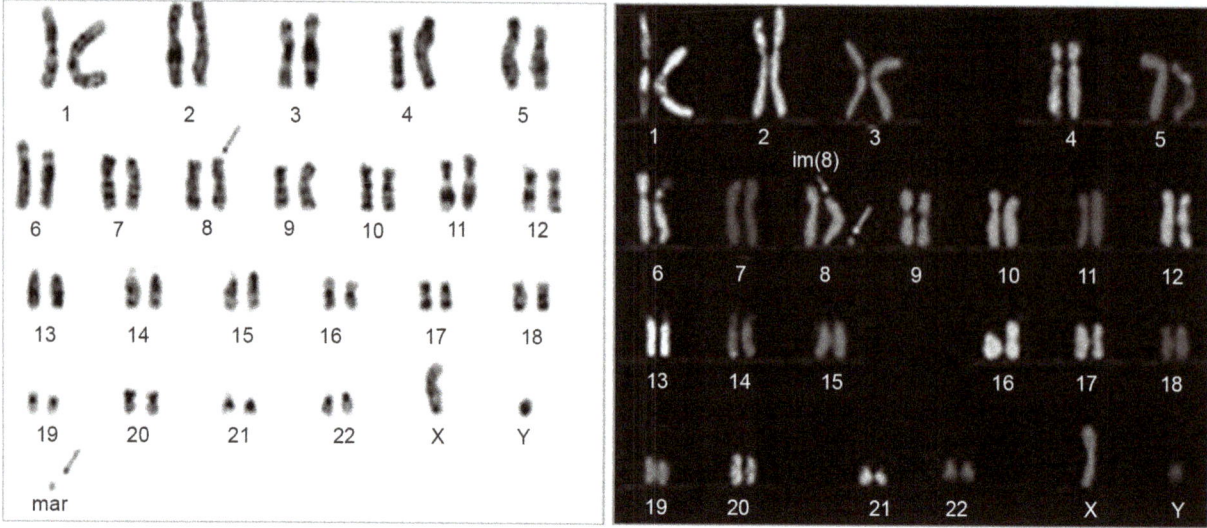

Fig. 2: Structure of chromosome in a karyotype.

peptide binding cleft facilitates presentation of self-antigen to autoreactive lymphocytes.

The MHC region and antigen processing: The MHC region situated on chromome 6 contributes to the risk of almost all autoimmune diseases. In humans, it is known as human leukocyte antigen (HLA). The exact mechanism of this causation is not known.

In RA, the MHC accounts for 33% of patients with genetic liability. Alleles at HLA-DRB1 contribute to this risk- DRB1*0401 carries an OR of 3. Genome Wide Association studies confirm the strong association with MHC variants, risk alleles confer an OR of around 2 to 3 as in homozygotes.

Systemic lupus erythematosus is strongly associated with alleles in class II region-HLA-DR2 (DRB1*1501) and DR3 (DRB1*0301). SLE is also associated with mutations in genes such as TNF, complement components C2, C4A and C4B. The HLA-B27 has a very strong association with AS with an OR of 200–300. In ankylosing spondylitis, HLA-B60 with an odds ratio of 3.6 and HLA-DR are involved.

Besides the MHC, two genes are involved in the etiopathogenesis of AS, namely-ARTS1 and IL-23R.

Interferon signaling in rheumatic diseases: Type 1 Interferons (IFN-α and IFN-β) are involved in the pathogenesis of SLE. IFN-α has multiple immunomodulatory actions; induction of dendritic cell differentiation, the upregulation of innate immune receptors like TLRs, the polarization of T cells towards TH1 phenotype and activation of B cells. Type 1 interferons are produced by all cells in response to viral infections **(Fig. 3)**.

Using a candidate gene approach targeting the IFN signaling pathway, the SNPrs2004640 in Interferon Regulating Factor 5 (IRF5) was found to be significantly associated with SLE (OR1.6).

In *IRF5* gene, a creation of a 5' Donor splice site in an alternative exon-1 thereby allowing the expression of several

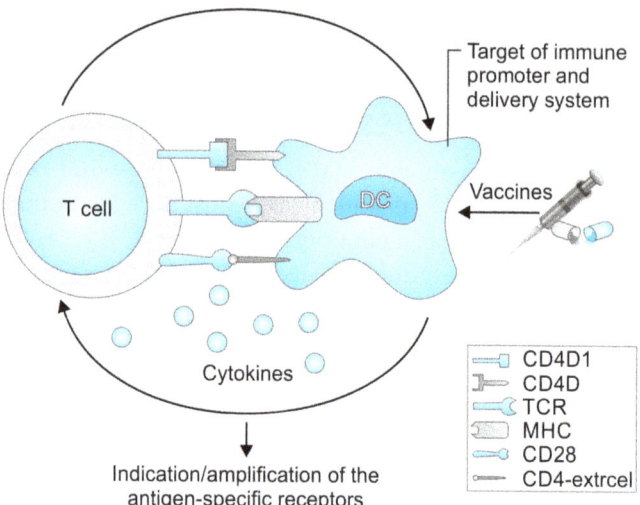

Fig. 3: Macrophage presenting antigen to T cell.

isoforms also a 30 base-pair-in-frame insertion or deletion variant of exon-6, a change in 3' untranslated region (3'UTR) and a CGGGG insertion-deletion (indel) polymorphism; the latter two affect the m-RNA stability causative mutations in rheumatic diseases.

The CGGGG indel allele carries risk for multiple sclerosis and inflammatory bowel disease.

TNF-associated signaling pathway: TNF-associated signaling pathway genes play a prominent role in the risk for SLE and RA.

The SNPrs10499194 in TNFAIP3 carries an OR of 1.33 for RA and rs5029939 an OR of 2.29 for SLE.

The complement system has long been known to be involved in the pathogenesis of RA.

Immunomodulatory adhesion molecule Integrin-AM: ITG_ AM variants are strongly associated with SLE. This mediates the adhesion of myeloid cells to endothelium via ICAM-1. It has a role in cell trafficking and phagocytosis.

Lymphocyte differentiation: Beyond the HLA region, strong genetic association of PTPN22 with RA has been suggested by the Candidate Gene Approach study. Based on linkage analysis identification of a susceptibility locus at 1p13. PTPN22 has remained the most consistent association mapped by GWA studies in RA. A role in SLE has also been identified. PTPN22 encodes lymphoid tyrosine phosphatase (LYP), a protein tyrosine phosphatase that inhibits T-cell receptor signaling, decreasing IL-2 production.

PTPN22 does not appear to be a risk factor for AS.

Polarization towards TH1 and TH17. phenotypes: STAT4 polarizes T cells towards TH1 and TH17 phenotypes which have the potential to promote autoimmunity STAT4 encodes signal transducer and activation of transcription factor-4 responsible for signaling by IL-12, IL-23 and Type 1 IFNs. There is convincing evidence that STAT4 is a risk locus for SLE in multiple racial groups.

According to WTCCC-AS study IL-23 is a risk gene in AS. IL-23 induces T cell towards TH17 differentiation, which is proinflammatory.

Interleukin-23 has been linked to psoriasis, ulcerative colitis and crohn's disease in GWA (Genome Wide Association) studies.

SINGLE GENE DISORDERS AND COMPLEX TRAITS

Single gene disorders are mainly due to error in one or both copies of a set of genes. Most single gene disease follow the Mendelian pattern of inheritance (**Figs. 4 to 6**).

- Autosomal recessive
- Autosomal dominant
- X-linked recessive
- X-linked dominant (rare).

For instance, familial Mediterranean fever is an autosomal recessive single gene disorder caused by a defect in the *MEFV* gene. Thus, if a person has errors in both copies of the gene, he or she is likely to be affected with the disease. It is presumed that both parents of the affected

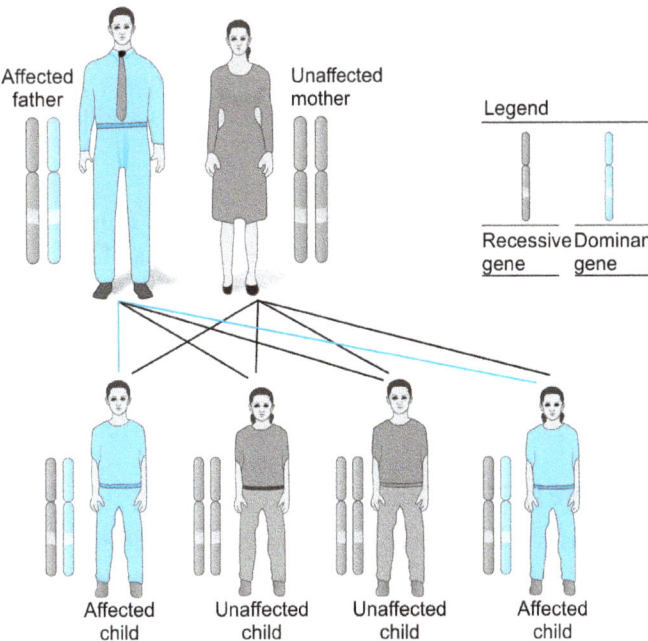

Fig. 5: Autosomal dominant inheritance.

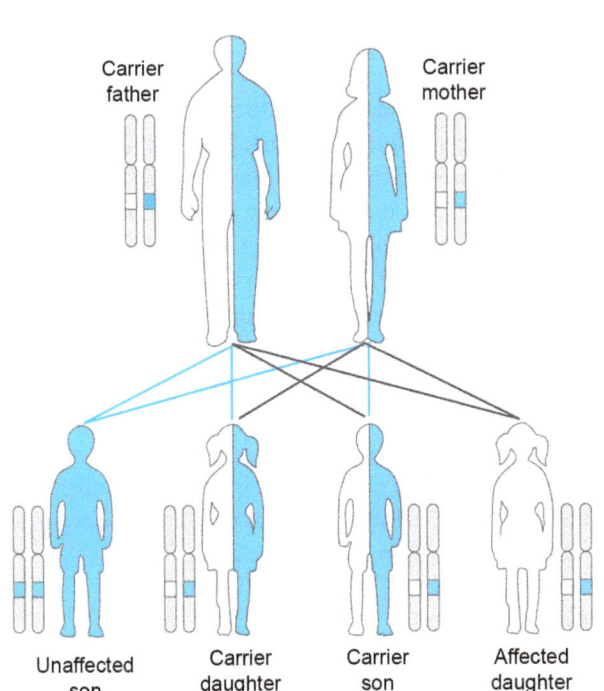

Fig. 4: Autosomal recessive inheritance.

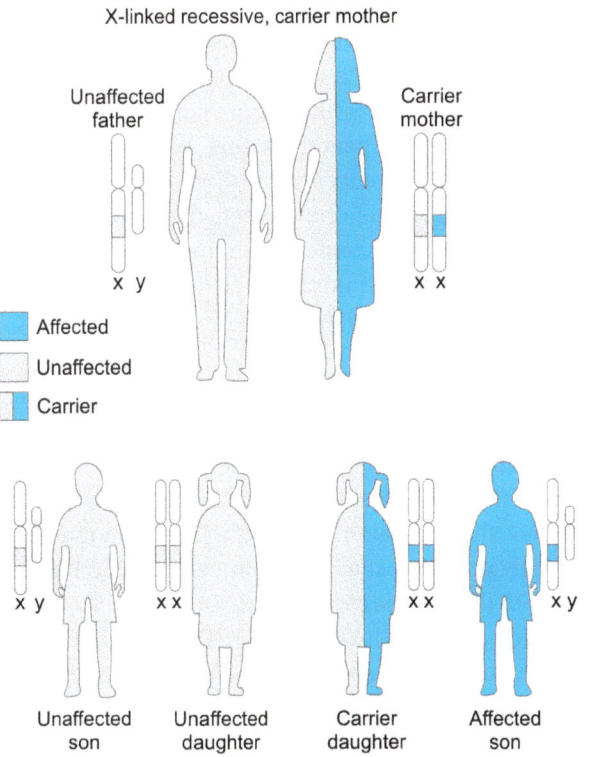

Fig. 6: X-linked recessive inheritance.

individual are carriers, which means they have error in one copy of the set of two copies of the *MEFV* gene. Carriers are heterozygotes and are usually unaffected. Affected persons are homozygotes. The risk of carrier parents having an affected child (homozygote for the mutation) is 1 in 4 or 25% for each pregnancy.

Here the MEFV mutation is responsible for causing the disease. At the same time, MEFV mutations carrying patients have additional susceptibility for Behçet's disease, ulcerative colitis and rheumatoid arthritis.

- *Ulcerative colitis*: An increased frequency of MEFV mutations has been found in persons with ulcerative colitis, especially those with episodic arthritis, and this may suggest a possible modifying effect of MEFV in the disease process.
- *Rheumatoid arthritis*: Mutations in *MEFV* gene, in particular the E148Q mutation, has been found to be an independent modifier of the clinical manifestations of RA. In RA, ulcerative colitis, and Behçet's disease, in contrast to familial Mediterranean fever, the *MEFV* gene error or polymorphism is not the sole cause of the disease; it interacts with other genes to predispose to ulcerative colitis or modify the clinical manifestation of RA.

GENETIC STUDIES

In diseases where autoimmunity has been implicated as the cause of the problem, familial aggregation is often observed, although its significance is still not clear. Segregation analysis is often compatible with autosomal dominant inheritance. Autoimmunity has been stated as an autosomal dominant trait.

More commonly, rheumatic diseases have a complex inheritance pattern which is not explained by simple Mendelian genetics; it is much more complex than was previously believed. Nongenetic factors, such as infections or smoking, too have an effect on the disease.

Various approaches have been designed to evaluate the contribution of genetic factors in the development of rheumatic disease. Autoimmune disorders are inherited as an autosomal-dominant trait.

FAMILY STUDY

The oldest approach is to study familial cases where the same or different autoimmune disease occurs in one family. An extensive pedigree will determine the affected family members and the pattern of inheritance. The members of the family probably share the same environmental factors along with the genetic variability.

Inheritance of HLADRB10101, DRB10401, DRB10404 increases the relative risk of RA. While HLADRB11101, DRB11501 protect the person against development of RA. Linkage analysis would then help to trace certain candidate genes causing the disease.

These candidate genes can be later tested to prove or disprove a hypothesis. However, genetic factors do not fully account for the incidence of RA thereby incriminating environmental factors in the causation of RA.

TWIN STUDY

Another useful approach is comparison between genetically identical, i.e., monozygotic twins; individuals with approximately 50% genes in common, such as dizygotic twins and siblings; and then unrelated individuals. If two individuals are unrelated, the overall degree of genetic similarity at polymorphic loci is relatively low with approximately <0.1% difference over the entire genome. The overall concordance rate for autoimmune disease is 15–30%. This means that 15–30 of the 100 probands with autoimmune disease who are monozygotic co-twins, will develop the disease. In SLE, the concordance rate is 5–10-folds greater in monozygotic twins than dizygotic twins. Lack of 100% concordance indicates that these diseases are a result of interacting genetic and environmental factors. The reverse is also true where only 2–5% of dizygotic twin or siblings will develop the disease. In these studies, the environmental factors are presumed to be the same.

It is also seen that family members of an individual with one autoimmune disease are predisposed to developing different autoimmune disease suggesting that common genes predispose to different forms of autoimmunity.

However, awareness of the Mendelian disease is important in this era of molecular biology as in very rare cases such a disease may underlie a common rheumatic condition; for example, gout, where the rare cause can be X-linked recessive disorder of hypoxanthine-guanine phosphoribosyltransferase (HGPRT) deficiency, also known as Lesch–Nyhan syndrome.

The process of identifying the genes which could be responsible for a disease can be through two approaches:

1. *Candidate gene study*: Hypothesized candidate genes are tested either by familial or animal studies. Prior studies would have linked the disease to a chromosome locus containing possible candidate genes. For instance, HLADR2 and HLADR3 confer a modest increased risk of SLE. SLE is more prevalent in individuals with C4,C1q,C1r or C2 complement deficiency. Probably in these patients clearance of circulating immune complexes (CIC) is defective. Men with Klinefelter syndrome are more prone to SLE.
2. *Positional cloning*: The protein product involved in the disease is known but the gene is unidentified. A genome-based scan helps to identify the gene.

HLA-B27

This is one of the protein products of the superfamily of genes (located at B locus) which comprises the MHC. HLA-B27 is found in about 8% of the healthy Caucasian population.

Variability in HLA-B27 allele frequency exists in different ethnic Indian populations. Studies conducted in India show a 5% prevalence in north Indian states as compared to 1% in south Indian states. Not all HLA-B27 positive individuals will develop AS.

Ankylosing spondylitis: Occurrence of the disease depends on other unknown factors, genetic factors, and environmental factors such as diet and ethnic origin. Interestingly, no association of HLA- B27 is seen in patients with spondyloarthritis in Africans or among Inuits.

Ankylosing spondylitis is the prototype of spondyloarthropathy. It is a chronic progressive inflammatory disorder involving sacroiliac joints, spine, and large peripheral joints. The chronic inflammatory process causes eventual fusion of the spine. The spondyloarthropathy spectrum includes a subset of psoriatic arthritis, reactive arthritis, arthritis associated with inflammatory bowel disease (IBD), and undifferentiated spondyloarthropathy. AS is one of the most common chronic rheumatic disease and is associated very strongly with the genetic marker HLA-B27. Many cases of RA are associated with IBD. About 50–75% of patients with both AS and IBD are HLA-B27 positive. Therefore, this molecule is supposed to play a central role in the pathogenesis of the disease. The subtypes of spondyloarthropathy are difficult to differentiate. Studies have suggested that a predominant shared component, including HLA-B27, predisposes to all phenotypic subsets, and that these subsets should be considered as various phenotypic expressions of the same disease.

While the role of HLA-B27 in clinical pathogenesis is established, molecular typing has made it possible to identify the subtypes that are more likely to cause spondyloarthropathy. Subtypes B*2706 and B*2709 probably play no pathogenic role, whereas other subtypes like B*2704 and B*2705 have a strong role in the pathogenesis of spondyloarthropathy. The difference in pathogenic consequences between certain subtypes of HLA B27 is explained by the presence of HLA-B40 in HLA-B27 positive individuals. HLA-B40 increases the risk for disease more than threefold.

Molecular typing has revealed that small differences exist between the pathogenic and nonpathogenic types in the amino acid residues 114 and 116 on the antigen-presenting groove of the molecule. The nonpathogenic molecule HLA-B*2706 has aspartic acid as compared to other amino acids seen in pathogenic molecules. This amino acid residue is situated on the rim between the D and the F pocket. The molecule B*2709 has histidine on position 116 on the bottom of the F pocket, which is unique. These studies have to continue and will help to reveal how these small differences can be responsible for the difference between health and disease.

HLA-B27 and its Clinical Relevance

This is a very useful test and it has a high negative predictive value. The association is strong with AS but all HLA-B27 positive individuals do not develop AS. Obviously, this is not the only contributing factor and there must be other genetic and environmental contributions which cause the disease. For example, Inuits do not develop AS despite being positive for HLA-B27; similarly, Africans are very unlikely to develop AS.

There are various methods of testing HLA-B27. These are serological and flow cytometry, though used in many centers, may not be accurate. However, molecular methods now being used are simple, accurate, and are able to identify the subtype, thereby making it more useful.

- Human leukocyte antigen is not only associated with autoimmune rheumatic diseases but also with certain autoantibodies, for example, anti-Ro and anti-La are autoantibodies most frequently encountered in SLE and Sjögren's syndrome Family members of an individual with RA are predisposed to different autoimmune diseases. MHC genes are located in chromosome 6p.
- Ankylosing spondylosis and IBD are strongly associated with HLA-B27. They are strongly associated with HLA-DR3 and DQ[1]

HLA and Other Autoimmune Disease Associations

The major susceptibility alleles associated with RA are the HLA-DR4 alleles DRB1*0401 and DRB1*0404. HLA-DR3 appears to be a general autoimmune haplotype, not only associated with insulin-dependent diabetes mellitus (IDDM) but also with SLE, Graves' disease, autoimmune hypothyroidism, and Addison's disease.

Toll-like receptors (TLRs) and TNF genes have been implicated in autoimmune disease susceptibility. For example, persons with SLE have an altered form of TLR-9 that reacts with the body's own DNA. TNF alpha-308 allele is associated with SLE. However, extensive studies are required to clarify the exact role of these genes.

Clearly, genes play a role in the pathogenetic mechanisms of rheumatic diseases. However, till further studies provide conclusive evidence as to the exact role of these genes, research and family studies should continue.

Physicians providing primary care, play a pivotal role in providing a meaningful direction to research by taking a thorough history (including family history) and applying the knowledge of medicine and genetics to identify families that can contribute to research. An attempt can be made to point out empiric risks for other family members who have relatives with rheumatic disease: this will depend on the type of disease and family members who are affected. Affected parents may be anxious about the risk of their offspring developing such diseases. They will need to be counseled with caution in such situations. No definite genes have been isolated which are known to cause disease in all those who have inherited it. The predisposition may be increased depending on the family history and other modifying genes that are inherited in that individual. The parents should be reassured and also educated. They could be directed to sources providing reliable information, advised to choose a healthy lifestyle, and adopt appropriate lifestyle modifications, and should be warned of the need for early intervention if the need arise. This will help in reducing the chances of developing the disease and its complications.

KEY POINTS

- Rheumatic diseases comprise a spectrum of diseases such as Sjögren's syndrome, Felty's syndrome, RA, AS, SLE, etc.
- Genetic factors do not fully account for the incidence of RA. It is a multifactorial disorder
- Family members of an individual with RA are predisposed to different autoimmune diseases.
- *MHC* genes are located in chromosome 6p.
- Ankylosing spondylosis and IBD are strongly associated with HLA-B27.

FURTHER READING

1. Begorich AB, Carlton VE, et al. Strong genetic association of PTPN22 with RA has been suggested by the Candidate Gene Approach study. Am J Hum Gen. 2004;75(2):330-7.
2. Brown MA, Kennedy LG, Darke C. Pile KD, et al. The effect of HLA-DR genes on the susceptibility to and severity of ankylosing spondylitis. Arthritis Rheum. 1998;41(3): 460-5.
3. Brown MA, Pile KD, Kennedy LG, Calin A, et al. HLA class 1 association of ankylosing spondylitis in the white population in the United Kingdom. Ann Rheum Dis. 1996; 55(4):268-70.
4. Clarke A, Vyse TJ. Genetics of rheumatic diseases. Pub Med. 2009;11(5):248.
5. Fernando MM, Stevens CR, Waish EC, et al. HLA-DR2 (DRB1*0301), defining the role of the MHC in autoimmunity, a review and pooled analysis. PLoS Genet. 2008;25:4(4): e1000024.
6. Graham RR, Cotsapas C, Davies L, Hacket R, et al. Genetic variants near TNFA1P3 on 6q23 are associated with SLE. Nat Genet. 2008; 40(9):1059-61.
7. Graham RR, Kuzyrev SV, Baechier EC. Reddy MV, et al. A common haplotype of interferon regulating factor5 (IRF5) regulates splicing and expression and is associated with increased risk of SLE. Nat Genet. 2006; 38(5):550-5
8. Graham RR, Kyogoku C, Sigurdsson S, Vlasova A. Three functional variants of IFN regulatory factor 5 (IRF-5) define risk and protective haplotypes for human lupus. Proc Natl Acad Sci. 2007;104(16):6758-63.
9. Imirzalioglu N, Dursum A, Tastan B, Soysal Y, Yakicier MC. MEFV gene is a probable susceptibility gene for Behçet's disease. Scand J Rheumatol. 2005;34:56-58.
10. Jayapal V. Fundamentals of Immunology: Rheumatic Diseases, 1st edition. New Delhi; Jaypee Brothers Medical Publishers; 2007. pp. 335-63.
11. Kastelein RA, Hunter CA, et al. WTCCC-AS study IL-23 is a risk gene in AS. IL-23 induces T-cell towards TH17 differentiation, which is proinflammatory. Annu Rev Immunol. 2007;25:221-42.
12. Lewis MJ, Botto M. Complement deficiencies in humans and animals links to autoimmunity. Autoimmunity. 2006;39(5): 367-78
13. Mathur AN, Chang HC, et al. STAT4 polarizes T cells towards TH 1 and TH17 phenotypes which have the potential to promote autoimmunity. J Immunol. 2007; 178(8):4901-7.
14. Rabinovich E, Livneh A, Langevitz P, Brezniak N. Shinar E, Pras M, et al. Severe disease in patients with rheumatoid arthritis carrying a mutation in the Mediterranean fever gene. Ann Rheum Dis. 2005;64: 1009-14.
15. Raychaudhuri S, Remmeri EF, Lee AT, Hacket R, et al. Common variants at CD 40 and other loci confer risk of rheumatoid arthritis. Nat Genet. 2008;40(10):1216-23.
16. Sigurdsson S, Gonning HH, Kristjansdottir G, Milanil, et al. Comprehensive evaluation of the genetic variants of interferon regulatory factor 5 (IRF5) reveals a novel 5bp length polymorphism as strong risk factor for SLE. Hum Mol Genet. 2008;17(6):872-81
17. Sigurdsson S, Nordmark G, Gonning HH, et al. Polymorphisms in the tyrosine kinase 2 and interferon regulatory factor 5 genes are associated with systemic lupus erythematosus. Am J Hum Genet. 2005;76(3): 528-37.
18. Watford WT, Hissong BD, et al. STAT4 encodes signal transducer and activation of transcription factor-4 responsible for signalling by IL-12, IL-23 and Type 1 IFNs. Immunol Rev. 2004;202:139-56.
19. Welcome Trust Case Control Consortium. IL23 has been linked to psoriasis, ulcerative colitis and Crohn's disease in GWA (Genome Wide Association) studies. Nature. 2007; 447(7145):661-78.

SECTION 2

Rheumatoid Arthritis in Orthopedic Rheumatology

- **Introduction of Orthopedic Rheumatology**
  Manish Khanna
- **Rheumatoid Arthritis: Etiopathogenesis, Clinical Features, and Management**
  Manish Khanna
- **Ultrasound in Early Inflammatory Arthritis**
  THS Bedi
- **Recent Advances in the Management of Rheumatoid Arthritis**
  Neeraj Jain
- **Biological Therapy**
  Shweta Agarwal
- **Surgical Considerations in Inflammatory Arthritis**
  Manish Khanna, Rashmi Chopra
- **Challenges in Arthroplasty in Rheumatoid Arthritis**
  Jitendra Chowdhary
- **Skin Manifestations in Orthorheumatology**
  Sunil Kumar Gupta

Introduction of Orthopedic Rheumatology

Manish Khanna

Orthopedic rheumatology, a term described in the literature, is a rapidly evolving medical surgical specialty, important and useful for orthopedic surgeons, occupied in surgical practices. New scientific discoveries related to this specialty are largely related to better understanding of immunology and pathogenesis of major rheumatological disorders which an orthopedic surgeon must be aware of.

Approximately 70% of Indian population live in villages and patients have been going to orthopedic surgeons for joint pain, hence, there has to be proper training for the management of the diseases (for both medical and surgical reasons). We very well know that the realistic goal of early management of polyarthritis could be achieved with early patient presentation and increased awareness both on the part of patient and the treating surgeon who must be up-to-date with the current practices.

In general, both rheumatologist and orthopedic surgeon treat problems of the musculoskeletal system but the rheumatologist does it mostly with medication and the orthopedic surgeon does it with surgery. But is surgery always required in various rheumatological disorders especially in the early stages? Why let an early arthritis progress to a severe arthritis where replacement is the only answer? The proper knowledge can cater the needs of mild to moderate arthritic joint.

For oversimplification: Orthopedic rheumatology caters the medical and surgical aspect of such diseases. The biggest challenge in the developing countries like India is limited number of specialists with rheumatological training especially in semiurban and rural areas. Awareness among orthopedic surgeons for proper treatment and newer development in this field should be there. We should create and develop international scientific relations with rheumatologists all over the world and favor as well as stimulate all efforts to do research work in this field.

It is a heartening fact that the Indian Orthopaedic Rheumatology Association (IORA) has matured over past 11 years into a well-progressive enlarging group of orthopedic professionals learning and practicing orthopedic rheumatology. IORA offers a unique forum for the exchange of scientific knowledge on the subject and its sincere efforts will render best services to the orthopedic fraternity. Orthopedic rheumatology represents this branch of medicosurgical knowledge at our National as well as International level and with such increasing awareness and interest in updating ourselves in this subject, the light at the end of the tunnel is indeed bright.

Rheumatoid Arthritis: Etiopathogenesis, Clinical Features, and Management

Manish Khanna

INTRODUCTION

Rheumatoid arthritis (RA) is a chronic systemic autoimmune inflammatory disease characterized by destructive symmetrical polyarthritis affecting small joints of hand and foot leading to radiological erosions and gradual deformities of joints. Pathologically, a chronic proliferative synovitis with villous hypertrophy, infiltrated by lymphocytes and plasma cells, is seen. It affects about 1–2% of population but prevalence varies depending on age and race. It is mainly prevalent in highly developed countries as USA and UK and the prevalence rate is slightly lower in developing countries.

ETIOLOGY AND PATHOGENESIS

Joint damage in RA is mediated through immunological mechanisms. For decades together, despite of intensive study and research work, the steps involved in pathogenesis of inflammation and joint erosions is still not clear and remains a mystery. The exact cause is unknown, many studies suggest that a blend of environmental, genetic factors, and even host factors is not sufficient for the full expression of disease.

- *Genetic factors*: Genes play a key role in susceptibility to RA and disease severity. Approximately 60% risk of developing RA can be associated by genetically class II major histocompatibility complex (MHC) genes, especially genes containing a specific 5 amino acid sequence in the hypervariable region of HLA-DR4.
- *Environmental factors*:
  - *Infectious agents*: Many virus and bacteria have been presumed to be the cause of RA in genetically susceptible individuals. Organisms, which can cause, are mycobacteria, streptococci, mycoplasma, and rubella. Repeated inflammatory insults especially through specialized receptors that recognize common molecules produced by pathogens, in a genetically susceptible individual might contribute to breakdown of tolerance and subsequent autoimmunity. Evidence of autoimmunity can be present in RA many years before the onset of clinical arthritis. Autoantibodies commonly associated are rheumatoid factor (RF) and anticyclic citrullinated peptide (anti-CCP) antibodies. These autoantibodies can recognize joint antigens such as type II collagen or systemic antigens such as glucose phosphate isomerase and thus contribute to synovial inflammation.

    Cytokines play a key role in the process of joint inflammation and the process includes interaction between proinflammatory and anti-inflammatory cytokines.
  - *Lifestyle factors*: There is an increased risk of developing RA with tobacco chewing and smoking. Increased exposure to crystalline silica has been associated with the likelihood of developing RA.
- *Host factors*: It has been observed that host immune factors have got a role in developing RA with autoimmune diseases such as type 1 diabetes and hypothyroidism.

In general, CD4 T cells are recognized to drive the inflammatory process. The synovium of joints affected by RA contains large numbers of activated T cells (CD4 T cells) and also contains macrophages and B lymphocytes.

CLINICAL FEATURES OF RHEUMATOID ARTHRITIS

Onset

Peak incidence seen in between 30 and 50 years, but RA can also occur in old age. Women are affected more than men 3:1. The greater prevalence of RA among women suggests that sex hormones estrogens play a role in development of the disease. But further there occurs an improvement in the condition of the disease during pregnancy and this is because the amount of circulating estrogen during pregnancy is just enormous. Within the first couple of months after the pregnancy, probably 90% of RA patients have a serious flare and have to go back on their medication.

In about 70% of patients, it appears insidiously as symmetrical arthritis over a period of weeks to months. The initial symptoms may be systemic or articular. In some individuals, fatigue, malaise, diffuse musculoskeletal pain, and swollen hands may be the first nonspecific complaints followed by gradual joint involvement. Some patients present with single joint involvement which then gradually progresses to involve other joints into a full blown later polyarthritis. Asymmetrical initial presentation with more symmetry developing later on in the course of disease is a common feature. The reason to this asymmetry of joints involvement as compared with other form of arthritis such as seronegative spondyloarthropathy is unknown.

Morning stiffness is a cardinal feature that usually appears even before pain. This is due to the accumulation of edematous fluid within the early inflamed tissue during inactivity/sleep and this fluid later disappears due to its absorption by lymphatics and venules following the activity of the muscles and joints in the morning. To be more specific, in RA this morning stiffness should persist for at least 30–45 minutes before disappearing. A similar phenomenon can occur if patient is inactive for a prolonged period during the day. It is rare for symptoms to remit completely in one set of joints while developing in another (this migrating pattern of arthritis is usually seen in rheumatic arthritis). Symptoms like low-grade fever, fatigue, anorexia, and weight loss may be present (weight loss is due to the catabolic effects of cytokines and due to an associated anorexia). Around 8–15% of patients have acute onset of symptoms which peak within few days and thus diagnosis of acute onset is difficult to make (sepsis or vasculitis must be ruled out in such cases). An intermediate type of onset in which symptoms develop over weeks occur in 15–20% patients.

Joint Involvement

Rheumatoid arthritis mainly involves the small joints of hand and foot. In hand, it affects mainly metacarpophalangeal (MCP) joints, proximal interphalangeal (PIP) joints, and wrist. Early synovitis of PIP joints gives the appearance of fusiform swelling (spindle shape appearance of the joint) **(Fig. 1)**.

Metatarsophalangeal (MTP) joints are involved in foot. Larger joints are generally involved after smaller joints.

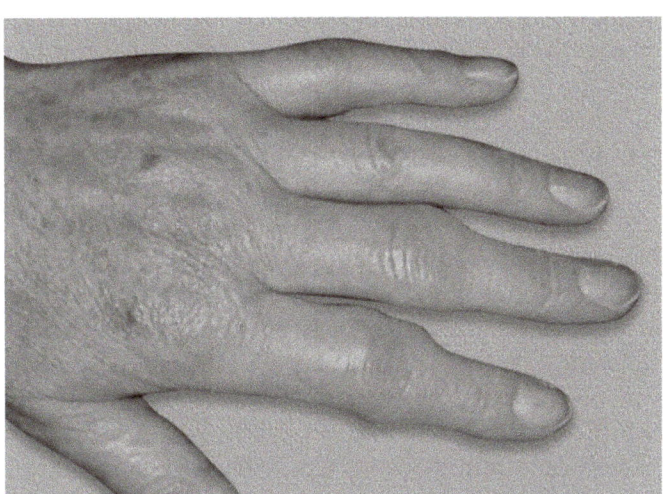

Fig. 1: Early synovitis of proximal interphalangeal joints.

Synovitis in larger joints is likely to remain asymptomatic for a longer duration than in smaller ones and a biopsy taken from an asymptomatic knee often shows histological evidence of synovitis. Other joints affected in decreasing order are as elbow, shoulder, ankle, knee, and hip. RA never affects thoracolumbar spine, also rarely affects sacroiliac (SI) joint but affects cervical spine at C1 and C2 junction leading to subluxation. Diagnostic clues that can be used to determine the patients in whom early arthritis may progress to classic RA and who may develop an alternative inflammatory arthritis, such as seronegative spondyloarthropathies or even may have spontaneous remission later on, are need to be worked up.

The importance of early disease management is obvious, as early treatment potentially could limit or prevent joint damage and even permit long-term remission. As approximately 30–40% patients with early synovitis have spontaneous remissions, accurate identification of patients with RA is a must, to avoid undertreatment and overtreatment. In a study, it was observed that some of the patients who could not be diagnosed as RA were placed under an "undifferentiated arthritis" category and such patients, at a later stage, may develop RA or even remain undifferentiated. Anti-CCP antibodies in particular are strongly associated with evolution of undifferentiated arthritis into RA and progression to erosive disease.

Older individuals, >65 years of age developing RA often present with stiffness, limb girdle pain, and diffuse boggy swelling of the hand and wrist. A clinical onset that mimics polymyalgia rheumatica also can occur in an elderly individual. Generally, elderly individuals who develop RA tend to have a more benign course of disease than younger patients. Also in elderly, there is lower frequency of positive tests for RF. The older patients have more rapid progression of damage to joint, indicating that osteoarthritis was responsible for a significant portion of the damage noted at the onset of disease. RA (even unilateral involvement) can occur with many other chronic diseases such as with poliomyelitis, meningioma, encephalitis, stroke, and cerebral palsy.

The signs of joint inflammation are pain, swelling, warmth, and painful limitation of joint movement.

Classical Deformities in Hands

- *Boutonniere's deformity* in which there is hyperflexion at the PIP joint and hyperextension at the distal interphalangeal joint **(Fig. 2)**.
- *Swan neck deformity* in which there occurs hyperextension at the PIP joint and hyperflexion at the distal interphalangeal joint **(Fig. 3)**.
- *Z deformity in thumb*: In this, there occurs fixed flexion and subsequent subluxation at metacarpophalangeal joint with hyperextension at the distal interphalangeal joint.

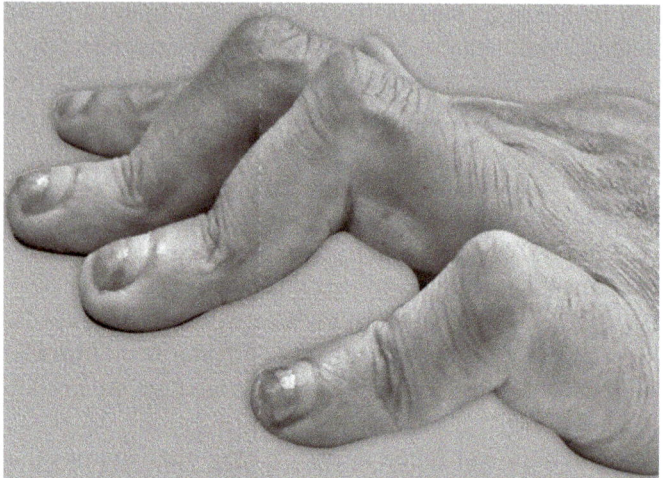

Fig. 2: Boutonniere's deformity.

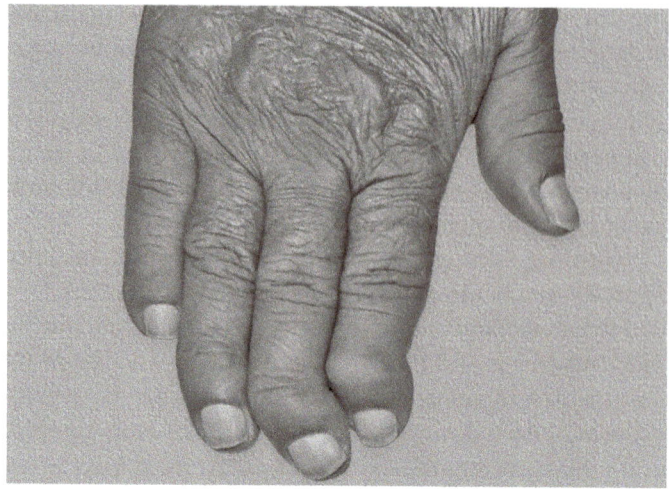

Fig. 3: Swan neck deformity.

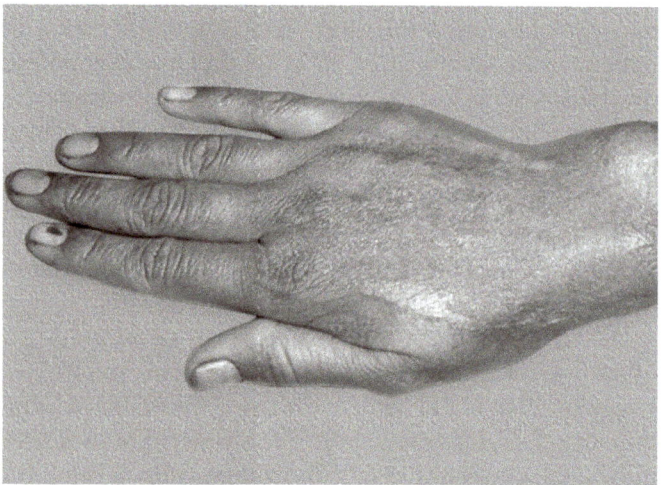

Fig. 4: Piano-key ulnar head deformity.

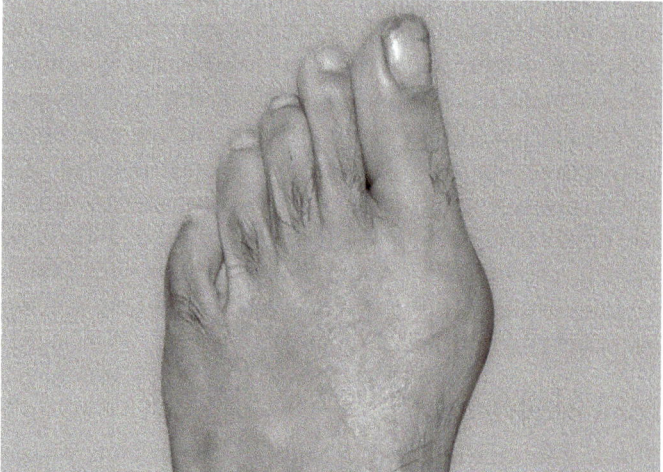

Fig. 5: Hallux valgus deformity.

- Gradual ulnar deviation of the fingers due to subluxation of MCP joints.
- Piano-key ulnar head due to secondary destruction of ulnar collateral ligament can be seen (**Fig. 4**).

Foot and Ankle

The ankle involvement is usually mild in RA, but damage can occur in severe progressive forms of the disease. Clinical evidence for ankle involvement is cystic swelling, anterior and posterior to the malleoli. Of those affected with foot and ankle disease, 90% have forefoot disease, 66% have subtalar joint involvement, and only about 9% have ankle disease. Due to subtalar joint involvement, valgus heel can be seen in RA.

Deformities of Forefoot

Hallux valgus deformity can be seen due to involvement of first MTP joints with medial displacement at the MTP joint and thus the lateral deviation of the first toe (**Fig. 5**). Actually this deformity starts with pathological changes in the ligamentous supporting structures on MTP joints resulting from the inflammation and later on, there occurs gradual progressive erosion of joint with remineralization and gradual blunt spur formation where the heads appear almost chewed due to advanced erosive disease. This erosive disease along with giving away of ligaments leads to metatarsal spread and thus produces laterally deviated forefoot called as *fibular deviation*. This is the most frequently encountered rheumatoid foot deformity which can be surgically corrected (**Fig. 6**).

Hallux valgus is defined when the first metatarsal and the base of first phalanx are at an angle >20°. As disease progress, the first toe tends to lie under the second and third toe (usually Bunion is formed medially over metatarsal head). Irritable MTP joints are the main sources of trouble. Due to plantar callosities along the plantar aspect of metatarsal heads, patients feel as there are pebbles in their shoes with grossly deformed toes (**Fig. 7**). One have to differentiate rheumatoid hallux valgus from idiopathic type. Hallux rigidus or arthritis of first MTP joint leading to stiffness and inability to dorsiflex is seen in 13% females and 7% males with RA.

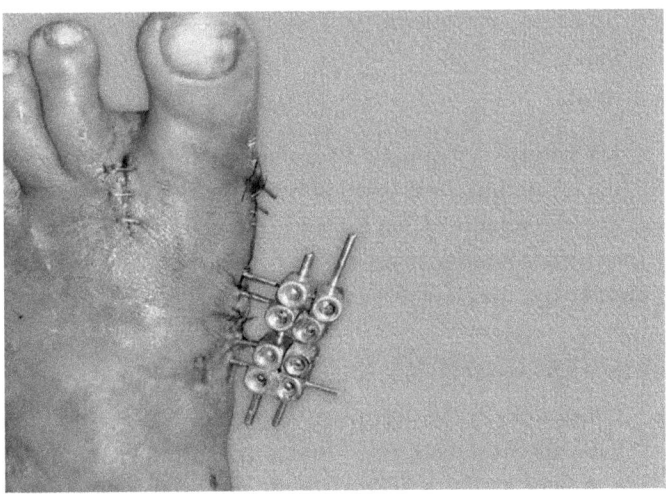

Fig. 6: Surgically corrected—perioperative image of the same patient in Figure 5.

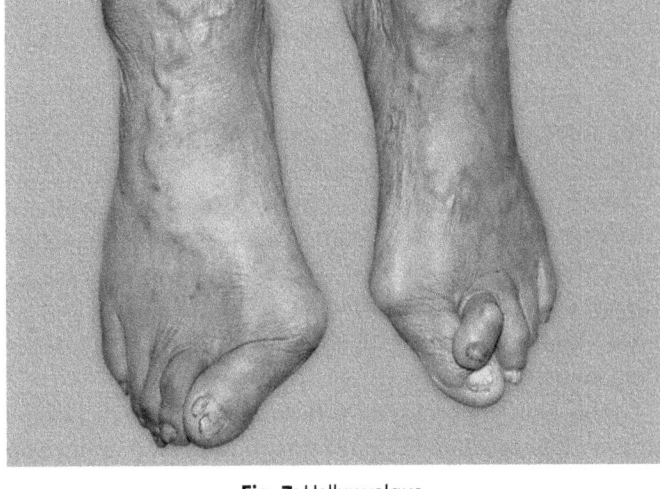

Fig. 7: Hallux valgus.

Deformities of Midfoot

The midfoot is not commonly involved in RA, but if it is, then talonavicular and naviculocuneiform joints are usually affected. As disease progresses, involvement of muscle and ligaments supporting the arches of foot occurs with further gradual involvement of talonavicular joint, resulting in pronation and eversion of the foot (pes planovalgus deformity).

Deformities of Hindfoot

Heel pain is slightly uncommon in RA. When tendo-Achilles insertion or plantar aponeurosis insertion at calcaneus is affected, then patients may complain of ill-defined heel pain (insertion of tendoachilles become inflamed and thickened.)

Rheumatoid nodules can develop in Achilles tendon at its insertion. Spontaneous rupture of tendon has been reported when diffuse granulomatous inflammation is present in the tendon.

Extra-articular Manifestations

Rheumatoid arthritis is a systemic disorder which manifests as extra-articular involvement in seropositive patients usually.

Rheumatoid Nodules

It is found in 20–30% of RA patients and presents as painless, firm nodules commonly found on extensor surface of forearm **(Fig. 8)**, olecranon, fingers, occiput, and Achilles tendon. Rarely found in heart, lungs, and vocal cords.

Rheumatoid Vasculitis

It is a rare complication seen in long-standing RA cases. Clinically, it presents as chronic nonhealing ulcers over leg. Palpable purpura on limbs and even on fingertips can be seen. Sometimes it causes vasculitis of nerves leading to painful neuropathy and even leading to paralysis.

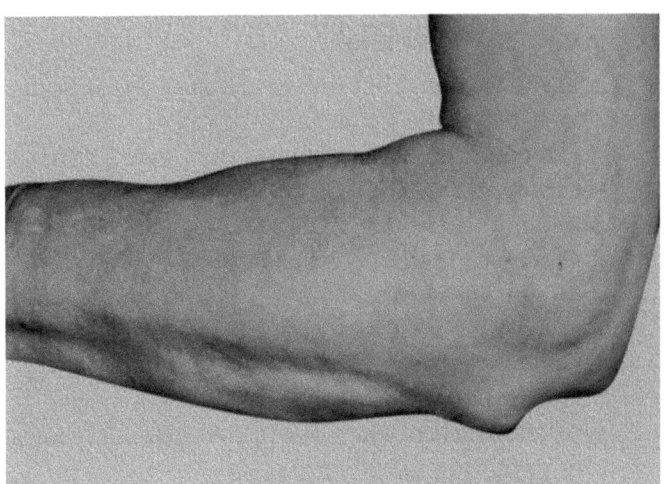

Fig. 8: Rheumatoid nodule.

Sjögren's Syndrome

It is the most common ocular manifestation in RA. It causes dryness of eyes and mouth. Dryness of mouth causes difficulty in swallowing, dental caries, and bad oral hygiene. It is also called as Sicca syndrome. Other ocular manifestations are episcleritis and scleritis.

Pulmonary Changes

Pulmonary changes are usually observed in advance stage of RA. It include pleuritis, pulmonary nodule, effusion, and interstitial lung disease (also called as rheumatoid lung). Patients slowly develop breathlessness, dry cough, and clubbing.

▮ DIAGNOSIS

According to old American College Rheumatology Criteria-1987 diagnosis of RA requires 4 out of 7 below-mentioned criteria, where the symptoms should be there for >6 weeks at least.
- Early morning stiffness lasting for an hour.
- Arthritis of 3 or 4 joints.

- Small joints of hand and foot should be involved.
- Arthritis should be symmetrical.
- Rheumatoid nodules should be present.
- Positive RF test to be present.
- Radiologically articular surface erosions, periarticular osteopenia should be present.

Problem with this ACR criteria was that it was not intended for diagnosis of routine clinical cases, but rather this criteria was primarily used to categorize the disease for research purposes. Clinically to wait to diagnose a patient until he/she fulfils the ACR criteria mostly results in worse outcome.

Joint working group of ACR and the European League against Rheumatism (EULAR) was thus formed to develop a new approach for classifying RA (Updated 2010 Criteria).

ACR/EULAR Definite RA Classification Criteria (Updated 2010 Criteria)

- Confirmed presence of synovitis in at least one joint
- Positive RF or anti-CCP antibody
- Elevated erythrocyte sedimentation rate (ESR) or C-reactive protein (CRP)
- Attaining a total score of at least 6 or more from the individual scores in four domains which are:
  1. Score-based algorithm: To add scores from Categories A to D
  2. Target population (who should be tested) Patients who:
     - Have at least 1 joint involved with definite clinical synovitis (swelling)
     - The synovitis not explained by any another disease.
  3. Score of >6/10 is needed for classifying a patient as having
  4. Definite RA:

A. Joint involvement:

1 Large joint	0
2–10 Large joints	1
1–3 Small joint (with or without involvement of large joint)	2
4–10 Small joints (with or without involvement of large joint)	3
>10 Joints (at least 1 small joint)	5

B. Serology (at least one test result is needed for classification):

Negative RF and negative anti-citrullinated protein antibodies (ACPA)	0
Low positive RF and low positive ACPA	2
High positive RF and high positive ACPA	3

C. Acute phase reactant (at least one test result is needed for classification):

Normal CRP and normal ESR	0
Abnormal CRP and abnormal ESR	1

D. Duration of symptoms:

<6 weeks	0
>6 weeks	1

A score of >6 is needed for classification of a patient as having definite RA. Although patients with a score <6 are not classifiable as having RA but their status should be reassessed from time to time as the criteria might be fulfilled cumulatively over a period of time.

INVESTIGATIONS

- *Laboratory tests*: Complete automated blood counts, liver function tests, renal function tests, urine analysis, and viral markers. Hypochromic normocytic anemia is frequently associated.
- *Acute phase reactants*: Raised ESR and raised CRP are features of active disease. ESR also rises in various conditions as anemia, infections, and also rises with age and is of limited value in the elderly. An elevated ESR in elderly patients should not prompt for further investigation in the absence of clinical findings. Elevated CRP suggests inflammatory arthritis and is a good indicator of disease activity and thus, serial measurements are useful.
- *Special tests*:
  - *Rheumatoid factor test:* It is a sensitive quantitative test to diagnose RA, but positive in 60–70% of RA patients only.
    Rheumatoid factor is an antibody that binds to the Fc portion of an immunoglobulin G (IgG) molecule. A negative RF does not rule out RA, rather the arthritis is seronegative RA. During the first year of onset of disease arthritis may be seronegative type (RF negative) but later on 70–80% of these patients may covert to seropositive arthritis (RF positive). False positive RF can be seen in other rheumatic diseases, chronic infections, and Sjögren's syndrome (70%). Even 10% of healthy population may have positive RF. Thus, this test is not very specific.
  - *Anticyclic citrullinated peptide:* Anti-CCP test is present in 70–80 % of all RA patients but is rarely positive in non-RA patients, giving its specificity of about 95% (can be false positive in active tuberculosis). Anti-CCP can be positive in early stage of RA or even before the onset of disease.
    In early cases of RA, clinical symptoms are sometime mild and nonspecific and patients may not fulfill definite ACR criteria. In early RA, the presence of anti-CCP with or without positive RF may be associated with more erosive disease which is aggressive in nature (a bad prognostic feature).
  - *Antinuclear antibody (ANA):* Although it is more commonly associated with connective tissue

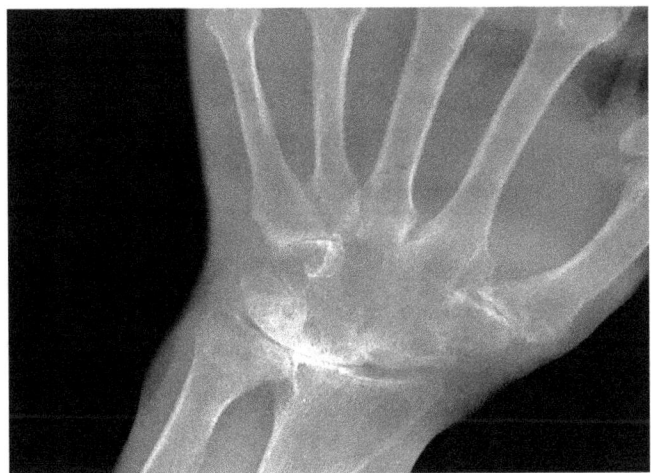

Fig. 9: Loss of joint space, bony destruction.

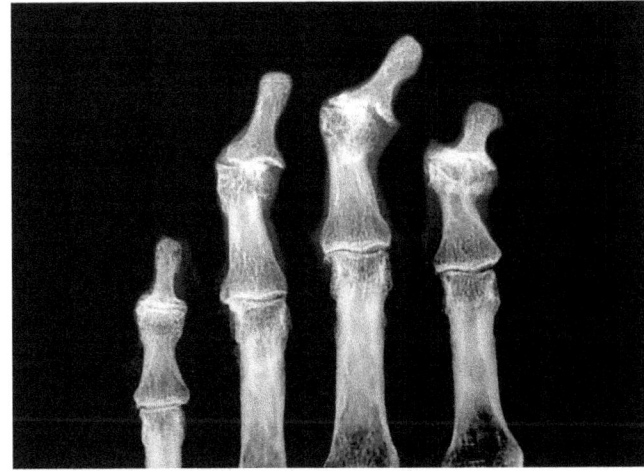

Fig. 10: Gradual sublaxation.

diseases as systemic lupus erythematosus (SLE), 30–40% of RA patients may have ANAs.
- *Synovial fluid analysis:* Analysis of synovial fluid can help to exclude other form of arthritis as gout and infections. Synovial fluid in RA is inflammatory in nature showing presence of white blood cell (WBC) count of 5,000–50,000/mm^3. Rarely, WBC count may exceed 100,000 (pseudo septic).

Radiological Features

- *Early*: Soft tissue swelling, juxta-articular osteoporosis, and erosions.
- *Late*: Loss of joint space, bony destruction (**Fig. 9**), and gradual subluxation (**Fig. 10**).

Magnetic Resonance Imaging

Magnetic resonance imaging (MRI) scans are more sensitive than X-rays for detecting the bone damage caused by RA. Not only the joint inflammation can be detected early by MRI, but also it can pick up the additional information about the tendinitis. For example, an MRI of the wrist may show tendinopathy as the earliest changes of RA.

Ultrasonography of the Joint

This is an effective way of showing joint inflammation before the X-ray shows the damage. It can show synovial thickening, erosions, and vascularity of synovial tissue.

■ MANAGEMENT

Drugs given in conventional therapy are:
- NSAIDs
- Conventional disease modifying antirheumatoid drugs (DMARDs)
- Corticosteroids
- Biological

Corticosteroids are given in early RA and in disease flare up. They can also be given in women developing RA in early pregnancy but again, for short durations only. RA with extra-articular manifestations are also the cases where steroids are added along with DMARDs. In general, if steroids are started, then it should be given for short durations and should be combined with DMARDs as well.

Disease-modifying antirheumatic drugs should be started as early as possible to minimize the joint damage. In fact, depending upon severity of disease, aggressive therapy can be planned. Prior to onset of therapy baseline investigations of liver function test, renal function test, and complete blood count should be done. History of pregnancy in young females must be taken. Monitoring of adverse reactions with DMARDs must be done. DMARDs usually take 3–6 months to act once started.

Common drugs used are: Methotrexate (MTX), hydroxy-chloroquine (HCQ), sulfasalazine (SSZ), and leflunomide.

Various drug regimens which are followed are:
- Monotherapy or
- Combination therapy.

Monotherapy

Single drug like MTX or HCQ or SSZ can be used.
- *Methotrexate* is considered as gold standard drug for mild and moderate cases. MTX inhibits dihydrofolate reductase, an enzyme involved in DNA synthesis. MTX has got both anti-inflammatory effect and cytostatic effect. In contrast to oncological conditions where it is used in higher doses, in RA MTX is used in low doses from 7.5 to 25 mg weekly. Starts with 7.5 mg/week, than slowly increase the dose up to 25 mg/week. The parenteral route of administration is preferred due to better bioavailability and tolerability. The anti-inflammatory effect of drug usually appear after a minimum duration of 4–6 weeks and it may further take up to 8 weeks to show its effect. Adverse reactions of MTX are nausea, vomiting, bone marrow suppression, and liver toxicity may be seen. Regular monitoring of blood counts, liver enzymes, and renal function should be done. If there is renal

impairment then the dose is decreased. The safety profile and tolerability of MTX is increased by adding approximately 1 mg per day of folic acid.
- *Sulfasalazine* alone is used in milder form of RA or when there is contraindication of MTX such as in cases of renal impairment, etc. Its effect comes not before 2–3 months after initiation of therapy. This molecule is linked to an antibiotic known as sulfapyridine with an anti-inflammatory agent called as 5-aminosalicylic acid. It has got a limited role in RA but since it has no teratogenicity effect so can be given in women planning pregnancy. Doses used are 1–2 g/day. Common adverse reactions which can be developed are dyspepsia, skin rashes, bone marrow suppression, and oligospermia. Counseling should be done whenever required in young males.
- *Hydroxychloroquine* is a drug used in the treatment of malaria and has got a limited use in treatment of active RA. It is given in mild form of RA. Contrast to MTX which reduces radiological progression of arthritis, HCQ has no proven impact on the radiological progression of disease. Its dose is 200–400 mg/day. It takes not less than 6–8 weeks to act then further takes weeks to reach its maximum activity. It is a safe drug, least toxic, and usually do not require any blood monitoring. Adverse effects in form of headache and dyspepsia may occur and long-term usage leads to retinal changes therefore, routine ophthalmological examination is mandated.
- *Leflunomide* is very toxic but potent drug to treat RA and should not be used in young females. Dose is 10–20 mg/day. It inhibits an enzyme involved in pyrimidine synthesis. The active metabolite of drug is long lasting (15–18 days) so elimination of molecule can be increased by cholestyramine whenever required. The safety profile is almost similar to MTX. Adverse reactions which can be seen are diarrhea, hypertension, skin rashes even alopecia, and liver toxicity.

Combination Therapy

It is indicated in moderate to severe arthritis, either using two or three drug combination.

MTX + HCQs or MTX + HCQs + SSZ or SSZ + HCQs or MTX + HCQ + LEF or MTX + LEF. LEF + SSZ

Later in combination therapy, one can opt for step-down therapy (from three drugs later can switch to two drugs or even one).

Biologicals

They are given when either DMARDs are not able to control the disease or when an aggressive form of arthritis is there. Drugs used are infliximab, rituximab, etanercept, and adalimumab.

COURSE OF DISEASE

Rheumatoid arthritis has a variable course of disease. There are now well-tested criteria for clinical remission. Definitions vary widely and can mean either absence of clinical and radiological signs of disease while the treatment is on, or a state with minimal or no disease activity after the therapy is withdrawn. The American College of Rheumatology criteria require absence of joint tenderness, fatigue, joint pain, joint swelling, and morning stiffness along with a normal ESR. In about 10–20% patients, arthritis progresses steadily despite DMARDs treatment. Limited remission may occur in pregnancy which may have a flare up (in 90% cases) after childbirth.

PROGNOSTIC FACTORS

A number of factors have been associated with poor prognosis which are:
- Early erosive disease
- Extra-articular involvement (including rheumatoid nodules)
- Positive RF
- Positive anti-CCP factor
- HLA-DR4
- Family history of RA
- Persistent synovitis despite treatment
- Persistently elevated ESR levels or even some time persistently elevated CPP levels
- Older age of onset of disease
- Low socioeconomic and educational level.

RECENT ADVANCES

Immunosuppressive capacities of mesenchymal stem cells have been evaluated in humans. Mesenchymal stem cell therapy is the future in the management of RA especially in severe disease refractory to standard current therapies.

KEY POINTS

- Approximately 60% risk of developing RA can be associated by genetically class II MHC genes.
- Many virus and bacteria have been presumed to be the cause of RA in genetically susceptible individuals.
- Morning stiffness lasting for 30–40 minutes is a cardinal feature that usually appears even before pain.
- In hand, it affects mainly MCP joints, PIP joints, and wrist.
- *Boutonniere's deformity* in which there is hyperflexion at the PIP joint and hyperextension at the distal interphalangeal joint.
- *Swan neck deformity* in which there occurs hyperextension at the PIP joint and hyperflexion at the distal interphalangeal joint.
- *Z deformity in thumb*: In this, there occurs fixed flexion and subsequent subluxation at metacarpophalangeal

joint with hyperextension at the distal interphalangeal joint.
- *Hallux valgus deformity* can be seen due to involvement of first MTP joints with medial displacement at the MTP joint and thus the lateral deviation of the first toe.
- The EULAR score of >6 is needed for classification of a patient as having definite RA.
- Anti-CCP test has a specificity of almost 95%.

FURTHER READING

1. Arernd WP. Physiology of cytokines pathways in rheumatoid arthritis. Arthritis Rheum. 2001;45:101-6.
2. Arnett FC, Edworthy SM, Bloch DA, Mcshane DJ, Fries JF, Cooper NS, et al. American Rheumatism Association 1987 revised criteria for the classification of rheumatoid arthritis. Arthritis Rhem. 1988; 31:315-24.
3. Calabro JJ. A critical evaluation of the diagnostic features of the feet in rheumatoid arthritis Arthritis Rheum. 1962;5:19-29.
4. Cush JJ. Rheumatoid arthritis. In: Clinical Symposia. East Hanover: Novartis. 1999; 51:2-41.
5. Fleming A, Crown JM, Corbett M, Wood PH. Early rheumatoid disease. II. Patterns of joint involvement. Ann Rheum Dis. 1976;35(4):361-4.
6. Grennan DM, Dyer PA, Clague R, Dodds W, Smeaton I, Harris R. Family studies in RA: the importance of HLA-DR4 and of genes for autoimmune thyroid disease. J Rheumatol. 1983;10(4):584-9.
7. Ingegnoli F, Pipitone N, Pitzalis C. Chemokines: key molecules in inflammation. J Ind Rheumatology. 2000;8:111-5.
8. Khanna D, Ranganath VK, Fitzgerald J, Park GS, Altman RD, Elashoff D, et al. Increased radiographic damage scores at the onset of seropositive rheumatoid arthritis in older patients are associated with osteoarthritis of the hands but not with more rapid progression of damage. Arthritis Rheum. 2005;52(8):2284-93.
9. Lindqvist E, Eberhardt K, Bendtzen K, Heinegard D, Saxne T. Prognostic laboratory markers of joint damage in rheumatoid arthritis. Ann Rheum Dis. 2005;64(2):196-201.
10. McQueen F, Beckley V, Crabbe J, Robinson E, Yeoman S, Stewart N. MRI evidence of tendinopathy in early rheumatoid arthritis predicts tendon rupture at six years. Arthritis Rheum. 2005;52(3):744-51.
11. Morel J, Combe B. How to predict prognosis in early rheumatoid arthritis. Best Pract Res Clin Rheumatol. 2005; 19(1):137-46.
12. Ostergaard M, Ejbjerg B, Szkudlarek M. Imaging in early rheumatoid arthritis. Role of MRI, ultrasonography, conventional radiography and CT scan. Best Pract Res Clin Rheumatol. 2005;19(1):91-116.
13. Pinals RS, Masi AT, Larsen RA. Preliminary criteria for clinical remission in rheumatoid arthritis. Arthritis Rheum. 1981;24:1308-5.
14. Price EJ, Venables PJ. The etiopathogenesis of Sjogren's syndrome. Semin Arthritis Rheum. 1995;25(2):117-33.
15. Rask MR. Achilles tendon rupture owing to rheumatoid disease: case report with a nine year follow up. JAMA. 1978;239:435-6.
16. Saag KG. Low dose corticosteroids therapy in rheumatoid arthritis, balancing the evidence. AM J Med. 1997;103:31s-39s.
17. Shmerling RH. Diagnostic test for rheumatic disease: clinical utility revisited. South Med J. 2005;98:704-11.
18. Silman AJ. Pearson JE. Epidemiology and genetics of rheumatoid arthritis. Arthritis Res. 2002:4(Suppl 3):s265-72.
19. Symmonds DP, Barkleed CR, Harrison BJ, Brennmar P, Barett EM, Scott BE, et al. Blood transfusion, smoking and obesity as risk factors for the development of rheumatoid arthritis: results from a primary case-based incident case control study in Norfolk, England. Arthritis Rheum. 1997; 40(II):1995-61.
20. Szekanecz Z, Koach AE. Cytokines. In: Harris ED, Sledge CB, Kelley WN. Kelley's Textbook of Rheumatology, 6th edition. WB Saunders Company; 2001. pp. 275-90.
21. Trieb K. Management of the foot in rheumatoid arthritis. J Bone Joint Surg Br. 2005;87(9):1171-7.
22. Turner S, Cherry N. Rheumatoid arthritis in workers exposed to silica in the pottery industry. Occup Environ Med. 2000;57(7): 443-7.
23. Weinblat ME, Kaplan H, Germain BF, Block S, Solomon SD, Merriman RC, et al. Methotrexate in rheumatoid arthritis. A five year prospective multicenter study. Arthritis Rheum. 1994;37(10):1492-8.
24. Weyand CM. New insights into the patho- genesis of rheumatoid arthritis. Rheumatology (Oxford). 2000;39(Suppl 1):3-8.
25. Yoghmai I, Rooholamini SM, Faunce HF. Unilateral rheumatoid arthritis: protective effects of neurologic deficits. Am J Roentgenol. 1977;1288:299-301.

Ultrasound in Early Inflammatory Arthritis

THS Bedi

■ INTRODUCTION

X-rays have been the mainstay of radiological assessment of joint diseases in the past with the use of nuclear scans, computed tomography (CT) scan, and magnetic resonance imaging (MRI) when required. Conventional radiography, however, is insensitive to early bone damage and almost completely insensitive and totally nonspecific to soft tissue assessment of articular disease processes. Early synovitis and erosions have as a result been totally missed.

The gold standard continues to be the MRI. There is however a large difference in not only the availability and cost of the two modalities but also the ability of each modality to show the disease process which cannot really be compared. However, in the last two decades now, musculoskeletal ultrasound (MSUS) has made significant strides from reluctant acceptance from rheumatologists and orthopedic doctors to now using this modality to its full advantage by not only referring patients for identification of disease process but also for follow-up and post-treatment. In Rheumatology Teaching Programs, MSUS is now a part of the teaching schedule with residents regularly manning the ultrasound units in India. Abroad, The European League Against Rheumatism (EULAR), a 70-year-old organization, regularly holds 3 levels of MSUS training for radiologists and those in rheumatology care and MSUS is regularly done in European Rheumatology Clinics. In orthopedic circles, there still seems to be an over indulgence for the MRI and a reluctance for MSUS both for rheumatology and nonrheumatology musculoskeletal disease especially in our country.

This acceptance has been possible due to technological improvements in machines as well as in higher frequency transducers. US is being used in the assessment of soft tissue disease, detection of fluid, cartilage, and bone surfaces. Due to better resolution, minute bone surface abnormalities may be depicted. Thus, destructive and/or reparative/hypertrophic changes on the bone surface may be seen before they are apparent on plain X-rays or even MRI. However, MSUS cannot penetrate bone; therefore, imaging of intra-articular disease is not possible. Also, due to "real-time" capability of US, this is the only modality allowing dynamic assessment of joint and tendon movements often leading to further assist in abnormality detection.

In the last two decades, numerous papers have reported MSUS to be many times more sensitive to plain radiography in the detection of soft tissue changes, detection of synovial effusion as well as detection of erosions, allowing earlier diagnosis. Tendon pathology, which may be the only and the earliest pathology identified in early inflammatory arthritis, is not identified on pain radiography and is readily identified on the MSUS. Ligament, muscle, peripheral nerve, and cartilage pathology apart from synovial effusion can also be readily demonstrated by MSUS. There is now use of MSUS to noninvasively diagnose and monitor not just joint and muscle disease but also nerve compression syndromes, scleroderma, vasculitis, and Sjögren's syndrome. Parotid gland assessment with high frequency transducers of the salivary glands is also very much in use now.

Needle guidance is improved by MSUS with use in steroid injection guidance, dry needling, joint aspirations, soft calcium deposit aspirations, synovial cyst aspirations, drug instillation in various bursae, etc. As the number of radiologists, rheumatologists, and orthopedic surgeons learning MSUS increases and the technical capabilities of MSUS improve, there is likely to be a better acceptance growing number of proven clinical indications for the application of MSUS in rheumatology practice. In a clinical setting, it is called the "Physician's extended finger."

PRACTICAL TIPS

- Ultrasound is more sensitive than X-rays for detection of early disease including early synovial disease and tendon disease.
- Ultrasound not to be used in isolation.
- X-rays are used primarily in chronic cases and MRI in cases of early ostitis.

■ IMAGING REQUIREMENTS

A dedicated musculoskeletal (MSK) radiology clinic usually has three probes, a low frequency (3–12 MHz) linear probe, a high frequency linear/hockey stick (8–18 MHz) linear probe, and a general curvilinear (1–7 MHz) probe for large joints or for deeper injections.

The higher the frequency of the probe, the better the resolution but lesser is the depth penetration. The lower the frequency, more is the depth penetration and lesser is the resolution. Phase array probes with tissue harmonic imaging and compound imaging is usually used. 3D/4D does not add to the diagnostic value though may add to the representative value of the images provided. Since MSUS has a small field of view, of a global presentation is impractical and hence is poorer than MRI in representation. "Extended field of view" is very useful in MSUS, as it allows a larger area to the represented as well as measured. The lower frequency probes up to 5 MHz are usually used for large joints as shoulder and hips which require more penetration. The size of the footprint is an important factor in examination technique. Transducers with a smaller footprint as in "hockey stick" probes are often better to visualize small joints of the hands and feet.

Ultrasound is the only modality, which readily allows us to see "real time" images which adds to the diagnostic capabilities.

Power and color Doppler are extremely useful in identifying even minute amount of blood flows, which increase in inflammation/infection and increase the confidence in diagnosing subtle changes.

Elastography has now been increasingly used in MSUS after being validated and clinically implemented in liver and breast diseases. Shear-wave elastography is used in tendon and muscle diseases to identify tears, masses, etc. However, technical difficulties like compression manner, reproducibility, and limited accuracy in measurements are still present and as a result hinders an adequate use of elastography in daily practice.

Ultrasound is an operator-dependent modality. Knowledge about the basic principles relevant to sound waves and a detailed knowledge of anatomy are mandatory. Although the procedure itself has no specific side effects, harm may result from incorrect acquisition and interpretation of images owing to operator inexperience.

PRACTICAL TIPS
- High-frequency linear probes (8–18 MHz) are the mainstay of most work with color and power Doppler application.
- Lower frequency probes for larger joints and deeper tissues.
- Highly operator-dependent with steep learning curve.

INDICATIONS

Musculoskeletal ultrasound was probably first used in identification of Baker's cyst and differentiation from thrombophlebitis. This was as early as 1972. Since then MSUS in rheumatology has grown tremendously to its present state. The indications today are:

- *Arthritis*:
  - *Joints*:
    - Synovial effusion
    - Synovial proliferation
    - Cartilage changes
    - Erosions
  - *Periarticular soft tissues*:
    - Tendon disease
    - Enthesitis
    - Bursal involvement
- *Nonarthritis*:
  - Infections
  - Hemarthrosis
- Soft tissue rheumatology
- Nerve involvement assessment
- Systemic rheumatoid disease assessment
- MRI contraindication.

IMAGING

Today no rheumatology practice is possible without imaging. It is an important part of the assessment, diagnosis, and follows up of patients of rheumatology. These are correlated with clinical history, physical examination, and laboratory tests. To reach a diagnosis various criteria are used by standardized American College of Rheumatology (ACR) criteria which may or may not involve radiology. The present state of USMS required a rethink of the various criteria at hand to better diagnose a rheumatology disease process.

Musculoskeletal ultrasound looks at the disease in the following areas described here.

SYNOVITIS

Most rheumatoid diseases affect the synovium. The presence of excess intra-articular fluid is secondary to synovitis. Sonography being exquisitely sensitive in detecting intra-articular fluid and there are now standards available for the same in most joints. MSUS is capable of detecting synovial fluid in excess of even 1 mm^2 **(Fig. 1)**. This technique is therefore potentially important in the management, diagnosis, monitoring, and the assessment of treatment efficacy. MSUS has been confirmed to be superior to clinical examination in the detection of effusion in small as well as large relatively easily palpable joints such as the knee joint. Musculoskeletal ultrasound started in the 1980s with the shoulder but the initial work on rheumatology was done on small joints of the hands and the wrist in patients of rheumatoid arthritis (RA). Traditionally, the pattern and location of synovitis of joints is an important aspect of most arthritis and may be diagnostic of the disease. In RA, synovitis of the metacarpophalangeal (MCP), metatarsophalangeal (MTP), and proximal interphalangeal (PIP) joints is primarily seen **(Fig. 2)**. The target joints in psoriatic arthritis are the distal interphalangeal (DIP) joints.

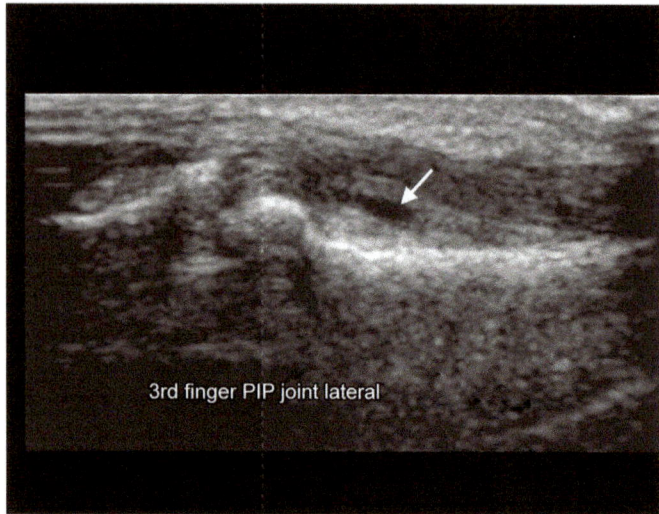

Fig. 1: Synovial fluid in the 3rd proximal interphalangeal (PIP) joint on the palmar aspect.

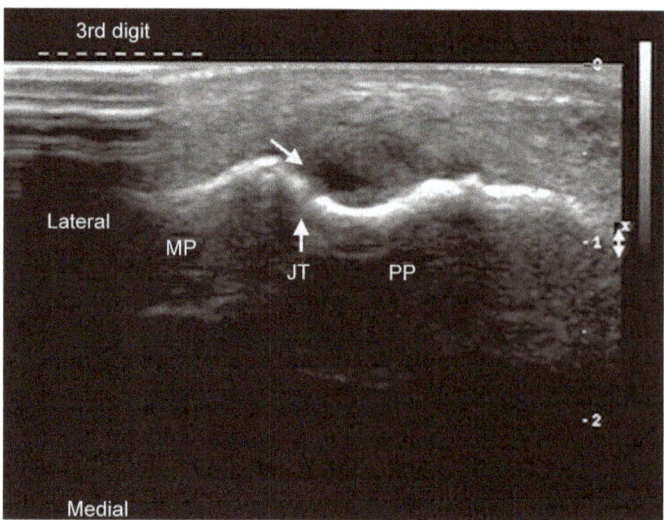

Fig. 2: Synovial effusion at the right 3rd carpo-metacarpal joint on the dorsal aspect. (MP: middle phalanx; JT: joint; PP: proximal phalanx)

However, in early disease, this typical pattern of involvement particular to a specific disease is not followed as was poorly understood prior to the use of MSUS. A bilaterally symmetrical disease may not present as one. At times, there may be exclusive tenosynovial involvement without joint involvement further confusing the traditional criteria for disease identification. Rather a few authors have questioned the classification of rheumatoid diseases.

As a result, in early disease, MSUS primarily assists the rheumatologist in confirming the presence or absence of disease or synovitis, synovial proliferation, tenosynovitis, sites and number of joints or tendons involved, amount of disease, and to assess whether there is any associated cartilaginous changes or erosions. Synovial proliferation is also easily seen with thickened synovium (**Fig. 3**). If the fluid in the joint cannot be compressed, it is usually to a thickened synovium. Color and/or power Doppler is routinely used to assess and grade the disease activity and burden. The thickened synovium may also show increased flow on Doppler application to differentiate it from only synovitis causing effusion. Proteinaceous material within the joint space may mimic the echotexture of synovial hypertrophy. Compression of the joint by the transducer and/or passive and active movements of the joint do not change the sonographic features if the echoes are generated by synovial pannus. Proteinaceous material, on the contrary, changes its distribution within the joint and generates different pictures after mechanical stress of the joint. In significant synovial proliferation a very irregular contour of the synovial membrane is seen with synechiae between the walls of the articular recesses in large joints.

The number of joints assessed in early disease change from practice to practice and from institute to institute. The DAS 28 (Disease Activity Count) is a well-accepted method to assess disease load. The 28-joint count includes

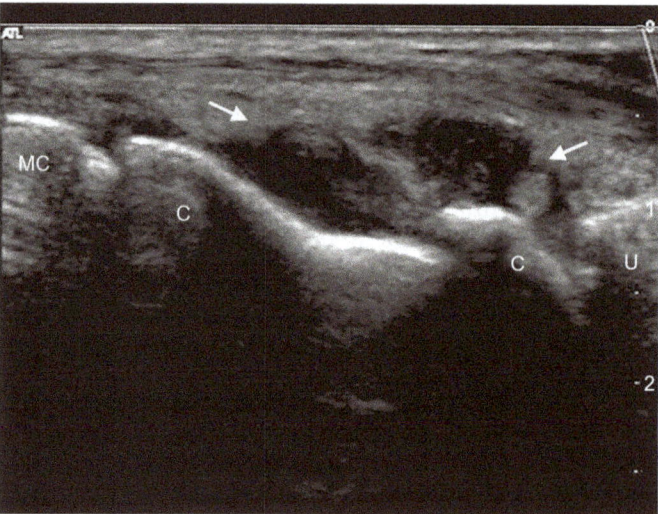

Fig. 3: Synovial effusion and proliferation at the carpal and carpo-metacarpal joints with synovial proliferation. (MC: metacarpal; C: carpal; U: ulna)

10 PIP and 10 MCP joints of the hands, 2 wrists, 2 elbows, 2 shoulders, and 2 knees. Later, studies have used a 42-joint count, which includes the 28-joint count and 10 MTP joints of the feet, hips, and ankles. Joints are assessed according to a Standard Protocol for Evaluation of Rheumatoid Arthritis (SPERA) not only for swelling and tenderness but also for motion limitations and deformity, which must be included to assess long-term outcomes.

In seronegative arthritis, involvements to the joint of interest are assessed only rather than the 42 joints as mentioned above and many diseases presentations may be monoarticular.

Musculoskeletal ultrasound has been confirmed to be superior to clinical examination in the detection of effusion, even in a large and relatively easily palpable joint such as the knee joint. MSUS is more sensitive than clinical examination and radiography in the detection of effusion in all peripheral small joints. If the presence of joint fluid is taken as the hallmark of inflammation, then the classification criteria of RA and the clinical diagnosis of mono-, oligo-, and polyarthritis will probably need to be re-evaluated in the future due to more widespread clinical use of US which may be a more accurate means of determining the number of inflamed joints.

Areas of acute disease show increased flow on Doppler application **(Fig. 4)**. A negative Doppler signal does not exclude the possibility of synovitis. Grading of synovial disease is also done with Doppler assessment. It is important that the quality of ultrasound devices is kept in mind while assessing the same.

Grading of the synovial disease is now done both with gray-scale as well as with color Doppler assessment. A EULAR-OMERACT (European League against Rheumatism-Outcome Measures Against Rheumatology) ultrasound taskforce was created for preparing a standardized, consensus-based scoring system for grading of RA **(Table 1)**. On gray scale imaging, Grade 1 was defined as a small anechoic line beneath the joint capsule, grade 2 as a capsule distension parallel to the joint area, and grade 3 as a pronounced convex distension of the joint capsule. On color/power Doppler, grade 1 was characterized by detection of single color signal, grade 2 by 1 confluent color signals of <50% of the synovial area, and grade 3 by color signals that filled 50% of the synovial area. It is as shown in **Figures 5A to C**.

Studies have been done by Ridden et al. and Hau et al. to estimate and visualize the efficacy of treatment with antitumor necrosis factor alpha in patients with RA using color Doppler and spectral Doppler ultrasonography to determine the possible changes in synovial perfusion post-treatment. These studies have shown that it is possible to see reduction in the number of color pixels in cases, post-treatment and correlates well with symptomatic improvement. In a few cases the sonographic improvement is seen even prior to the symptomatic improvement. Similar improvements are seen with steroid injection. In a study by Filippucci et al., in 70% patients' improvement of both gray scale and power Doppler was found post-treatment with steroids.

It is important to understand the limitations of MSUS in the evaluation of joint effusions. MSUS cannot yet accurately differentiate whether a fluid collection is inflammatory, infectious, or hematogenous **(Fig. 6)** in most cases and aspiration of fluid—which is more successful with MSUS guidance—remains the gold standard.

TENDON DISEASE

In the two decades, MSUS has become the gold standard for examination of tendons. Tenosynovial effusion, tenosynovial proliferation, and tendon tears are routinely detected by MSUS **(Fig. 7)**. Clinical examination of tendon involvement is poorer than joint involvement and may not even be used as criteria by rheumatologist to estimate the disease load. MSUS is still far superior to MRI in the detection of longitudinal split tendon tear, subluxing tendon, and snapping tendon and has the advantage of allowing dynamic tendon examination assessing impingements, etc. MSUS also demonstrates focal or diffuse tendonitis, calcified tendonitis, partial and full thickness tears, and tendon xanthomas. X-rays obviously do not show tendon disease and MRI is far too costly.

Synovial involvement of the tendon sheath is not uncommon in seropositive arthritis and is known as

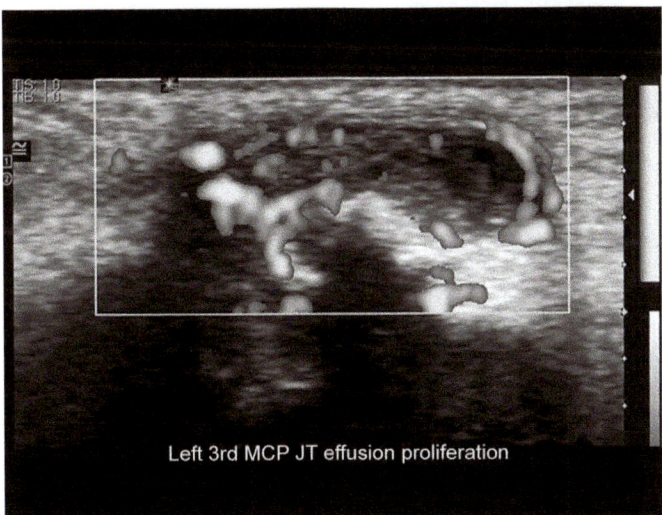

Fig. 4: Synovial effusion and proliferation at the 3rd metacarpophalangeal joint (MCP joint) showing increased flow on Doppler application.

TABLE 1: EULAR-OMERACT combined scoring system for grading synovitis in rheumatoid arthritis.

Grade	Clinical finding	Description
0	Normal joint	No GS-detected SH and no PD signal (within the synovium)
1	Mild synovitis	Grade 1 SH and ≤Grade 1 PD signal
2	Moderate synovitis	Grade 2 SH and ≤Grade 2 PD signal or Grade 1 SH and a Grade 2 PD signal
3	Severe synovitis	Grade 3 SH and ≤Grade 3 PD signal or Grade 1 or 2 SH and a Grade 3 PD signal

Proposed combined power Doppler ultrasound (PDUS) (GS and PD) scoring system graded from 0 to 3 describing the criteria for the individual grades in relation to the GS SH and Doppler signal. The higher of the two determines the final combined score.
(EULAR: European League Against Rheumatism; GS: gray scale; OMERACT: Outcome Measures in Rheumatology; PD: power Doppler; SH: synovial hypertrophy)

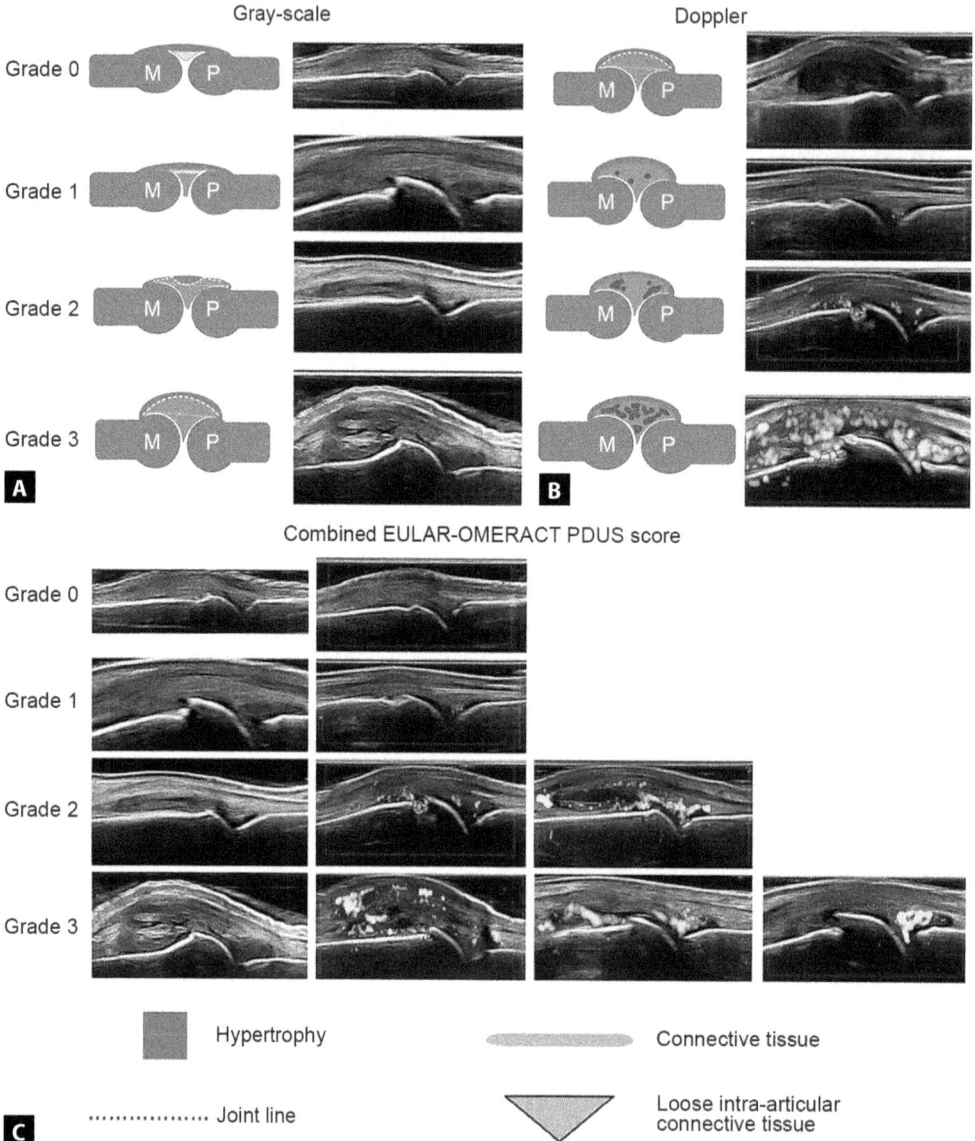

Figs. 5A to C: (A) Schematic drawing of the individual grades of hypoechoic SH for GS alone. For each grade is also shown the corresponding GS image. (1) None=Grade 0: no SH independently of the presence of effusion; (2) minimal=Grade 1: SH with or without effusion up to level of horizontal line connecting bone surfaces M and P; (3) moderate=Grade 2: SH with or without effusion extending beyond joint line but with upper surface convex (curved downwards) or hypertrophy extending beyond joint line but with upper surface flat; (4) severe=Grade 3: SH with or without effusion extending beyond joint line but with upper surface flat or convex (curved downwards); (B) Schematic drawing of the individual grades for Doppler activity. For each grade is also shown the corresponding ultrasound image. (1) None=Grade 0: no Doppler activity; (2) minimal=Grade 1: up to three single Doppler spots or up to one confluent spot and two single spots or up to two confluent spots; (3) moderate=Grade 2: greater than Grade 1 but <50% Doppler signals in the total GS background; (4) severe=Grade 3: greater than Grade 2 (>50% of the background GS); (C) EULAR-OMERACT score for PDUS synovitis combining gray-scale SH and PD signal. Normal joint=Grade 0: no gray-scale-detected SH and no PD signal (within the synovium); minimal synovitis=Grade 1: Grade 1 SH and ≤Grade 1 PD signal; moderate synovitis=Grade 2: Grade 2 SH and ≤Grade 2 PD signal or Grade 1 SH and a Grade 2 PD signal; severe synovitis=Grade 3: Grade 3 SH and ≤Grade 3 PD signal or Grade 1 or 2 synovial hypertrophy and a Grade 3 PD signal. (EULAR: European League Against Rheumatism; GS: gray-scale; fx2: hypertrophy; fx3: joint line; fx4: loose intra-articular connective tissue; M: metacarpal head; P: proximal phalangeal bone; OMERACT: Outcome Measures in Rheumatology; PD: power Doppler; SH: synovial hypertrophy)

tenosynovitis. It is less common in seronegative arthritis. Tendon involvement may present prior to joint involvement in RA and at times may be the only imaging abnormality identified. A swollen joint, for example the wrist joint, may not be due to joint effusion but due to tenosynovitis. MSUS helps differentiate the cause of swelling by clearly showing if it is joint effusion or overlying tenosynovitis **(Fig. 8)**.

Synovial disease involves tendons, which have a synovial sheath, and is particularly common in RA and involves the tendons of the flexor digitorum superficialis and profundus tendons, flexor carpi ulnaris and radialis as well as the extensor digitorum **(Fig. 9)**. The flexor digitorum superficialis and profundus tendons are probably the most common tendons involved in the hands in psoriatic arthropathy giving a typical "sausage digit" appearance **(Fig. 10)**. Areas of active disease show increased flow on Doppler application.

Musculoskeletal ultrasound can also identify partial and complete tears in tendons as has been used for years in

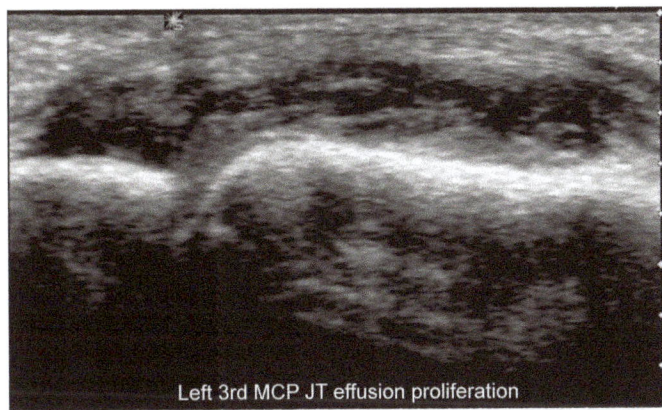

Fig. 6: Synovial effusion at the left 3rd metacarpophalangeal joint (MCP joint), due to systemic lupus erythematosus (SLE), with synovial proliferation.

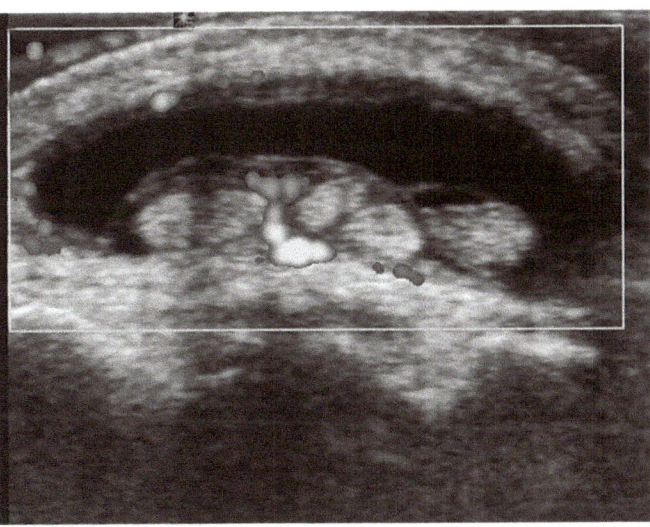

Fig. 7: Fluid in the tendon sheath of the left extensor digitorum in rheumatoid arthritis with increased flow on color Doppler application—tenosynovitis.

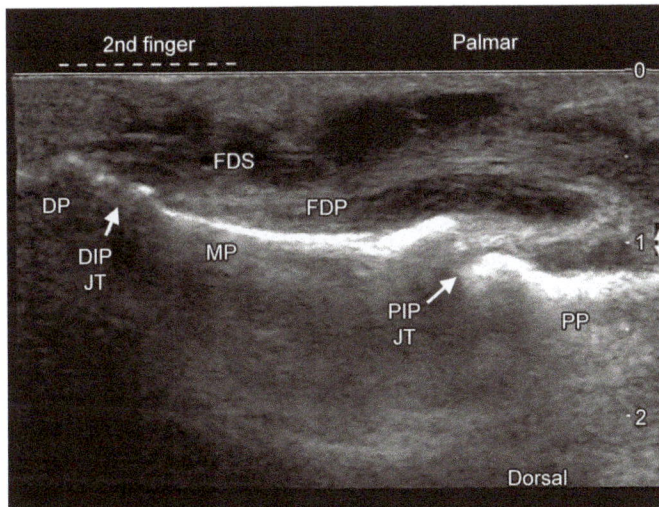

Fig. 8: Finger swelling at MCP joint. Cause clearly identified as tenosynovial effusion and proliferation of the flexor digitorum superficialis and profundus tendons. (FDS: flexor digitorum superficialis; DIP JT: distal interphalangeal joint; MP: middle phalanx; PIP JT: proximal interphalangeal joint; PP: proximal phalanx; MCP: metacarpophalangeal)

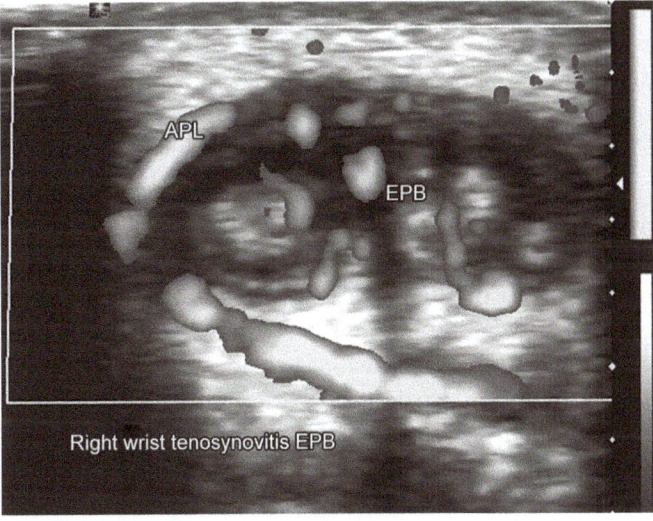

Fig. 9: De Quervain's tenosynovitis of abductor pollicis longus and extensor pollicis brevis. Power Doppler showing active disease. (APL: abductor pollicis longus; EPB: extensor pollicis brevis)

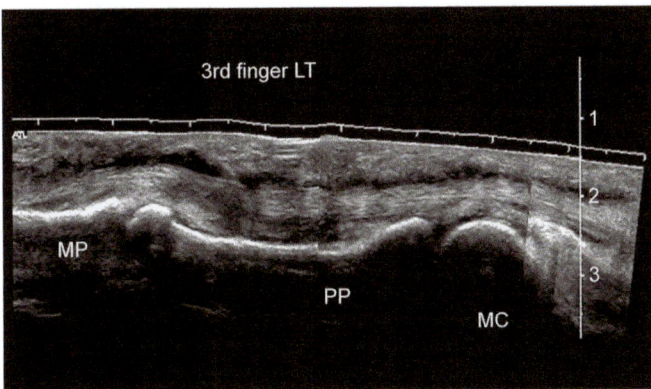

Fig. 10: Sausage finger to tenosynovial effusion of the left 3rd finger flexor digitorum superficialis and profundus tendons.

shoulder and tendo-Achilles sonography. In the last decade, MSUS is now used to study most tendons of the upper and lower limbs.

Although ultrasound is sensitive in identification of tendon disease, like synovitis, it is nonspecific. Correlation with biochemical parameters and history is important to come to a diagnosis.

CARTILAGE CHANGES

Early cartilage changes can be detected sonographically as thinning of the articular cartilage. Normal weight bearing cartilage ranges from 1.2 to 1.9 mm in thickness. The cartilage in the wrists and hands is thinner. Nonvisualization of the

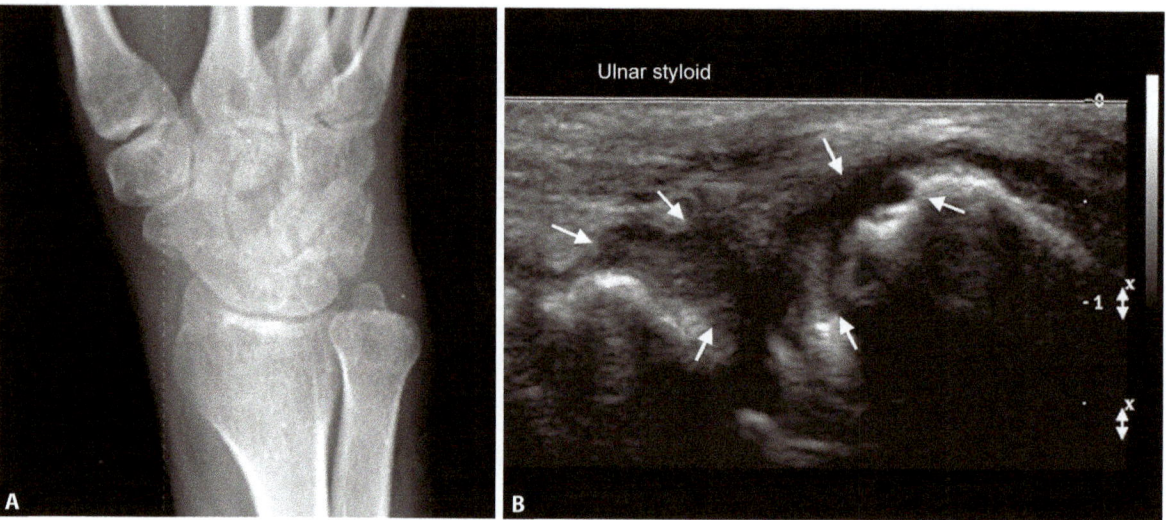

Figs. 11A and B: (A) X-ray showing suspicious erosion at the distal ulna; (B) Erosion at the distal ulna with surrounding synovial effusion and proliferation.

cartilage is not an ominous sign as it may not be always seen. However, an irregular thinning or thickening of the cartilage is abnormal **(Figs. 11A and B)**. The knee is another common site for assessment of cartilage damage.

EROSIONS

It is every rheumatologist's desire to identify the diagnosis and to treat the patient prior to erosion which may become irreversible. At times the identification of erosions at specific sites leads to the diagnosis. In many clinics even today, X-rays are used to identify the erosions and have proved to less sensitive as all erosions are not identified on X-ray unless the X-ray beam is at 90° to the erosion site. Moreover, there is the question of interobserver agreeability to the same erosions which on various studies has proven not to be sensitive. Digital X-rays have helped partially in the manner.

Ultrasound, which has a high spatial resolution, does not share these problems in identifying presence of erosions. Numerous studies in the last 20 years have shown sonography has been proved to be valuable in early diagnosis of erosions. It has multiplanar capabilities which allows a more complete assessment of the bone surfaces sparing those surfaces where the transducer cannot be properly applied to the assessment areas as in the web spaces of the hands and feet. All erosions are confirmed on two planes 90° to each other. One should be careful to not label all the indentations seen in a bone as erosions.

Erosions are identified as loss of cortical bone with crater-like defects in the bone surface along the edges of the articular cartilage affecting the so-called bare areas of the bone **(Figs. 11A and B)**. In RA, pannus is seen as a hypoechoic soft tissue mass filling these erosions and in the surrounding joint cavity with or without bulge of the joint capsule. Color and power Doppler usually show an intense increase in flow at the site especially in active disease. In acutely inflamed joints with erosions, it is not uncommon to a vascular pedicle supplying the pannus up to the erosion crater **(Figs. 12A and B)**.

Magnetic resonance imaging is however the gold standard for erosion assessment. Small erosions of the carpal bones may be difficult to interpret on sonography due to normally irregular carpal bone surface. MRI shows more abnormalities in this area. Bone marrow edema and cartilaginous changes which are the earliest bony changes in RA not seen on sonography and are best seen on MRI. Subarticular cysts are completely missed on sonography.

CRYSTAL DEPOSIT DISEASE

Calcium pyrophosphate dihydrate (CPPD) deposition disease is the third most common inflammatory arthritis and its incidence increases with age. Initially, CPPD diagnosis was based on the presence of typical crystal deposits at conventional radiology (CR) and synovial fluid analysis (McCarty criteria). With the use of sonography and its ability to identify crystals in joints, the task force of EULAR after systematic review of the literature, concluded that US can demonstrate CPP crystals in peripheral joints with high accuracy and can be used in the diagnosis of CPPD.

Calcium pyrophosphate dihydrate calcifications are hyperechoic deposits that presented as tiny hyperechoic spots, punctuate spots, linear deposits, or band-like deposits which may be in the articular fibrocartilage, tendons, and synovial fluid.

Gout is also now has ultrasound probably as the first radiological investigation. The acceptance of the "double contour sign" by the 2014 joint EULAR/ACR revised criteria for gout is an important further acceptance of ultrasound in early rheumatologic joint diseases. Gout crystal deposition can be identified on ultrasound as hyperechoic irregular echogenicity of the articular surface of the hyaline cartilage

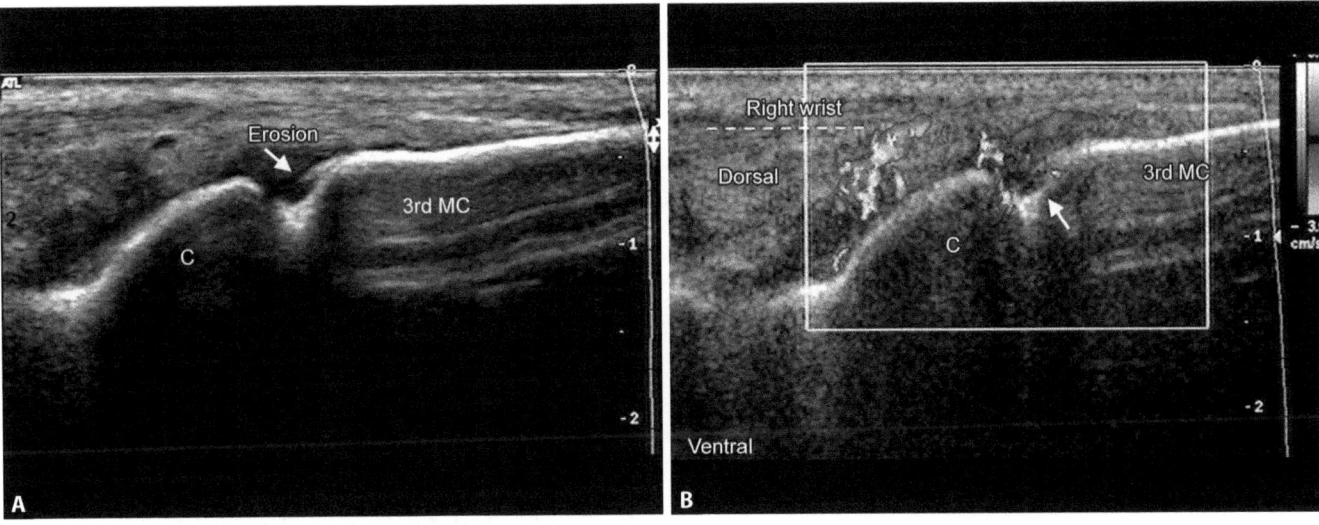

Figs. 12A and B: In acutely inflamed joints with erosions, it is not uncommon to a vascular pedicle supplying the pannus up to the erosion (taken from my previous paper in IJRI). (C: carpal; MC: metacarpal)

(double contour sign), hyperechoic aggregates suggestive of tophi within the joint or along tendons, and floating hyperechoic foci within the joint space which have the appearance of a snowstorm.

BURSA

Bursitis is a common disease entity in joint diseases. In the shoulder, the subacromial-subdeltoid bursitis may be the only finding identified sonographically. The Baker's cyst is seen in chronic cases.

ENTHESITIS

Enthesitis, the inflammation of the origin and insertion of ligaments, tendons, aponeuroses, annulus fibrosis, and joint capsules, is not an acute process and tends to be seen more in seronegative cases.

KEY POINTS

- Ultrasound is indispensible in the early inflammatory arthritis clinic, it is the rheumatologist's extended finger or like a stethoscope.
- It identifies synovial disease, tendon disease, and early erosions much earlier than X-rays which has been the mainstay of investigation.
- Early synovitis and erosions easily picked up and can be graded to assess load of disease.
- Typical pattern of disease (example bilaterality in RA) may not be seen as sensitivity of ultrasound to pick up early synovitis and tenosynovitis is very high.
- Tendon involvement may be the first radiological sign of disease especially in cases of seropositive arthritis.
- Cartilage loss and erosions better picked up on ultrasound than X-rays.
- May help in confirming diagnosis in crystal deposit diseases without the use of joint aspiration for crystals.
- Dynamic assessment of tendons allows better assessment in chronic cases with tendon tears and splits.
- Much better than clinical examination for identifying bursa and enthesitis.
- Only radiological investigation which is real-time so helps in injections and interventions.
- Ultrasound cannot differentiate the cause of disease, i.e., between inflammatory, infective, and hematogenous.
- Not much use in chronic cases except for identifying acute on chronic disease.
- It is to be used in association with X-rays and MRI.

FURTHER READING

1. Backhaus M, Burmester G-R, Gerber T, Grassi W, Machold KP, Swen WA, et al. Guidelines for musculoskeletal ultrasound in rheumatology. Ann Rheum Dis. 2001; 60:641-9.
2. Backhaus M, Kamradt T, Sandrock D, Loreck D, Fritz J, Wolf KJ, et al. Arthritis of the finger joints: a comprehensive approach comparing conventional radiography, scintigraphy, ultrasound, and contrast-enhanced magnetic resonance imaging. Arthritis Rheum. 1999;42:1232-45.
3. Balint PV, Kane D, Wilson H, McInnes IB, Sturrock RD. Ultrasonography of entheseal insertions in the lower limb in spondyloarthropathy. Ann Rheumat Dis. 2002;61:905-10.
4. Bedi THS, Bagga RN. Ultrasound in rheumatology. Indian J Radiol Imaging. 2007;17: 299-305.
5. Campbell RS, Grainger AJ. Current concepts in imaging of tendinopathy. Clin Radiol. 2001;56:253-67.
6. Carpenter JR, Hattery RR, Hunder GG, Bryan RS, McLeod RA. Ultrasound evaluation of the popliteal space. Comparison with arthrography and physical examination. Mayo Clin Proc. 1976;51:498-503.
7. D'Agostino MA, Terslev L, Aegerter P, Backhaus M, Balint P, Bruyn GA, et al. Scoring ultrasound synovitis in rheumatoid arthritis: a EULAROMERACT ultrasound taskforce—Part 1: definition and development of a standardized, consensus-based scoring system. RMD Open. 2017;3:e000428.
8. Filippucci E, Farina A, Carotti M, Salaffiand F, Grassi W. Grey scale and power Doppler sonographic changes induced by

intra-articular steroid injection treatment. Ann Rheum Dis. 2004;63:740-3.
9. Frediani B, Filippou G, Falsetti P, Lorenzini S, Baldi F, Acciai C, et al. Diagnosis of calcium pyrophosphate dihydrate crystal deposition disease: ultrasonographic criteria proposed. Ann Rheumat Dis. 2005;64:638-40.
10. Fuchs HA, Brooks RH, Callahan LF, Pincus T. A simplified twenty-eight joint quantitative articular index in rheumatoid arthritis. Arthritis Rheum. 1989;32:531-7.
11. Grassi W, Cervini C. Ultrasonography in rheumatology: an evolving technique. Ann Rheum Dis. 1998;57:268-71.
12. Grassi W, Filippucci E, Farina A, Cervini C. Sonographic imaging of tendons. Arthritis Rheum. 2000;43:969-76.
13. Grassi W, Filippucci E, Farina A, Salaffi F, Cervini C. Ultrasonography in the evaluation of bone erosions. Ann Rheum Dis. 2001; 60:98-104.
14. Grassi W, Lamanna G, Farina A, Cervini C. Synovitis of small joints: sonographic guided diagnostic and therapeutic approach. Ann Rheum Dis. 1999;58:595-7.
15. Grassi W, Okano T, Filippucci E. Use of ultrasound for diagnosis and monitoring of outcomes in crystal arthropathies. Curr Opin Rheumatol. 2015;27(2):147-55.
16. Grassi W, Tittarelli E, Pirani O, Avaltroni D, Cervini C. Ultrasound examination of metacarpophalangeal joints in rheumatoid arthritis. Scand J Rheumatol. 1993;22:243-7.
17. Grassi W, Tittarelli E, Pirani O, Avaltroni D, Cervini C. Ultrasound examination of metacarpophalangeal joints in rheumatoid arthritis. Scand J Rheumatol. 1993;22:243-7.
18. Hau M, Kneitz C, Tony HP, Keberle M, Jahns R, Jenett M. High-resolution USG detects a decrease in pannus vascularization of small finger joints in patients with rheumatoid arthritis receiving treatment with soluble anti-tumor necrosis factor alpha receptor. Ann Rheum Dis. 2002;61:55-8.
19. Kane D, Balint PV, Sturrock RD. Ultrasonography is superior to clinical examination in the detection and localization of knee joint effusion in rheumatoid arthritis. J Rheumatol. 2003;30:966-71.
20. Kane D, Grassi W, Sturrock R, Balint PV. A brief history of musculoskeletal ultrasound: 'From bats and ships to babies and hips'. Rheumatology. 2004;43:931-3.
21. Kane D, Grassi W, Sturrock R, Balint PV. Musculoskeletal ultrasound—a state of the art review in rheumatology. Part 2: Clinical indications for musculoskeletal ultrasound in rheumatology. Rheumatology. 2004;43:829-38.
22. Klauser AS, Miyamoto H, Bellmann-Weiler R, Feuchtner GM, Wick MC, Jaschke WR. Sonoelastography: musculoskeletal applications. Radiology. 2014;272(3):622-33.
23. McGonagle D, Gibbon W, O'Connor P, Blythe D, Wakefield R, Green M, et al. A preliminary study of bone erosion in early rheumatoid arthritis. Rheumatol. 1999;38:329-31.
24. Pincus T, Brooks RH, Callahan LF. A proposed standard protocol to evaluate rheumatoid arthritis (SPERA) that includes measures of inflammatory activity, joint damage, and long-term outcomes. J Rheumatol. 1999;26:473-80.
25. Ridden C, André B, Marcelis S, Kaye O, Mathy L, Bonnet V, et al. Rheumatoid hand joint synovitis: gray-scale and power Doppler US quantifications following anti-tumor necrosis factor-alpha treatment: pilot study. Radiology. 2003;229:562-9.
26. Schmidt WA, Schmidt H, Schicke B, Gromnica-Ihle E. Standard reference values for musculoskeletal ultrasonography. Ann Rheum Dis. 2004;63(8):988-94.
27. Sokka T, Pincus T. Eligibility of patients in routine care for major clinical trials of anti-tumor necrosis factor alpha agents in rheumatoid arthritis. Arthritis Rheum. 2003;48:313-8.
28. Szkudlarek M, Klarlund M, Narvestad E, Court-Payen M, Strandberg C, Jensen KE, Thomsen HS, et al. Ultrasonography of the metacarpophalangeal and proximal interphalangeal joints in rheumatoid arthritis: a comparison with magnetic resonance imaging, conventional radiography and clinical examination. Arthritis Res Ther. 2006;8(2):R52.
29. Szkudlarek M, Klarlund M, Narvestad E, Court-Payen M, Strandberg C, Jensen KE, et al. Ultrasonography of the meta-carpophalangeal and proximal interphalangeal joints in rheumatoid arthritis: a comparison with magnetic resonance imaging, conventional radiography and clinical examination. Arthritis Res Ther. 2006;8(2):R52.
30. Wakefield RJ, Gibbon WW, Emery P. The current status of ultrasonography in rheumatology. Rheumatology (Oxford). 1999;38:195-8.
31. Wakefield RJ, Gibbon WW, O'Csonnor P. High resolution ultrasound: a superior method to radiography for detecting cortical bone erosions in rheumatoid arthritis. Br J Rheumatol. 1998;7:S197.
32. Wakefield RJ, Green MJ, Marzo-Ortega H, Conaghan PG, Gibbon WW, McGonagle D, et al. Should oligoarthritis be reclassified? Ultrasound reveals a high prevalence of subclinical disease. Ann Rheum Dis. 2004;63:382-5.
33. Wakefield RJ, Green MJ, Marzo-Ortega H, Conaghan PG. Should oligoarthritis be reclassified? Ultrasound reveals a high prevalence of subclinical disease. Ann Rheumat Dis. 2004;63:382-5.
34. Witt M, Mueller F, Nigg A, Reindl C, Leipe J, Proft F, et al. Relevance of grade 1 gray-scale ultrasound findings in wrists and small joints to the assessment of subclinical synovitis in rheumatoid arthritis. Arthritis Rheum. 2013; 65(7):1694-701.

Recent Advances in the Management of Rheumatoid Arthritis

Neeraj Jain

The treatment armamentarium for rheumatoid arthritis (RA) has substantially expanded over the last two decades. Early diagnosis and prompt treatment initiation is essential, which will aid to facilitate optimal care and favorable outcomes in patients with RA. The current management strategy in RA mainly aim at remission or, at least, low disease activity, with rapid adaptation of treatment if therapeutic target is not attained. Thus, adopting a *treat-to-target approach* helps in preventing progression of joint damage and optimize physical function status, and work-related quality of life and social participation **(Fig. 1)**.

Management of RA mainly consists of combination of pharmacotherapy and lifestyle modification interventions. There are five major classes of drugs that are currently being used—analgesics, non-steroidal anti-inflammatory drugs (NSAIDs), glucocorticoids, non-biologic and biologic disease-modifying antirheumatic drugs (DMARDs). Current recommendations from clinical practice guidelines suggest that clinicians should start biologic drugs, if patients have suboptimal response, or are intolerant to one or two conventional disease modifying drugs [methotrexate (MTX), sulfasalazine (SSZ), leflunomide and hydroxychloroquine (HCQ)]. Commonly, a combination of these drugs is used in the treatment of RA. However, advancement in research have made it possible now to target specific elements in the immune system (e.g., cytokines, B cells, and T cells), which plays a crucial role in the pathogenesis of RA.

CONVENTIONAL MANAGEMENT OF RHEUMATOID ARTHRITIS WITH NSAIDs AND CORTICOSTEROIDS

Conventional treatment approach mainly aims to relieve pain and decrease inflammation. Fast-acting conventional treatment options include NSAIDs such as acetylsalicylate, naproxen, ibuprofen, and etodolac. Aspirin is one of the oldest NSAIDs administered for joint pains. However, aspirin at higher doses are associated with side effects such as hearing loss, tinnitus and gastric intolerance. Commonly used NSAIDs in RA treatment are listed in **Table 1**.

There are NSAIDs which have comparable efficacy, and which act by inhibiting cyclooxygenase (COX), preventing the synthesis of prostaglandins, prostacyclin and thromboxanes. Commonly reported side effects with these medications include nausea, abdominal pain, ulcers, and gastrointestinal (GI) bleeding. However, these side effects are commonly managed when taken along with food, or with antacids, proton pump inhibitors, or misoprostol. It is important to note that several COX inhibitors have been withdrawn from market due to cardiovascular safety concerns. However, celecoxib and etoricoxib are still available for use. Celecoxib has demonstrated lesser risk of GI side effects.

Corticosteroids, are another class of drugs used in RA management, which are more potent anti-inflammatory drugs than NSAIDs. But, these drugs are associated with greater side effects. Hence, corticosteroids are administered for short duration and at low doses, especially during exacerbations or flares of RA. For managing local symptoms of inflammation, intra-articular (IA) injections of corticosteroid can be used, which act by preventing phospholipid release and decreasing actions of eosinophils. This helps to decrease inflammation. Side effects of IA injections of corticosteroid include weight gain, bone thinning, diabetes, and immunosuppression. Gradual dose tapering with improvement can minimize the associated side effects. It is crucial to note that injected or oral corticosteroids should not be discontinued abruptly as it can result in hypothalamic-pituitary-adrenal axis (HPA) suppression or flares of RA.

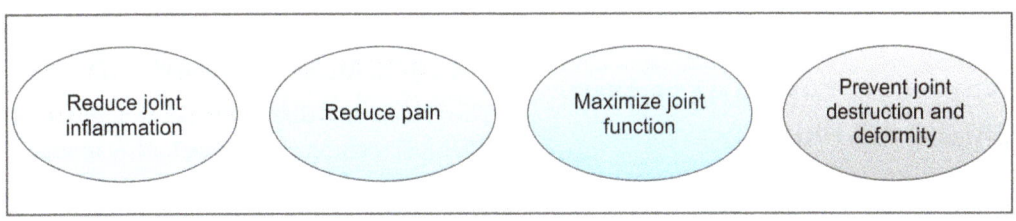

Fig. 1: Major goals for the treatment of rheumatoid arthritis (RA).

TABLE 1: Commonly prescribed NSAIDs in the management of rheumatoid arthritis.

Short-acting NSAIDs	Long-acting NSAIDs
• Ibuprofen	• Naproxen
• Diclofenac	• Celecoxib
• Ketoprofen	• Meloxicam
• Indomethacin	• Nabumetone
	• Piroxicam

(NSAIDs: nonsteroidal anti-inflammatory drugs)

MANAGEMENT OF RHEUMATOID ARTHRITIS WITH CONVENTIONAL SYNTHETIC DMARD

Therapeutic goal for treatment with conventional synthetic DMARDs is to promote remission by slowing or stop the progression of joint destruction and deformity. Commonly used conventional synthetic DMARDs *(non-biologic DMARDs)* in the management of RA include MTX, SSZ, leflunomide, and HCQ.

Methotrexate is the initial choice of treatment among conventional DMARDs, and there is a need to conduct regular blood tests due to its side effects such as liver problems, cirrhosis, and bone marrow deterioration. Compared to other DMARDs, MTX is more effective and has lower side effects with dose flexibility (dosage adjustment can be done as required). Studies have shown that about 60% of patients with RA may experience mild toxicity; but more than 70% of them continue treatment with it at the end of the first year making it superior to other non-biologic DMARDs.

Hydroxychloroquine, an antimalarial drug, can be considered for long-term treatment of rheumatoid arthritis. Hydroxychloroquine acts by decreasing the secretion of monocyte-derived proinflammatory cytokines. Common side effects include problems in the GI tract, skin, and central nervous system. At higher doses, use of HCQ can affect the eyes.

Sulfasalazine is another DMARD that has been used for the treatment of RA when combined with anti-inflammatory drugs. Exact mechanism of action of SSZ in RA has not been defined. It is thought that sulfapyridine, a reduced form of the SSZ post-administration, may reduce secretions of interleukin 8 (IL-8) and monocyte chemoattractant protein (MCP). Common side effects include GI and central nervous system symptoms as well as rash. Other immunosuppressive medications used in RA management include azathioprine, cyclophosphamide, chlorambucil, and cyclosporine, especially for patients with very aggressive RA or complications of the disease.

NEWER THERAPIES IN THE MANAGEMENT OF RHEUMATOID ARTHRITIS

Biological disease-modifying anti-rheumatic drugs (bDMARDs), also referred as biologics or biosimilars, represent the newer class of drug in the rheumatologic armamentarium. Biologics are found to be rapidly effective in delaying the progression of joint damage that results due to RA. Hence, they are clinically defined as "direct" or "targeted" therapies. Biologics that inhibits the action of tumor necrosis factor (TNF) include etanercept, infliximab, adalimumab, golimumab, and certolizumab pegol. These medications are recommended, if patients do not respond to *conventional synthetic DMARDs*. These medications are often used in combination with other DMARDs, especially MTX. Moreover, TNF inhibitors are contraindicated in patients with congestive heart failure of demyelinating diseases.

Anakinra binds to IL-1, and can be used in combination with other DMARDs or as monotherapy. However, it is not used as frequently due to its lower response rate than other biologics. Also, when TNF-inhibitors fail, rituximab can be a treatment option in RA, which helps in depletion of B cells. Rituximab is also reported to be effective in managing complications of RA, such as vasculitis and cryoglobulinemia. Furthermore, patients who were not effectively treated with traditional DMARDs can be treated with abatacept.

Novel biosimilars have been developed that inhibit IL-6 and Janus kinase (JAK). Sarilumab is the newest biologic for approved by FDA in 2017 for the treatment of RA. Tocilizumab is another biologic that blocks IL-6 and is used in those who have not been effectively treated with traditional DMARDs. In contrast to IL-6 inhibitors, sirukumab, a monoclonal antibody that selectively binds to the cytokine, has been developed for RA patients who had failed conventional DMARDs with good therapeutic response.

Januse kinase inhibitors are the promising class of oral therapy in the management of RA. They play an integral role in cell signaling in immune cells, and it controls the response to may cytokines. Recently, in 2017 European Medicines Agency has approved two JAK inhibitors—tofacitinib and baricitinib in the treatment of RA. Tofacitinib is indicated for patients with moderate to severe active RA. It may be used in combination with methotrexate or another conventional synthetic DMARDs or as monotherapy. Baricitinib has been approved as monotherapy or in combination with methotrexate, for the treatment of adult patients with moderate to severe active RA who have responded inadequately to, or who are intolerant to one or more DMARDs. Few JAK inhibitors are in pipeline such as Filgotinib, Upadacitinib and Peficitinib.

CLINICAL RECOMMENDATIONS

The European Alliance of Associations for Rheumatology (EULAR) recommendations for the management of RA with synthetic and biological disease-modifying antirheumatic drugs: 2019 update are given in **Flowchart 1**.

Chapter 8: Recent Advances in the Management of Rheumatoid Arthritis

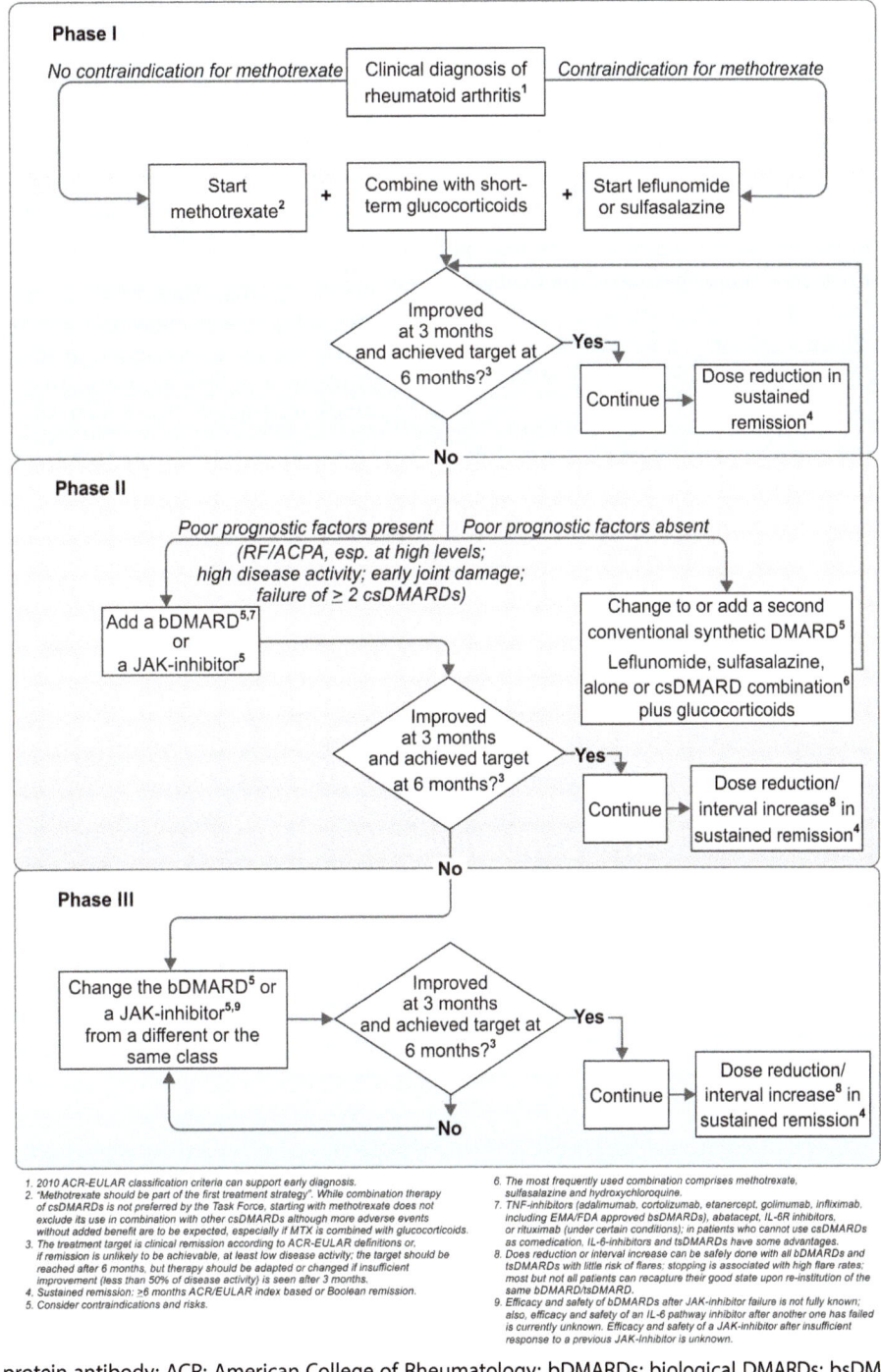

Flowchart 1: 2019 update of the EULAR RA management recommendations.

1. 2010 ACR-EULAR classification criteria can support early diagnosis.
2. "Methotrexate should be part of the first treatment strategy". While combination therapy of csDMARDs is not preferred by the Task Force, starting with methotrexate does not exclude its use in combination with other csDMARDs although more adverse events without added benefit are to be expected, especially if MTX is combined with glucocorticoids.
3. The treatment target is clinical remission according to ACR-EULAR definitions or, if remission is unlikely to be achievable, at least low disease activity; the target should be reached after 6 months, but therapy should be adapted or changed if insufficient improvement (less than 50% of disease activity) is seen after 3 months.
4. Sustained remission: ≥6 months ACR/EULAR index based or Boolean remission.
5. Consider contraindications and risks.
6. The most frequently used combination comprises methotrexate, sulfasalazine and hydroxychloroquine.
7. TNF-inhibitors (adalimumab, cortolizumab, etanercept, golimumab, infliximab, including EMA/FDA approved bsDMARDs), abatacept, IL-6R inhibitors, or rituximab (under certain conditions); in patients who cannot use csDMARDs as comedication, IL-6-inhibitors and tsDMARDs have some advantages.
8. Dose reduction or interval increase can be safely done with all bDMARDs and tsDMARDs with little risk of flares; stopping is associated with high flare rates; most but not all patients can recapture their good state upon re-institution of the same bDMARD/tsDMARD.
9. Efficacy and safety of bDMARDs after JAK-inhibitor failure is not fully known; also, efficacy and safety of an IL-6 pathway inhibitor after another one has failed is currently unknown. Efficacy and safety of a JAK-inhibitor after insufficient response to a previous JAK-inhibitor is unknown.

(ACPA: anticitrullinated protein antibody; ACR: American College of Rheumatology; bDMARDs: biological DMARDs; bsDMARD: biosimilar DMARDs; csDMARDs: conventional synthetic DMARDs; DMARDs: disease-modifying antirheumatic drugs; EMA: European Medicines Agency; EULAR: European League Against Rheumatism; FDA: Food and Drug Administration; IL-6R: interleukin 6 receptor; JAK: Janus kinase; MTX: methotrexate; RA: rheumatoid arthritis; RF: rheumatoid factor; TNF: tumor necrosis factor; tsDMARDs: targeted synthetic DMARDs)

■ KEY POINTS

- Adopting a *treat-to-target approach* helps in preventing progression of joint damage and optimize quality of life.
- Commonly prescribed NSAIDs for pain relief and anti-inflammatory properties are divided into short and long acting.
- Corticosteroids are administered for short duration and at low doses, especially during exacerbations or flares of rheumatoid arthritis.
- Methotrexate is the initial choice of treatment among conventional DMARDs.
- Biologics that inhibits the action of TNF include etanercept, infliximab, adalimumab, golimumab, and certolizumab pegol.

FURTHER READING

1. Bullock J, Rizvi SAA, Saleh AM, Gaston KJ. Rheumatoid arthritis: a brief overview of the treatment. Med Princ Pract. 2018;27(6):501-7.
2. Burmester GR, Pope JE. Novel treatment strategies in rheumatoid arthritis. Lancet. 2017;389(10086):2338-48.
3. Kucharz EJ, Stajszczyk M, Kotulska-kucharz A, Batko B, Brzosko M, Jeka S, et al. Tofacitinib in the treatment of patients with rheumatoid arthritis: position statement of experts of the Polish Society for Rheumatology. Reumatologia. 2018;56(4):203-11.
4. Kumar P, Banik S. Pharmacotherapy options in rheumatoid arthritis. Clin Med Insights Arthritis Musculoskelet Disord. 2013;6:35-43.
5. Mahajan TD, Mikuls TR. Recent advances in the treatment of rheumatoid arthritis. Curr Opin Rheumatol. 2018;30:1-7.
6. Markham A. Baricitinib: first global approval. Drugs. 2017;77(6):697-704.
7. Rivellese F, Lobasso A, Barbieri L, Liccardo B, de Paulis A, Rossi FW. Novel Therapeutic approaches in rheumatoid arthritis: role of Janus kinases inhibitors. Curr Med Chem. 2019;26(16):2823-43.
8. Smolen JS, Aletaha D, Barton A, Burmester GR, Emery P, Firestein GS, et al. Rheumatoid arthritis. Nat Rev Dis Primers. 2018;4:18001.
9. Smolen JS, Landewé RBM, Bijlsma JWJ, Burmester GR, Dougados M, Kerschbaumer A, et al. EULAR recommendations for the management of rheumatoid arthritis with synthetic and biological disease-modifying antirheumatic drugs: 2019 update. Ann Rheum Dis. 2020;79(6):685-99.

9. Biological Therapy

Shweta Agarwal

INTRODUCTION

Various rheumatic diseases are believed to arise from dysregulation of immune system. T cells, B cells and various cytokines have been shown to play an important role in pathogenesis of these disorders and hence have attracted researchers as target molecules for development of antirheumatic therapies. There is enough evidence of upregulation of proinflammatory cytokines such as tumor necrosis factor (TNF), interleukin (IL)-1 and IL-6 in rheumatoid synovium. Drugs targeting these inflammatory mediators have shown considerable efficacy in controlling disease activity as well as in arresting radiological progression in various trials, thus establishing their role in management of rheumatic diseases. This chapter focuses on role of the following anticytokine agents and cell-targeted therapies in rheumatoid arthritis (RA) and ankylosing spondylitis (AS).

Anticytokine Agents

- *Anti-TNFα drugs*: Infliximab, Etanercept, Adalimumab, Golimumab, Certolizumab pegol.
- *Interleukin (IL)-1 blockers*: Anakinra, Canakinumab, Rilonacept.
- *IL-6 blockers*: Tocilizumab, Sarilumab, Sirukumab.
- *IL-17 blockers*: Secukinumab, Ixekizumab, Brodalimumab.

Cell-targeted Biologics

- *Anti-CD 20 agent*: Rituximab
- *Costimulation modulator*: Abatacept.

TUMOR NECROSIS FACTOR INHIBITORS

Tumor necrosis factor is mainly produced by activated macrophages in RA and plays a key role in its pathogenesis by various mechanisms including induction of other proinflammatory cytokines (IL-1, IL-6) and chemokines (IL-8); enhancement of leukocyte migration; activation of various cell types and induction of the synthesis of acute phase reactants. This makes TNF an attractive target in management of RA and AS. TNF inhibitors bind to both soluble and membrane forms of TNF and thus block its proinflammatory actions.

- *Infliximab*: Infliximab is a chimeric mouse-human monoclonal antibody composed of constant region of human immunoglobulin (Ig) G coupled to variable regions of murine antibody. It has proven efficacy in RA and AS. It is administered as intravenous infusion over, atleast, 2 hours at 0, 2, 6 weeks followed every 8 weeks, doses being 3–5 mg/kg.
  - *Rheumatoid arthritis*: A pivotal study, anti-TNF Trial in RA with Concomitant Therapy (ATTRACT) proved efficacy of infliximab in RA. The study enrolled 428 patients with advanced disease on a constant dose of methotrexate (MTX). They were randomly given infusions of placebo, 3 mg/kg or 10 mg/kg of infliximab at 0, 2 and 6 weeks followed every 4 or 8 weeks. Infliximab and MTX treatment was found to be significantly better than MTX alone in terms of ACR responses, tender and swollen joint counts, pain scores and CRP levels. In the Active-Controlled Study of Patients receiving Infliximab for the treatment of Rheumatoid Arthritis of Early onset (ASPIRE) trial, infliximab plus MTX showed significant improvement in disease activity in patients with early RA (<3 years). It also showed favorable effects of infliximab on radiological progression when used early in disease. The BEST study confirmed that adding infliximab to MTX in early stage not only improves clinical disease activity but also halts radiological progression. It even induced drug free remission in few patients.

  Dose used in RA is 3 mg/kg IV infusion combined MTX at 0, 2 and 6 weeks followed by every 8 weeks. Dose can be increased to 10 mg/kg if required and the frequency may be increased to every 4 weeks in patients with incomplete response. Formation of human anti-chimeric antibodies (HACA) may lead to secondary failure of response to infliximab. Combining it with MTX can minimize infliximab immunogenicity leading to improved and prolonged efficacy.

- *Ankylosing spondylitis*: Various studies have demonstrated the statistically significant improvement in disease related indices for AS such as Bath Ankylosing Spondylitis Disease Activity Index (BASDAI), Bath Ankylosing Spondylitis Functional Index (BASFI), Bath Ankylosing Spondylitis Metrology Index (BASMI), anemia, CRP levels and sleep quality in patients receiving infliximab. The incidence of enthesitis and anterior uveitis was also found to be significantly decreased during third year of treatment with infliximab.

  Recommended dose of infliximab in AS is 5 mg/kg with or without MTX at 0, 2 and 6 weeks followed every 8 weeks.

- *Etanercept*: Etanercept is a fusion protein where recombinant TNF receptor is coupled to Fc component of human IgG1. It binds to TNF and lymphotoxin-α inhibiting their function. Etanercept is administered subcutaneously in a dose of 25 mg twice a week or 50 mg once a week as monotherapy or in combination with MTX.
  - *Rheumatoid arthritis*: The ERA (early rheumatoid arthritis) trial provided evidence in favor of etanercept monotherapy when compared to MTX monotherapy in terms of clinical features, inflammatory markers, physical function, and quality of life indices. Etanercept has even been shown to reduce radiographic progression. The TEMPO study demonstrated the superiority of the combination of etanercept and MTX over the two drugs alone. The COMET study further emphasized the benefits of combination therapy.
  - *Ankylosing spondylitis*: Etanercept showed significant improvements in BASDAI, BASFI and BASMI scores in AS in various studies as early as 2 weeks after starting the therapy. Patients even had improvement in spinal inflammation on MRI. After stopping etanercept relapses occurred at a mean interval of 6 weeks though reinstitution of therapy led to similar results as found on the initial usage of therapy. Most patients were able to discontinue NSAIDs completely.

- *Adalimumab*: Adalimumab is a recombinant, human, anti-TNF IgG1 monoclonal antibody. It binds to both soluble and transmembrane forms of TNF thus inhibiting binding of TNF to its receptors. It is used subcutaneously in doses of 40 mg every other week either as monotherapy or in combination with MTX.
  - *Rheumatoid arthritis*: ARMADA trial showed ACR20 responses in significantly higher number of patients of RA receiving adalimumab with MTX compared to placebo with MTX. PREMIER trial further emphasized that radiographic progression in patients with RA was significantly less in those receiving adalimumab with MTX than those on either adalimumab or MTX alone.
  - *Ankylosing spondylitis*: The ATLAS trial evaluated the long-term efficacy and safety of adalimumab in AS. Significantly higher number of patients receiving adalimumab showed ASAS20 response as compared with those receiving placebo at week 12 and 24. Adalimumab proved to be safe and well tolerated and it also significantly reduced sacroiliac and spinal inflammation as assessed by MRI.

- *Golimumab*: Golimumab is a genetically engineered, human IgG1, monoclonal, anti-TNF antibody. It is administered subcutaneously in the doses of 50 mg once a month with or without MTX.

  In GO-FORWARD study, patients of RA with active disease, despite being on stable doses of MTX, were enrolled. Golimumab in combination with MTX was found to be superior in improving clinical features as well as inflammation as demonstrated by MRI. In GO-RAISE study, golimumab was evaluated in patients with active AS on stable doses of sulfasalazine, low doses corticosteroids or NSAIDs. Significantly better results were found with golimumab at 14 and 24 weeks in terms of ASAS20 and ASAS40 responses as well as MRI-detected spinal inflammation.

- *Certolizumab pegol*: Pegylated certolizumab is a Fab fragment of recombinant humanized monoclonal anti-TNF antibody fused to a PEG moiety. It is administered subcutaneously at doses of 400 mg at 0, 2 and 4 weeks followed by 200 mg every other week. The dose of 400 mg is administered as 200 mg at two different sites at the same time.

  Its efficacy in RA, in combination with MTX, was evaluated in RAPID (Rheumatoid Arthritis Prevention of structural Damage)-I and RAPID-II trials. Along with the sustained improvements in RA signs and symptoms it also showed significant reduction in radiological progression.

  It was also found to be significantly efficacious in patients with AS in terms of better BASDAI, BASFI and BASMI scores as well as reduced spinal and sacroiliac inflammation.

Adverse Effects of TNF Inhibitors

Infections: A meta-analysis of nine clinical trials of TNF inhibitors revealed that patients receiving TNF inhibitors were at higher risk of developing serious infection. The pharmacovigilance studies have also revealed increased incidence of serious infections in patients receiving TNF inhibitors. Furthermore, TNF inhibitors can mask the initial symptoms and signs of infection making it even more important for the clinician to remain watchful. Opportunistic infections particularly disseminated and extrapulmonary tuberculosis (TB) are of maximum concern. Most of the cases of TB were found within first few months of initiation of therapy and were attributed to the reactivation of latent TB leading to mandatory screening for latent TB before initiation of anti-TNF therapy. Currently, it recommends that PPD (purified protein derivative) skin testing and chest radiograph are done before initiating anti-TNF therapy. If PPD is positive without evidence of active infection, treatment with isoniazid for 9 months is recommended, preferably starting a month before initiating anti-TNF therapy.

Malignancy: Risk of certain malignancies including lymphoma and lung cancer appear to be increased in patients of RA but receiving anti-TNF therapy does not seem to increase the risk any further.

Autoimmune disorders: Around 10–15% of patients receiving anti-TNF therapy develop antibodies to double stranded DNA though only around 0.2–0.4% develop symptoms of drug induced lupus. These symptoms improve after discontinuation of therapy.

Demyelinating syndromes: Cases of multiple sclerosis and peripheral demyelinating disease have been reported in patients on anti-TNF therapy though the risk appears very small.

Infusion and injection site reactions: Infusion reactions associated with infliximab are usually mild and transient. They consist of mainly headache and nausea and can be controlled by slowing the rate of infusion and giving antihistamines or acetaminophen. Injection site reactions occurring with other agents usually consist of erythematous and urticarial lesions which rarely lead to discontinuation of therapy. Reactions usually decrease with time even with continued dosing.

Antigenicity: Antibodies to anti-TNF agents may develop with time leading to decrease in efficacy. Concomitant use of MTX can decrease immunogenicity of anti-TNF drugs.

Monitoring

Before starting therapy: Every patient should be evaluated for active and latent tuberculosis [tuberculin skin test, chest radiograph, Interferon Gamma Release Assay (IGRA) for *M. tuberculosis*] and for hepatitis B and C viruses.

During therapy: Patient should be monitored for any sign or symptom of infection, malignancy or demyelinating disease. Complete blood count can be done intermittently. Repeat testing for tuberculosis has been recommended annually.

Pregnancy and Lactation

Tumor necrosis factor inhibitors are classified as US FDA Pregnancy category B. Thus, their use in pregnancy is recommended only if it is clearly required. Transfer of the drug to fetus is possible and may require monitoring accordingly. Anti-TNF agents are not recommended to be used during lactation.

INTERLEUKIN-1 BLOCKERS

Interleukin-1 (IL-1) is one of the key mediators of inflammation. Members of IL-1 family include IL-1α, IL-1β and the naturally occurring IL-1 receptor antagonist (IL-1Ra). They bind to two cell surface receptors: type I (IL-1RI) and type II (IL-1RII). Animal models of arthritis have shown the therapeutic potential of IL-1 blockade. Human studies in moderate to severe RA show only modest efficacy as compared to that with TNF inhibitors. These drugs are also being investigated for use in acute gout, osteoarthritis and graft versus host disease.

- *Anakinra*: Anakinra is a recombinant, nonglycosylated homolog of IL-1R and blocks the activity of IL-1 by competitively inhibiting IL-1 binding to IL-1RI receptor. In patients of RA, it is recommended at doses of 100 mg/day, subcutaneously. Anakinra can be used alone or in combination with MTX but is not recommended for use along with TNF inhibitors.
- *Canakinumab*: Canakinumab is a human monoclonal antibody which acts selectively against IL-1β. For patients having weight more than 40 kg, it is given in doses of 150 mg every 8 weeks, subcutaneously. Patients weighing between 15 and 40 kg are administered drug at dose of 2 mg/kg. It is also approved for systemic onset juvenile idiopathic arthritis.
- *Rilonacept*: Rilonacept is a fusion protein consisting of extracellular domains of human IL-1 receptor and Fc portion of human IgG1. It has very high affinity for IL-1 and is specific for IL-1β and IL-1α. It is given subcutaneously with a loading dose of 320 mg followed by 160 mg once weekly.

Adverse Events

Injection site reactions were the most common adverse events in the studies but they were usually mild and transient. Infections were uncommon and were mainly bacterial infections like cellulitis and pneumonia. Other adverse events reported were neutropenia, headache, nausea, diarrhea, sinusitis, influenza like syndrome and abdominal pain. Combination of anti-TNF agents and IL-1 blockers was found to increase rates of infection and serious infection and is thus not recommended. Patients on anti-IL-1 therapy should be monitored for infection. Neutrophil count should be checked prior to starting therapy, monthly for 3 months and every 4 months thereafter. These agents should be used in pregnancy only if clearly indicated and should be avoided in lactation.

■ INTERLEUKIN-6 BLOCKERS

Interleukin-6 is secreted by various cell types such as monocytes, T and B lymphocytes and fibroblasts. Its levels in serum and synovial tissue are found to be raised in inflammatory arthritis like RA and PsA and are directly proportional to the levels of CRP and disease activity. IL-6 has multiple effects on various aspects of immune system to initiate inflammation making it an attractive target for treatment of RA.

- *Tocilizumab*: Tocilizumab is a recombinant humanized IgG1 monoclonal antibody against human IL-6 receptor which competes with IL-6 to bind with IL-6 receptor and thus blocks its actions. It is approved for use alone or in combination with MTX in patients with RA in whom anti-TNF agents have failed. It is administered as intravenous infusion over one hour every 4 weeks at the doses of 8 mg/kg maximum being 800 mg per infusion.
- *Sarilumab*: Sarilumab is a human monoclonal antibody against IL-6 receptor. It is given subcutaneously every 2 weeks in doses of 150 mg or 200 mg.
- *Sirukumab*: It is a human monoclonal anti-IL-6 antibody effective in RA at doses of 100 mg subcutaneously every 2 weeks.

Adverse Events

Infections are a concern with IL-6 blockers. The most commonly reported infections were upper respiratory infections and nasopharyngitis. Higher doses were associated with serious infections such as cellulitis, pneumonia, diverticulitis, gastroenteritis and herpes zoster. Only rare cases of opportunistic infection have been reported. Transient elevation of liver enzymes was commonly seen after tocilizumab infusion. Lipid profile was found to be altered in patients receiving tocilizumab. Neutropenia, thrombocytopenia and rare events of gastrointestinal perforation, malignancy and demyelinating disorders have also been reported in clinical trials. Hypertension has been reported during infusion and headache and skin reactions within 24 hours of infusion with tocilizumab. A few patients developed antibodies to tocilizumab and very few developed hypersensitivity reaction leading to withdrawal of treatment.

Patients should be evaluated for tuberculosis and other infections before starting therapy. Liver enzymes should be done prior to starting therapy and every 4–8 weeks during treatment. Lipid levels, neutrophil count and platelet count should also be monitored.

Tocilizumab is not recommended to be used in combination with other biologic DMARDs. It is recommended that patient's vaccination status is up to date before starting anti-IL-6 therapy but no live vaccination is allowed along with the therapy. Tocilizumab is a Pregnancy Category C drug and should be used in pregnancy only if benefits justify risk to fetus and should be avoided during lactation.

■ INTERLEUKIN-17 BLOCKERS

Interleukin-17 levels are found to be raised in serum and synovial fluid of RA patients. IL-17 inhibitors have a modest efficacy in patients with RA but their efficacy in psoriasis has been found to be dramatic.

- *Secukinumab*: It is a humanized anti-IL-17 monoclonal antibody approved for RA, psoriatic arthritis and AS. It can be given, subcutaneously at a dose of 10 mg/kg at 0, 2, and 4 weeks, followed by 150 mg every 4 weeks, to the patients of RA following anti-TNF failure.
- *Ixekizumab*: It is also an anti-IL-17 monoclonal antibody found to be safe and effective for treatment of PsA.
- *Brodalimumab*: It is IL-17 receptor subunit A monoclonal antibody approved for treatment of PsA.

■ ANTI-CD20 AGENT

B-lymphocytes play an important role in acquired immunity. The surface antigen, CD20, plays a key role in B-cell activation. CD20+ B cells constitute the predominant population of cells in synovial tissue of patients with RA and thus can be targeted for therapeutic role.

Rituximab is a chimeric mouse-human monoclonal antibody against the extracellular domain of CD20 antigen. It selectively lyses B cells expressing CD20 by antibody-dependent, cell-mediated cytotoxicity and by initiating apoptosis of B cells. Rituximab has been found to be effective in patients of RA who had inadequate response to anti-TNF agents or were intolerant to them. It has been found to be maximally effective in seropositive patients. It is administered as two intravenous infusions of 1 g each at interval of 2 weeks with a premedication of 100 mg of methylprednisolone along with once a week oral MTX. This cycle of two infusions can be repeated every 6–12 months. Infusion reactions can occur with rituximab but usually are mild to moderate and can be minimized by prior use of methylprednisolone. Infection and serious infections have been reported to be—6 events per 100 patient-years over 5 courses. Progressive multifocal leukoencephalopathy is rarely reported in patients of RA following treatment with rituximab.

Other anti-CD 20 agents such as *ocrelizumab* and *ofatumumab* are under investigation.

■ COSTIMULATION MODULATOR

Activated T cells play key role in pathogenesis of RA. Successful T-cell activation requires multiple signals making costimulation an essential step in the induction of adaptive immunity. Costimulatory signal is provided by interaction between CD80 or CD86 on antigen-presenting cells and CD28 on T cells.

Abatacept is a fully human fusion protein consisting of extracellular portion of CTLA-4 (cytolytic T lymphocyte-associated protein 4) and the Fc fragment of IgG-1. It binds to CD80 and CD86 on antigen-presenting cells preventing their binding to CD28 on T cells and thus blocking costimulation and adequate activation of T cells and consequently resulting in reduction in auto-immune activity and inflammation.

In a phase III trial, abatacept trial in treatment of anti-TNF inadequate (ATTAIN) responders, abatacept was administered at doses of 10 mg/kg along with fixed dose of MTX in patients of RA who responded inadequately to anti-TNF agents. Significantly greater improvement was reported in ACR response criteria and quality of life (QoL). Abatacept is administered as intravenous infusion of 10 mg/kg, over 30 minutes, at 0, 2, 4 weeks and 4 weekly thereafter. It can be combined with MTX but not with other biologic agents because of increase in incidence of serious adverse events when combined with other biologicals.

■ FUTURE TREND

Biological response modifiers available currently have remarkably changed the goals of management in autoimmune disorders. They not only control disease activity but also decrease radiological progression of disease, improve quality of life and patient's functional ability. Cost remains a major hurdle in their use in India but with the advent of health insurance, we may look forward toward a better management of autoimmune diseases with the help of biological agents.

■ KEY POINTS

- Anti-TNFα drugs such as infliximab, etanercept, adalimumab, golimumab and certolizumab pegol block the proinflammatory action of TNF which is implicated in RA and AS.
- Infliximab is a chimeric mouse-human monoclonal antibody with proven efficacy in RA and AS. It is administered as intravenous infusion over, at least, 2 hours at 0, 2, 6 weeks followed every 8 weeks, doses being 3–5 mg/kg.
- Etanercept is a fusion protein where recombinant TNF receptor is coupled to Fc component of human IgG1. It is administered subcutaneously in a dose of 25 mg twice a week or 50 mg once a week as monotherapy or in combination with MTX.
- Adalimumab is a recombinant, human, anti-TNF IgG1 monoclonal antibody which is used subcutaneously in doses of 40 mg every other week either as monotherapy or in combination with MTX.
- Golimumab is a genetically engineered, human IgG1, monoclonal, anti-TNF antibody. It is administered subcutaneously in the doses of 50 mg once a month with or without MTX.
- Pegylated certolizumab is a Fab fragment of recombinant humanized monoclonal anti-TNF antibody fused to a PEG moiety. It is administered subcutaneously at doses of 400 mg at 0, 2 and 4 weeks followed by 200 mg every other week.
- Antibodies to anti-TNF agents may develop with time leading to decrease in efficacy. Concomitant use of MTX can decrease immunogenicity of anti-TNF drugs.
- Patients receiving TNF inhibitors are at higher risk of developing serious infection. Opportunistic infections particularly disseminated and extrapulmonary tuberculosis (TB) are of maximum concern.
- Every patient should be evaluated for active and latent tuberculosis before starting anti-TNF therapy. Patient should be monitored for any sign or symptom of infection, malignancy or demyelinating disease during therapy.
- Interleukin-1 blockers such as anakinra, canakinumab, rilonacept have modest efficacy in RA.
- Anakinra is a recombinant, nonglycosylated homolog of IL-1R used in patients of RA at doses of 100 mg/day, subcutaneously, alone or in combination with MTX.
- Canakinumab is a human monoclonal antibody approved for systemic onset juvenile idiopathic arthritis whereas rilonacept is a fusion protein.
- Patients on anti-IL-1 therapy should be monitored for infection. Neutrophil count should be checked prior to starting therapy, monthly for three months and every 4 months thereafter. These agents should be used in pregnancy only if clearly indicated and should be avoided in lactation.
- IL-6 blockers such as tocilizumab, sarilumab, sirukumab are used as second line biologicals in RA. Patients should be evaluated for tuberculosis and other infections before starting therapy. Liver enzymes should be done prior to starting therapy and every 4–8 weeks during treatment. Lipid levels, neutrophil count and platelet count should also be monitored.
- Secukinumab is a humanized anti-IL-17 monoclonal antibody approved for RA, psoriatic arthritis and AS. Ixekizumab and brodalumab are other IL-17 blockers approved for PsA.
- Rituximab is a chimeric mouse-human monoclonal antibody which selectively lyses B cells expressing CD20 by antibody-dependent, cell-mediated cytotoxicity. It has been found to be effective in patients of RA especially seropositive. Infusion reactions, infections and progressive multifocal leukoencephalopathy have been reported after use of rituximab.
- Abatacept is a fully human fusion protein which blocks costimulation and adequate activation of T cells and consequently results in reduction in autoimmune activity and inflammation. It can be used in RA in combination with MTX.

FURTHER READING

1. Blanco FJ, Moricke R, Dokoupilova E, Codding C, Neal J, Anderrson M, et al. Secukinumab in active rheumatoid arthritis: A phase III randomized, double-blind, active comparator- and placebo-controlled study. Arthritis Rheumatol. 2017;69(6):1144-53.
2. Bongartz T, Sutton AJ, Sweeting MJ, Buchan I, Matteson EL, Montori V. Anti-TNF antibody therapy in rheumatoid arthritis and the risk of serious infections and malignancies: systematic review and meta-analysis of rare harmful effects in randomized controlled trials. JAMA. 2006;295(19):2275-85.
3. Brandt J, Khariouzov A, Listing J, Haibel H, Sörensen H, Grassnickel L, et al. Six-month results of a double-blind, placebo-controlled trial of etanercept treatment in patients with active ankylosing spondylitis. Arthritis Rheum. 2003;48(6):1667-75.
4. Braun J, Baraliakos X, Brandt J, Listing J, Zink A, Alten R, et al. Persistent clinical response to the anti-TNF-alpha antibody infliximab in patients with ankylosing spondylitis over 3 years. Rheumatology. 2005;44(5):670-6.
5. Braun J, Brandt J, Listing J, Zink A, Alten R, Burmester G, et al. Long-term efficacy and safety of infliximab in the treatment of ankylosing spondylitis: an open, observational, extension study of a three-month, randomized, placebo-controlled trial. Arthritis Rheum. 2003;48(8):2224-33.
6. Braun J, Brandt J, Listing J, Zink A, Alten R, Golder W, et al. Treatment of active ankylosing spondylitis with infliximab: a randomised controlled multicentre trial. Lancet. 2002; 359(9313):1187-93.
7. Breedveld FC, Weisman MH, Kavanaugh AF, Cohen SB, Pavelka K, van Vollenhoven R, et al. The PREMIER study: a multicenter, randomized, double-blind clinical trial of combination therapy with adalimumab plus methotrexate versus methotrexate alone or adalimumab alone in patients with early, aggressive rheumatoid arthritis who had not had previous methotrexate treatment. Arthritis Rheum. 2006;54(1):26-37.
8. Bresnihan B, Alvaro-Gracia JM, Cobby M, Doherty M, Domljan Z, Emery P, et al. Treatment of rheumatoid arthritis with recombinant human interleukin-1 receptor antagonist. Arthritis Rheum 1998;41(12): 2196-204.
9. Cohen SB, Emery P, Greenwald MW, Dougados M, Furie RA, Genovese MC, et al. REFLEX trial group. Rituximab for rheumatoid arthritis refractory to anti-tumor necrosis factor therapy: results of a multicenter, randomized, double-blind, placebo-controlled, phase III trial evaluating primary efficacy and safety at twenty-four weeks. Arthritis Rheum. 2006;54:2793-806.
10. Davis JC, van der Heijde DM, Braun J, Dougados M, Cush J, Clegg DO, et al. Recombinant human tumor necrosis factor receptor (etanercept) for treating ankylosing spondylitis: a randomized, controlled trial. Arthritis Rheum. 2003; 48(11):3230-6.
11. Davis JC, van der Heijde DM, Braun J, Dougados M, Cush J, Clegg D, et al. Sustained durability and tolerability of etanercept in ankylosing spondylitis for 96 weeks. Ann Rheum Dis. 2005;64(11):1557-62.
12. Davis JC, van der Heijde DM, Dougados M, Woolley JM. Reductions in health-related quality of life in patients with ankylosing spondylitis and improvements with etanercept therapy. Arthritis Rheum. 2005; 53:494-501.
13. Emery P, Fleischmann R, Filipowicz-Sosnowska A, Schechtman J, Szczepanski L, Kavanaugh A, et al. DANCER study group. The efficacy and safety of rituximab in patients with active rheumatoid arthritis despite methotrexate treatment: results of a phase IIB randomized, double-blind, placebo-controlled, dose-ranging trial. Arthritis Rheum. 2006;54(5):1390-400.
14. Feldman M, Brennan FM, Maini RN. Role of cytokines in rheumatoid arthritis. Annu Rev Immunol. 1996;43:28-38.
15. Feldman M, Eliot MJ, Woody JN. Anti-tumor necrosis factor-α therapy of rheumatoid arthritis. Adv Immunol. 1997; 64:283-350.
16. Fleischmann RM, Halland AM, Brzosko M, Burgos-Vargas R, Mela C, Vernon E, et al. Tocilizumab inhibits structural joint damage and improves physical function in patients with rheumatoid arthritis and inadequate responses to methotrexate: LITHE study 2-year results. J Rheumatol. 2013; 40(2):113-26.
17. Fleischmann RM, Tesser J, Schiff MH, Schechtman J, Burmester GR, Bennet R, et al. Safety of extended treatment with anakinra in patients with rheumatoid arthritis. Ann Rheum Dis. 2006;65(8):1006-12.
18. Genovese MC, Bathon JM, Martin RW, Fleischmann RM, Tesser JR, Schiff MH, et al. Etanercept versus methotrexate in patients with early rheumatoid arthritis: two-year radiographic and clinical outcomes. Arthritis Rheum. 2002;46(6):1443-50.
19. Genovese MC, Cohen S, Moreland L, Lium D, Robbins S, Newmark R, et al. Combination therapy with etanercept and anakinra in the treatment of patients with rheumatoid arthritis who have been treated unsuccessfully with methotrexate. Arthritis Rheum. 2004;50(5):1412-9.
20. Genovese MC, Fleischmann RM, Kivitz AJ, Rell-Bakalarska M, Martincova R, Fiore S, et al. Sarilumab plus methotrexate in patients with active rheumatoid arthritis and inadequate response to methotrexate: results of a phase III study. Arthritis Rheumatol. 2015;67(6):1424-37.
21. Genovese MC, Schiff M, Luggen M, Becker JC, Aranda R, Teng J, et al. Efficacy and safety of the selective co-stimulation modulator abatacept following 2 years of treatment in patients with rheumatoid arthritis and an inadequate response to anti-tumour necrosis factor therapy. Ann Rheum Dis. 2008;67(4):547-54.
22. Hernandez-Cruz B, Garcia-Arias M, Ariza Ariza R, Martin Mola E. Rituximab in rheumatoid arthritis: a systematic review of efficacy and safety. Reumatol Clin. 2011; 7(5):314-22.
23. Inman RD, Davis JC Jr, van der Heijde D, Diekman L, Sieper J, Kim SI, et al. Efficacy and safety of golimumab in patients with ankylosing spondylitis: results of a randomized, double-blind, placebo-controlled, phase III trial. Arthritis Rheum. 2008;58(11):3402-12.
24. Kavanaugh A, Cohen S, Cush J. The evolving use of TNF inhibitors in rheumatoid arthritis. J Rheumatol. 2004; 31:1881-4.
25. Kekow J, Moots RJ, Emery P, Durez P, Koenig A, Singh A, et al. Patient-reported outcomes improve with etanercept plus methotrexate in active early rheumatoid arthritis and the improvement is strongly associated with remission: the COMET trial. Ann Rheum Dis. 2010;69(1):222-5.

26. Keystone E, van der Heijde D, Mason D Jr, Landewé R, Vollenhoven RV, Combe B, et al. Certolizumab pegol plus methotrexate is significantly more effective than placebo plus methotrexate in active rheumatoid arthritis: findings of a fifty-two-week, phase III, multicenter, randomized, double-blind, placebo-controlled, parallel-group study. Arthritis Rheum. 2008;58(11):3319-29.
27. Keystone EC, Genovese MC, Klareskog L, Hsia EC, Hall ST, Miranda PC, et al. Golimumab, a human antibody to tumour necrosis factor {alpha} given by monthly sub-cutaneous injections, in active rheumatoid arthritis despite methotrexate therapy: the GO-FORWARD Study. Ann Rheum Dis. 2009;68(6):789-96.
28. Koch AE, Kunkel SL, Strieter RM. Cytokines in rheumatoid arthritis. J Invest Med. 1995;43:28-38.
29. Korth-Bradley JM, Rubin AS, Hanna RK, Simcoe DK, Lebsack ME. The pharmacokinetics of etanercept in healthy volunteers. Ann Pharmacother. 2000;34(2):161-4.
30. Lambert RJ, Salonen D, Rahman P, Inman RD, Wong RL, Einstein SG, et al. Adalimumab significantly reduces both spinal and sacroiliac joint inflammation in patients with ankylosing spondylitis: a multicenter, randomized, double-blind, placebo-controlled study. Arthritis Rheum. 2007;56(12):4005-14.
31. Landewe R, Braun J, Deodhar A, Dougados M, Maksymowych WP, Mease PJ, et al. Efficacy of certolizumab pegol on signs and symptoms of axial spondyloarthritis including ankylosing spondylitis: 24-week results of a double-blind randomised placebo-controlled Phase 3 study. Ann Rheum Dis. 2014;73(1):39-47.
32. Lipsky PE, van der Heijde DM, St Clair EW, Furst DE, Breedveld FC, Kalden JR, et al. Infliximab and methotrexate in treatment of rheumatoid arthritis. Anti-Tumor Necrosis Factor Trial in Rheumatoid Arthritis with Concomitant Therapy Study Group. N Engl J Med. 2000;343(22):1594-602.
33. Maini R, St Clair EW, Breedveld F, Furst D, Kalden J, Wesman M, et al. Infliximab (chimeric anti-tumour necrosis factor alpha monoclonal antibody) versus placebo in rheumatoid arthritis patients receiving concomitant methotrexate: a randomised phase III trial. ATTRACT Study Group. Lancet. 1999;354:1932-9.
34. Maini RN, Breedveld FC, Kalden JR, Smolen JS, Davis D, Macfarlane JD, et al. Therapeutic efficacy of multiple intravenous infusions of anti-tumor necrosis factor alpha monoclonal antibody combined with low-dose weekly methotrexate in rheumatoid arthritis. Arthritis Rheum. 1998;41(9):1552-63.
35. Maini RN, Taylor PC, Szechinski J, Pavelka K, Bröll J, Balint G, et al. Double-blind randomized controlled clinical trial of the interleukin-6 receptor antagonist, tocilizumab, in European patients with rheumatoid arthritis who had an incomplete response to methotrexate. Arthritis Rheum. 2006; 54(9):2817-29.
36. Malaviya AN, Kapoor S, Garg S, Rawat R, Shankar S, Nagpal S, et al. Preventing tuberculosis flare in patients with inflammatory rheumatic diseases receiving tumor necrosis factor-alpha inhibitors in India-An audit report. J Rheumatol. 2009;36(7):1414-20.
37. Nahakara H, Song J, Sugimoto M, Hagihara K, Kishimoto T, Yoshizaki K, et al. Anti-interleukin-6 receptor antibody therapy reduces vascular endothelial growth factor production in rheumatoid arthritis. Arthritis Rheum. 2003;48(6):1521-9.
38. Nash P, Kirkham B, Okada M, Rahman P, Combe B, Burmester GR, et al. SPIRIT-P2 study group. Ixekizumab for the treatment of patients with active psoriatic arthritis and an inadequate response to tumor necrosis factor inhibitors: results from the 24-week randomized, double-blind, placebo-controlled period of the SPIRIT-P2 phase 3 trial. Lancet. 2017;389(10086):2317-27.
39. Nishimoto N, Hashimoto J, Miyasaka N, Yamamoto K, Kawai S, Takeuchi T, et al. Study of active controlled monotherapy used for rheumatoid arthritis, an IL-6 inhibitor (SAMURAI): evidence of clinical and radiographic benefit from an X-ray reader-blinded randomised controlled trial of tocilizumab. Ann Rheum Dis. 2007;66(9):1162-7.
40. Olsen NJ, Stein CM. New drugs for rheumatoid arthritis. N Engl J Med. 2004;350:2167-79.
41. Reichert JM. Antibodies to watch in 2017. MABS. 2017;9(2):167-81.
42. Smolen JS, Beaulieu A, Rubbert-Roth A, Ramos-Remus C, Rovensky J, Alecock E, et al. Effect of interleukin-6 receptor inhibition with tocilizumab in patients with rheumatoid arthritis (OPTION study): a double-blind, placebo-controlled, randomised trial. Lancet. 2008;371(9617):987-97.
43. Smolen JS, Han C, van der Heijde DM, Emery P, Bathon JM, Keystone E, et al. Active-Controlled Study of Patients Receiving Infliximab for the Treatment of Rheumatoid Arthritis of Early Onset (ASPIRE) Study Group. Ann Rheum Dis. 2009;68(6):823-7.
44. Smolen JS, Kay J, Doyle MK, Landewe R, Matteson EL, Wollenhaupt J, et al. Golimumab in patients with active rheumatoid arthritis after treatment with tumor necrosis factor inhibitors (Go-AFTER): a multicentre, randomized, double-blind, placebo-controlled, phase III trial. Lancet. 2009; 374:210-21.

Surgical Considerations in Inflammatory Arthritis

Manish Khanna, Rashmi Chopra

INTRODUCTION

The purpose of this chapter is to present an approach to the surgical considerations in patients who do not respond completely to conservative modality of management. There are numerous considerations which must be addressed before proceeding to surgery including current serum levels, etc. Imaging studies such as radiographs, computerized tomography scans, radionucleotide scans, and occasionally magnetic resonance imaging of the concerned joint are crucial to decide the extent of damage. Recent onset rheumatoid arthritis (RA) (RA, disease duration of less than 2 years) usually does not produce that severely damaged joint than produced in established RA cases (disease duration of more than 2 years).

When surgery is offered, explain that the main expected benefits are:
- Pain relief
- Improvement and/or prevention of further deterioration of joint function
- Improvement and or prevention of deformity

Surgical management is offered in any of following conditions which do not respond to optimal nonsurgical management:
- Persistent pain due to joint damage or other identifiable soft tissue cause worsening joint function
- Progressive deformity
- Progressive localized synovitis
- Nerve compression (e.g., carpal tunnel syndrome)

Do not let concerns about the long-term durability of prosthetic joints influence decisions to offer joint replacements to younger people.

While continuation of methotrexate in the perioperative period is probably safe, data on the other disease-modifying antirheumatic drugs (DMARDs) are sparse. Leflunomide therapy should be given with care in view of its long drug half-life.

More data on the perioperative use of the modern targeted agents are also needed. Preliminary evidence shows that the risks of perioperative infections under treatment with tumor necrosis factor (TNF)-blocking agents are low. Thus, interruption of anti-TNF therapy in the perioperative period, can be kept limited.

After fingers and toes joint involvement, the next commonly involved joints in RA are shoulders, wrist, knee, and ankles. Monocompartmental arthritis of the knee is one of the common indications for deformity correction surgery provided the disease progression has stopped.

COMMON SURGICAL PROCEDURES

- *Synovectomy*: Partial synovectomy is indicated in patients where joint destruction is minimal and if the main cause of pain and swelling is synovitis not responding to conservative treatment (usually done in knee and ankle). In elbow along with synovectomy, radial head excision can be attempted in severe cases. In wrist dorsal synovectomy with or without resection of distal end of ulna can be attempted.

  In 1990s, several publications cast doubt on arthroscopic debridement for knee arthritis as a tool for routine practice. But now it is very much clear that routine arthroscopic debridement has not much role in disease prognosis.

- *Osteotomy*: If articular surface of hip or knee is partially damaged then osteotomy can be planned usually with age of patient below 60. In seronegative arthropathies spinal osteotomy to correct spine deformity can be done.

- *Arthrodesis*: This gives a long-term pain relief with loss of movement in that fused joint. Nevertheless, the stress may cause secondary osteoarthritis (OA) in the adjacent joints unless they are able to compensate for the loss of movement. Lack of movement after fusion of the wrist can be absorbed at the elbow and shoulder without significant functional improvement, but fusion of the hip puts lot of strain on the spine and knee.

  Arthrodesis thus tends to be done for peripheral joints as wrist, ankle, interphalangeal (IP) joints of hands and feet if nothing else much can be done. In these joints the functional loss is less disabling and arthroplasty is little less reliable.

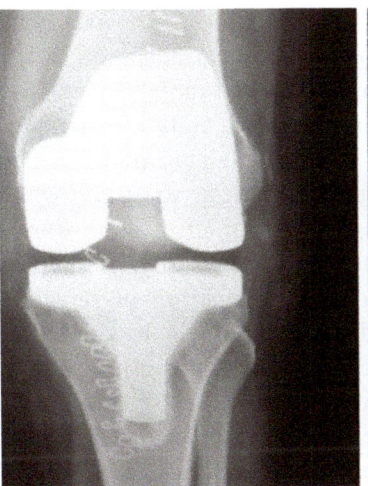
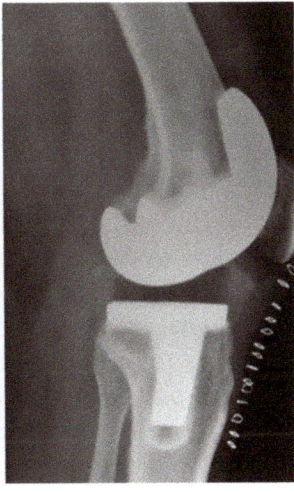

Fig. 1: Radiograph showing total knee replacement in rheumatoid knee.

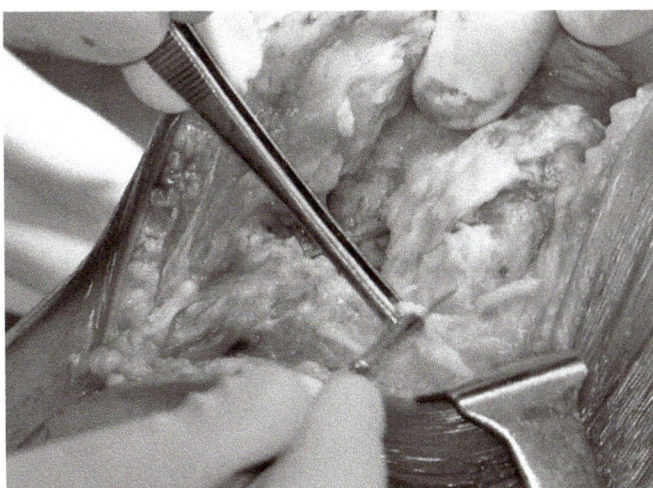

Fig. 2: Proper soft tissue balancing.

- *Arthroplasties*: Arthroplasties of hip, knee (**Fig. 1**) ankle shoulder is indicated in advanced diseases causing severe pain and incapacitating disability due to stiffness and instability. In knee, soft tissue balancing in such cases is very important (**Fig. 2**).

RHEUMATOID TENOSYNOVITIS ABOUT ANKLE

The most commonly affected tendons are flexor hallucis longus, tibialis posterior below the medial malleolus, tendon tibialis, anteriorly the tibialis anterior and below the lateral malleolus the peronei. Diagnostic rheumatoid lesions may be demonstrable in synovial biopsy.

Surgical decompression may be effective in such cases. The surgical approach is made through curvilinear incision 1 cm posterior to medial malleolus.

Ankle Arthrodesis

For over 40 years ankle arthrodesis is the mainstay for end stage arthritis for which numerous techniques and approaches exist. Unfortunately it results in 60–70% loss of sagittal movement as well as decreased movement in subtalar joint.

Selection of the surgical techniques should be based on the underlying disorder. Usually external fixators are preferred if severe osteopenia is there and also when preexisting septic joint state is there. Arthroscopic arthrodesis should be reserved for patients with minimal deformity. Patients with significant ankle deformity should be managed by open arthrodesis. Clinically walking speed is decreased by 16% and in addition to other complications, an increased incidence of arthritis in hindfoot and midfoot joints has been observed. Complications usually associated with ankle arthrodesis are malunion, syndesmotic nonunion, infection resulting in wound complications and rarely neurological injury.

SURGERY FOR RHEUMATOID HAND AND WRIST

The surgical procedures commonly required can be grouped as prophylactic surgeries and reconstructive surgeries. Prophylactic surgery as the name suggests, may delay the joint and tissue destruction by reducing the disease activity and by removing the inflamed granulation tissue. These surgeries are synovectomy, tenosynovectomy and tendon balancing surgeries. Reconstructive procedures are performed in advanced disease and include tendon transfer, arthroplasty and arthrodesis.

Wrist Joint

A stable and painless wrist is essential to achieve successful outcome from the more distal surgeries.

The tendon sheath involvement can cause swelling over the dorsum or volar aspect of wrist. If the tenosynovitis is not responding to medications or causing significant swelling surgery is indicated. Dorsal tendons are accessed through a dorsal longitudinal/slightly curved approach (**Fig. 3**). The extensor retinaculum is elevated as a V or U-shaped radially based flap. Each affected compartment is opened in a systematic manner and inflamed tenosynovium is excised using sharp dissecting scissors. The wrist joint can be accessed through a flap or transverse incision of the capsule. Joint synovium removed with a rongeur. The distal radioulnar joint (DRUJ) can be accessed and necessary intervention such as synovectomy, excision of osteophyte or removal of head of ulna can be performed. Early hand movement is recommended with a resting splint in extension state of metacarpophalangeal joint (MCPJ) and the wrist in the neutral position.

Volar tenosynovitis can cause symptoms of carpal tunnel syndrome or flexor tendon attrition and subsequent rupture. Volar tenosynovectomy is performed through a volar incision. The cutaneous and muscular branches of the median nerve should be protected. Wrist splinted in neutral with early finger movements.

Wrist radiographs in RA can show some typical pattern of affection. The distal ulna and scaphoid are commonly involved and lead to rotatory instability of the scaphoid, loss of carpal height, ulnar and volar translation of the carpus, dorsal subluxation of ulna and radial deviation of the metacarpals **(Figs. 4 and 5)**. In the authors experience patients present late with established deformities limiting the role of preventive surgeries such as wrist and DRUJ synovectomy. These can be performed through dorsal approach as described earlier. Limited fusions such as radiolunate fusion have shown good long-term preservation of the wrist joint. DRUJ disease can be dealt with either Darrach's procedure (excision of distal ulna) or Sauvé-Kapandji procedure (Fusion of the DRUJ with distal ulnar osteotomy). For painful, debilitating, and severely deformed wrist the choice is between total wrist arthroplasty or wrist arthrodesis. Arthrodesis preferred due to better results and cost effectiveness. In authors' experience, total wrist fusion using a dorsal plate or Steinmann pin is a reliable procedure. Wrist is fused in neutral or up to 15 degrees of extension. Total wrist replacement is preferred in patients with low demands and who have bilateral wrist involvement with one side treated with fusion and other with replacement.

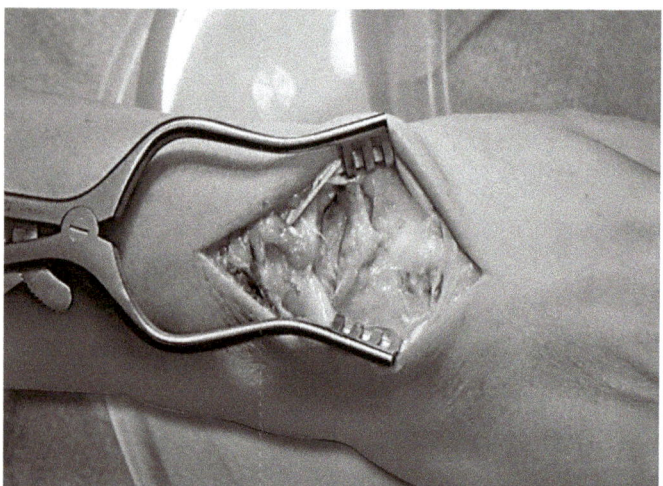

Fig. 3: Dorsal approach to the wrist.

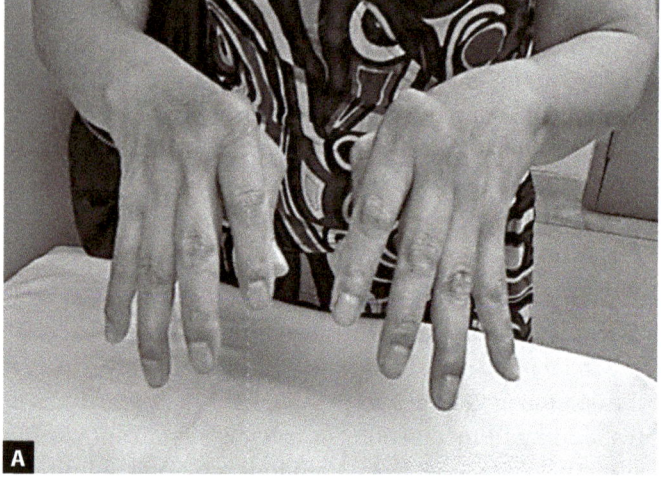
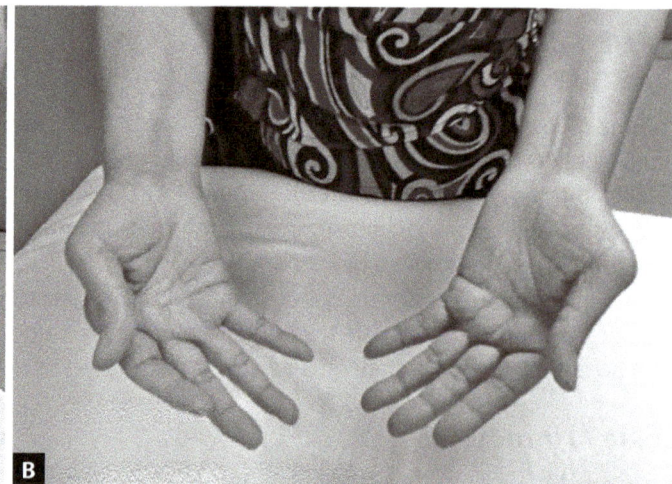

Figs. 4A and B: Metacarpophalangeal joint (MCPJ) disease in rheumatoid arthritis (RA) with subluxation, ulnar deviation.

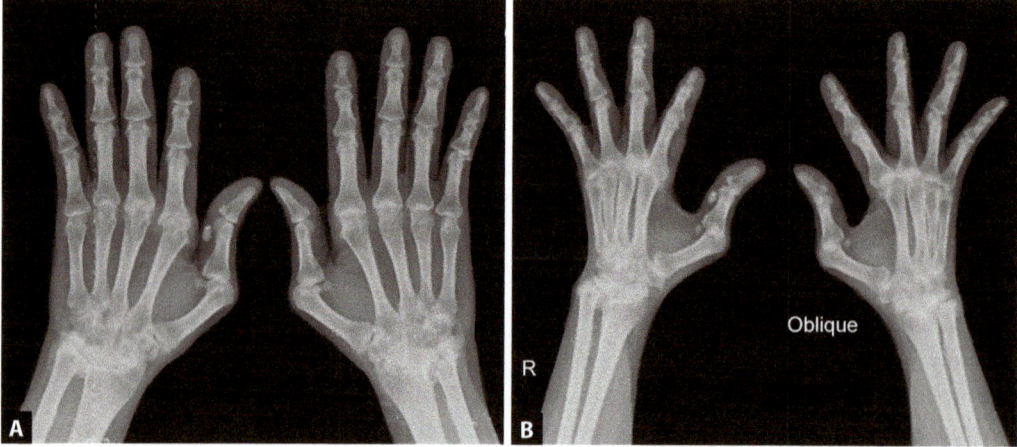

Figs. 5A and B: Rheumatoid arthritis (RA) hand—bilateral wrist and metacarpophalangeal joint (MCPJ) disease. Patient had stable, mobile and painless wrist. Note the volar subluxation of the proximal phalanges.

Metacarpophalangeal Joints

The typical deformity is that of volar displacement of the bases of the proximal phalanges with ulnar deviation of the digits. The patients are unable to actively extend the MCP joints as the long extensors slip into the ulnar side of the joints and prevent extension **(Figs. 4 and 5)**.

Prophylactic surgery such as synovectomy and tendon realignment can be useful and help slow down the progression of the deformities. The author prefers to do these procedures through the dorsal approach, by using a separate longitudinal incision for each MCPJ. A single transverse incision can also be used for multiple joints. Extensor retinaculum and capsule opened through radial longitudinal incision. Synovectomy performed using a Rongeur. Soft tissue balance is achieved by release of the ulnar intrinsic muscles and double breasting of the extensor apparatus on the radial side to realign and centralize the extensor tendon.

In advanced disease, with chronically subluxed MCPJ the articular cartilage is damaged. Silastic MCPJ arthroplasty is widely accepted procedure for severe MCPJ arthritis. This was described and popularized by Swanson in 1972. Satisfactory long-term results have been reported in terms of function and appearance. The author has achieved very good results with silastic MCPJ arthroplasty. The approach is dorsal as described earlier. Good postoperative rehabilitation with static and dynamic splinting plays a vital role in successful outcome **(Figs. 6 to 8)**.

Use of MCPJ excision arthroplasty is limited to patients with severe deformities and concerns with personal hygiene. MCPJ arthrodesis is not useful as it significantly limits the motion of the whole digit.

Interphalangeal Joints

Digital tenosynovitis affects the synovial sheath of the long flexors. Due to the limited space available for the tendons in the fibro-osseous canal, patients may present with triggering of fingers, stiffness or tendon rupture. Flexor tenosynovectomy is performed through zig-zag incisions. The annular pulleys are preserved to prevent bow stringing. Intratendinous nodules, if present, are excised and the defect repaired with fine nonabsorbable sutures. Early and differential finger motion is the key to prevent adhesions.

Two most common deformities of the fingers in RA are: (1) Boutonniere and (2) Swan neck deformities as described earlier in the chapter. Boutonniere deformity is a result of affection of the proximal interphalangeal joint (PIPJ).

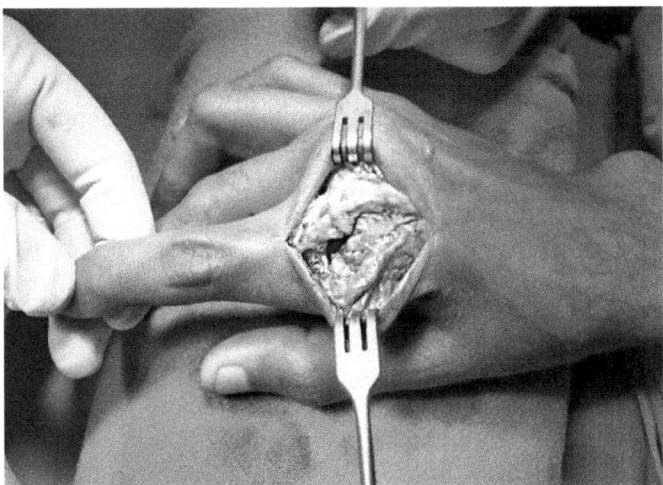

Fig. 6: Dorsal approach to metacarpophalangeal joint (MCPJ).

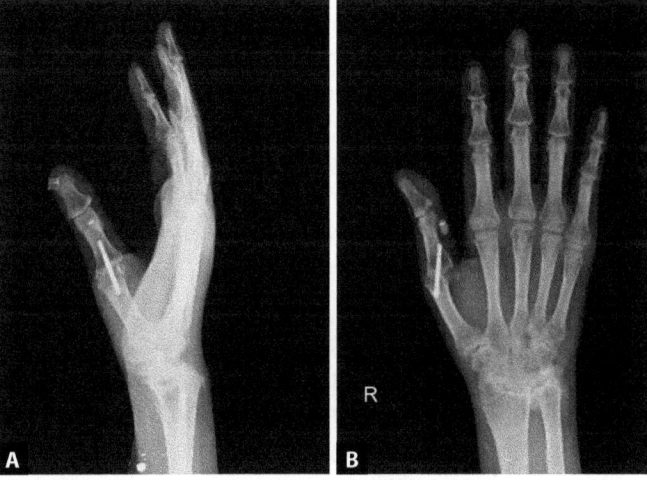

Figs. 7A and B: Digital metacarpophalangeal joint (MCPJ) arthroplasty with arthrodesis of the thumb MCPJ using headless screw.

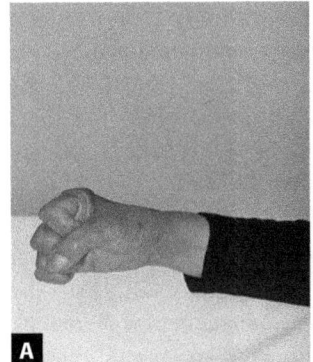 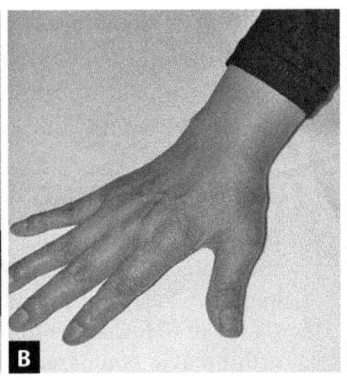 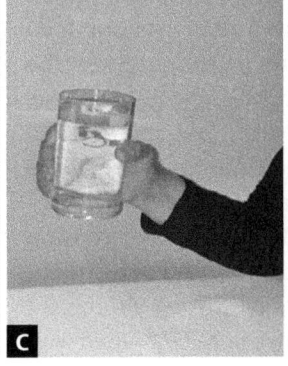 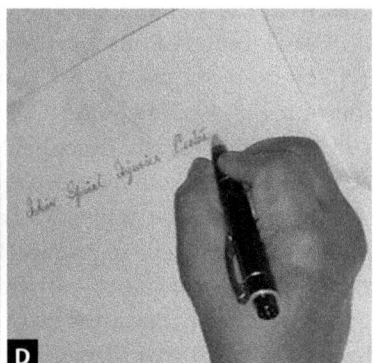

Figs. 8A to D: Hand function 4 months postoperatively.

Synovitis of the PIPJ can lead to attenuation of the central extensor slip and the lateral bands fall volarward thereby acting as the flexors of the PIPJ and extensors of the distal interphalangeal joint (DIPJ). Synovectomy may help in early stages and is performed through a curved dorsal or lateral incision. Early and differential motion is advised. Soft tissue reconstruction procedures such as tightening of the lax central slip and dorsal mobilization of the lateral bands of the extensor expansion can be performed. In advanced cases with damaged articular cartilage, PIPJ fusion or arthroplasty is performed. Author prefers arthrodesis as it provides a stable and pain-free joint. Through a dorsal curved approach the joint is fused in a functional position using a headless compression screw or K wires. 6 weeks of splintage is advised. The MCPJ and DIPJ are mobilized early.

The management of flexible swan neck deformities is directed towards treating the joint responsible for the deformity. In MCPJ pathology, the apparent swan neck deformity corrects after the correction of MCPJ deformity. At the level of PIPJ, flexor digitorum superficialis (FDS) tenodesis is the simple procedure of author's choice. Through a zig-zag incision over the proximal phalanx, a slip of FDS (attached distally) is harvested and stitched onto itself after passing through a slit in A2 pulley. Stitching onto the A1 pulley is also described. Other procedures such as mobilization of the lateral bands and Littler oblique retinacular ligament reconstruction are also useful. In advanced stages, arthrodesis or arthroplasty are the reconstructive procedures of choice.

The preferred surgical treatment for painful arthritic DIPJ is fusion. This can be performed through T-shaped dorsal incision and fixation with K wires or headless screw. 6 weeks of protective splintage is advised.

Thumb

Boutonniere deformity is the most common deformity of the thumb in RA presenting with MCPJ flexion and interphalangeal joint (IPJ) hyperextension. If the deformity is flexible with no arthritis, reconstruction of the extensor apparatus with synovectomy is the procedure of choice. In severe deformity, MCPJ fusion works best if the carpometacarpal joint (CMCJ) and DIPJ are flexible. In many cases, both CMCJ and MCPJ are involved. Author has obtained satisfactory outcome by excision arthroplasty of the trapezium with fusion of the MCPJ using a headless screw. MCPJ arthroplasty is also described.

Swan neck deformity, the second common deformity is due to hyperextension at the MCPJ and flexion at IPJ. CMCJ pathology leads to this deformity. In early stages excision arthroplasty of the trapezium with or without ligament reconstruction is the author's procedure of choice. In advanced stages, the above procedure can be combined with MCPJ fusion **(Figs. 7A and B)**.

Radial deviation of the MCPJ is a result of MCPJ pathology (Gamekeeper's thumb). In early stages, treated by synovectomy and ulnar collateral ligament reconstruction. MCPJ arthrodesis/arthroplasty is reserved for advanced arthritis.

If the IPJ is treated with fusion, surgeon should try and preserve the MCPJ motion.

Tendon Rupture/Transfer

Tendon ruptures are common in RA and occur due to abrasion of the tendon due to friction over an osteophyte/joint, e.g., DRUJ or attrition of the tendon due to synovial invasion. Tendons commonly affected are long extensors, commonly extensor digiti minimi (EDM) and extensor digitorum communis (EDC) to the little finger due to the osteophytes of distal ulna (Vaughan-Jackson syndrome). The EDC to ring finger may follow. Most of these ruptures are detected late and tendons are weakened therefore direct repair is not possible. Extensor indicis proprius (EIP) transfer is the procedure of choice. FDS of ring finger can also be used.

Flexor pollicis longus (FPL) tendon is prone to rupture due to friction over the eroded scaphoid (Mannerfelt syndrome). Repair using a tendon graft or transfer using brachioradialis or FDS of index finger is performed.

Considering the complexity of deformities and multiple joints and soft tissues involved in patients with RA, it is needless to say that good preoperative assessment with consideration of patients' needs can help the surgeon to plan appropriate surgery and achieve desired outcomes.

■ KEY POINTS

- Surgical management is offered in any of following conditions which do not respond to optimal nonsurgical management.
- Persistent pain due to joint damage and progressive deformity are common indications for surgery in RA.
- Synovectomy, arthrodesis, arthroplasties and osteotomies are common surgical procedures performed in joints affected with RA.
- DRUJ disease can be dealt with either Darrach's procedure (excision of distal ulna) or Sauvé–Kapandji procedure (fusion of the DRUJ with distal ulnar osteotomy.)
- Tendon transfer surgeries are also done in surgical management of RA.

■ FURTHER READING

1. Borisch N, Haussmann P. Radiolunate arthrodesis in the rheumatoid wrist: a retrospective clinical and radiological long-term follow-up. J Hand Surg Br. 2002;27:61-72.
2. Cavaliere CM, Chung KC. A systematic review of total wrist arthroplasty compared with total wrist arthrodesis for rheumatoid arthritis. Plast Reconstr Surg. 2008;122:813-25.

3. Chung KC, Burns PB, Kim HM, Burke FD, Wilgis EF, Fox DA. Long-term follow up for rheumatoid arthritis patients in a multicenter outcomes study of silicone metacarpophalangeal joint arthroplasty. Arthritis Care Res (Hoboken). 2012;64(9): 1292-300.
4. Chung KC, Pushman AG. Current concepts in the management of the rheumatoid hand. J Hand Surg Am. 2011;36(4):736-47.
5. Coester LM, Saltzman CL, Leupold J, Pontarelli W. Long term results following ankle arthrodesis for post traumatic arthritis. J Bone Surg Am. 2001;83A(2):219-28.
6. De Smet L. The distal radioulnar joint in rheumatoid arthritis. Acta Orthop Belg. 2006;72(4):381-6.
7. Feldon P, Terrono AL, Nalebuff EA, Millender LH. Rheumatoid Arthritis and Other Connective Tissue Diseases. In: Green DP, Hotchkiss RN, Pederson WC, Wolfe SW (Eds). Operative Hand Surgery, 3rd edition. New York: Elsevier; 2017. pp. 2049-136.
8. Hintermann B, Nigg BM. Influence of arthrodesis on kinematics of the axially loaded ankle complex during dorsiflexion/plantarflexion. Foot Ankle Int. 1995;16(10): 633-6.
9. Kozlow JH, Chung KC. Current concepts in the surgical management of rheumatoid and osteoarthritic hands and wrists. Hand Clin. 2011;27(1):31-41.
10. Pieringer H, Stuby U, Biesenbach G. Patients with rheumatoid arthritis undergoing surgery: how should we deal with antirheumatic treatment? Semin Arthritis Rheum. 2007;36:278-86.
11. Potter TA, Kuhns JG. Rheumatoid tenosynovitis. J Bone Joint Surg. 1958; 40A:1230.
12. Swanson AB. Flexible implant arthroplasty for arthritic finger joints: rationale, technique and results of treatment. J Bone Joint Surg. 1972;54(03);435-544.
13. Thompson JS, Littler JW, Upton J. The spiral oblique retinacular ligament (SORL). J Hand Surg Am. 1978;3:482-7.

11. Challenges in Arthroplasty in Rheumatoid Arthritis

Jitendra Chowdhary

INTRODUCTION

Knee replacement surgery one of the most successful surgeries. In rheumatoid arthritis, the scenario changes with issues of medications, systemic involvement and bone deformities, defects, and porosis. The percentage of knee replacement in rheumatoid arthritis has come drastically down in all registry data due to awareness of the disease, early start of medication, better drugs and good patient compliance. We need to be aware of the possible early and late complications in these patients to get good results and better long-term survival. The data shows if principles are followed and with better perioperative management the results are promising.

CHALLENGES

- Knee
- Comorbidities and other joint involvement
- Disease-modifying antirheumatic drugs (DMARDs) and biologics.

Challenges in Knee

- Bone deformities ranges from valgus, fixed flexion, rotational and combination
- *Bone defects*: Contained with surrounding shell of bone and uncontained
- *Osteoporosis*: Varied amount of porosis in the same femur with hard and soft on femur and tibia
- *Synovitis*: Simple villi to gross synovial thickening
- Cartilage issues pertaining patella.

Other Joint Involvement

Small joints of hand involvement, shoulder, elbow, and hip should be clearly analyzed as postoperative ambulation for first few weeks will be with support.

Associated diabetes and hypertension should be well in control for good post-recovery and wound healing.

Medication

DMARDs: There has a lot of literature supporting in earlier days for stopping of drugs and contrary too, for reasons of flare up of disease.

The American Academy providing guidelines for the medications to continue and stop before surgery according to their half-life to avoid wound complications and disease flare up **(Table 1)**.

SURGERY

Preoperative Assessment

- Physician to look after respiratory system and cardiovascular system
- Anesthetist to preoperative assessment to see for spinal issues and decide spinal or general anesthesia and anticipate the problems of spine deformity in giving spinal anesthesia or intubation (cervical spine) in general anesthesia
- Hemoglobin to build up before surgery by giving hematinics and delaying surgery till patient hemoglobin percent is above 11 g

TABLE 1: Preoperative advice for medication.

Medication	Comments
NSAIDs	Discontinue 5 half-lives before surgery. Aspirin should be stopped 7–10 days before surgery
Corticosteroids	Individualized based on the magnitude of surgery and the severity of patient's illness
Methotrexate	Continue perioperatively for all procedures. Consider withholding 1–2 doses for patients with poorly controlled diabetes; the elderly; and patients with liver, renal, or lung disease
Leflunomide	Withhold 1–2 days before surgery and restart 1–2 weeks later or withhold 2 weeks before surgery and restart 3 days later
Sulfasalazine	Withhold 1 day before surgery and restart 3 days later
Hydroxychloroquine	Continue for all procedures
TNF antagonist	Withhold etanercept for 1 week, and plan surgery for the end of the dosing interval for adalumimab and infliximab. Restart 10–14 days postoperatively
IL-1 antagonist	Withhold 1–2 days before surgery and restart 10 days postoperatively

(NSAIDs: nonsteroidal anti-inflammatory drugs; TNF: tumor necrosis factor; IL-1: interleukin-1)

- C-reactive protein (CRP) values are going to be high, there is no literature supporting cut-off value of CRP to be fit for surgery.

Operative Planning (Figs. 1 to 5)

- Assessment of knee deformities
- Knee range of motion (ROM), deformities, osteoporosis, and ligament laxity is noted
- Knee ROM if less accordingly patient positioning is decided and care is taken for patella tendon avulsion by putting a pin on the tendon
- Valgus knee lateral condyle defect is seen, then it is usually more medial side of tibia is cut contrary to osteoarthritis
- Or femoral posterolateral condyle may be defective, care is taken to check epicondylar line and then decide external rotation of femur on that
- *Fixed flexion deformity*: It is better to do standard cuts than posterior capsule release. If still fixed flexion deformity, the additional 2 mm of femoral distal cut can be planned. The limit of distal cut is attachments of the collaterals on epicondyle
- Ligaments after surgery has to be aligned and be on the tighter side contrary to osteoarthritis as ligaments tend to stretch out
- Patella if diseased and thickness above 24 mm then replacement is advised. Be cautious on soft patella and fracturing or crushing patella
- Synovium has to be excised precisely and postoperative drains are the must after synovectomy.

Bone Defects (Figs. 6 and 7)

- Contained bone defects are managed with bone grafting and extension rods in implants

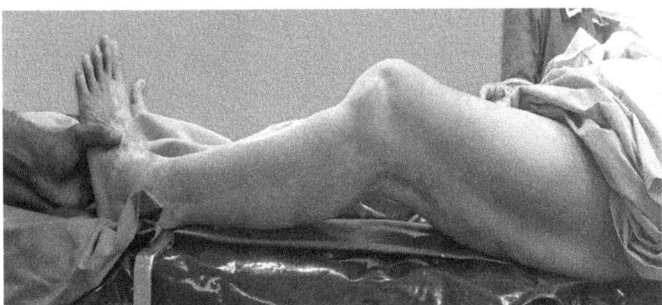

Fig. 1: Fixed flexion deformity of knee.

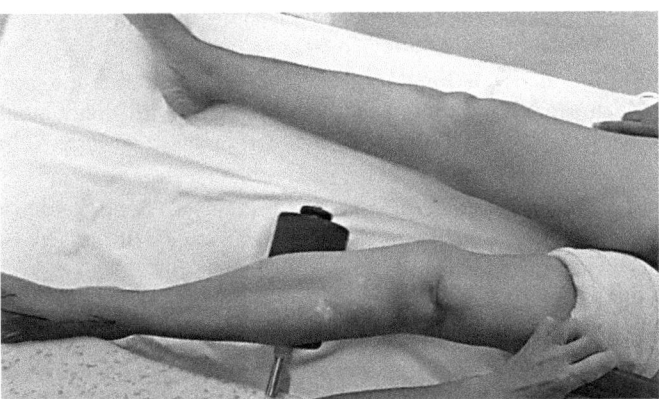

Fig. 2: Genu valgum left knee.

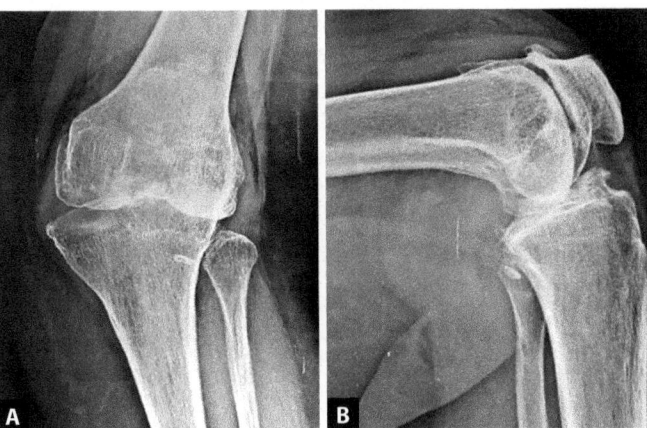

Figs. 3A and B: Valgus knee. Osteoporosis ranges from mild to severe and differential meaning soft one condyle and hard other condyle.

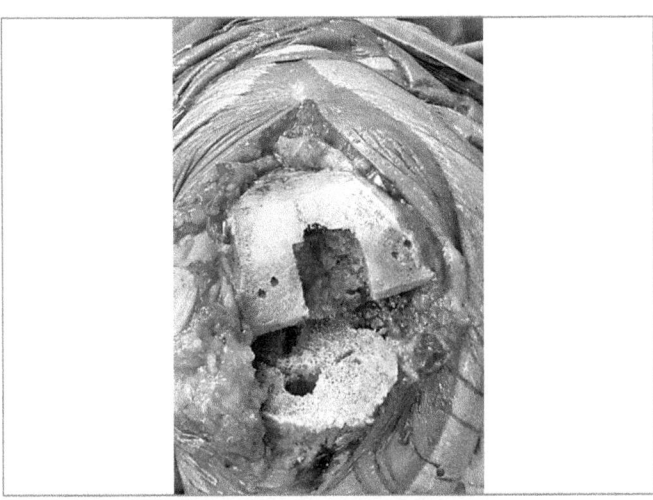

Fig. 4: Femoral condyle split while introducing intramedullary guide.

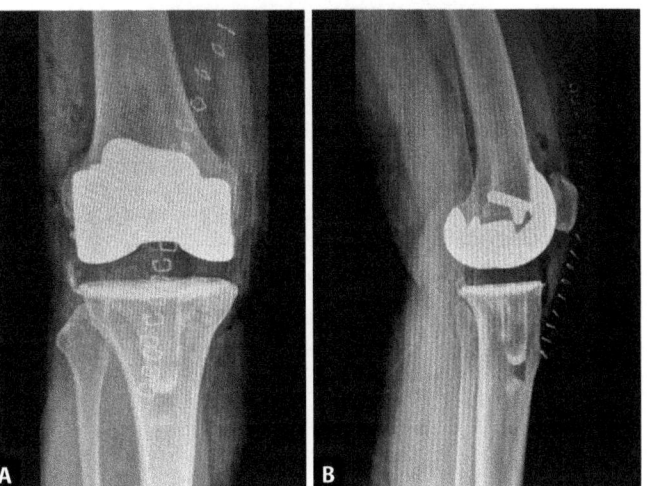

Figs. 5A and B: Femoral condyle split fracture managed with cross screw.

- Cautions about intraoperative fractures which needs fixation. So necessary armamentarium should be ready
- Bilateral total knee replacement remains debatable (with the thought on gross deformities where both knee can be planned or patient has to wait till both knee deformities are corrected).

Postoperative Protocol

- Proper wound care for soft skin
- Drains removed after 24–48 hours
- The degree of osteoporosis will decide weight bearing with support
- Postoperative medication including routine drugs we can start on DMARDs after 2 weeks

FURTHER READING

1. Chmell MJ, Scott RD. Total knee arthroplasty in patients with rheumatoid arthritis. An overview. Clin Orthop Relat Res. 1999;365:54-60.
2. da Silva E, Doran MF, Crowson CS, O'Fallon WM, Matteson EL. Declining use of orthopedic surgery in patients with rheumatoid arthritis? Results of a long-term, population-based assessment. Arthritis Rheum. 2003;49:216-20.
3. Dalury DF, Ewald FC, Christie MJ, Scott RD. Total knee arthroplasty in a group of patients less than 45 years of age. J Arthroplasty. 1995;10:598-602.
4. Grennan DM, Gray J, Loudon, J, Fear S. Methotrexate and early postoperative complications in patients with rheumatoid arthritis undergoing elective orthopaedic surgery. Ann Rheum Dis. 2001;60:214-7.
5. Kristensen O, Nafei A, Kjaersgaard-Andersen P, Hvid I, Jensen J. Long-term results of total condylar knee arthroplasty in rheumatoid arthritis. J Bone Joint Surg Br. 1992;74:803-6.
6. Lee JK, Choi CH. Knee. Surg Relat Res. 2012;24(1):1-6.
7. Poss R, Thornhill TS, Ewald FC, Thomas WH, Batte NJ, Sledge CB. Factors influencing the incidence and outcome of infection following total joint arthroplasty. Clin Orthop Relat Res. 1984;182:117-26.
8. Rodriguez JA, Saddler S, Edelman S, Ranawat CS. Long-term results of total knee arthroplasty in class 3 and 4 rheumatoid arthritis. J Arthroplasty. 1996;11:141-5.
9. Saag KG, Teng GG, Patkar NM, Anuntiyo J, Finney C, Curtis JR, et al. American College of Rheumatology 2008 recommendations for the use of nonbiologic and biologic disease-modifying antirheumatic drugs in rheumatoid arthritis. Arthritis Rheum. 2008;59:762-84.

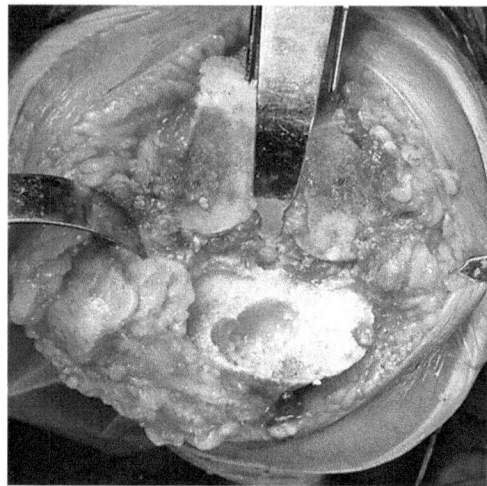

Fig. 6: Tibial defect.

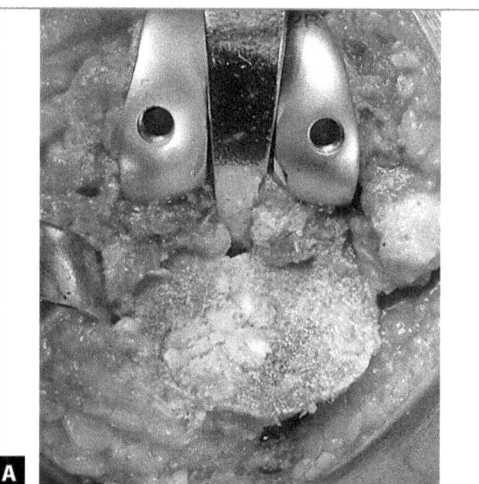

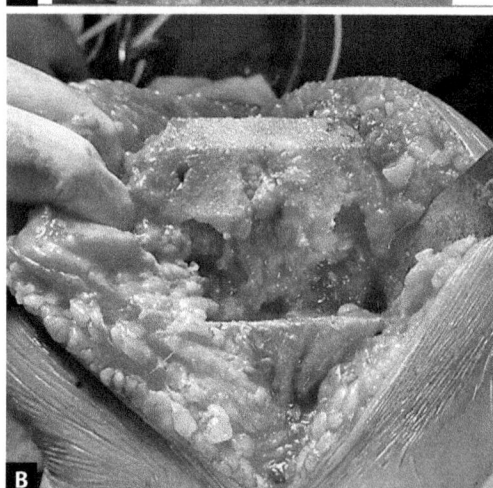

Figs. 7A and B: Femoral posterior condyle defects.

12. Skin Manifestations in Orthorheumatology

Sunil Kumar Gupta

INTRODUCTION

The skin is the largest body organ. Every system of the body if diseased, directly or indirectly manifest on skin. Orthopedic is one of the important in them. Most of patients suffering from dermatologic condition are associated with orthorheumatic problem too or vice versa. For example, ganglion cysts, which are encountered by the orthopedics and dermatologists both but its pathologies such as leprosy and carpal tunnel syndrome are missed by both. At the same time, pathologies such as notalgia paresthetica and brachioradial pruritus are not well characterized and are seldom described; more seldom still in routine dermatologic practice. These disorders often necessitate prompt recognition in order to properly refer for definitive treatment as well as to avoid unnecessary diagnostic procedures. The aim of this chapter is to identify dermatologic diseases with orthopedic presentations and discuss the diagnosis and treatment of these pathologies.

CUTANEOUS MANIFESTATIONS OF ORTHOPEDIC DISORDERS

Localized Itch

Notalgia Paresthetica

It is also known as subscapular pruritus and classified as a chronic sensory neuropathy. It is more common in middle aged women. It is clinically present with a chronic itch, sometimes accompanied by burning pain, numbness, and hyperesthesia in the T2-T6 region on the back and is thought to be secondary to the compression of the posterior rami of the T2-T6 nerve roots. Degenerative cervical spine disease as commonly seen in Pott's spine has also been implicated in notalgia paresthetica of corresponding dermatomes. A subscapular hyperpigmented patch overlying the affected area, thought to be secondary to the scratching of the affected pruritic area can be appreciated on examination **(Fig. 1)**. Most important therapy is the management of basic etiology. Other treatment modalities include transcutaneous electrical nerve stimulation, topical capsaicin, gabapentin, oxcarbamazepine, local anesthetic nerve block, botulinum toxin, narrow-band UVB, and nerve decompression.

Brachioradial Pruritus

Brachioradial pruritus generally present with chronic itch over the dorsolateral part of the upper arm or sometimes the lateral aspect of the proximal forearm. It occurs at any age with either sex or more common on tropics where ultraviolet (UV) radiations are more. The most important orthopedic cause is cervical spinal disease involving the compression of the C5-C8 cervical nerve roots besides UV radiation damage. Cervical disk herniation and cervical radiculopathy, confirmed by imaging, are important pathology. Medical managements include simple ice cube application in acute cases with topical capsaicin, oral gabapentin, carbamazepine and nonsteroidal anti-inflammatory drugs. Orthopedic management includes cervical spine manipulation and ventral cage fusion with cage implantation.

Cutaneous Rash

Implant-induced Contact Dermatitis

Foussereau and Laugier in 1966 first described the allergic contact dermatitis to metallic orthopedic implants. It is clinically present with erythematous pruritic papules and plaques at implanted area or as generalized maculopapular

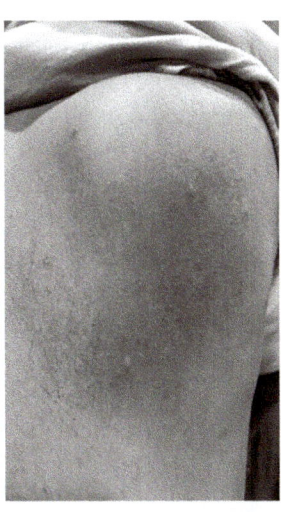

Fig. 1: Notalgia paresthetica, showing hyperpigmented patch over interscapular region due to scratching.

rash with itching. The cell-mediated response to released metal ions has been demonstrated in relation to nickel, cobalt, chromium, tantalum, titanium, and vanadium, with nickel being most commonly implicated. Metal implantation allergy is highly unpredictable due to variable reaction of metal into the body. Recently, the incidence of knee-replacement dermatitidis has been steadily decreasing, likely secondary to the decreased use of metal-on metal and increased use of metal-on-plastic prostheses. Options for metal allergy testing include patch testing, intradermal testing, lymphocyte transformation testing, leukocyte migration inhibitor testing. Leukocyte migration test is the most sensitive test for orthopedic implants. Recently preoperatively surgically imbedded subcutaneous metal implantation sensitivity test was reported (done preoperatively to assess sensitivity). A careful history of past surgeries and verification of the material component of the implanted prostheses remains an integral part of a workup of dermatitis of unknown origin.

Subcutaneous Cyst

Ganglion

It is the most common soft tissue mass of hands and sometimes feet. It is more common in female than male at the age of third to fifth decade. The presentation is one of soft, rubbery, compressible, transilluminating subcutaneous nodules, most commonly found on the dorsal aspect of the wrist, with attachment to underlying tissue. Ganglions are mostly asymptomatic but sometimes present pain if present at wrist joint due to frequent movement. The etiology of ganglion cysts is not well-understood, with herniation or leakage of synovial tissue and fluid leading to irritation and formation of a pseudocapsule as possible explanations. The common causes of ganglions are trauma, carpal tunnel syndrome, rheumatoid arthritis (RA), and leprosy. It is very common in tennis players. Reports of multiple ganglion cysts appearing at multiple sites has led to a proposed genetic susceptibility to the development of this condition. Basic diagnostic tool for ganglion is ultrasound but gold standard test is MRI with high signal intensity T2-weighted images. Aspiration of the cyst yielding gelatinous material is diagnostically confirmatory. As most cysts are asymptomatic, and have been shown to resolve spontaneously in 50% of cases, intervention is often not necessary. If ganglion is painful and hinders the daily activity then active management is indicated. Treatments include intralesional steroid injection, sclerotherapy and orthoscopic resection.

Baker's Cyst

It is a common complication of arthritic degenerated knee joint such as osteoarthritis of the knee, rheumatologic diseases affecting the knee (RA, SLE), and systemic conditions such as hypothyroidism and sarcoidosis. Baker's cysts are true cysts and are lined with synovium.

Patients with Baker's cysts present with a fluctuant popliteal mass or swelling, which is often painful and exacerbated by activity. Extension of the knee worsens symptoms, a phenomenon explained by the valve-like mechanism in the communicating tract between the cyst and joint space, trapping the fluid in the cyst space. Alteration of cyst size with flexion and extension, known as Foucher sign, is a pathognomonic finding. Ultrasonography is the choice of diagnostic tool. Treatments include aspiration and surgical resection. Serious complications occur if not treated and that include partial occlusion of the popliteal artery leading to lower leg ischemia and lower leg and ankle swelling from vein compression by a dissecting or enlarging cyst mimicking deep vein thrombosis. Rupture of popliteal cysts is also problematic with reports of posterior tibial nerve entrapment and resulting pain and hypoesthesia. Posterior and anterior compartment syndromes are also reported.

Subcutaneous Nodules

Subungual Exostosis

It was first described by Dupuytren in 1817. It is not uncommon nowadays due to increase reporting. Though subungual exostosis occurs on the digits of both the upper and lower extremities, the pathology is more commonly observed on the foot, especially the hallux. The lesion presents as a firm, raised, and painful solitary nodule. The most common site is the lateral and anterior nail fold, near the free edge of the nail with a pathognomonic loosened raised nail plate often present. It affects people in the second and third decades of life, though 16% of the cases are in the pediatric population. The exact etiology is not known but consider as benign osteocartilaginous tumor secondary to microtrauma. The common differentials are subungual verruca, granuloma pyogenicum, glomus tumor, melanotic whitlow, enchondroma, and chondrosarcoma. Diagnosis is best established via radiographic imaging; that reveals a terminal calcifying projection and the cortex and medulla of the outgrowth are continuous with the parent bone. Surgical excision is the choice of treatment.

Digital Fibromatosis

Digital fibromatosis is a spectrum of disorders that presents as red/pink subcutaneous nodules measuring up to 2 cm in size. Attached to underlying tissues, these lesions usually appear on the extensor surfaces of the fingers and toes, sparing the thumb and big toe. It is quite common in children that are why also known as infantile digital fibromatosis. Infantile myofibromatosis, a histologic subtype, occurs 80% of the time before the age of 2 years and may present with lesions in the bone and viscera.

Palmoplantar Fibromatosis

Palmar fibromatosis is known as Dupuytren's contracture while plantar fibromatosis is known as Ledderhose disease. It is clinically present as asymptomatic volar nodules **(Fig. 2)**. It is secondary to a proliferation and accumulation of differentiated fibroblasts, fibrocytes, and myofibroblasts that leads to the deposition of abnormal fibrous tissue in the fascial layers. It is genetically inherited and common in Caucasians. It is commonly seen after 60 years of age. Diabetes mellitus, alcoholic liver disease, tobacco use, and long-term use of anticonvulsants can precipitate palmoplantar fibromatosis. Treatment modalities are calcium channel blockers and intralesional injection of triamcinolone, Botox toxin, collagenase and imiquimod with variable results. Radiation therapy has proven to cure or even relieve the symptoms of palmoplantar fibromatosis.

Piezogenic Pedal Papules

Piezogenic pedal papules are very common in general population. Patient is typically presents with multiple papules or small subcutaneous nodules on foot which appear when weight is applied on the foot and disappear when the foot does not bear weight. This occurs due to connective tissue weakness. Diagnosis is made with the help of characteristic clinical findings with aid of ultrasonography. Treatment is conservative in most cases, with surgical intervention sometimes undertaken for painful lesions or with cosmetic therapeutic goals. In cases of painful papules, pain control techniques such as electroacupuncture have been found to be effective.

Tibialis Anterior Muscle Herniation

Tibialis anterior muscle herniation is not very uncommon. It occurs due to defect in the fascial layer near the anterior tibialis muscle. It is clinically present as asymptomatic, soft, skin colored nodules that are compressible on palpation. With muscle contraction, the subcutaneous nodules generally retract or become invisible, but sometimes increase in size. A biopsy may be necessary to differentiate the herniation from lipomas, leiomyomas, schwannomas, dermatofibromas and even histoid leprosy although, unlike muscle herniations, these lesions do not have positional variability. Diagnosis is confirmed with the help of dynamic ultrasonography. Tibialis anterior muscle herniation is treated surgically but it should be avoid in asymptomatic condition as surgery may lead to compartment syndrome.

CUTANEOUS MANIFESTATIONS OF AUTOIMMUNE RHEUMATIC DISORDERS

Systemic Lupus Erythematosus

Systemic lupus erythematosus (SLE) includes specific and nonspecific cutaneous features with multisystem involvement. Specific cutaneous features include malar rash, discoid rash and photosensitivity while nonspecific skin lesions such as vasculitis or vasculopathic changes and a myriad other skin lesions may also occur in these diseases. Discoid rash of SLE typically present with asymptomatic, erythematous, indurated scaly plaques with lilac color border. Center of the lesion is atrophied and covered with a scale which when remove shows minute tacks on the undersurface (Carpet tack sign). Malar rash is a butterfly shaped erythema covering the malar area of the face and bridge of the nose **(Fig. 3)**. It has waxing and waning course and leave hyperpigmentation when resolve mimicking melasma. Nonspecific skin lesions in SLE are noncicatricial diffuse alopecia, recurrent oral ulceration, telangiectasia and purpura.

In SLE, arthralgia is more frequent than arthritis and arthritis is classically described as nonerosive, involving mainly the wrists, knees, shoulders, and hands. However, 5%

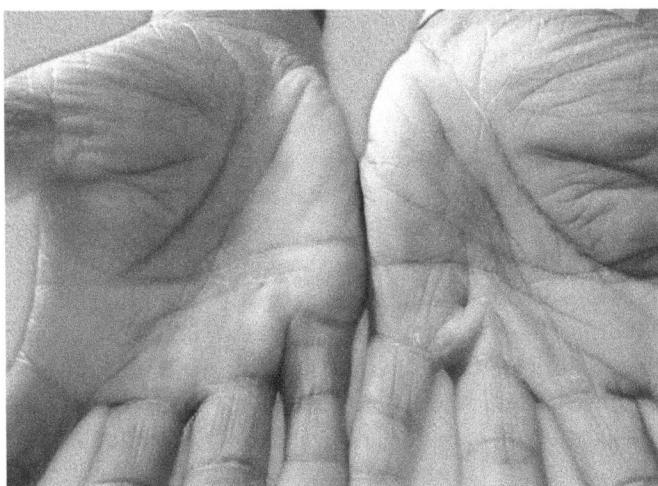

Fig. 2: Dupuytren's contracture showing volar nodules due to palmar fibromatosis.

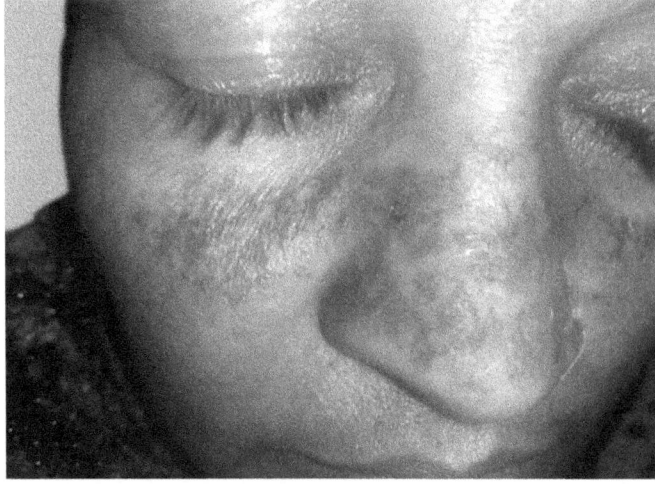

Fig. 3: Malar rash of systemic lupus erythematosus (SLE).

cases of SLE may be associated with a correctable nonerosive deformity of the hand joints known as *Jaccoud arthritis*. Internal organ involvement should be specifically examined, both from a diagnostic and therapeutic point of view. Serological tests are often required to confirm or rule out the diagnosis. Diagnosis is made by American Association of Rheumatology (ARA) criteria and lupus specific blood investigations. Treatments are basically sun protection and immunosuppressives including high dose of oral steroid, hydroxychloroquine, methotrexate, azathioprine and mycophenolate mofetil.

Systemic Sclerosis

Systemic sclerosis (SSc) is multisystem disorder involve skin, renal, lung, gastrointestinal (GI) tract, heart, and joints. It is classified in diffuse cutaneous systemic sclerosis (dSSc) and limited cutaneous systemic sclerosis (lSSc). Skin become sclerosed with matt-like telangiectasia on face and salt and pepper such as pigmentary changes are seen **(Fig. 4)**. Sclerotic changes are more marked in dSSc. Facial skin sclerosis with loss of furrows gives the appearance of "mask like facies". The lower eyelid cannot be retracted. Perioral rhagades give rise to purse string appearance to the mouth.

Fingers and toes become shiny, atrophic and semiflexed with thinning of overlying skin due to sclerodactyly. Peripheral vasculopathy results into stellate scarring at the tip of fingers.

CREST syndrome is a part of lSSc characterized by *Calcinosis, Raynaud's phenomenon, Esophageal dysmotility, Sclerodactyly* and *Telangiectasia*. It has better prognosis.

There is an erosive arthropathy, with "pestle and mortar" deformity of the distal interphalangeal joints. Osteopoikilosis, and osteolysis both are reported in systemic sclerosis.

Diagnosis of SSc is made with the help of typical clinical features and detection of specific antibody tests. Treatment is generally supportive to improve quality-of-life.

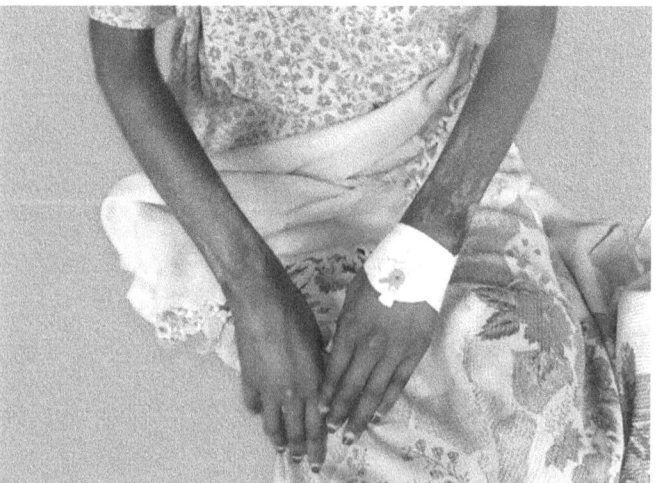

Fig. 4: Systemic sclerosis showing paper-and-salt pigmentation with sclerodactyly.

Vasodilators, viz. calcium channel blockers and xanthinol nicotinate are used to prevent Raynaud's phenomenon. D-Penicillamine is used as antisclerotic agent but its role is controversial. Physiotherapy is advised from beginning to avoid contracture.

Rheumatoid Arthritis

It is one of the most common conditions presenting with both the cutaneous and articular involvement. RA is a systemic inflammatory disorder which has an insidious onset and has significant extra-articular manifestations. RA clinically present with joint effusion, pain, erythema, and stiffness. Joint stiffness and pain is aggravated in the morning or after long inactivity. There is bilateral symmetrical involvement of small joints of hands and feet preferentially the wrist, ankle and proximal interphalangeal joints and sparing the distal interphalangeal joints which differentiate it from psoriatic arthritis (PsA). Axial skeleton is also involved but sparing the lumbar region that differentiates RA from other arthritis. Synovitis can lead to tethering of tissue with loss of movement and erosion of the joint surface. Some of the specific hand deformities include ulnar deviation, swan neck deformity, boutonniere deformity, and Z-thumb deformity and notably, these are fixed deformities.

In RA skin becomes atrophic with easy bruisability and nails may become brittle with multiple longitudinal ridging. Specific cutaneous lesions in RA are rheumatoid nodules, accelerated nodulosis, interstitial granulomatous disease, neutrophilic dermatosis in the form of pyoderma gangrenosum and cutaneous vasculitis.

Rheumatoid nodules are the most common extra-articular manifestations of RA and are seen in approximately 25% of the patients with RA. They appear as solitary or multiple skin-colored nodules ranging in size from a few millimeters to several centimeters and are usually situated on areas of repetitive trauma such as the olecranon, extensor forearms, occiput, fingers, and heel. They are typically situated within the deep subcutaneous tissue, and rarely, they may also involve the internal organs.

Accelerated rheumatoid nodulosis occur in patients on long-term treatment with methotrexate. It is more common in males and may be seen in patients with no pretreatment history of rheumatoid nodules. The lesions are more commonly found on the hands, especially on the metacarpophalangeal and proximal interphalangeal joints.

Interstitial granulomatous dermatitis is an uncommon condition, seen in middle-aged women with severe RA and rheumatoid factor positivity. Clinically, the lesions present symmetrically on the axilla, trunk, and inner portions of the thighs as erythematous to violaceous papules, nodules, and plaques, which may be tender or associated with a burning sensation. Erythematous to violaceous indurated linear cords (the rope sign) are characteristic.

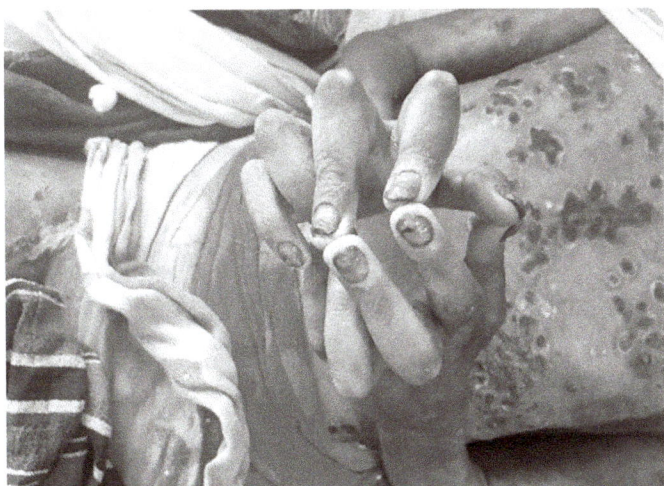

Fig. 5: Rheumatoid arthritis with pyoderma gangrenosum.

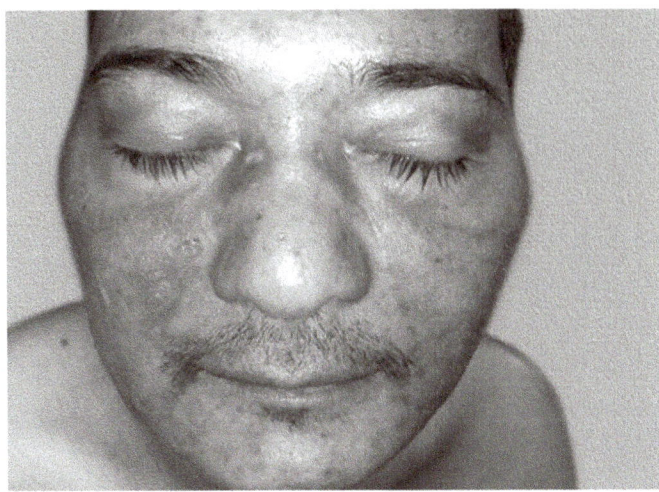

Fig. 6: Heliotrope rash of dermatomyositis.

Ulcerative type of pyoderma gangrenosum (Fig. 5) is the most common neutrophilic dermatosis associated with RA and clinically present with painful cribriform ulcer with bluish margin on the trauma prone site of the body and heal with scar formation.

Skin manifestations are the common presenting features of rheumatoid vasculitis and include petechiae, palpable purpura, digital infarcts, ulcer and peripheral gangrene. It may cause acute, painful, punched-out leg ulcers to appear along the lateral malleolus or the pretibial region.

Dermatomyositis

A multisystem disorder mainly affecting skin, muscle and blood vessels in which characteristic erythematous and edematous changes in the skin are usually associated with muscle weakness and inflammation. The characteristic cutaneous findings in dermatomyositis are facial erythema, heliotrope rash and Gottron's papules. Erythema is present on face which is not photosensitive. Heliotrope rash is characterized by purple erythematous, edema of upper and lower eye lids (Fig. 6). Purplish erythema is also present on neck, shoulders, and upper back known as Shawl sign. Accentuation of erythema on interphalangeal joints is known as Gottron's sign. Multiple violaceous papules are present on the interphalangeal and elbow joints which are slightly itchy (Gottron's papules) (Fig. 7).

A mild inflammatory arthritis may occur, but erosive arthritis is rare although a rheumatoid picture can occur. Patients with arthritis frequently have pulmonary involvement.

Diagnosis is confirmed by biopsy. High doses of oral steroids and immunosuppressives are used to manage the condition.

Sjögren's Syndrome

The disease is caused by an immune-mediated inflammation of exocrine glands, and involves salivary, lacrimal and

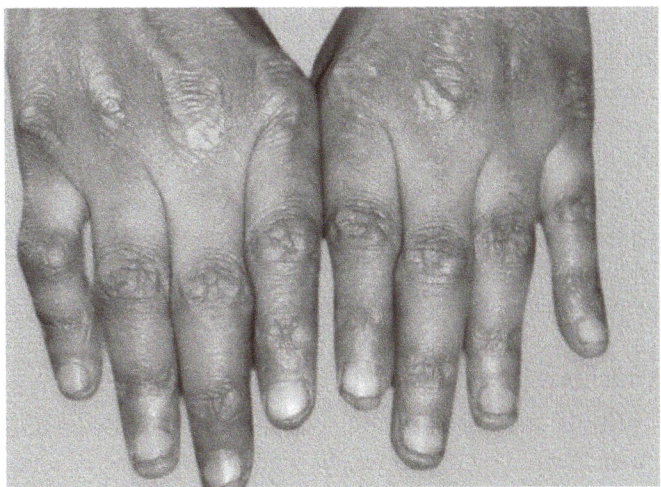

Fig. 7: Gottron's papules in dermatomyositis.

sweat glands. The most common features of the condition are dryness and atrophy of the conjunctiva and cornea (keratoconjunctivitis sicca), and a dry mouth (xerostomia). Annular polycyclic erythematous papulosquamous lesions are characteristic cutaneous findings. Mild articular symptoms occur in 83%, with mild synovitis.

Systemic Vasculitis

The microscopic polyangiitis (MPA), Wegener granulomatosis (WG), and Churg-Strauss syndrome (CSS), polyarteritis nodosa (PAN), Henoch-Schönlein purpura and Behçet's disease are important vasculitis which involve skin and joint both. The typical pattern of joint involvement is migratory and oligoarticular, often involving large joints, but polyarthritis is also observed.

In cases of medium vessel vasculitis (PAN), the skin manifestations that are common include nodules, ulcers, livedo reticularis, and digital infarctions. MPA, WG and CSS present with more diverse skin manifestations with papulonecrotic punched out ulcerations (Fig. 8).

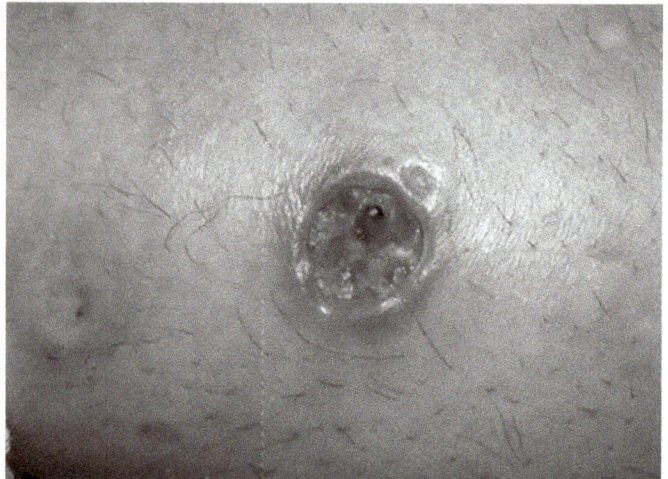

Fig. 8: Typical punched out ulcer of systemic vasculitis.

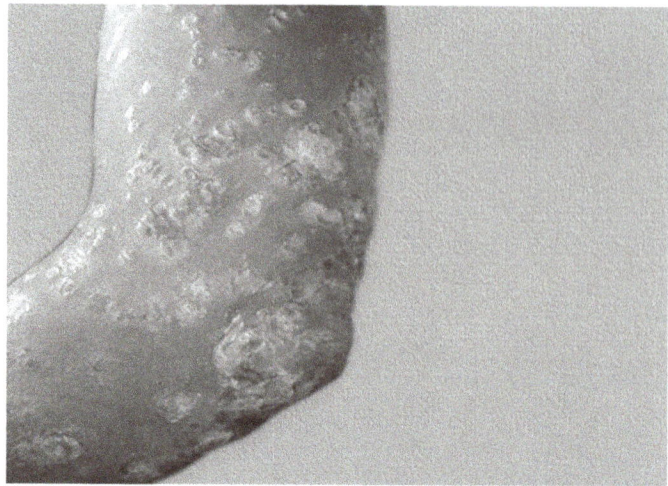

Fig. 9: Typical scaly plaques of psoriasis.

In HSP (now termed IgA vasculitis) joints, kidney and gut also involved with skin. Ankle and knee joints are most commonly involved and the arthritis is usually nondeforming and self-limiting. Cutaneous lesions are palpable purpura on the dependent pat of the body.

Behçet's disease usually presents with recurrent oral aphthous ulceration, genital erosions and uveitis. Skin lesions include papulopustular lesions, pseudofolliculitis, acneiform eruptions, and erythema nodosum-like lesions.

Psoriasis

Psoriasis is a chronic papulosquamous disorder of skin characterized by erythematous plaque covered with silver colored scales and has relapsing and remitting course **(Fig. 9)**. When scales of the lesion is removed with the help of a glass slide it removes such as candle wax (Grattage sign) and after complete removal of the scales, there are pinpoint bleeding on the surface of lesions (Auspitz's sign). Skin lesions precede joint involvement in 70-80% of the cases by approximately 10 years. However, in 15% of the patients, arthritis and psoriasis begin simultaneously, and in an additional 15%, arthritis precedes psoriasis by as long as 15 years. Nail involvement in the form of coarse pits, oil drop spots, and subungual hyperkeratosis are more frequent in psoriatic patients with associated PsA and has been seen in 60-80% of the patients **(Fig. 10)**. Therefore, nail changes in a patient with psoriasis should prompt a search for joint disease.

Psoriatic arthritis is a seronegative (negative rheumatoid factor and negative anti-CCP), predominantly peripheral spondyloarthropathy, which occurs in up to 40% of the patients with moderate to severe psoriasis. The arthropathy in psoriasis is heterogeneous; and according to the Moll and Wright classification, is classified as peripheral mono or asymmetric oligoarthritis, symmetric oligoarthritis mimicking RA, arthritis mutilans, as well as an axial disease predominantly affecting the spine. The symmetrical type

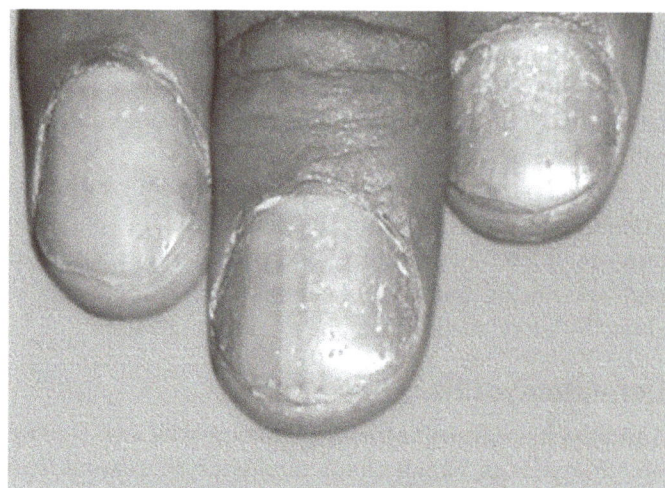

Fig. 10: Coarse pits in psoriatic nails.

is especially difficult to differentiate from RA, however, the distal interphalangeal joint involvement, presence of dactylitis and enthesitis helps to diagnose PsA.

Reiter's Disease

Now it is known as reactive arthritis due to development of inflammatory arthritis after exposure to an infectious agent (usually *Chlamydia*, *Shigella*, *Yersinia*, *Salmonella*, and *Campylobacter* species). It presents usually in a young male, with the symptomatic triad of arthritis, urethritis, and conjunctivitis. An acute onset asymmetrical oligoarthritis, predominantly involving the lower extremities, is the major presenting symptom, often associated with constitutional symptoms such as fever.

Skin and mucocutaneous lesions are commonly observed. Keratoderma blennorhagicum is one of the characteristic findings, which is described as a papulosquamous rash, which begins as clear vesicles on erythematous bases and progresses to papules, and nodules **(Fig. 11)**. These lesions are found on the soles of the feet, palms, trunk, or scalp.

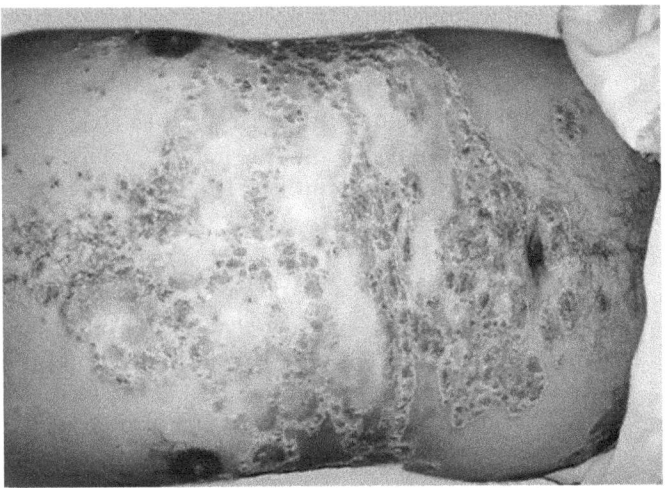

Fig. 11: Keratoderma blennorhagicum, papulosquamous lesions of Reiter's syndrome.

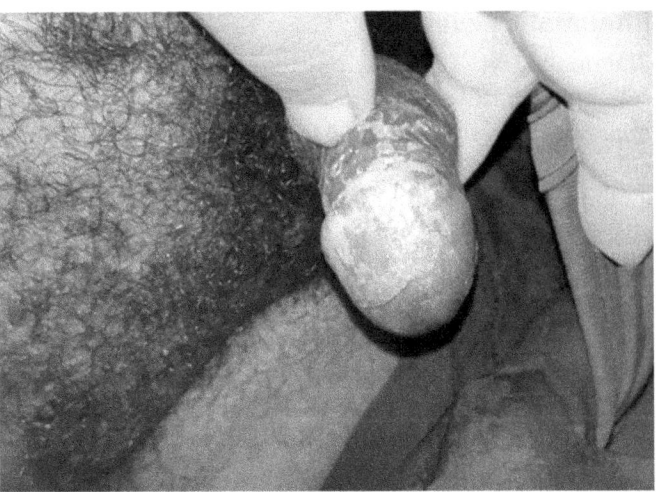

Fig. 12: Circinate balanitis in Reiter's syndrome.

Annular erythematous papulosquamous lesions are also present on glans penis termed as circinate balanitis (Fig. 12).

CUTANEOUS MANIFESTATIONS OF CRYSTAL ARTHROPATHIES

Gout and Pseudogout

Gout is a disease characterized by deposition of monosodium urate crystals in the joints or synovial fluid with or without hyperuricemia, renal insufficiency, or nephrocalcinosis. In acute gouty arthritis, the first metatarsophalangeal joint most commonly (podagra) affected. In chronic tophaceous gout, crystals are found in skin, cartilages, and tendons of various sites. The tophi may be confused with rheumatoid nodules and aspiration or biopsy might prove helpful in differentiating them.

Pseudogout is caused by calcium pyrophosphate crystals and termed calcium pyrophosphate dihydrate crystal deposition (CPPD). The presentation may be diverse and may be asymptomatic; acute crystal arthritis mimicking gout, while chronic crystal inflammatory arthritis mimicking RA. Unlike gout, most common joints affected are the knee and the wrist joints.

ARTHRITIS IN CUTANEOUS INFECTIONS

Leprosy

Leprosy is caused by *Mycobacterium leprae*. The cardinal features of leprosy are hypopigmented or erythematous and anesthetic patch with thickened and tender cutaneous nerve trunk and demonstration of acid fast bacilli (Fig. 13). Leprosy patches are varies in number from single to more than 20 and its size also varies from a tiny papule to a large geographic size and shape. During type 1 reaction in leprosy, all the lesions become erythematous and tender with severe neuritis while in type 2 reaction; crops of erythematous tender subcutaneous nodules appear with high grade fever.

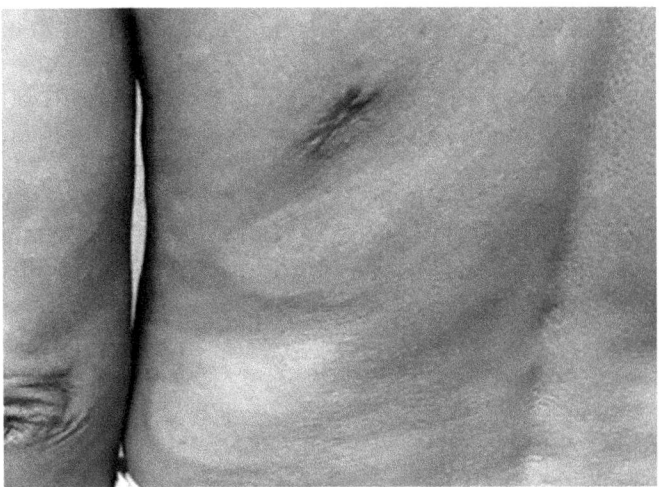

Fig. 13: Hypopigmented anesthetic patches of leprosy.

Leprosy affects joint directly in lepromatous cases where joint effusion occur due to infiltration of synovium by *M. leprae*. In leprosy, arthritis occurs in type 1 and type 2 lepra reaction both. It may also manifest in the form of Charcot's arthropathy or as isolated tenosynovitis or tenosynovitis associated with arthritis or neuropathy.

Lyme Disease

Infection with *B. burgdorferi* results in a multisystem disorder. The cutaneous hallmark of Lyme disease is erythema migrans (EM), a slowly enlarging annular lesion initially starting from the site of the tick bite and later spread to involve the whole body. In the late stage variable sized atrophic papule and plaques developed, known as acrodermatitis chronica atrophicans. Intermittent episodes of arthritis develop during the course of disease and even several weeks or months after the infection, and despite adequate antimicrobial therapy. Sometimes Lyme arthritis can lead to cartilage and bone erosion with permanent joint dysfunction.

Rheumatic Fever

Rheumatic fever generally precipitates after streptococcal sore throat. It is typically present with acute onset of painful migratory polyarthritis in 80% of cases. Commonly knee, ankle, shoulders, and elbow joints are involved. Erythema marginatum is the typical skin lesions in rheumatic fever and characterized by asymptomatic, evanescent, erythematous, semicircular plaques. Erythema marginatum is seen only in 10–25% of cases. Another important skin lesion in rheumatic fever is subcutaneous nodules, which are present on palms, wrist and forearms. Signs of carditis must be looked for at the time of presentation. Sydenham's chorea is rare and even if present is usually a late manifestation.

Sexually Transmitted Infection and HIV/AIDS

Arthralgia and arthritis are present in syphilis, gonorrhea, non-gonococcal urethritis and in HIV/AIDS.

Though syphilis is now rare but joints are involved in both type of syphilis including acquired and congenital. In congenital syphilis, Parrot' syphilitic osteochondritis (in infant) "Clutton's joints" (older children) are the common syphilitic arthritis. Sabre shin is one of the characteristic bone deformities in congenital syphilis with other characteristic lesions such as Hutchinson's teeth, saddle nose and papulovesicular rash. In acquired syphilis, arthritis occur either in synovial or osseous forms in tertiary stage in association with syphilitic gumma.

Gonococcal arthritis may be localized septic arthritis, or as a part of bacteremia, seen in disseminated gonococcal infections. The dermatitis arthritis syndrome seen in bacteremia refers to the triad of maculopapular skin rash, tenosynovitis, and polyarthritis. Non-gonococcal urethritis sometimes complicates with septic arthritis due to mycoplasma or urea-plasma infections.

HIV/AIDS may be associated with joint manifestations in the form of seronegative arthritis, and synovitis. Generalized morbilliform rash is associated with HIV infection.

KEY POINTS

- Dermatology and rheumatology are two specialties that deal with significant overlap. So both specialties should involve in a case of orthorheumatic condition with skin lesions.
- Orthopedic disorders commonly present with localized pruritus (notalgia paresthetica, brachioradial pruritus), rash (implant induced contact dermatitis and neurodermatitis), papules and nodules (Piezogenic pedal papules, Subungual exostosis and Palmoplantar fibromatosis) and cysts (ganglion).
- Autoimmune rheumatological conditions, viz. systemic lupus erythematosus, systemic sclerosis, rheumatoid arthritis, and mixed connective tissue disorders are generally present with features of cutaneous vasculitis such as retiform purport, ecchymosis, punched out ulcers and photo rash.
- Some of the important dermatological conditions such as psoriasis, leprosy with Lepra reaction and Reiter's disease masquerade with arthritis and related disorders.
- Even sexually transmitted disease such as HIV/AIDS, gonorrhea and syphilis involve the bones and joints and presents with arthralgia/arthritis.

FURTHER READING

1. Aggarwal K, Gupta S, Jain VK, et al. Subungual exostosis. Indian J Dermatol Venereol Leprol. 2008;74(2):173-4.
2. Bayat A, Alansar A, Hajeer AH, Shah M, Watson JS, Stanley JK, et al. Genetic susceptibility in Dupuytren's disease: lack of association of a novel transforming growth factor beta(2) polymorphism in Dupuytren's disease. J Hand Surg Br. 2002;27(1):47-9.
3. Binder A, Folster-Holst R, Sahan G, Koroschetz J, Stengel M, Mehdorn HM, et al. A case of neuropathic brachioradial pruritus caused by cervical disc herniation. Nat Clin Pract Neurol. 2008;4(6);338-42.
4. Eisenberg E, Barmeir E, Bergman R. Notalgia paresthetica associated with nerve root impingement. J Am Acad Dermatol. 1997;37(6):998-1000.
5. Gawkrodger DJ. Metal sensitivities and orthopaedic implants revisited: the potential for metal allergy with the new metal-on-metal joint prostheses. Br J Dermatol. 2003; 148(6):1089-93.
6. Goodkin R, Wingard E, Bernhard JD. Brachioradial pruritus; cervical spine disease and neurogenic/neuropathic [corrected] pruritus. J Am Acad Dermatol. 2003;48(4): 521-4.
7. Gupta SK, Singh KK, Lalit M. Comparative therapeutic evaluation of different topicals and narrow band ultraviolet B therapy combined with systemic methotrexate in the treatment of palmoplantar psoriasis. Indian J Dermatol. 2011;56:165-70.
8. Handa S, Dogra S, Prasad R. Metal sensitivity in a patient with a total knee replacement. Contact Dermatitis. 2003; 49(5):259-60.
9. Savk E, Savk O, Bolukbasi O, Culhaci N, Dikicioğlu E, Karaman G, et al. Notalgia paresthetica; a study on pathogenesis. Int J Dermatol. 2000;39(10):754-9.
10. Savk E, Savk SO. On brachioradial pruritus and notalgia paresthetica. J Am Acad Dermatol. 2004;50(5):800-1.
11. Sayah A, English JC 3rd. Rheumatoid arthritis: a review of the cutaneous manifestations. J Am Acad Dermatol. 2005;53:191-209.
12. Shinawi M, Hicks J, Guillerman RP, Jones J, Brandt M, Perez M, et al. Multiple ganglion cysts (cystic ganglionosis): an unusual presentation in a child. Scand J Rheumatol. 2007;36(2):145-8.
13. Thyssen JP, Menn T, Schalock PC, Taylor JS, Maibach HI. Pragmatic approach to the clinical work-up of patients with putative allergic disease to metallic orthopaedic implants before and after surgery. Br J Dermatol. 2011;164(3):473-8.
14. Veien NK, Svejgaard E. Lymphocyte transformation in patients with cobalt dermatitis. Br J Dermatol. 1978;99(2):191-6.
15. Wallengren J. Self-healing photo-neuropathy and cervical spinal arthrosis in four sisters with brachioradial pruritus. J Brachial Plex Peripher Nerve Inj. 2009;4:21-3.
16. Woodrow SL, Brereton-Smith G, Handfield-Jones S. Painful piezogenic pedal papules: response to local electro-acupuncture. Br J Dermatol. 1997;136(4):628-30.
17. Ziff M. The rheumatoid nodule. Arthritis Rheum. 1990;33:761-7.

SECTION 3

Spondyloarthropathies in Orthopedic Rheumatology

- **Ankylosing Spondylitis**
  Manish Khanna, Shantanu Lahkar
- **Surgical Management in Ankylosing Spondylitis**
  Md Neshar Ansari, Rajiv Lakhotia, Abhinandan Reddy M
- **Other Spondyloarthropathies**
  Bhaskar Borgohain, Kashif A Ahmed, Shantanu Lahkar

Ankylosing Spondylitis

Manish Khanna, Shantanu Lahkar

INTRODUCTION

Ankylosing spondylitis (AS) is a form of chronic inflammatory arthritis characterized by sacroiliitis, enthesitis, and a marked propensity for sacroiliac joint and spinal fusion. AS is a condition in the spondyloarthritis (SpA) family of diseases, which share several clinical, genetic, and immunologic features. AS is distinguished in this family by universal involvement with sacroiliac joint inflammation or fusion, and more prevalent spinal ankylosis.

Symptoms of AS start in young age and usually affect men. Patients of AS usually present with severe stiffness in the morning and back pain, which can improve with activity. AS may at times affect peripheral joints. The gene called *HLA B27* increases the risk of developing this condition, however only 2% (1 out of 50) of HLA B27 positive individuals develop AS during their lifetime.

Spondyloarthropathy is the name for a family of chronic inflammatory rheumatic diseases that cause progressive arthritis often predominantly involving the sacroiliac joints and the spinal column. By definition spondyloarthropathy, is a chronic, multisystem inflammatory disorder involving primarily the sacroiliac (SI) joints and the axial skeleton. Because these disorders are not associated with positive rheumatoid factor or other serologic autoantibody abnormalities, they have often been traditionally labeled under the umbrella term "seronegative" spondyloarthropathy.

The most common spondyloarthritis is AS, which affects mainly the spine. Other spondyloarthropathies include:
- Undifferentiated spondyloarthropathy (USpA) which affects mainly the spine and pelvic joints
- Peripheral spondyloarthritis, affecting mostly the extremity joints
- Reactive arthritis (formerly known as Reiter's syndrome)
- Psoriatic arthritis
- Enteropathic arthritis/spondylitis associated with inflammatory bowel diseases/IBD (ulcerative colitis and Crohn's disease).

Ankylosing spondylitis is the prototype of the spondyloarthropathies presenting with inflammation of the axial skeleton, peripheral arthritis, and enthesitis. The basic pathological lesion occurs at the entheses (i.e., the sites of attachment to bone of ligaments, tendons, and joint capsules. Enthesitis or enthesopathy is the basic pathological lesion of AS. The disease process usually starts at the sacroiliac joints.

GENETICS AND EPIDEMIOLOGY

In ankylosing spondylitis, the usual onset of disease is from the late teens to age 40 years. It is characteristically associated with the HLA-B27 antigen as well as a familial aggregation. The age of onset of the symptoms of AS is approximately 25 years in HLA-B27 positive and 28 years in HLA-B27 negative patients. It is predominantly seen in males and the male-female ratio is roughly 3:1.

Interestingly, HLA-B27 antigen is present in 7% of the general population and only 1% of individuals eventually develop ankylosing spondylitis. Ankylosing spondylitis develops in 15–20% of the HLA-B27 positive individuals if they have a first-degree relative with AS. Hence, HLA B27 cannot be considered a screening or diagnostic test for AS. HLA-B27 is present in 90–95% of patients with ankylosing spondylitis, 60–90% of patients with reactive arthritis, 50–60% of patients with psoriatic arthritis or inflammatory bowel disease and spondylitis, and 80–90% of children with juvenile ankylosing spondylitis. There is a possibility of unknown environmental factor triggering AS in genetically predisposed persons. It has been postulated that endogenic component (HLA-B27) and exogenous component (*Klebsiella/Yersinia* antigen) may trigger the disease process. People with inflammatory bowel disease also tend to have a higher probability of having ankylosing spondylitis and psoriasis. Drugs tested for one also may be effective against the other in both Crohn's disease and ankylosing spondylitis. Two genes have also been linked to ankylosing spondylitis: *ARTS1 and IL23R*, both of which influence immune function. AS is more common in whites with the highest prevalence in northern Europe and the lowest in sub-Saharan Africa.

PATHOLOGY

The pathology is inflammation at the enthesis or subchondral bone with bone marrow edema, lymphocytic infiltrates, increased osteoclast density and increased microvascular density that are typical findings in acute inflammation. Enthesopathy means inflammation occurring at the insertion sites of tendons, ligaments and joint capsules to bone. Enthesopathy results in new bone formation and subsequent calcification and ossification in these regions. Pathological changes tend to occur along the Sharpey's fibers, associated with erosion and eburnation of the subligamentous bone. The primary pathology of enthesitis involves chronic immune inflammation, including participation of the CD4+ and CD8+ group of T lymphocytes and macrophages. Cytokines, particularly Tumour necrosis factor α (TNFα) and Transforming growth factor β (TGFβ) participate in the inflammatory process that eventually lead to fibrosis and ossification at the sites of enthesitis. TNFα is a proinflammatory cytokine that is involved in the pathogenesis and inflammatory response of AS and related SpA, in addition to psoriasis, and inflammatory bowel disease.

In the spine, enthesitis results in invasion of the margins of the disk by hyperemic granulation tissue arising from subchondral bone. They replace the disk fibers with new bone. Formation of bony bridges between adjacent vertebrae (syndesmophytes) and progressive ossification of extraspinal joint capsules and ligaments are characteristic of the disease.

In the synovial joints, a proliferative chronic synovitis indistinguishable from rheumatoid arthritis may occur; however, subchondral bone and cartilage are invaded by reactive tissue originating from the bone. Capsular fibrosis and bony ankylosis tend to occur. Unlike rheumatoid arthritis, pannus formation is not a classical feature of spondyloarthropathies.

■ CLINICAL FEATURES

Classically AS is a young male and onset after 50 years is unusual. A small subset of patients (15%) have a juvenile onset before age of 16 years, but in developing countries this form of AS is more common (up to 40%). General symptoms include those related to inflammatory back pain, peripheral enthesitis, arthropathy, and constitutional and organ-specific extra-articular manifestations. Inflammatory back pain is the most common and the first manifestation in approximately 75% of patients. Symptoms are usually insidious in onset occurring over months or years, generally with at least 3 months of symptoms before presentation with characteristic stiffness and fatigue. Fever and weight loss may occur during periods of active disease. Limitation of chest expansion relative to age and sex-matched individuals support diagnosis of spondyloarthropathy.

New criteria to define inflammatory back pain have been proposed; when 2 of the 4 criteria are present. These criteria include the following: (1) morning stiffness that lasts more than 30 minutes; (2) improvement of back pain with exercise but not rest; (3) nocturnal back pain during second half of the night only; (4) alternating buttock pain. The spinal disease starts in the sacroiliac joints (bilateral lumbosacral region). Most patients have mild chronic disease or intermittent flares with periods of remission. The spinal disease is rarely persistently active. The disease progresses proximally from the lumbosacral spine with ossification of the annulus fibrosus that results ultimately in the advanced form called "the bamboo spine".

The peripheral musculoskeletal involvement in AS is in about 30–50% of all patients. Peripheral enthesitis involves inflammation at the site of insertion of ligaments and tendons. This often progresses from erosion, osteitis to ossification, resulting in telltale radiological signs of periosteal new bone formation. Sites commonly involved are the Achilles tendon insertion, the insertion of the plantar fascia on the calcaneus or the metatarsal heads, the base of the fifth metatarsal head, the tibial tuberosity, the superior and inferior poles of the patella, and the iliac crest. Other sites of involvement include the greater trochanter, ischial tuberosity, costochondral junctions, distal scapula, lateral epicondyle, and distal ulna.

Hip involvement is usually seen in the first decade of the disease; typically bilateral and nearly symmetrical. Radiological signs include uniform loss of joint space like in osteoarthritis. There is axial migration of femoral head (called "Mushrooming") which may eventually get ankylosed resulting in grossly limited range of motion and flexion-abduction deformities. Shoulder joint is involved in 30% of cases and is usually bilateral. There are surface erosions at superolateral aspect of humerus and uniform loss of joint space. Other joints may be involved, including the shoulder girdle (glenohumeral, acromioclavicular, and sternoclavicular joints), costovertebral joints, costosternal junctions, manubriosternal joints, symphysis pubis, and temporomandibular. Enthesopathy is seen at coracoclavicular ligament attachment. AS may need to be differentiated from reactive arthritis, psoriatic arthritis, spondyloarthropathy associated with inflammatory bowel disease, undifferentiated spondyloarthropathy, Forestiers disease, Scheuermann disease, Whipple disease and Behçet disease.

■ PHYSICAL FINDINGS IN SPINE

In early stages of the disease, indirect evidence of sacroiliitis and spondylitis may be observed; including tenderness of the sacroiliac joints (elicited by either direct pressure approximately 2.5 cm below the PSIS or indirectly on pelvic compression test) or a limited range of spine motion documented commonly by Schober's test. With progression of the disease in the spine, there is loss of lumbar lordosis and accentuated thoracic kyphosis and in advanced stages there is stiffness of the spine with stooped posture. In AS, the solid column of bone below atlas may place increased stresses at craniovertebral junction. It along with additional effect of inflammation of transverse ligament, or associated effect of hyperemia on its bony attachments, may result in atlantoaxial subluxation or dislocation which may be stable without significant symptoms.

Radiological examination shows "squared" vertebral bodies due to calcification on the entheses. In later stages, bony bridges (syndesmophytes) form between adjacent vertebrae, there is ossification of spinal ligaments and, in late disease; there may be complete fusion of the vertebral column (bamboo spine). Spinal osteopenia is also common.

Juvenile Ankylosing Spondylitis

In approximately 10–20% of all cases, symptom onset occurs before age 16 years with a male-to-female ratio of 3:1. Enthesitis is prominent early in the course of the disease, while spinal symptoms and limitation of motion may not be present until several years later. Peripheral arthritis, especially in the lower extremities, and dactylitis are more common in children than in adults. Systemic manifestations (e.g., fever, weight loss, anemia, and leukocytosis) occur at disease onset in children more frequently than in adults. Initial radiography findings of the sacroiliac regions and spine are often normal or difficult to interpret in children which make definitive diagnosis difficult. The presence of *HLA-B27* would support the diagnosis in such cases.

DIAGNOSTIC CRITERIA
Modified New York Criteria

The modified New York criteria serve as the basis for the ASAS ("Assessment in AS") international working group/EULAR (the European League against Rheumatism) recommendations. The radiographic presence of sacroiliitis is a necessary condition for diagnosis. The presence of a grade ≥II bilaterally or Grade III or IV unilaterally satisfies the New York criteria for the diagnosis of AS. Besides sacroiliitis, the patient must exhibit 2 of the following 3 clinical criteria for a diagnosis of AS to be established: (1) low-back pain and stiffness ≥3 months with palliation by exercise and no relief with rest; (2) limitation of lumbar spinal motion in sagittal and coronal planes; and (3) limitation of chest expansion relative to age- and sex-matched individuals. Schober's test is commonly used bedside to assess lumbar spine mobility in sagittal plane.

In plain X-rays, the severity of sacroiliac joint disease may be divided into 4 grades. Grades I and II represent initial joint space widening, followed by joint space narrowing and the indistinctness of the sacroiliac joint. Grades III and IV involve bone destruction and ultimate fusion of the sacroiliac joint. Although the limitations of the New York criteria include their conservative reliance on a sacroiliitis that may tend to overlook other dimensions of the disease, the overwhelming majority of randomized controlled trials involving AS rely on this criteria. Squaring of the vertebral body is often the first distinct radiological feature in AS. Among the routine blood tests, ESR is elevated in over 70% cases of AS and this may be a useful adjunct to corroborate an initial working diagnosis. Radiographic features may take years to develop, which limit these classification criteria by potentially excluding patients early in the disease course when optimum treatment may have most favorable outcomes. In more recent classification, the designation "nonradiographic axial SpA" encompasses patients who have chronic back pain and features suggestive of SpA but who do not meet the radiographic criteria for AS.

TREATMENT
Medical Treatment

There is no cure for ankylosing spondylitis, but treatment is available to help relieve the symptoms. Treatment can also help delay or prevent the process of ankylosis of the spine. In most cases, treatment involves a combination of counseling, exercise, physiotherapy (hydrotherapy, etc.) and medication. Managing patients of AS is a team work and a team responsibility. It involves Orthopedic surgeon, Rheumatologist, Physiotherapist, Occupation therapist, General physicians, Family physician, and the patients' family. Best results may be obtained when Orthopedic surgeon and Rheumatologist work in tandem as both sides of a coin. The goals of treatment of AS (and non-radiographic axial SpA) are to reduce symptoms, maintain spinal flexibility and normal posture, reduce functional limitations, maintain work ability, and decrease disease complications. The mainstays of treatment have been nonsteroidal anti-inflammatory drugs (NSAIDs) and exercise, with the additional use of slow-acting anti-rheumatic drugs (SAARDs) in patients with peripheral arthritis. Over the past 15 years, the availability of tumor necrosis factor inhibitors (TNFi) has greatly altered the treatment approach. More recently, additional biologic agents have been developed. With more new treatment options, recommendations are evolving to help optimize care of these patients. Treatment decisions should always involve education of the patient as to anticipated benefits and potential harms. Although there are clinical similarities between AS and non-radiographic axial SpA, experts considered these conditions separately so far.

The NSAIDs improve the symptoms of the disease. Indomethacin may be more effective than other NSAIDs; although this has not been proven conclusively. Cyclooxygenase-2 (COX-2) inhibitors appear to be as effective as nonselective NSAIDs. Sulfasalazine, a disease modifying anti-rheumatoid drug (DMARD), has been shown to be useful in ankylosing spondylitis, particularly in reducing spinal stiffness, peripheral arthritis, and ESR values, but no definite evidence shows that spinal mobility, enthesitis, or physical function is benefited.

Pharmacologic Therapy

Agents used in the treatment of AS include the following:
- NSAIDs
- Sulfasalazine/DMARD
- TNFα antagonists (The Biologics and Biosimilars)
- Short-term corticosteroids used occasionally and in extra-articular manifestations.

Considerable progress has taken place in the therapy of spondyloarthropathies in the last decade. TNFα inhibitors like monoclonal antibodies or soluble receptors (now referred as *biologics*) are the first representative disease modifying drugs indicated in patients with AS. The TNFi have been shown to be effective in the treatment of ankylosing spondylitis, and etanercept, infliximab, and adalimumab are now approved therapies. These agents are very effective with fairly rapid onset of action (2 weeks) and have been shown to reduce inflammatory activity of spinal disease as assessed with MRI. TNFα is a proinflammatory cytokine that is involved in the pathogenesis of AS and related SpA, in addition to psoriasis, and inflammatory bowel disease. The detection of an abundance of TNF messenger RNA has been documented in synovial biopsies from sacroiliac joints in patients with AS. Recently, it has been demonstrated that the TNFα blocking agents infliximab, etanercept, and adalimumab have a prompt effect on almost all features of AS. These agents may suppress disease activity, improve physical function, and slow disease progression particularly in those cases refractory to NSAIDs and physical therapy. Before TNFα blocking agents are considered and used in AS, the mainstay of first-line therapy remains NSAIDs, sulfasalazine and physiotherapy followed by hip replacement surgery for advanced hip arthritis selectively in failed cases.

The TNFi approved by the US FDA for use in patients with ankylosing spondylitis are:
- Infliximab, which is given intravenously (by IV infusion) every 6–8 weeks at a dose of 5 mg/kg
- Etanercept, given by an injection of 50 mg under the skin once weekly
- Adalimumab, injected at a dose of 40 mg every other week under the skin
- Golimumab, injected at a dose of 50 mg once a month under the skin.

American College of Rheumatology (ACR) and others (2015) after evidence based study conditionally recommends that no particular TNFi was preferred except in patients with concomitant inflammatory bowel disease or recurrent iritis, in whom TNFi monoclonal antibodies should be used. The main limitations of biological therapies are their high cost and risk of opportunistic infections including risk of pulmonary tuberculosis due to immunosuppression.

Therefore, their risk-benefit and cost-benefit analysis must be individualized. When the disease has advanced and cartilage and enthesis degeneration is significant, biologics are of little help. Cost and affordability besides pretreatment screening for tuberculosis are concerns in Indian context.

NICE Guidelines

The National Institute for Health and Care Excellence (NICE) has produced useful guidance about the use of anti-TNF medication for AS. The NICE guidelines states that adalimumab, etanercept and golimumab may only be used if the following criteria are met: (1) a diagnosis of ankylosing spondylitis has been confirmed; (2) the level of pain is assessed twice (using a simple scale that patients fill in) 12 weeks apart and confirms that patient's condition has not improved; (3) Patient's Bath Ankylosing Spondylitis Disease Activity Index (BASDAI) is tested twice, 12 weeks apart, and confirms that the condition has not improved (BASDAI is a set of measures devised by experts to evaluate patient's condition by asking a number of questions about their symptoms); (4) when treatment with two or more NSAIDs for 4 weeks at the highest possible dose has not controlled patient's symptoms. After 12 weeks of treatment with anti-TNF medication, patient's pain score and BASDAI will be tested again to see whether they have improved enough to make continuing treatment worthwhile. If they have, treatment should continue and they should be tested every 12 weeks. If there is not enough improvement after 12 weeks, they should be tested again at a later date or the treatment should be stopped.

Evidence-based Treatment Recommendations in Ankylosing Spondylitis (ACR)

The treatment recommendations in ankylosing spondylitis are given in **Box 1**.

Treatment with SAARD sulfasalazine or high dose pamidronate could be considered mainly for patients with contraindications to TNFi or those who decline (or cannot afford) treatment with TNFi. Treatment with high-dose pamidronate was associated with improved patient-reported outcomes compared to low-dose pamidronate in systematic review and deserves further study. Sulfasalazine may provide a small beneficial effect on spinal pain but not on other outcomes, and had a higher risk of side effects than placebo. Although treatment with sulfasalazine did not improve peripheral joint counts, small benefit was seen in a composite measure of peripheral arthritis symptoms. Sulfasalazine could be considered for those with prominent peripheral arthritis. Selected patients with both NSAIDs and sulfasalazine-refractory active inflammatory disease may respond well to TNFi. Anakinra, a recombinant human interleukin-1 (IL-1) receptor antagonist, may be effective in treatment-resistant ankylosing spondylitis. It has also been

Box 1: Treatment recommendations in ankylosing spondylitis.

- In adults with active AS, we strongly recommend treatment with NSAIDs over no treatment with NSAIDs
- In adults with active AS despite treatment with NSAIDs, we strongly recommend treatment with TNFi over no treatment with TNFi
- In adults with active AS, we do not recommend any particular TNFi as the preferred choice, except for patients with concomitant inflammatory bowel disease or recurrent iritis
- In adults with AS and inflammatory bowel disease, we strongly recommend treatment with TNFi monoclonal antibodies over treatment with etanercept
- In adults with active AS, we strongly recommend against treatment with systemic glucocorticoids
- In adults with active AS, we strongly recommend treatment with physical therapy over no treatment with physical therapy
- In adults with AS and advanced hip arthritis, we strongly recommend treatment with total hip arthroplasty over no surgery
- In adults with active nonradiographic axial SpA despite treatment with NSAIDs, we conditionally recommend treatment with TNFi over no treatment with TNFi

(NSAIDs: nonsteroidal anti-inflammatory drugs; AS: ankylosing spondylitis; TNFi: tumor necrosis factor inhibitors)

shown that active juxta-articular bony inflammation ("bone edema"), as detected by magnetic resonance imaging (MRI), can be suppressed by biological agents, and it is hoped that this kind of treatment will also favorably influence long-term outcome, including reduction or prevention of radiologic progression. Recent data also show that AS patients with a short disease duration and good functional status are more likely to respond to TNFα blocking agents than patients with long-standing disease and impaired function. Thus, an early and reliable diagnosis of AS has now become an important and very relevant issue.

Bisphosphonates may be useful for preventing osteoporosis in addition to other disease modifying drug treatment and regular physiotherapy. It may also reduce aseptic osteolysis after cemented hip arthroplasty. Bisphosphonates are known to inhibit osteoclasts, improve osteoporotic bone density measurements, and prevent fractures. It suppresses pro-inflammatory cytokines such as IL-1, TNFα and IL-6, and show anti-inflammatory properties in arthritic conditions.

The gold standard for measuring and evaluating disease activity in ankylosing spondylitis is the Bath Ankylosing Spondylitis Disease Activity Index (BASDAI). Scores of 4 or greater suggest suboptimal control of disease, and patients with scores of 4 or greater are usually good candidates for either a change in their medical therapy or for enrollment in clinical trials evaluating new drug therapies directed at ankylosing spondylitis. Extra-articular manifestations such as uveitis, inflammation of the aortic vales may need treatment.

Physiotherapy

Regular and supervised physiotherapy (PT) and postural training is of paramount importance to reduce morbidity, complications and maintain function. Rest is recommended in the acute stage of the disease. Chest physiotherapy to maintain good vital capacity to control restrictive lung disease is essential.

Cochrane review found that

- An individual home-based or supervised exercise program is better than no intervention.
- Supervised group physiotherapy is better than home exercises.
- Combined inpatient SpA-exercise therapy followed by group physiotherapy is better than group physiotherapy alone.
- Evidence of at least short-term positive effects of physiotherapy, in particular exercise, in AS.

Spinal extension and deep-breathing exercises help to maintain spinal mobility, encourage erect posture and promote chest expansion. Using a firm mattress with a thin pillow reduces the tendency of thoracic kyphosis. Hydrotherapy and swimming are also beneficial. Immobilization of the spine is undesirable since it may hasten ankylosis and osteoporosis.

Surgical Treatment Options

Surgery is indicated when the disease has advanced; causing significant deformity and disability to such an extent that it is affecting activities of daily living. Surgery may also be indicated for managing complications.

The following procedures can be used in the surgical management of AS when medical management has failed.

- *Joint replacement*: Patients with significant involvement of the hips may benefit from total hip arthroplasty.
- *Vertebral osteotomy*: Patients with fusion of the cervical or upper thoracic spine leading to gross kyphosis may benefit from extension osteotomy of the cervical spine.

Surgically associated hip disease has to be considered before addressing spinal disease. Patients may need total hip replacement (THR) to provide a painless, mobile and stable joint to improve function in severe arthritis. Since patients are young with relatively good bone stock, cementless or hybrid THR are usually preferable. The hip joint may be ankylosed and after doing osteotomy of the femoral neck, it may be difficult to remove the femoral head necessitating piecemeal removal or direct reaming of the head after completing the neck osteotomy to get the acetabular exposure. In selected cases surface replacement arthroplasty with due care to avoid osteoporotic femoral neck fracture during surgical dislocation is necessary; conversion to conventional THR should be kept open as an option. DMARDs may need to be discontinued or modified briefly prior to surgery. DMARDs can resumed again after wound healing following surgery with due discussion with the rheumatologist. Heterotopic ossification with loss of range of motion may particularly be common after total joint replacement in AS, and postoperative NSAIDs (e.g., indomethacin) may reduce its risk. Generally, the outcome of a well performed total joint replacement in AS patients is quite satisfactory.

Spine surgery is occasionally useful in correcting spinal deformities in AS. Vertebral osteotomy may be performed to correct spinal deformities, but significant neurologic complications may occur. About 10% of patients with AS who have severe bony changes may need such spine surgery. The loss of lumbar lordosis can be corrected by multiple posteriorly based wedge osteotomies (Smith Peterson procedure), by decancellation procedure of L3 or L4 or pedicle subtraction osteotomy based at L3 and L4. Decancellation of the vertebral body shortens the spinal column and dreaded complication of rupture of calcified aorta and death may be avoided. After completion of osteotomy, spine is fused in correct position along with appropriate pedicle screw rod system. However, the pedicular screws should be inserted before the corrective osteotomy gap is closed.

Severe kyphosis at cervical spine may be quite disabling in neglected and advanced cases due to reduction in the visual field and inability to see forward. Walking on stairs or crossing a road may become dangerous or impossible. Thorough preoperative assessment of deformities and measuring the so-called chin-eyebrow to floor angle are helpful for planning. Optimum Chin brow to vertical angle is 10 degree: the patient can still look down at a desk and see steps well. Relative contraindications are poor general condition, and significant scarring of major blood vessels. Cervical osteotomy is performed between C7-T1, to avoid injury to vertebral artery that enters the foramina of C6. After the removal of posterior element and neural decompression, the kyphotic deformity is gently corrected with gentle extension of head and internal fixation or halo vest for immobilization.

NATURAL HISTORY OF SPINE IN ANKYLOSING SPONDYLITIS

A small cohort of treated patients develops gross spinal fusion or classical ankylosis. This may result in severe kyphosis with associated limited motion; often including the cervical spines. The fused spine is more susceptible to fracture, even with trivial trauma. Occasionally the hip and shoulder joints develop severe arthropathy, requiring joint replacement. Extra-articular manifestations, e.g., recurrent uveitis, cardiovascular involvement, pulmonary involvement, and amyloidosis, etc., rarely result in significant morbidity or even mortality. The speed at which spinal ankylosis progresses is slower in female patients, but women patients suffer more morbidity due to AS. Fortunately, female patients tend to be younger than the males and have shorter average disease duration.

MORTALITY/MORBIDITY

A few patients develop chronic progressive disabling diseases due to spinal inflammation leading to fusion, often with thoracic kyphosis. Erosive disease involving peripheral joints, especially the hips and shoulders are not uncommon and can add to further disability. Patients with spinal fusion are prone to spinal fractures that may result in neurologic deficits. Spinal fractures may need fixation surgically using pedicular screw rod system and instrumented fusion. Most functional loss in ankylosing spondylitis occurs during the first 10 years of illness.

The existing criteria, namely the modified New York Criteria, require advanced radiographic changes to be present in the sacroiliac joints and this may lead to dilemma and delay in establishing early diagnosis and initiating optimum treatment. In rare cases with severe long-standing ankylosing spondylitis significant extra-articular manifestations such as cardiovascular disease, including cardiac conduction defects and aortic regurgitation; pulmonary fibrosis; neurologic sequelae (e.g., cauda equina syndrome); or amyloidosis may develop.

PROGNOSIS

Ankylosing spondylitis generally carry a good prognosis. Patients often require long-term anti-inflammatory therapy. Morbidity can occur related to spinal and peripheral joint involvement or, rarely, extra-articular manifestations. Poor prognostic indicators include peripheral joint involvement, young age of onset, elevated ESR, and poor response to NSAIDs. The risk of mortality increases in patients with severe long-standing disease and significant extra-articular manifestations. In recent years, there have been two major developments in the management of AS that make earlier diagnosis possible and offer the hope of alleviating pain and preventing structural changes that result in loss of function. These developments include the use of magnetic resonance imaging (MRI) to visualize the inflammatory changes in the sacroiliac joint and the axial spine, and the demonstration that TNF blocking agents are highly efficacious in reducing spinal inflammation and possibly in slowing radiographic progression.

ACKNOWLEDGMENT

This chapter quotes extensively from the texts of: Borgohain B, Lahkar S. Ankylosing spondylitis. In: Kulkarni GS (Eds). Textbook of Orthopedics and Trauma; 3rd edition. New Delhi: Jaypee Brothers Medical Publishers (P) Ltd.; 2016. pp. 502-8.

FURTHER READING

1. Akgul O, Ozgocmen S. Classification criteria for spondyloarthropathies. World J Orthop. 2011;2(12):107-15.

2. American College of Rheumatology. (2012). Spondyloarthritis (Spondyloarthropathy). [online] Available from http://www.rheumatology.org/Practice/Clinical/Patients/Diseases_And_Conditions/Spondylarthritis_ (Spondylarthropathy)/. [Last accessed May, 2021].
3. Anderson JJ, Baron G, van der HD, Felson DT, Dougados M. Ankylosing spondylitis assessment group preliminary definition of short-term improvement in ankylosing spondylitis. Arthritis Rheum. 2001;44:1876-86.
4. Appel H, Loddenkemper C, Miossec P. Rheumatoid arthritis and ankylosing spondylitis - pathology of acute inflammation. Clin Exp Rheumatol. 2009;27(4 Suppl 55):S15-9.
5. Bhan S. Ankylosing spondylitis. In: Kulkarni GS (Eds). Textbook of Orthopedics and Trauma, 2nd edition. New Delhi: Jaypee Brothers Medical Publishers (P) Ltd.; 2008. pp. 113, 873-8.
6. Borgohain B, Lahkar S. Ankylosing spondylitis. In: Kulkarni GS (Eds). Textbook of Orthopedics and Trauma; 3rd edition. New Delhi: Jaypee Brothers Medical Publishers (P) Ltd.; 2016. pp. 502-8.
7. Brandt J, Haibel H, Cornely D, Golder W, Gonzalez J, Reddig J, et al. Successful treatment of active ankylosing spondylitis with the anti-tumor necrosis factor alpha monoclonal antibody infliximab. Arthritis Rheum. 2000;43:1346-52.
8. Brandt J, Khariouzov A, Listing J, Haibel H, Sörensen H, Grassnickel L, et al. Six-month results of a double-blind, placebo-controlled trial of etanercept treatment in patients with active ankylosing spondylitis. Arthritis Rheum. 2003;48:1667-75.
9. Braun J, Baraliakos X, Golder W, Brandt J, Rudwaleit M, Listing J, et al. Magnetic resonance imaging examinations of the spine in patients with ankylosing spondylitis, before and after successful therapy with infliximab: evaluation of a new scoring system. Arthritis Rheum. 2003;48:1126-36.
10. Braun J, Bollow M, Remlinger G, Eggens U, Rudwaleit M, Distler A, et al. Prevalence of spondylarthropathies in HLA-B27 positive and negative blood donors. Arthritis Rheum. 1998;41:58-67.
11. Braun J, Sieper J. Ankylosing spondylitis. Lancet. 2007; 369:1379-90.
12. Calin A, Porta J, Fries JF, Schurman DJ. Clinical history as a screening test for ankylosing spondylitis. *JAMA*. 1977;237(24):2613-4.
13. Clegg DO, Reda DJ, Mejias E, Cannon GW, Weisman MH, Taylor T, et al. Comparison of sulfasalazine and placebo in the treatment of psoriatic arthritis: a Department of Veterans Affairs cooperative study. Arthritis Rheum. 1996;39:2013-20.
14. Cutolo M, Seriolo B, Pizzorni C, Mease PJ, Callis Duffin K. Methotrexate in psoriatic arthritis. Clin Exp Rheumatol. 2002;20: S76-S80.
15. Dagfinrud H, Kvien TK, Hagen KB. Physiotherapy interventions for ankylosing spondylitis. Cochrane Database Syst Rev. 2008;23(1):CD002822.
16. Davis J Jr, van der Heijde D, Braun J. Recombinant human tumor necrosis factor receptor (etanercept) for treating ankylosing spondylitis: a randomized, controlled trial. Arthritis Rheum. 2003;48:3230-6.
17. Dhaon BK. Ankylosing spondylitis. In: Kulkarni GS (Ed). Textbook of Orthopedics and Trauma, 1st edition. New Delhi: Jaypee Brothers Medical Publishers (P) Ltd.; 1999. pp. 122, 872-4.
18. Fraser SM, Hopkins R, Hunter JA, Neumann V, Capell HA, Bird HA. Sulphasalazine in the management of psoriatic arthritis. BJR. 1993;32:923-5.
19. Gorman JD, Sack KE, Davis JC Jr. Treatment of ankylosing spondylitis by inhibition of tumor necrosis factor alpha. N Engl J Med. 2002;346:1349-56.
20. Keane J, Gershon S, Wise RP, et al.: Tuberculosis associated with infliximab, a tumor necrosis factor alpha-neutralizing agent. N Engl J Med. 2001;345:1098-104.
21. Maksymowych WP, Inman RD, Gladman D, Thomson G, Stone M, Karsh J, et al. Spondyloarthritis Research Consortium of Canada (SPARCC): Canadian Rheumatology Association Consensus on the use of anti-tumor necrosis factor-alpha directed therapies in the treatment of spondyloarthritis. J Rheumatol. 2003;30: 1356-63.
22. Maksymowych WP, Jhangri GS, Fitzgerald AA, LeClercq S, Chiu P, Yan A, Skeith KJ, et al. A six-month randomized, controlled, double-blind, dose-response comparison of intravenous pamidronate (60 mg versus 10 mg) in the treatment of nonsteroidalantiinflammatory drug-refractory ankylosing spondylitis. Arthritis Rheum. 2002;46:766-73.
23. Maksymowych WP, Jhangri GS, LeClercq S, Skeith K, Yan A, Russell AS. An open study of pamidronate in the treatment of refractory ankylosing spondylitis. J Rheumatol. 1998; 25:714-7.
24. Marzo-Ortega H, McGonagle D, O'Connor P, Emery P. Efficacy of etanercept in the treatment of the entheseal pathology in resistant spondylarthropathy: a clinical and magnetic resonance imaging study. Arthritis Rheum. 2001;44:2112-7.
25. Melis L, Elewau D. Progress in spondylarthritis. Immuno-pathogenesis of spondyloarthritis: which cells drive disease? Arthritis Res Ther. 2009;11(3):233.
26. Nicholas J Sheehans. The ramifications of HLA-B27. J R Soc Med. 2004;97(1):10-4.
27. Perez Alamino R, Maldonado Cocco JA, Citera G, Arturi P, Vazquez-Mellado J, Sampaio-Arros PD, et al. Differential features between primary ankylosing spondylitis and spondylitis associated with psoriasis and inflammatory bowel disease. J Rheumatol. 2011;38:1656-60.
28. Rudwaleit M, Baraliakos X, Brandt J, Sieper J, Braun J. Magnetic resonance imaging (MRI) of the spine and the sacroiliac joints (SIJ) in ankylosing spondylitis (AS) before and during therapy with the anti-TNF agent etanercept. Ann Rheum Dis. 2004;63(Suppl 1):397.
29. Rudwaleit M, Listing J, Brandt J, Braun J, Sieper J. Prediction of a major clinical response (BASDAI 50) to tumour necrosis factor blockers in ankylosing spondylitis. Ann Rheum Dis. 2004;63:665-70.
30. Sampaio-Barros PD, Costallat LT, Bertolo MB, Neto JF, Samara AM. Methotrexate in the treatment of ankylosing spondylitis. Scand J Rheumatol. 2000;29:160-2.
31. Shaikh SA. Ankylosing spondylitis: recent breakthroughs in diagnosis and treatment. J Can Chiropr Assoc. 2007;51(4): 249-60.
32. Singh D. Ankylosing spondylitis: an update. North East Orthoscan. 2011;7(3):43-8.
33. Van den Bosch F, Kruithof E, Baeten D, De Keyser F, Mielants H, Veys EM. Effects of a loading dose regimen of three infusions of chimeric monoclonal antibody to tumour necrosis factor alpha (infliximab) in spondyloarthropathy: an open pilot study. Ann Rheum Dis. 2000;59:428-33.

34. Van den Bosch F, Kruithof E, Baeten D, Herssens A, de Keyser F, Mielants H, et al. Randomized double-blind comparison of chimeric monoclonal antibody to tumor necrosis factor alpha (infliximab) versus placebo in active spondylarthropathy. Arthritis Rheum. 2002;46:755-65.
35. Van den Linden SM, Valkenburg HA, Jongh BM, Cats A. The risk of developing ankylosing spondylitis in HLA-B27 positive individuals: a comparison of relatives of spondylitis patients with the general population. Arthritis Rheum. 1984; 27(3):241-9.
36. Van der Horst B, Irene E. Clinical aspects of ankylosing spondylitis. In: Ankylosing Spondylitis: Diagnosis and Management. New York: Taylor and Francis; 2006. pp. 45-70, 129-136.
37. Van der Linden S, van Tubergen A, Hidding A. Physiotherapy in ankylosing spondylitis: what is the evidence? Clin Exp Rheumatol. 2002;20:S60-S64.
38. Ward MM, Deodhar A, Akl EA, Lui A, Ermann J, Gensler LS, et al. American College of Rheumatology/Spondylitis Association of America/Spondyloarthritis Research and Treatment Network 2015 recommendations for the treatment of ankylosing spondylitis and nonradiographic axial spondyloarthritis. Arthritis Care Res (Hoboken). 2016;68:151-66.
39. Ware JE Jr, Sherbourne CD. The MOS 36-item short-form health survey (SF 36): conceptual framework and item selection. Med Care. 1992;30:473-83.
40. Zink A, Braun J, Listing J, Wollenhaupt J. Disability and handicap in rheumatoid arthritis and ankylosing spondylitis-results from the German rheumatological database. J Rheumatol. 2000;27:613-622.
41. Zochling J, Smith EU. Seronegative spondyloarthritis. Best Pract Res Clin Rheumatol. 2010;24:747-56.
42. Zochling J, van der Heijde D, Dougados M, Braun J. Current evidence for the management of ankylosing spondylitis: a systemic literature review of the ASAS/EULAR management recommendations in ankylosing spondylitis. Ann Rheum Dis. 2006;65:423-32.

14. Surgical Management in Ankylosing Spondylitis

Md Neshar Ansari, Rajiv Lakhotia, Abhinandan Reddy M

INTRODUCTION

Ankylosing spondylitis (AS) is an inflammatory condition of the spine usually presenting in 2nd and 3rd decade. The usual symptoms are pain followed by stiffness. Because of the inflammatory process joints become arthritic and eroded followed by autofusion. Sacroiliac joint and spine are involved and not uncommonly peripheral joints. Hips and shoulder are most frequently involved peripheral joints in AS and 35% of patient may have these joints involved at some stage of disease.

PATHOLOGY

Enthesis: The primary sites of ossification occur in the axial skeleton and are usually the spinal entheses, sites of ligaments/tendon insertion to the spine and sacroiliac joints. Apophyseal joints, intervertebral disks and anterior and anterolateral attachment of ligaments to outer annulus are site of enthesopathy in spine. Initially invasion of the anterior corners of the vertebrae leads to the squaring off of the vertebral bodies and formation of erosions. Healing of these erosions occurs by woven bone which eventually matures into lamellar bone. Because of this process of healing by ossification of anterior longitudinal ligament and annulus fibrosis lead to vertically oriented marginal syndesmophyte. The end-stage is formation of "bamboo spine".

Muscle: Studies suggest that paraspinal volume is decreased in AS patients even without deformity compared with age and spinopelvic alignment matched non-AS patients with chronic back pain. Further reduction occurs with development of kyphotic deformity. Histopathological changes include atrophy of type II muscle fibers and excess of perifiber connective tissue.

Bone: Both osteoporosis and osteopenia are common in AS. Osteoporosis in AS is possibly because of cytokine-induced and inflammatory changes. Immobility is another causative factor. In the early course of disease AS patients with low BMD may develop compression fracture and development of kyphotic deformity. As the disease progresses BMD is increased because of extensive enthesopathy but overall bone is weak and brittle. Once the bone is completely ankylosed there is increased possibility of transvertebral and transdiscal fractures rather compression fracture.

PATHOGENESIS OF DEFORMITY

The disease process starts in the sacroiliac joint and then progressively ascend to involve thoracolumbar and then cervical spine. When the disease involves lumbar spine, because of inflammation there is paraspinal spasm leading to loss of lumbar lordosis. Its natures attempt to offload the inflamed facet joint. Initially it starts as a compensatory process but gradually as the facet joint becomes ankylosed these deformity becomes fixed leading to fixed thoracolumbar deformity. Involvement of cerical spine leads to formation of "chin on chest deformity". Because of kyphotic deformity, global sagittal balance of spine is offset leading to positive sagittal vertical axis. Abnormal sagittal balance leads to abnormal excessive loading of anterior vertebral bodies leading to wedging of vertebra and further accentuation of thoracolumbar kyphotic deformity (TLKD). Muscle atrophy occurs because of inactivity and disease process and is one of the factors in evolution of deformity as they are at mechanical disadvantage in holding up the trunk.

Characteristic deformity of AS: TLKD (round back deformity) with chin on chest deformity.

Compensatory mechanism in TLKD: The chief disability of patient with TLKD is difficulty in maintaining a forward gaze. To maintain forward gaze compensation must occur at cervical spine above and pelvis and lower extremities below. However, there is not much scope of compensation at cervical spine because of associated chin on chest deformity. Therefore, major compensation occurs at pelvis.

Maintenance of upright stance with minimum expenditure requires normal lumbar lordosis and pelvic parameters. Reduction in lumbar lordosis is compensated by pelvic retroversion which can be measured radiographically as pelvic tilt. Once maximum compensation is achieved, further compensation occurs in lower extremity with hip extension. Since there is a limit to maximum hip extension possible therefore compensation that can occur at pelvis is limited. Some compensation occurs at knee by flexion and dorsiflexion at ankle. The result of these compensation produces a "crouched stance" with apparent flexion at hip (actually hip is maximally extended) and knee.

INDICATIONS FOR SURGICAL MANAGEMENT IN ANKYLOSING SPONDYLITIS

- Deformity
- Andersson lesion
- Spinal fracture.

Deformity Correction

Kyphotic deformity produces sagittal malalignment because of which there is difficulty in maintaining forward gaze and patient gaze is fixed to floor. Because of inability to see above horizon there is difficulty in interpersonal communication, eating, personal hygiene, crossing the road, etc. Patient may also show intestinal problem because of compression of abdominal viscera by rib margin.

Aim of deformity correction in AS:
- To restore forward gaze by correcting chin-brow vertical angle (CBVA)
- Restoration of sagittal balance
- To restore pelvis to neutral position.

Radiological Parameters

Cervical lordosis: Cervical lordosis is angle subtended between superior endplate of C2 and inferior endplate of C7 **(Fig. 1)**.

C7 sagittal vertical axis: Vertical plumbline is drawn from center of C7 vertebral body **(Fig. 2)**. The distance is measured in millimeters from the posterosuperior corner of sacrum. It is considered positive if pumbline falls in front of sacrum and negative if it falls behind sacrum.

Chin-brow vertical angle: Patient is made on stand with hip and knee extended and neck in neutral position **(Fig. 3)**. A line is drawn joining the chin and brow of patient. The angle subtended between this line and vertical axis is chin-brow vertical angle.

Thoracic kyphosis: Thoracic kyphosis is angle subtended between superior endplate of T4 to inferior endplate of T12. Normal value ranges from 10° to 40°.

Pelvic incidence: Midpoint of sacral endplate is localized and from this midpoint a line perpendicular to endplate is drawn. A second line is drawn joining this point to midpoint of femoral head. The angle subtended between these two lines is pelvic incidence. This is a morphologic parameter and is not changed by orientation of pelvis in space. So, for a given individual, this remains fixed after skeletal maturity **(Fig. 4)**.

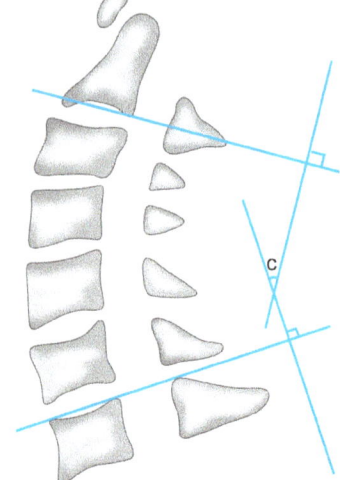

Fig. 1: Cervical lordosis.

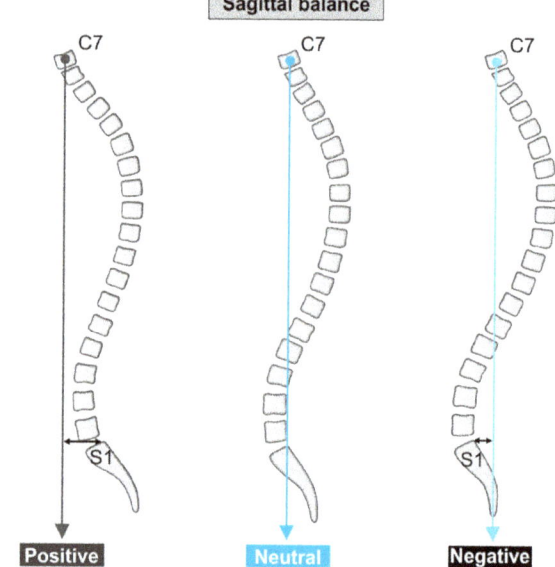

Fig. 2: C7 sagittal vertical axis.

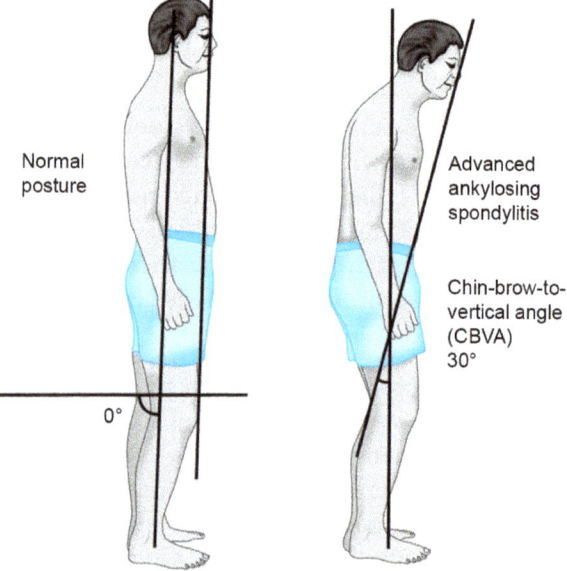

Fig. 3: Chin-brow vertical angle.

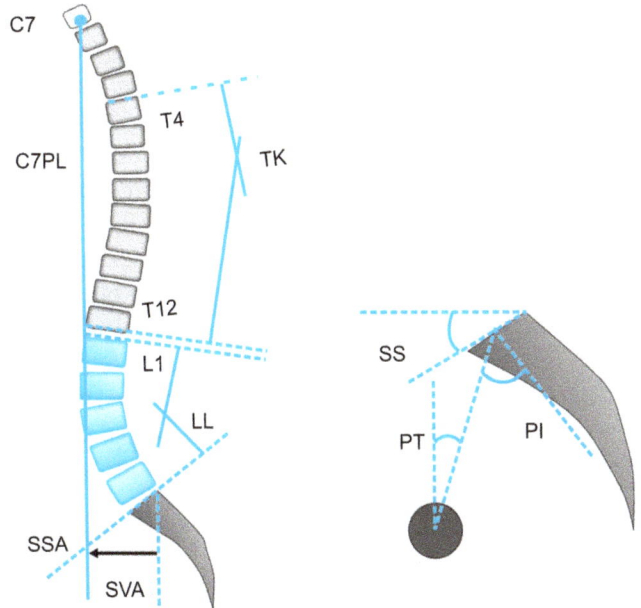

Fig. 4: Measurement of spinopelvic parameters. (C7PL: C7 plumbline; SVA: sagittal vertical axis; TK: thoracic kyphosis; LL: lumbar lordosis; SS: sacral slope; PT: pelvic tilt; PI: pelvic incidence)

Sacral slope: It is the angle formed between horizontal reference line and sacral endplate.

Pelvic tilt: A line is drawn from midpoint of sacral endplate to femoral head. Angle subtended between this line and a vertical reference line passing through center of femoral head is pelvic incidence (PI). This is not a fixed parameter and is influenced by orientation of pelvis in space. PI decreases in anteversion and retroversion.

Preoperative Planning

Careful examination of patient in standing, seating, and supine position is to be done to determine the major component of deformity. Deformity at hip joints corrects on moving from standing to seating position and in which case hip arthroplasty to be considered first. If deformity is present in sitting position and corrects in supine position then lumbar osteotomy is usually indicated. If deformity persists even in supine position then the patient has "chin on chest deformity", i.e., in cervicothoracic region and osteotomy in this area is indicated.

Radiographic assessment: A whole spine AP and lateral radiograph with neck in neutral position and hips in fully extended position is needed. The radiograph allows measurement of various parameters and CBVA. An AP pelvis X-ray is also essential to see condition of hip and arthroplasty to be considered first before planning to correct deformity in case hip joints are involved.

Preoperative Planning for Measuring Osteotomy Angle

Optimal CBVA to be achieved after surgery has been shown to be between 10° and 20°. In this position patient can see both the floor as well as forward gaze is possible. Correction to 0° is not advisable in such case though the forward gaze is achieved but the patient cannot see the floor leading to difficulty in walking.

Determination of Osteotomy Angle

- *X-ray trace and cutout method*: Spinal curvature is traced and then wedge is cutout from vertebra to be osteotomized with apex at anterior longitudinal ligament. The superior and inferior end plates are then approximated. After approximation if the CBVA is restored then the wedge angle is amount of correction needed.
- *Patient is made to stand such that forward gaze* is restored with hips extended and flexion at knees. The osteotomy angle can be estimated by dividing the angle made at knees by half.
- Computer-based software such as ASKyphoplan and Surgimap

Location of Osteotomy—there are Certain Factors which Need to be Considered

- The correction is traditionally performed at the site of the patient's most significant radiographic deformity.
- For thoracolumbar kyphosis, the osteotomy is usually at the lumbar spine for lesser chance of neurological complications and more effective correction of sagittal malalignment. Compared to osteotomy at thoracic levels there is less chance of neurological complication as spinal cord has already ended at T-11, and canal is spacious. More effective correction of sagittal malalignment is because long- lever arm is available for correction with distal osteotomy.
- The thoracic osteotomy correction is limited by the ankylosis of the costa- vertebral joints, narrow spinal canal and presence of spinal cord at this level increasing the chance of neurological deterioration.
- The cervical osteotomy is performed at the C7 to T1 level to avoid injury to the vertebral artery. Also the spinal canal diameter normally is greatest at this level.

Types of Osteotomy (Fig. 5)

There are basically three types of osteotomy which has been described for correction of deformity in AS. They are extension type osteotomy namely:
1. Smith–Peterson opening wedge osteotomy
2. Pedicle subtraction osteotomy and
3. Polysegmental dorsal wedge osteotomy.

Smith–Peterson opening wedge osteotomy: It is an opening wedge osteotomy. This is a V-shaped osteotomy in coronal plane with intersection point of "V" in midline. Osteotomy involves resection of articular process bilaterally and removal of ample amount of lamina and flavum followed by

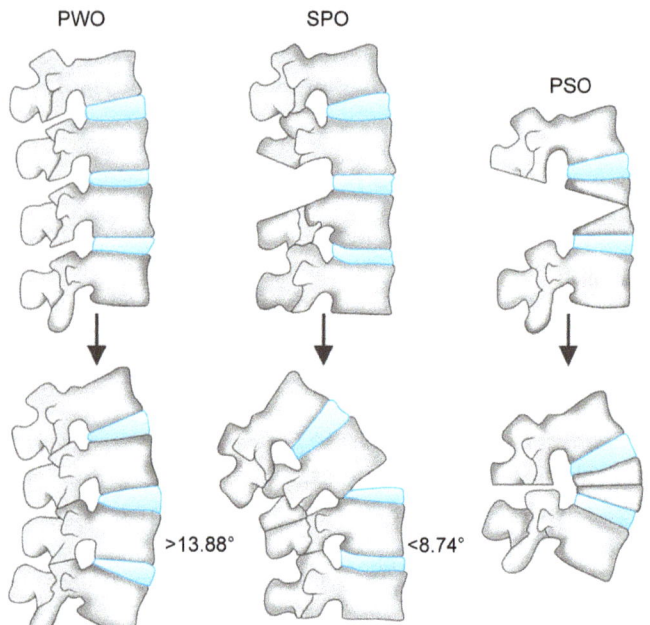

Fig. 5: Different types of osteotomy. (PWO: polysegmental wedge osteotomy; SPO: Smith–Peterson osteotomy; PSO: pedicle subtraction osteotomy)

closure of osteotomy. In this process, there is lengthening of anterior column by forceful extension causing osteoclasis and shortening of posterior column with axis of correction at posterior margin of intervertebral disk. Osteotomy is closed by closing over instrumentation. Ideally three levels of fixation both proximally and distally are needed. Because of anterior lengthening anterior bone gap is created. If osteotomy does not heal favorably then bone grafting may be needed.

Acute lordotic correction has been presumably associated with aortic rupture, superior mesenteric artery syndrome, paraplegia and cauda equina syndrome.

Polysegmental wedge osteotomy: It is a modification of SPO. It is a multilevel osteotomy in which osteotomy is performed at interlaminar space and is extended laterally into facet at approximately 30° to horizontal. The entire facet joint complex is removed though the amount of bone removed is less compared to SPO. The pivot of correction is posterior column. About 10° kyphosis correction is possible at each level. Approximately 1 mm of bone removed posteriorly leads to 1° correction at disk space. The kyphosis is then gently corrected with help of contoured rods. Because of more harmonious correction of deformity there is less risk of vascular and neurologic complication associated with SPO.

- *Pedicle subtraction osteotomy*: PSO allow greater angular correction by removal of wedge of corticocancellous bone from the posterior aspect of the vertebral body in combination with removal of articular processes, transverse processes, and pedicles. The wedge is then closed with anterior cortex acting as hinge. There is no anterior bony gap. Because of bone on bone contact anteriorly by osteotomy closure there is better rate of union. The degree of correction by PSO is 30° for single level and two-level PSO can achieve 60–80° correction. PSO is usually done at L2 or L3 as it is near to apex of deformity, longer lever-arm for correction of sagittal malalignment, and less risk of neurological deficit as osteotomy is below level of conus medullaris. Distal osteotomy at L4 or L5 is not preferred because it is far from deformity and also less points are available for distal fixation. If two-level PSO is warranted then usually done at T12-L2 or L1-L3. The technical expertise required for PSO is more than SPO, with more time needed as well as intraoperative blood loss. Still PSO is favored over SPO because lethal complications of aortic rupture seen with SPO.
- *Complications:* Increased blood loss and dural injury, neurological deficit, wound healing problem, implant failure are the complications seen.

Conclusion

Patients of AS with global sagittal malalignment due to either kyphotic deformity or cervical deformity are severely disabled due to difficulty in maintaining a forward gaze. Patients can experience significant benefits from correction of these deformities. However, spinal reconstructive surgery in AS patients is challenging because of demanding techniques for deformity correction and associated factor like osteopenia. However, technical advances in surgical techniques, instrumentation, neurophysiologic monitoring, and medical management have reduced the risk of intraoperative complications and have made surgeries in ankylotic spine a safer option. The location of osteotomy is based on clinical and radiological measurements and lumbar closing type osteotomy being safest and simple. The ultimate aim of surgery is to restore forward gaze and center C7 plumb line over sacrum.

Andersson Lesion

Andersson lesion is a localized discovertebral or vertebral lesion which was first described in 1937 by Andersson. Prevalence is highly variable and in literature has been described from 1 to 28%. Various other names has been used to describe Andersson lesion such as "destructive vertebral lesion", "spondylodiscitis", "diskitis", "sterile diskitis", "pseudarthrosis" or "(stress-) fracture".

Clinical Features

The most common symptom is back pain, some may develop neurological symptoms, and some lesions may remain asymptomatic. Middle-aged males are most commonly involved. However, nature of this pain is different from inflammatory pain of AS. The back pain in AS is diffuse, dull aching that aggravates with rest and improves on activity.

However, the pain of AL is sharp, localized, worsens with activity, and improves with rest. Neurological symptoms may be present in form of radiculopathy or myelopathy. Clinical examination reveals tenderness at site of lesion.

The thoracolumbar junction is most commonly involved area of spine because of it being a transitional zone with high stress risers.

Etiology

Various theories have been put forward to explain the pathogenesis. Most favored out of them being is either traumatic or inflammatory. Based on etiology, Bron has attempted to classify lesion into three types. They are:
1. Localized lesion which are almost always inflammatory.
2. Extensive lesion without fractured posterior elements. These are transdiscal lesion and without fusion of facet joints. These lesions result from combination of mechanical and inflammatory causes.
3. Extensive lesion with fractured posterior element. These have been proposed due to mechanical factors and can be either transdiscal or transvertebral.

Pathology

Tissues from lesion on histopathology showed hemorrhage, fibrous tissue, small amounts of callus, and sclerosis of the adjacent vertebral bone similar to microscopic appearance at site of nonunion of long bone.

Radiology

X-ray: Plain radiographs are initial imaging study of choice. Osteolytic destruction with a surrounding zone of reactive sclerosis and vertebral osteophytes is suggestive of AL. Dihlmann et al. suggested that AL can be differentiated radiologically from an inflammatory spondylodiscitis by the demonstration of a circumscribed defect in one or two neighboring vertebral bodies with varying degrees of narrowing of the intervening disc space, angular kyphosis of the affected spinal segment and an area of reactive sclerosis in the vertebral cancellous bone surrounding the defect. The spinal lesion can be confined to vertebral body (transvertebral), through the disk (transdiscal), or both (discovertebral).

Computed tomography (CT) imaging: CT is superior to radiographs in determining the extent of lesion. CT shows vertebral or discovertebral osteolysis with surrounding reactive sclerosis. Fracture of posterior elements and nonfusion of facet joints are also accurately demonstrated on CT. Axial images can provide information regarding extent of spinal stenosis.

MRI: MRI is considered best imaging modality with highest sensitivity. On T1-weighted images lesion show decreased intensity in disk space and vertebral bodies with increased signal intensity after enhancement with contrast medium. T2-weighted images show increased signal intensity. MR images provide additional information on anterior longitudinal ligament disruption, vertebral translation, abnormal dural enhancement, epidural lesions and spinal canal stenosis. It can also be used to differentiate from infectious spondylitis and primary or metastatic tumor.

Management

There are no clear-cut guidelines to approach AL. However, conservative management is first step in management. Conservative management includes rest, braces and anti-inflammatory medications. Though plaster immobilization in halo-jacket has been used, success is least likely and also duration of immobilization is ambiguous in literature. AL is more likely to heal in upper thoracic spine as the presence of an intact sternal–rib complex provides stability and might prevent kyphosis. This sternal–rib complex has been described as "the fourth column". At more mobile, cervical and thoracolumbar level, healing is less likely with conservative management. Healing is impaired even with plaster immobilization as the spine acts as fractured long bone with persistent motion at AL site. Medical management is in form of anti-inflammatory drugs. Newer therapy with biologics such as anti-TNF factor such as infliximab, etanercept and adalimumab are available. Exercise program advocated in AS is contraindicated after development of AL.

Surgical management is indicated in following situations: (1) neurological deficit, (2) instability threatening neurological deficit, and (3) progressively worsening pain and deformity. Surgical stabilization and fusion is the mainstay of management. In presence of neurological symptoms decompression is always indicated. Approach can be either anterior, posterior or combined anterior and posterior. Out of all these approach posterior approach is least morbid and is usually preffered. Long segment posterior stabilization is preferred because of poor bone quality due to osteoporosis compromising the bone holding capacity of screws **(Figs. 6A to E)**. Usually anterior procedure is not required as AS have good bone healing capability and lesion heal if stabilized adequately. If AL is associated with coexisting deformity then deformity correction can be done simultaneously.

Conclusion

A strong clinical suspicion helps in diagnosis of AL if there is change in nature of pain or rapid exacerbation of deformity. Radiological investigations aid diagnosis. Once AL is identified prompt management should be started such as to prevent neurological complication. Long segment posterior stabilization is the treatment of choice as bone heals well in AS because of good bone-forming capacity.

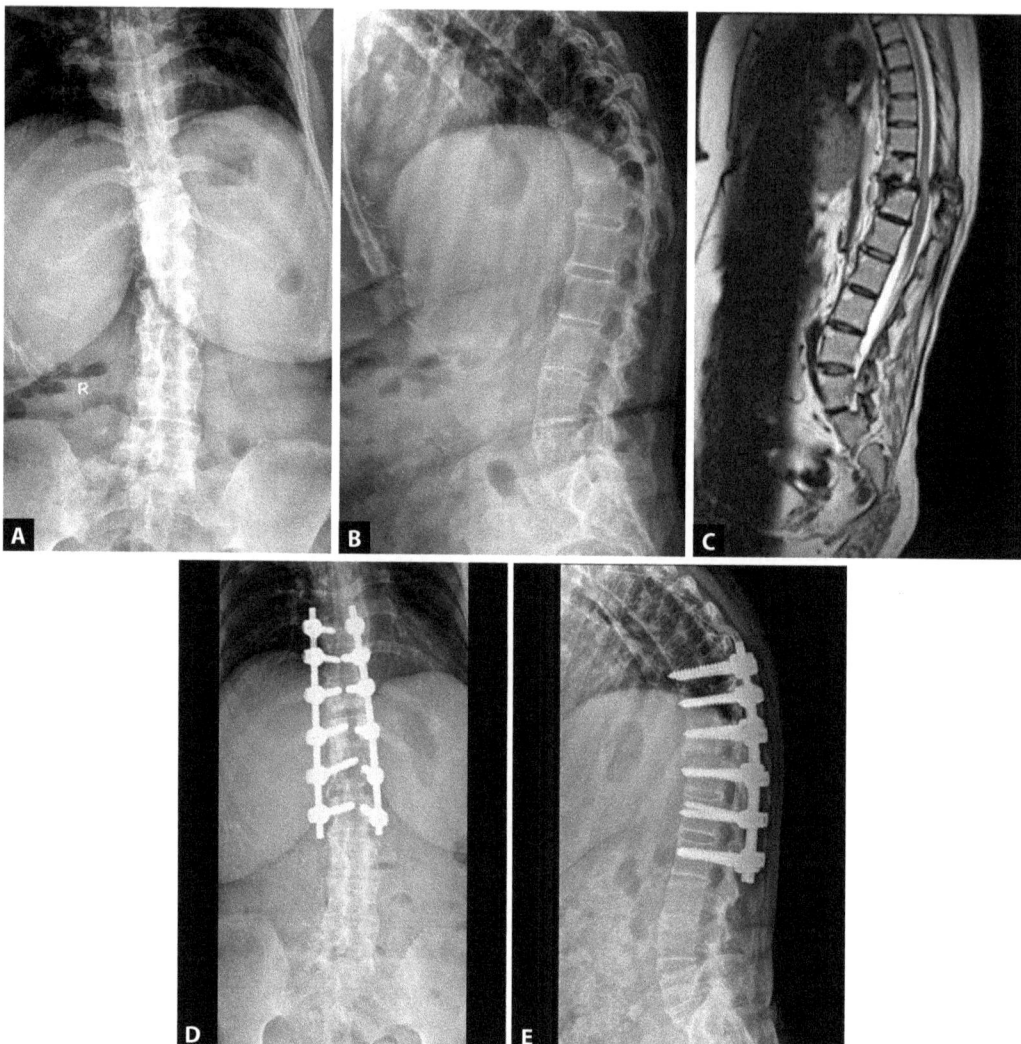

Figs. 6A to E: A 47-year-old female sustaining Andersson at T11-12. (A) Anteroposterior (AP) X-ray; (B) Lateral X-ray; (C) T2W-MRI; (D) AP X-ray after posterior stabilization; and (E) Lateral X-ray after posterior stabilization.

Spinal Fracture in Ankylosing Spondylitis

The inflammatory process in AS causes autofusion by ligamentous ossification and syndesmophytosis resulting in a classic "bamboo spine" which is stiff and brittle. Patients with AS have four times increased risk of spinal fracture and it can occur with even trivial trauma. The increased risk of spinal fracture is due to altered biomechanics and vertebral osteoporosis. Biomechanically, the rigid spine acts as continuous rigid axial support which is unable to dissipate energy even from trivial trauma. Susceptibility to fracture is further increased by impaired mobility, peripheral arthritis poor posture and impaired balance. There are basically two types of vertebral fracture, viz., compression fracture and three column injuries. Vertebral compression fracture leads to characteristic kyphotic deformity. The three column injuries though less are more clinically relevant.

Mechanism of injury: Majority of these fractures occur due to low-energy trauma. Hyperextension is most commonly observed mechanism of injury.

Site of injury: Lower cervical spine is most frequently involved followed by thoracolumbar junction. Factors such as small vertebral bodies, oblique articular facets, increased mobility and the mobility of the skull on it predispose lower cervical spine to fractures.

Transdiscal versus transvertebral fracture: Transdiscal fracture alone or in combination with transvertebral fracture is comparatively more common than isolated transvertebral fracture. Fracture through intervertebral disk is more common as it is the weakest part of ankylosed spine. Also these fractures extend through all three column of vertebral column rendering it to be unstable and susceptible to neurological deficit.

Neurological deficit: The incidence of neurological deficit in spinal fractures in AS patient has been reported up to 60%. AS patients with spinal fracture have 11 times increased risk of developing neurological deficit. This increased rate of neurological deficit may be attributed to overall increased risk of fracture and also some AS-specific cause. In AS, the ligaments are ossified, which gets fractured along with bone.

Therefore, they are not able to provide any structural support in a fractured AS spine. Fracture displacement can occur when a patient with deformity sustain fracture and he is strapped to a spine board causing hyperextension at fracture site, precipitating neurological deficit in patient who earlier had no deficit. Hematomas can be the cause of secondary neurological deficit. They occur in these patients because of bleeding from osteoporotic bone or from scarred epidural vessels adjacent to a fracture.

Radiography

Plain X-ray: Plain radiographs can be used as screening tool, but it is neither sensitive nor specific. The most common site of fracture, i.e., lower cervical spine is poorly visualized because of shoulder girdle overlap. Plain radiographs misses fracture because of abnormal spinal structure due to ossified ligaments, surrounding osseous growth, osteoporosis and poor outlining of disk space.

CT scan: It is the investigation of choice. CT requires a shorter scanning time and better bony details are available for surgical planning. The location of fracture as well as fracture morphology can be seen. Transdiscal fracture is seen as widening of intervertebral disk whereas fracture through vertebral body is seen as lucency.

MRI: MRI is superior to CT in showing better soft tissue details, bone marrow, and spinal cord. Whenever spinal cord injury is present, MRI is warranted as it readily identifies epidural hematoma, any other extradural compression or cord edema. It can also differentiate acute fracture from old fracture. Disadvantage is its time taking and difficult to get patient with deformity inside gantry.

Treatment: Treatment starts at site of injury. As soon as fracture is suspected in a patient of AS, patient should be immobilized in position of comfort according to deformity present. Patient should not be stabilized on standard spine board which is flat. Such positioning causes hyperextension at fracture site and neurological deficit may develop. If a patient is awake he may guide positioning according to his comfort. Preferably the patient should be initially immobilized in a halo vest in the preinjury alignment. Management of these fractures are challenging because of increased risk of displacement and precipitation of neurological deficit. Also management is complicated by associated comorbidities. Undisplaced or minimally displaced fracture can be managed conservatively. But as we know, these fractures are highly unstable three columnar injury with propensity for neurological deterioration, surgical management with long fixation and fusion is preferred.

Nonoperative Management

Nonoperative management consists of halo vest application and external orthosis. They can be advised in nondisplaced fractures. But there are many factors because of which nonoperative management is not ideal. External orthosis are difficult to apply because of associated deformities. Poorly fitted orthosis can force spine to lose its preinjury alignment and cause neurological deficit. These fractures are three column unstable injury with high probability of fracture displacement. Undisplaced fracture gets displaced because of long lever arm of fractured segment and fulcrum at fracture site. Because of this rate of nonunion is also increased. Studies show that the rate of complication as well as mortality is more in conservatively managed patient compared to surgical management.

Operative management: Surgical management should be the choice of management in unstable fractures. Necessary preoperative planning is very important. Awake fiberoptic nasotracheal intubation assisted general anesthesia is standard of care. Precautions should be taken during positioning. Whenever available neuromonitoring to be used to prevent new neurological deficit.

Cervical spine fracture: Two factors need to be considered while deciding fixation of spinal fracture in ankylosing spondylitis. First the long lever arm acting at fracture site and associated osteoporosis. Therefore, isolated anterior fixation is biomechanically weak and therefore posterior only or combined posteroanterior fixation to be considered. The choice of fixation can be arrived upon by determining if fracture is transdiscal or transcorporeal.

In transdiscal fracture endplates are intact and good bony apposition is possible. In such cases, only posterior fixation with three levels of fixation above and below fracture segment should be done. Distally fixation should not end at cervicothoracic junction. In such cases, fixation should extend to thoracic segment.

In transcorporeal fracture as the fracture passes through the cancellous bone of body of vertebra, there is tendency for body to collapse and create an anterior bony gap **(Figs. 7A to F)**. Major gaps need to be reconstructed anteriorly especially at cervicothoracic junction. Minor gap of anterior column are likely to heal with posterior fixation alone. Whenever needed anterior surgery is not simple because of associated cervical deformity which makes access difficult.

Thoracolumbar fractures: Posterior long segment fixation with pedicle screws (three to four segments) fixation above and below fracture is used. There is always chance of fracture site opening. This is prevented by adequate positioning with help of bolsters avoiding lordosing frame (Jackson frame). If anterior fracture gap remains after posterior fixation and is significant then anterior approach bone grafting is advisable. The role of laminectomy is controversial in patients with intact neurological symptoms. They add to instability and decrease fusion bed area **(Figs. 8A to E)**. Some surgeon

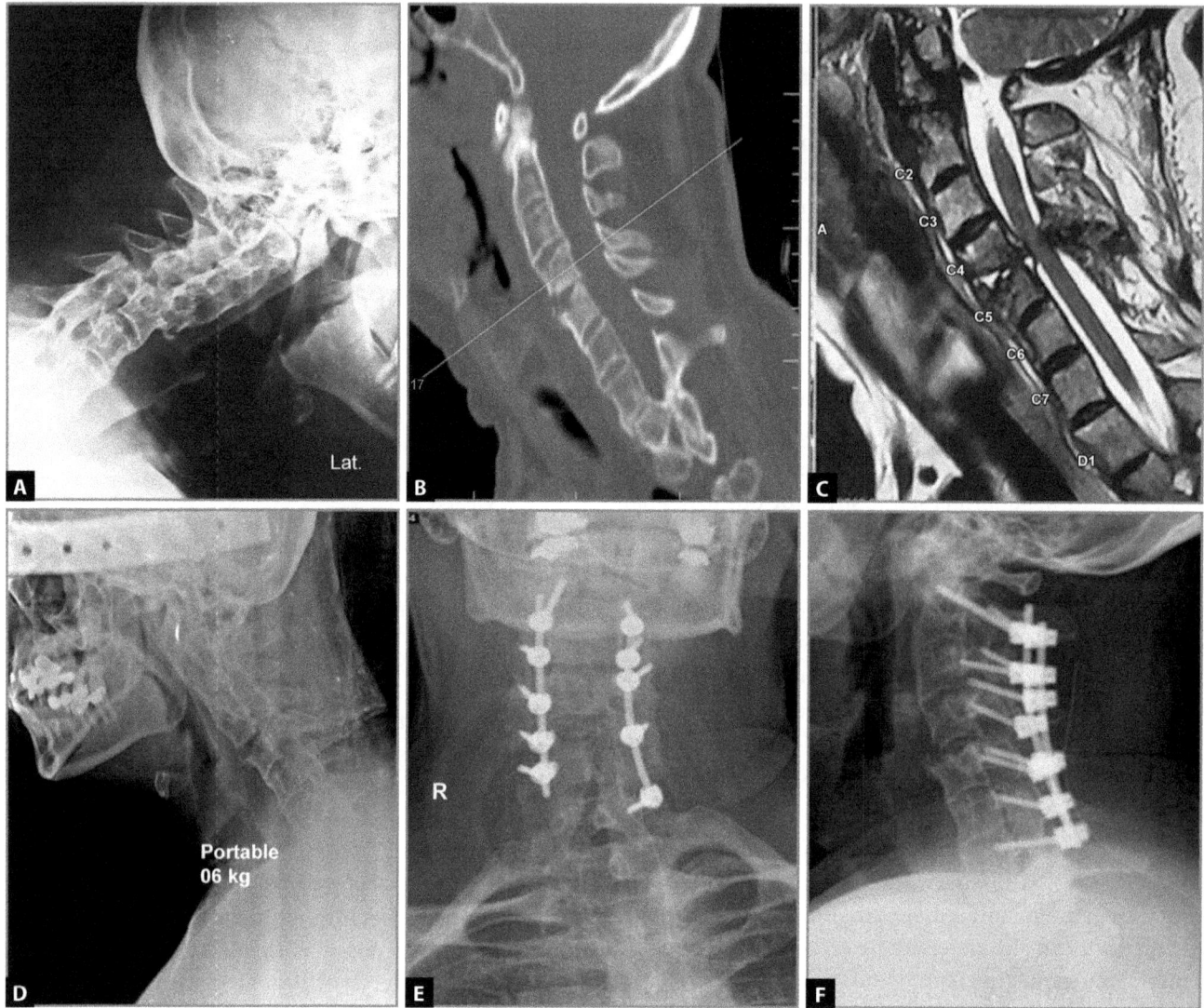

Figs. 7A to F: A 48-year-old male sustaining transdiscal fracture at C4-C5 level. (A) X-ray; (B) CT-scan; (C) T2-MRI; (D) Postreduction X-ray with Halo; (E and F) Postoperative X-ray after lateral mass fixation.

routinely advise as it provides should decompression should epidural hematoma develop.

Complications: The complication rate in fracture in ankylosing spondylitis patient is more than spinal fracture in general population. The complications described are pseudarthrosis, neurological deficit, deep venous thrombosis with pulmonary embolism and pneumonia. Aortic dissection, aortic pseudoaneurysm and tracheal rupture are potentially lethal complication which has been reported. The rate of complication and mortality in ankylosing spondylitis is more in conservatively managed patient compared to surgically managed patient.

Conclusion: Fracture in ankylosing spondylitis is unstable with high risk of neurological deficit. The complication rate in conservatively managed patient is more than surgically managed patient. In consideration with above surgical management, long posterior fixation is the choice of management.

ANESTHETIC IMPLICATIONS

The anesthesiologist should review the anesthetic plan based on extent of disease focused in four main aspects: extent of upper airway involvement, pulmonary restrictive pathology, extent of cardiac dysfunction, and access to the neuroaxis.

The range of movements of all joints should be evaluated to minimize damage during positioning of the patient. The preoperative investigations are ordered as per the severity of the disease including lung function tests, imaging of the cervical spine and arterial blood gas analysis. The potential for conduction defects mandates an electrocardiogram (ECG). An echocardiogram is required to assess the severity of the valvular disease associated with AS.

There is no clear consensus regarding the management of anti-TNFα blockers in the perioperative period. The Dutch Society for Rheumatology advocated stopping the anti-TNFα about 4.5 times the half-life of the medication prior to surgery in view of increased risk of bacterial infections in

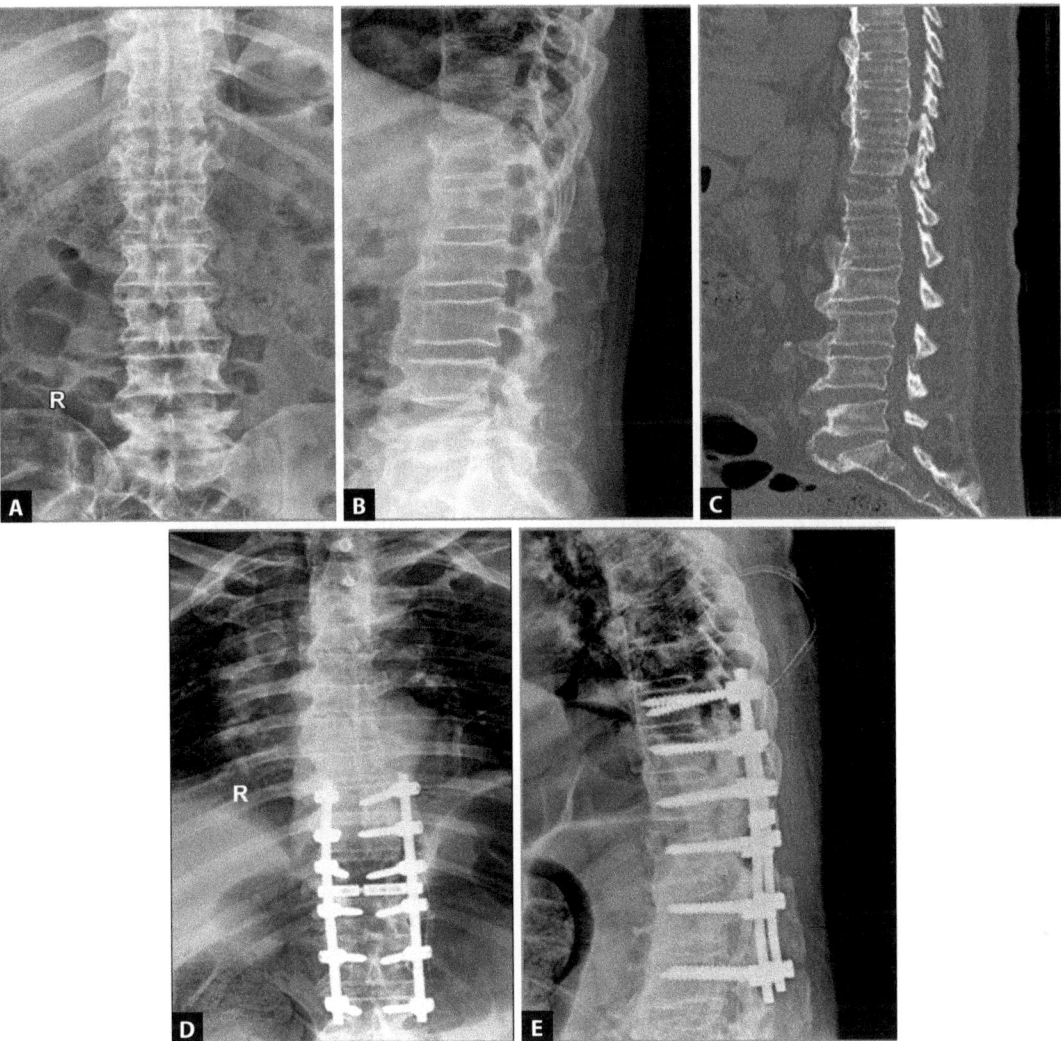

Figs. 8A to E: A 53-year-old male sustaining T11-T12 sustaining transdiscal fracture. (A) Anteroposterior X-ray; (B) Lateral X-ray; (C) CT scan; (D and E) X-ray images after posterior stabilization T9-L2.

the postoperative period. This recommendation is under debate. Prospective studies are needed to address this issue.

Respiratory insufficiency and limitation of chest expansion increase the incidence of pulmonary complications and the need for mechanical ventilation in the intensive care unit (ICU). The hypotension associated with spinal anesthesia is poorly tolerated in patients with defects in aortic valve, hence better avoided. External cardiac massage may be ineffective in a patient with rigid thoracic wall. X-ray of lumbar spine is useful to evaluate the feasibility of subarachnoid block. Nevertheless, neuroaxis blocks are technically difficult owing to decreased articular flexibility and ossification of interspinal spaces. These difficulties concomitantly increase the risk of complications, viz., spinal cord hematoma postepidural anesthesia as well as accidental intraosseous injection in caudal anesthesia precipitating seizures.

Precautionary steps should be undertaken for gastric protection due to rampant use of NSAIDs in patients of AS. Physiological changes of pregnancy in a patient with disease manifestations of AS render anesthesia administration more challenging. AS with accentuated kyphoscoliosis and rigidity is a relative contraindication for videolaparoscopic abdominothoracic surgery.

AIRWAY MANAGEMENT

Functional limitation of range of movement of neck in flexion hinders tracheal intubation compounded further when temporomandibular joint is involved. Evaluation of neck mobility, X-rays of cervical spine lateral and in maximal extension is mandatory. The criteria that predict difficult airways, viz. Mallampati grading, Wilson index, thyromental distance, sternomental distance, and mouth opening should be reviewed. Cricoarytenoid arthritis with dyspnea, stridor and fixation of the vocal cords may rarely occur. Preoperative indirect laryngoscopy can be helpful in assessing difficult intubation in affected cases. Excessive neck extension in the presence of chronic cervical kyphosis increases the risk of neurological injury. Bony encroachments on the vertebral artery may predispose vertebrobasilar insufficiency during extension of neck. Iatrogenic injuries during emergency intubation include dislocation of C6 vertebra and quadriparesis. Fixed flexion deformities render tracheostomy treacherous. Neck supports under anesthesia are advocated and forcible movements under neuromuscular blockade prohibited.

Awake fiberoptic intubation (AFOI) is the safest option, whence on indirect laryngoscopy larynx is not visualized or in the presence of chin on chest deformity. AFOI is aided with instillation of local anesthetic in the mucous membrane, infiltration of the superior laryngeal nerves, and transcricothyroid instillation of local anesthetic. Retrograde intubation is another possible option if fiberoptic intubating scope is not available. Patients with severe flexion deformities make laryngeal mask airway (LMA) a difficult proposition as the angle of oropharynx axis may kink the LMA and obstruct positioning over trachea. The intubating laryngeal mask (ILM) may be a useful device in such patients. However, mouth opening of <1.2 cm or presence of fixed extension deformity or large cervical osteophytes preclude the use of LMA. Videolayngoscope can be useful for improved visualization of the larynx and facilitate nasotracheal intubation in patients of AS.

FURTHER READING

1. Alaranta H, Luoto S, Konttinen YT. Traumatic spinal cord injury as a complication to ankylosing spondylitis. An extended report. Clin Exp Rheumatol. 2002;20(1):66-8.
2. Baek HJ, Shin KC, Lee YJ, Kang SW, Lee EB, Yoo CD, et al. Clinical features of adult-onset ankylosing spondylitis in Korean patients: patients with peripheral joint disease (PJD) have less severe spinal disease course than those without PJD. Rheumatology (Oxford). 2004;43(12):1526-31.
3. Ball J. Enthesopathy of rheumatoid and ankylosing spondylitis. Ann Rheum Dis. 1971;30(3):213-23.
4. Bok DH, Kim J, Kim TH. Comparison of MRI-defined back muscles volume between patients with ankylosing spondylitis and control patients with chronic back pain: age and spinopelvic alignment matched study. Eur Spine J. 2017;26(2):528-37.
5. Braun J, Sieper J. Ankylosing spondylitis. Lancet. 2007; 369:1379-90.
6. Bridwell KH, DeWald RL. The Textbook of Spinal Surgery, 3rd edition. Philadelphia: Lippincott Williams and Wilkins; 2011. pp. 1343.
7. Bron JL, de Vries MK, Snieders MN, van der Horst-Bruinsma IE, van Royen BJ. Discovertebral (Andersson) lesions of the spine in ankylosing spondylitis revisited. Clin Rheumatol. 2009;28:883-92.
8. Calin A, Robertson D. Spondylodiscitis and pseudarthrosis in a patient with enteropathic spondyloarthropathy. Ann Rheum Dis. 1991;50:117-9.
9. Campagna R, Pessis E, Feydy A, Guerini H, Thévenin F, Chevrot A, et al. Fractures of the ankylosed spine: MDCT and MRI with emphasis on individual anatomic spinal structures. Am J Roentgenol. 2009; 192(4):987-95.
10. Cawley MI, Chalmers TM, Kellgren JH, Ball J. Destructive lesions of vertebral bodies in ankylosing spondylitis. Ann Rheum Dis. 1972;31(5):345-58.
11. Chan FL, Ho EK, Fang D, Hsu LC, Leong JC, Ngan H. Spinal pseudarthrosis in ankylosing spondylitis. Acta Radiol. 1987;28(4):383-8.
12. Chang KW, Tu MY, Huang HH, Chen HC, Chen YY, Lin CC. Posterior correction and fixation without anterior fusion for pseudoarthrosis with kyphotic deformity in ankylosing spondylitis. Spine (Phila Pa 1976). 2006;31:E408-13.
13. Chhabra HS. Management of Spine Fractures. New Delhi: Wolters Kluwer; 2015.
14. Detwiler KN, Loftus CM, Godersky JC, Menezes AH. Management of cervical spine injuries in patients with ankylosing spondylitis. J Neurosurg. 1990;72(2):210-5.
15. Dihlmann W, Delling G. Disco-vertebral destructive lesions (so-called Andersson lesions) associated with ankylosing spondylitis. Skeletal Radiol. 1978;3:10-6.
16. Finkelstein JA, Chapman JR, Mirza S. Occult vertebral fractures in ankylosing spondylitis. Spinal Cord. 1999;37(6):444-7.
17. Fox MW, Onofrio BM, Kilgore JE. Neurological complications of ankylosing spondylitis. J Neurosurg. 1993;78(6):871-8.
18. Hehne HJ, Zielke K, Böhm H. Polysegmental lumbar osteotomies and transpedicled fixation for correction of long-curved kyphotic deformities in ankylosing spondylitis. Report on 177 cases. Clin Orthop Relat Res. 1990;258:49-55.
19. Kanter AS, Wang MY, Mummaneni PV. A treatment algorithm for the management of cervical spine fractures and deformity in patients with ankylosing spondylitis. Neurosurg Focus. 2008;24(1):E11.
20. Kouyoumdjian P, Guerin P, Schaelderle C, Asencio G, Gille O. Fracture of the lower cervical spine in patients with ankylosing spondylitis: retrospective study of 19 cases. Orthop Traumatol Surg Res. 2012;98(5):543.
21. Lafage R, Ferrero E, Henry JK, Challier V, Diebo B, Liabaud B, et al. Validation of a new computer-assisted tool to measure spino-pelvic parameters. Spine J. 2015;15(12): 2493-502.
22. Lai HY, Chen IH, Chen A, Hwang FY, Lee Y. The use of the Glidescope for tracheal intubation in patients with Ankylosis Spondylitis. Br J Anaesth. 2006;97:419-22.
23. Langlois S, Cedoz JP, Lohse A, Toussirot E, Wendling D. Aseptic discitis in patients with ankylosing spondylitis: a retrospective study of 14 cases. Jt Bone Spine. 2015;72(3):248-5.
24. Leone A, Marino M, Dell'Atti C, Zecchi V, Magarelli N, Colosimo C. Spinal fractures in patients with ankylosing spondylitis. Rheumatol Int. 2016;36(10):1335-46.
25. Liu H, Yang C, Zheng Z, Ding W, Wang J, Wang H, et al. Comparison of Smith-Petersen osteotomy and pedicle subtraction osteotomy for the correction of thoracolumbar kyphotic deformity in ankylosing spondylitis: a systematic review and meta-analysis. Spine. 2015;40(8):570-9.
26. Mountney J, Murphy AJ, Fowler JL. Lessons learned from cervical pseudoarthrosis in ankylosing spondylitis. Eur Spine J. 2005;14: 689-93.
27. Mullaji AB, Upadhyay SS, Ho EKW. Bone mineral density in ankylosing spondylitis. J Bone Joint Surg. 1994;76B:660-5.
28. Nederlandse Verenigingvoor Reumatologie. Medicijnen: Hettoepassen van TNF blockade in debehandling van reumatoide arteritis. Dutch Society for Rheumatology; 2003.
29. Obradov M, Schonfeld DH, Franssen MJ, de Rooy DJ. Andersson lesion in ankylosing spondylitis. JBR-BTR 2001; 84(2):71.
30. Popitz MD. Anesthetic implications of chronic disease of the cervical spine. Anesth Analg. 1997;84:672-83.

15 Other Spondyloarthropathies

Bhaskar Borgohain, Kashif A Ahmed, Shantanu Lahkar

INTRODUCTION

It is comprehensible that seronegative spondyloarthropathies (SpA) are a group of overlapping disorders and they share certain clinical and genetic relationship. Traditionally these spondyloarthropathies are considered as "seronegative" because serological antibody markers are absent. Instead it is classical to find familial tendencies, frequent positive association with HLA-B27, asymmetrical oligoarthritis with enthesitis, axial spondylitis and sacroiliitis. However, extra-articular manifestations like rheumatoid nodules are absent. Uveitis are not uncommon though. Unlike rheumatoid arthritis, these group of arthropathies have a male preponderance except for psoriatic arthritis which is equally distributed between males and females.

JUVENILE ANKYLOSING SPONDYLITIS

Onset of symptoms in juvenile ankylosing spondylitis may occur before 16 years of age in a small minority (10–20% of all cases). A male to female ratio of 3:1 in this age group is noteworthy. Enthesitis is the most prominent early finding and often described under enthesitis-related arthritis (ERA). However, spinal symptoms or restriction of joint motion may not be obvious for years. Asymmetrical peripheral oligoarthritis, especially involving joints of the lower limbs and dactylitis are common. Systemic manifestations (fever, weight loss, anemia, and leukocytosis) tend to occur at the onset of the disease. Extra-articular manifestations are usually absent.

In juvenile ankylosing spondylitis, it is unusual to find any radiological findings in spine or sacroiliac joints (SI) initially. Hence, making a definitive diagnosis of juvenile ankylosing spondylitis in children may be quite challenging. Therefore, the presence of HLA-B27 is supportive of a diagnosis. Familial juvenile form of ankylosing spondylitis with a positive HLA-B27 report may regrettably progress to classical adult AS form with age.

Some children with pre-radiographic stage of classic spondyloarthropathy with back pain but not fulfilling the classical criteria of juvenile ankylosing spondylitis, are considered to be undifferentiated SpA (USpA). Most USpAs have fewer extra-articular manifestations. Even sacroiliitis or spondylitis tends to be very mild or absent despite years of active disease. Only MRI may pick up the mild unilateral and more rarely bilateral sacroiliac joint involvement in USpA.

Treatment of juvenile ankylosing spondylitis involves nonsteroidal anti-inflammatory drugs (NSAIDs), disease-modifying anti-rheumatic drugs (DMARDs), biologics, and intra-articular and oral glucocorticoids taking into consideration comorbidities and patient values and preferences. However, the DMARDs are unlikely to resolve the spinal component of the disease.

PSORIATIC ARTHRITIS

Psoriasis is an autoimmune disorder primarily involving the skin. However, psoriatic arthritis (PsA) does occur in about 15% of patients with psoriasis. The exact etiology is unknown but it is likely that the immune system is activated in such a pattern that it results in production of antibodies that attacks the joints in return. Arthritis usually occurs a decade after onset of skin psoriasis. However, in a small minority, arthritis may precede skin lesions. PsA is often a chronic arthritis and can affect any joint. Symptoms may vary from person to person. Clinical psoriatic arthritis may range from mild occasional flare ups to persistent joint inflammation leading to serious joint damage.

Psoriatic arthritis is usually diagnosed between 30 and 50 years of age, but it can begin as early as childhood. Men and women are equally at risk of developing psoriatic arthritis. Patients presenting with joint manifestations before the skin lesions can make the diagnosis a difficult one. Psoriatic arthritis may easily be confused with other diseases, often leading to misdiagnoses as gout, rheumatoid arthritis or even osteoarthritis. Fatigue and anemia are common in patients of psoriatic arthritis. Notably, children with psoriatic arthropathy are at risk of developing uveitis and this must not be missed.

Psoriatic arthritis may affect any of the joints of the skeleton, often presenting as symmetrical polyarthritis or asymmetrical oligoarthritis. Distal interphalangeal joint (DIPJ) involvement is classical of psoriatic arthropathy;

making it distinct from rheumatoid arthritis. The affected fingers and toes often get deformed and appear to be like swollen sausages. This condition is referred to as dactylitis. Finger and toe nail dystrophy (onycholysis or pitting with erythematous border) are often clinically evident. PsA may involve the spine (psoriatic spondylitis) as well.

Enthesitis is a typical hallmark of psoriatic arthritis. Psoriatic enthesitis can cause pain at insertion sites of tendons, for instance at the back of the heel achillies tendonitis. Such enthesitis may occur in the sole of the foot, around the elbows or in any other areas of the body producing corresponding pain. About 40% of the psoriatic arthritis patients may have family history of psoriasis or arthritis, suggesting possible influence of heredity. Psoriatic arthritis may be triggered by infection mediated immune activation, e.g., following streptococcal sore throat. Just like its skin counterpart psoriatic arthritis can have lifelong chronicity with bouts of wax and wane of the disease. The presentation of this disease can vary from person to person and can also affect different locations in the same body over time.

A clinical diagnosis of psoriatic arthritis is based on involvement of swollen joints with associated skin and nail changes. The *CASPAR* criteria (*classification criteria for psoriatic arthritis*) has been popular for making a clinical diagnosis reliable **(Table 1)**. The CASPAR criteria for the diagnosis of PsA are found to be simple and highly specific (99%) but a bit less sensitive (91%) than the Vasey and Espinoza criteria.

Radiological investigations are required to assess the degree of joint involvement. Presence of asymmetrical sacroiliitis and fewer syndesmophytes are considered classical. Shortening of the digits (called telescoping) are not uncommon. A classical case may involve the DIPJ leading to a "pencil in cup deformity" in radiographs. Various signs of enthesitis, periostitis, osteolysis, dactylitis, juxta-articular new bone formation or small joint ankylosis can be seen. In order to rule out common arthritis like gout and rheumatoid arthritis blood investigations can be done. In patients with psoriatic arthritis, blood tests may reveal high ESR and mild anemia. In extensive psoriasis serum uric acid may be elevated. Rarely anti CCP antibody may be positive. Occasionally skin biopsies are needed to confirm the diagnosis of psoriasis.

Early diagnosis of PsA is important to avoid damage to joints. The disease is practically treated in the same line as ankylosing spondylitis. Hydroxychloroquine (HCQS) is usually avoided as it can cause a flare of psoriasis. Fortunately treatments are effective for most people. Physical activity helps maintain joint movement. Treatment also largely depends on the number of joints involved as well as the severity of symptoms. In mild diseases only NSAIDs for joint pain and topical applications for skin lesions are required. In resistant cases Methotrexate (MTX) and TNF inhibitors (TNFi) are found to be effective. Surgery is reserved for joint salvage.

REACTIVE ARTHRITIS (REITER'S SYNDROME)

Reactive arthritis as the name suggests is a condition that occurs as a reaction to an infection in the body. It is also referred to as Reiter's syndrome. Usually genitourinary or sexually transmitted infections like that of *Chlamydia trachomatis* can predispose to this condition. Many a times gastrointestinal infections caused by *Salmonella* contaminated foods can also lead to this type of arthritis and is referred to as gastrointestinal Reiter's syndrome. Reactive arthritis is characterized by asymmetrical inflamed large joints and affects mostly young men, between the ages of 20 and 40 years. About 80% of people with the tendency to develop this disease have the special gene marker HLA-B27.

Reactive arthritis basically manifests as a classical triad of arthritic symptoms, urinary tract symptoms and conjunctivitis. Symptoms typically last 3–12 months, but may develop into chronic disease in a small percentage of people. However, each individual may experience symptoms differently. Symptoms may include: Joint pain and inflammation that often affect the knees, feet, and ankles, enthesopathy, which may cause heel pain or the shortening and thickening of the fingers, heel spurs, spondylitis and sacroiliitis. Nonarthritic symptoms in men are increased urinary output, burning micturition, urethral discharge and prostatitis. In women, there may be inflamed cervix, inflamed urethra, causing a burning micturition, salpingitis and vulvovaginitis. Ocular symptoms such as red eyes, painful and irritated eyes blurry vision, conjunctivitis and uveitis.

Reactive arthritis is a clinical diagnosis and hence can be confirmed based on medical history and symptomatology. There is a need to rule out other clinical conditions, such as rheumatoid arthritis and lupus. Other tests may include: X-ray to look for spondylitis, sacroiliitis or damage to the joint, raised ESR and tests for bacterial infections like *Chlamydia* in urine and Salmonella in stool samples and synovial fluid analysis after an arthrocentesis.

TABLE 1: The *CASPAR* criteria (*classification criteria for psoriatic arthritis*).

Criteria	Point value
Skin psoriasis:	
• Present	2
• Previously present	1
• Family history (if patient not affected)	1
Nail lesion (onycholysis, pitting, hyperkeratosis)	1
Dactylitis (present or past with documentation by rheumatologist)	1
Negative rheumatoid factor	1
Juxta-articular new bone formation on radiograph	1

Specific treatment for reactive arthritis usually includes antibiotics to treat the infection that is causing the reactive arthritis symptoms. Treatment involves NSAIDs for mild early disease. Rest to reduce pain and inflammation and exercise to strengthen muscles and improve joint function are essential. Corticosteroids may be used to reduce inflammation. Immunosuppressive medications, such as MTX to suppress inflammation is reserved for in more serious or chronic disease.

ENTEROPATHIC ARTHRITIS: INFLAMMATORY BOWEL DISEASE-ASSOCIATED ARTHROPATHY

Inflammatory bowel disease-associated arthropathy is considered a subtype of seronegative SpA. It can present with axial or peripheral arthropathy. Peripheral arthritis has found to be non-erosive and the oligoarticular variant has been strongly associated with intestinal manifestations. However, axial arthritis is less likely to have intestinal complaints and patient can present with inflammatory back pain (spondylitis or sacroiliitis). HLA-B27 is associated with the axial form of the disease.

While there have been advances in identifying predisposing genetic factors and in elucidating pathophysiology of inflammatory bowel disease (IBD), the mechanisms surrounding the development of arthritis in IBD remain unclear.

Treatment of IBD is not always sufficient for control of arthritis. Oligoarticular peripheral arthritis usually parallel the course of IBD, treatment of IBD may resolve this type of arthritis.

Axial and polyarticular arthritis need special attention during treatment as it is not dependent on intestinal disease activity of IBD. While treatment with biologic agents is promising, there is no current optimal therapy of IBD-associated arthropathy. In IBD associated arthropathy the role of hydroxychloroquine and azathioprine is doubtful.

Immunomodulatory therapy is indicated in patients with peripheral manifestations like dactylitis and enthesitis. Sulfasalazine may be effective in treating peripheral arthritis and has activity for ulcerative colitis bowel inflammation, although it is not particularly effective for axial disease. MTX has been found to be useful in coeliac disease rather than in ulcerative colitis. TNFi have been found to be effective for IBD patients who are steroid dependent or refractory to conventional treatment. Presently the best anti-TNF therapy in IBD is Infliximab.

FURTHER READING

1. American College of Rheumatology. Psoriatic Arthritis. [online] Available from www.rheumatology.org/Practice/Clinical/Patients/Diseases_And_Conditions/Psoriatic_Arthritis. [Last accessed June, 2021]
2. Arvikar SL, Fisher MC. Inflammatory bowel disease associated arthropathy. Curr Rev Musculoskelet Med. 2011;4(3):123-31.
3. Johns Hopkins Medicine. Reactive Arthritis (Reiter's Syndrome). [online]. Available from: www.hopkinsmedicine.org/health library/conditions/arthritis and other rheumatic diseases/reactive_arthritis_reiters_syndrome 85,P00064 [Last accessed June, 2015]
4. Maksymowych WP, Inman RD, Gladman D, et al. Spondyloarthritis Research Consortium of Canada (SPARCC): Canadian Rheumatology Association Consensus on the use of anti-tumor necrosis factor-alpha directed therapies in the treatment of spondyloarthritis. J Rheumatol. 2003;30:1356-63.
5. National Institute of Arthritis and Musculoskeletal and Skin Diseases. [online] Available from www.niams.nih.gov [Last accessed June, 2021]
6. Taylor W, Gladman D, Helliwell P, Marchesoni A, Mease P, Mielants H. Classification Criteria for Psoriatic Arthritis: Development of New Criteria from a Large International Study. Arthritis and Rheumatism. 2006;54(8):2665-73.
7. Zochling J, van der Heijde D, Dougados M, et al. Current evidence for the management of ankylosing spondylitis: a systemic literature review of the ASAS/EULAR management recommendations in ankylosing spondylitis. Ann Rheum Dis. 2006;65:423-32.

SECTION 4

Crystal-induced Inflammation, Disorders of Cartilage and Bone in Orthopedic Rheumatology

- **Crystal Deposition Disorders**
  Omkarnath Gudapati
- **Osteoarthritis: Etiology, Pathogenesis, and Management**
  Venus Khanna, Manju Agrawal, Alok Chandra Agrawal
- **Osteoporosis**
  SS Jha, Lalit Kishore
- **Osteomalacia**
  SS Jha, Rahul Ranjan
- **Paget's Disease of Bone**
  SS Jha, Rahul Ranjan

16 Crystal Deposition Disorders

Omkarnath Gudapati

INTRODUCTION

Polarizing light microscopy used during synovial fluid analysis in 1961 by McCarty and Hollander, and subsequent application of other crystallographic techniques, such as electron microscopy, energy-dispersive elemental analysis, and X-ray diffraction, have allowed to identify the roles of different microcrystals, including monosodium urate (MSU), calcium pyrophosphate dihydrate (CPPD), calcium hydroxyapatite (apatite), and calcium oxalate (CaOx), in inducing acute or chronic arthritis or periarthritis **(Fig. 1)**.

Endogenous crystals shown to be pathogenic include monosodium urate (gout), CPPD, and basic calcium phosphate (hydroxyapatite). Exogenous crystals, such as corticosteroid ester crystals and talcum, and the biomaterials such as polyethylene and methyl methacrylate, may also induce joint disease. Silicone, polyethylene, and methyl methacrylate are used in prosthetic joints, and their debris that accumulates with long use and wear-tear may result in local arthritis and failure of the prosthesis. Endogenous and exogenous crystals produce disease by triggering the cascade that results in cytokine-mediated cartilage destruction. The possible musculoskeletal manifestations of crystal-induced arthritis are listed in **Tables 1 and 2**.

GOUT

Man is the only mammal to spontaneously develop hyperuricemia and gout, as only humans lack uricase, the enzyme responsible for the degradation of uric acid in other mammals. This, in combination with a high reabsorption rate of filtered urate, predisposes humans to hyperuricemia and gout, which is the common end point of a group of disorders that produce hyperuricemia.

Definition

Gout is a disorder of purine metabolism characterized by hyperuricemia, deposition of MSU crystals in joints and periarticular tissues and recurrent attacks of acute synovitis. Such deposits are commonly known as *tophi*. Late changes include cartilage degeneration resulting in a painful gouty arthritis, renal dysfunction, and uric acid urolithiasis.

Fig. 1: Sites of hand or wrist involvement in various arthritis. (CMC: carpometacarpal; DIP: distal interphalangeal; MCP: metacarpophalangeal; OA: osteoarthritis; PIP: proximal interphalangeal; RA: rheumatoid arthritis; SLE: systemic lupus erythematosus)

TABLE 1: Classification of crystal-induced arthritis.

Endogenous crystals	Exogenous crystals
• Monosodium urate (MSU)	• Corticosteroid ester crystals
• Calcium pyrophosphate dehydrate (CPPD)	• Cholesterol crystals
	• Talcum
• Basic calcium phosphate (hydroxyapatite)	• Polyethylene
	• Silicone
• Calcium oxalate (CaOx)	• Methyl methacrylate

TABLE 2: Musculoskeletal manifestations of crystal-induced arthritis.

• Acute mono- or polyarthritis	• Destructive arthropathies
• Bursitis	• Pseudorheumatoid arthritis
• Tendinitis	• Pseudoankylosing spondylitis
• Enthesitis	• Spinal stenosis
• Tophaceous deposits	• Crowned dens syndrome
• Peculiar type of osteoarthritis	• Carpal tunnel syndrome
• Synovial osteochondromatosis	• Tendon rupture

Historical Milestones

The term "gout", derived from the Latin "gutta" (drop), was introduced in the 13th century AD, and points to the belief that a poison falling drop by drop into the joint causes the disease.

- Early best description can be found in the works of Hippocrates.
- In 1st century AD, Seneca mentioned the familial nature of gout.
- In 3rd century AD, Galen described the tophi.
- In 1679, Van Leeuwenhoek was the first identified crystals microscopically in a tophus.
- In 1683, Sydenham gave the description of the classic symptoms of acute attack.
- In 1774, Scheele discovered uric acid.
- In 1797, Wollaston demonstrated uric acid in Tophi.
- In 1859, Garrod described "thread test" (the amount of uric acid is increased in the blood of gouty patients).
- In 1896, Huber reported the radiological description.
- In 1899, His and Freudweiler showed that injected synthetic MSUM crystals induce inflammatory response.
- In 1913, Folin and Danis described the measurement of serum urate concentration.
- In 1936, Cohen described efficacious use of colchicine.
- In 1950, Talbot, Gutman and Yu demonstrated uricosuric effect of probenecid.
- In 1961, McCarty and Hollander, first reported constant presence of monosodium urate monohydrate (MSUM) crystals in gouty joint fluid.
- In 1963, Hitchings and Elion described the usefulness of allopurinol, a xanthine oxidase inhibitor in role of gout.
- In 2003, Bosly et al., Rasburicase has been shown to lower urate levels more effectively than allopurinol.
- In 2009, Pascual et al., Febuxostat is a novel xanthine oxidase inhibitor that was recently approved for the treatment of hyperuricemia in patients with gout.

Disorders of Purine Metabolism: Hyperuricemia and Gout

Humans convert adenosine and guanosine to uric acid. Adenosine is first converted to inosine by adenosine deaminase. In mammals other than higher primates, uricase converts uric acid to the water-soluble product allantoin. Due to lack of uricase in humans, the end product of purine catabolism is uric acid. Gout is a metabolic disorder of purine catabolism. Gout is caused by excess of uric acid. Hyperuricemia can result from increased production or decreased excretion of uric acid or from a combination of the two processes. Sustained hyperuricemia clinical manifestations including gouty arthritis urolithiasis, and renal dysfunction are shown in **Figure 2**.

Hyperuricemia is defined as plasma (or serum) urate concentration >405 μmol/L (6.8 mg/dL). The risk of developing gouty arthritis or urolithiasis increases with higher urate levels. Causes of hyperuricemia are described in **Table 3**.

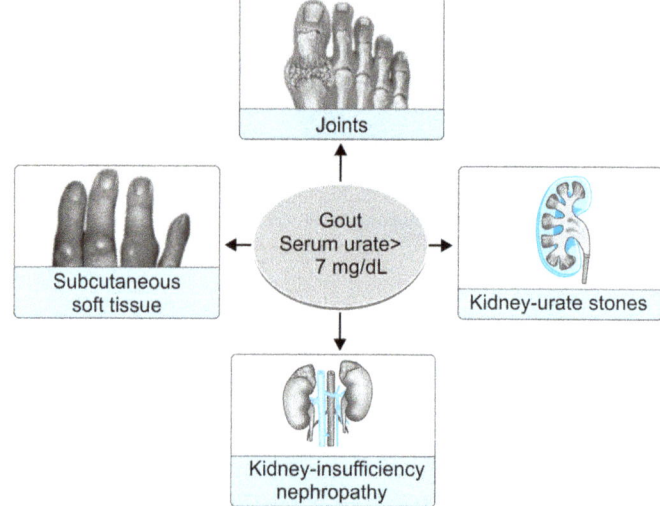

Fig. 2: Hyperuricemia—gout, a heterogeneous group of diseases.

TABLE 3: Classification of hyperuricemia.

Overproduction of uric acid

• Primary idiopathic	• Paget's disease
• HPRT deficiency	• Glycogenosis III, V, and VII
• PRPP synthetase overactivity	• Rhabdomyolysis
• Hemolytic processes	• Exercise
• Lymphoproliferative diseases	• Alcohol
• Myeloproliferative diseases	• Obesity
• Polycythemia vera	• Purine-rich diet
• Psoriasis	

Under excretion of uric acid

• Primary idiopathic	• Hypothyroidism
• Renal insufficiency	• Toxemia of pregnancy
• Polycystic kidney disease	• Bartter's syndrome
• Diabetes insipidus	• Down syndrome
• Hypertension	• Drug ingestion
• Acidosis	– Salicylates (>2 g/day)
– Lactic acidosis	– Diuretics
– Diabetic ketoacidosis	– Alcohol
• Starvation ketosis	– Levodopa
• Berylliosis	– Ethambutol
• Sarcoidosis	– Pyrazinamide
• Lead intoxication	– Nicotinic acid
• Hyperparathyroidism	– Cyclosporine

Combined mechanism (overproduction and under excretion)

• Glucose-6-phosphatase deficiency	• Alcohol
• Fructose-1-phosphate aldolase deficiency	• Shock

(HPRT: hypoxanthine-guanine phosphoribosyltransferase; PRPP: phosphoribosylpyrophosphate)

Classification

Gout is classified into "primary" and "secondary" forms. Primary gout occurs in 90% cases in the absence of any obvious cause. Secondary gout occurs in 10% of cases due to prolonged hyperuricemia (acquired disorders) **(Box 1)**.

Primary Gout

Primary gout is an inborn error of metabolism due to overproduction of uric acid and is mostly related to increased synthesis of purine nucleotides **(Fig. 3)**. The following are the important metabolic defects (enzymes) associated with primary gout:

PRPP synthetase: PRPP synthetase is under feedback control by purine nucleotides (ADP and GDP). However, variant forms of PRPP synthetase, which are not subjected to feedback regulation, have been detected, which leads to the increased production of purines.

Box 1: Classification of gout.

Primary gout or idiopathic gout (90% of cases)
1. Overproduction of uric acid (Phosphoribosyl transferase deficiency) diet
   Unknown enzyme defects (80–90%)
   Known enzyme defects (e.g., partial HGPRT deficiency, rare)
2. Abnormality of urine excretion (reduced excretion of uric acid with normal production)

Secondary gout (10% of cases) **(Fig. 3)**
Overproduction of uric acid with increased urinary excretion
1. Increased nucleic acid turnover (e.g., leukemias and other aggressive neoplasms)
2. Inborn errors of metabolism (e.g., complete HGPRT deficiency)
3. Reduced excretion of uric acid with normal production: Chronic renal disease

PRPP glutamyl amidotransferase: Lack of feedback control of PRPP glutamyl amidotransferase by purine nucleotides also leads to their elevated synthesis.

HGPRT deficiency: HGPRT is an enzyme of purine salvage pathway, and its defect causes Lesch–Nyhan syndrome, which is associated with increased synthesis of purine nucleotides by a two-fold mechanism. Firstly, decreased utilization of purines (hypoxanthine and guanine) by salvage pathway, resulting in the accumulation and diversion of PRPP for purine nucleotides. Secondly, the defect in salvage pathway leads to decreased levels of IMP and GMP causing impairment in the tightly controlled feedback regulation of their production.

Glucose-6-phosphatase deficiency: Type I glycogen storage disease (von Gierke's), glucose 6-phosphate cannot be converted to glucose due to the deficiency of glucose 6-phosphatase. This leads to the increased utilization of glucose 6-phosphate by hexose monophosphate shunt (HMP shunt) resulting in elevated levels of ribose 5-phosphate and PRPP and, ultimately, purine overproduction. Von Gierke's disease is also associated with increased activity of glycolysis. Due to this, lactic acid accumulates in the body which interferes with the uric acid excretion through renal tubules.

Elevation of glutathione reductase generates more NADP+ which is utilized by HMP shunt. This causes increased ribose 5-phosphate and PRPP synthesis.

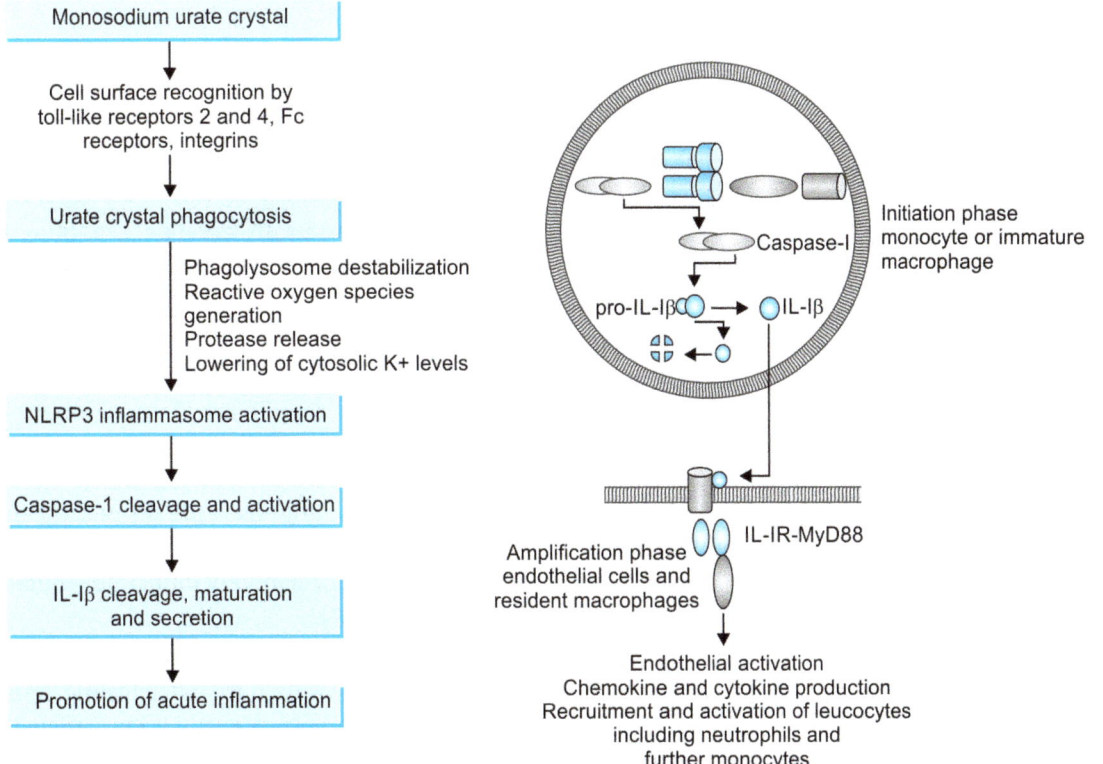

Fig. 3: Monosodium urate crystals as an endogenous danger signal.

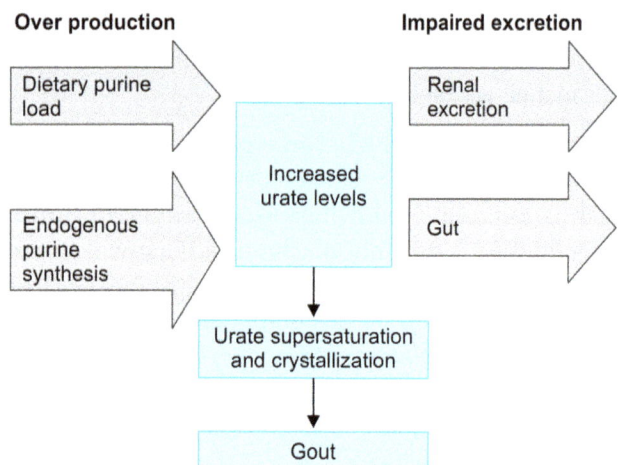

Fig. 4: Pathogenesis of secondary gout: Increased synthesis or decreased excretion of uric acid.

TABLE 4: Criteria for diagnosis of gout.	
Rome criteria	*New York criteria*
• Serum urate concentration >7 mg/ 100 mL in males, >6 mg/100 mL in females • Painful joint swelling, with abrupt onset, clearing in 1–2 weeks initially • Presence of urate crystals in synovial fluid • Presence of a tophus	• Chemical or microscopic demonstration of urate crystals in the synovial fluid or in the tissues • Presence of two or more of the following criteria • Two attacks of painful limb joint swelling with abrupt onset, remitting in 1–2 weeks initially • A single such attack involving the great toe • Response to colchicine, with major decrease in inflammation in 48 hours • Presence of a tophus

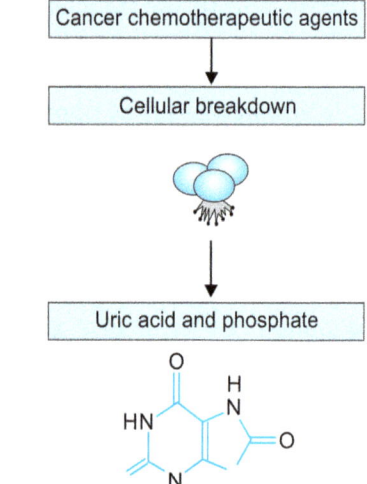

Fig. 5: Pathogenesis of secondary gout: Increased degradation of nucleic acids.

The first three above-mentioned enzymes are directly involved in purine synthesis. The remaining two indirectly regulate purine production.

Secondary Gout

Secondary hyperuricemia is due to various diseases causing increased synthesis or decreased excretion of uric acid. Increased degradation of nucleic acids (hence more uric acid formation) is observed in various cancers (leukemias, polycythemia, lymphomas, etc.) psoriasis and increased tissue breakdown (trauma, starvation, etc.) **(Figs. 4 and 5)**. The disorders associated with impairment in renal function cause accumulation of uric acid which may lead to gout **(Table 4)**.

Pathogenesis of Gout

Sodium urate is deposited as crystals on the surface of articular cartilage **(Flowchart 1)**. Then articular cartilage is eroded through and the subchondral bone is replaced in well circumscribed punched out areas by the crystalline deposits. A pannus of granulation tissue grows over the articular surface, invades and replaces the cartilage and may bridge the joint to the opposite articular surface producing a fibrous ankylosis.

The irregularity of joint surface leads to a secondary degenerative arthritis. Further urate salts are deposited in synovial membrane, periarticular soft tissues and the subcutaneous tissues. Acute attack of gout occurs when urate crystals trigger a marked inflammatory response. In acute gout, the predominant synovial fluid cell is the neutrophil and it is thought to provide maximum of the pro-inflammatory stimulus. Urate crystals have their initial interaction with physiological synovial cell types like cells of monocyte. Macrophage lineage (type A synoviocyte); fibroblast-like (type B) synoviocyte and possibly mast cells.

In the first acute attack of gout, synovial proliferation with phagocytosis of urate crystals has been demonstrated, which is associated with vascular congestion and an inflammatory infiltrate.

Monosodium urate crystals are phagocytozed by macrophages and activate the NALP3 inflammasome (A multiprotein complex that includes the protease "Caspase-1") **(Fig. 6)**. This inflammasome activated caspase-1 in turn cleaves and activates several cytokines, most notably IL-1-beta and IL-18.

IL-1-beta express adhesion molecule and synthesize neutrophil chemokine CXCL8, which is essential for localization of neutrophils at the site of acute inflammation. Repeated attacks of acute arthritis eventually lead to chronic arthritis and the formation of tophi in the inflamed synovial membrane **(Fig. 7)**.

Genetic contribution to gout is thought to be mainly through hyperuricemia, but genes affecting the inflammatory threshold may also play a role. It is likely there is a polygenic component in most patients, although a predominant contribution from single gene (e.g., putative renal urate

Chapter 16: Crystal Deposition Disorders

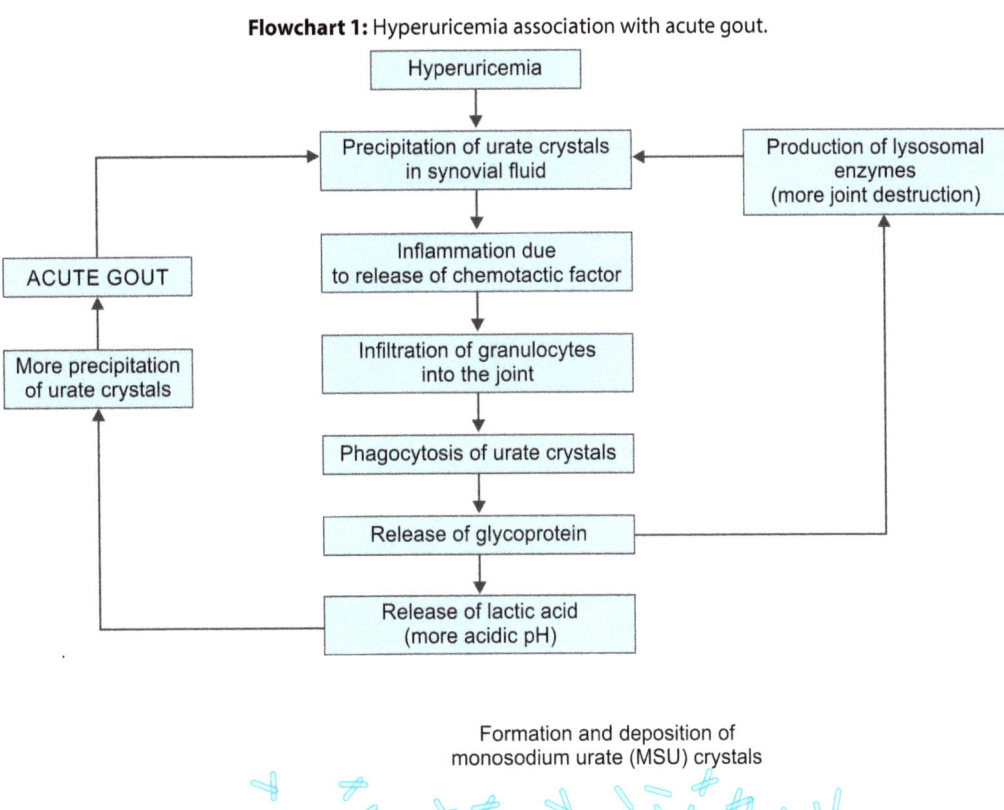

Flowchart 1: Hyperuricemia association with acute gout.

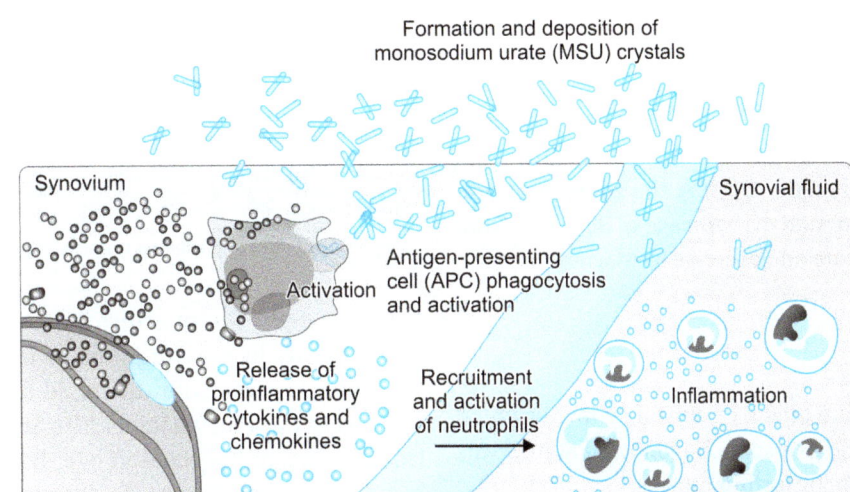

Fig. 6: Pathogenesis of acute gout: Activation of phagocyte by membrane—active crystals thereby activate compliment—generates chemotactic fragments, attracting neutrophils into the area-making inflammation.

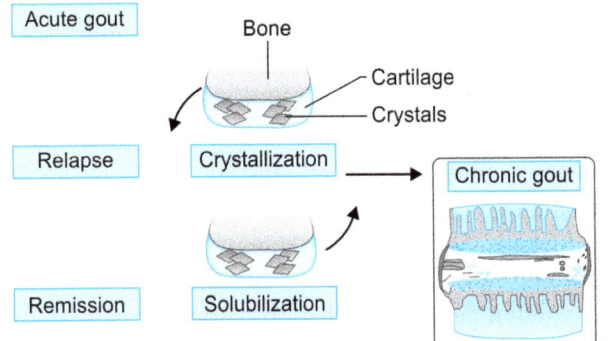

Fig. 7: Pathogenesis of gouty arthritis: Deposition of urate crystals in the joints-acute or chronic inflammation of the affected joint.

transporter mutation). URAT1 (urate transporter 1 gene) has an important role in the reabsorption process.

Lesch–Nyhan syndrome: Complete lack of hypoxanthine-guanine phosphoribosyl transferase (HGPRT) occurs is uncommon X-linked syndrome.

Microscopic Features of Gout

The urate crystal deposits are surrounded by an inflammatory reaction, fibrous tissue, and giant cells. Acute arthritis is characterized by a dense neutrophilic infiltrate that permeates the synovium and synovial fluid. MSU crystals are frequently found in the cytoplasm of the neutrophils and are arranged in small clusters in the synovium. Synovium is edematous and congested also contains scattered lymphocytes, plasma cells and macrophages.

Tophi are the pathogenic hallmark of gout formed by large aggregations of urate crystals surrounded by an intense

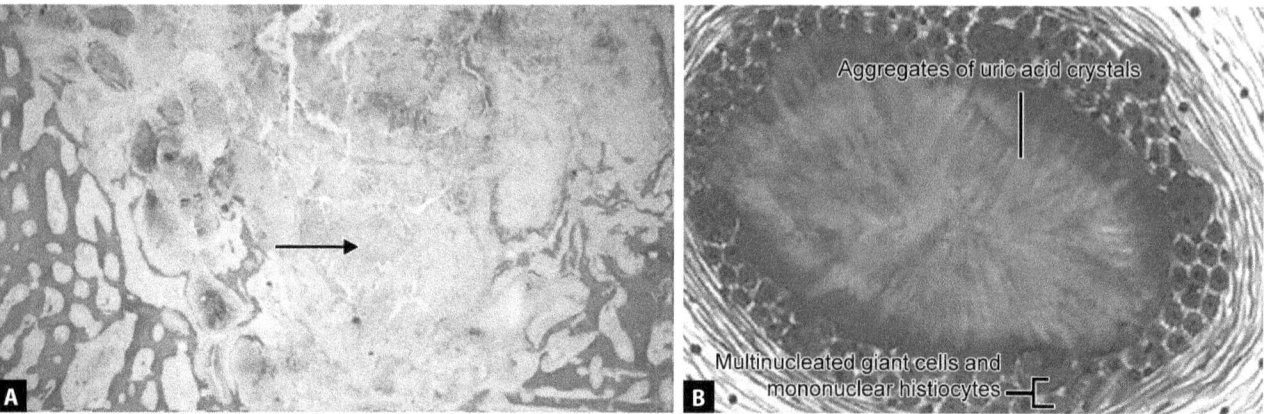

Figs. 8A and B: Gouty tophus: Aggrigates of uric acid crystals, which typically elicit a foreign body reaction with numerous multinucleated giant and mononuclear histiocytes surrounding the crystals. In properly fixed tissue (100% alcohol) the uric acid crystals show birefringent under polarized light.

inflammatory reaction of macrophages, lymphocytes and large foreign body giant cells, which may have completely or partially engulfed masses of crystals **(Figs. 8A and B)**.

In kidney: Lots of urate crystals are spread throughout the cortex and linear streaks through the medulla and production of uric acid renal stones.

Epidemiology

Gout occurs most frequently in adult men, with a peak incidence in the fifth decade. Gout is the most common inflammatory arthritis in men over the age of 30 years. Gout rarely occurs in men before adolescence or in women before menopause.

Clinical Features

Gout presents as an acute attack of crystal synovitis which clears completely in a week or so, to be followed at intervals of weeks, months or years by further attacks.

Important predisposing or risk factors for an acute gout: Gout is associated with hyperuricemia. Gouty attacks are triggered not by a particular level of uric acid but typically by acute changes in the level of uric acid. These are multifactorial and have a hereditary basis, age of the individual and duration of hyperuricemia. Other conditions causing hyperuricemia include obesity and hyperlipidemia in general, hypertension, alcoholism, drugs, such as diuretics (e.g., thiazides), cyclosporine, ethambutol, lead toxicity, rapid weight reduction, recent surgery and infections.

The most common joints affected include the first metatarsophalangeal joints (podagra) **(Fig. 9)**, the dorsum of the foot, the ankle, the knee, and occasionally the joints of the upper extremity.

The presentation of gout is divided into four stages:

Stage 1—Asymptomatic hyperuricemia: Symptoms are usually not present, although a small percentage of patients develop urinary calculi.

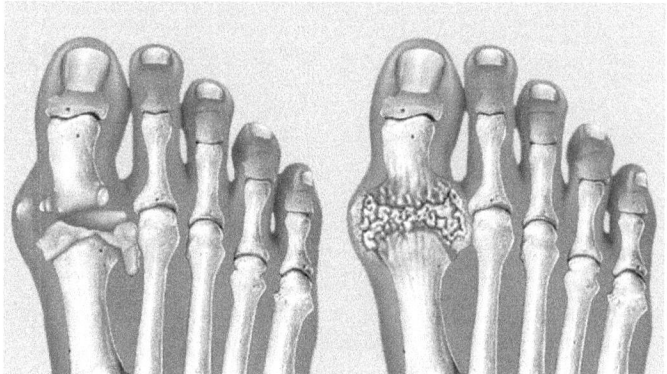

Fig. 9: Gout affecting the first metacarpopharyngeal joint (Podagra).

Stage 2—Acute gouty arthritis: It occurs usually in men, and typically in smaller joints or in the olecranon bursa. This stage is heralded by the rapid onset of severe pain and swelling of the affected joints. The first metatarsophalangeal (MTP) joints are affected in over half of initial attacks and eventually in up to 90% of patients with gout. Other sites commonly affected are other joints in the foot, the ankle, and the knee *(polyarticular gout)* **(Figs. 10A to E)**. When the hand is affected, the swelling may be quite significant. Almost 90% of initial attacks are monoarticular. The affected joints are markedly erythematous, more so than in other types of noninfectious arthritis. Tendons and bursae may be affected. Although mild attacks resolve within a few days, more severe attacks require several weeks to resolve completely. Patients are occasionally systemically ill, and may even appear septic.

Common precipitants of acute attack include aggressive introduction of hypouricemic therapy, alcohol or shellfish binges, sepsis, myocardial infarction, other acute severe illness, sudden cessation of hypouricemic therapy, trauma, surgery, and dehydration.

Drugs that worsen or precipitate gout include: Aspirin (low dose), cyclosporine, chemotherapeutic cytotoxics, diuretics (especially thiazides), ethambutol, ethanol, levodopa, nicotinic acid, pyrazinamide and tacrolimus.

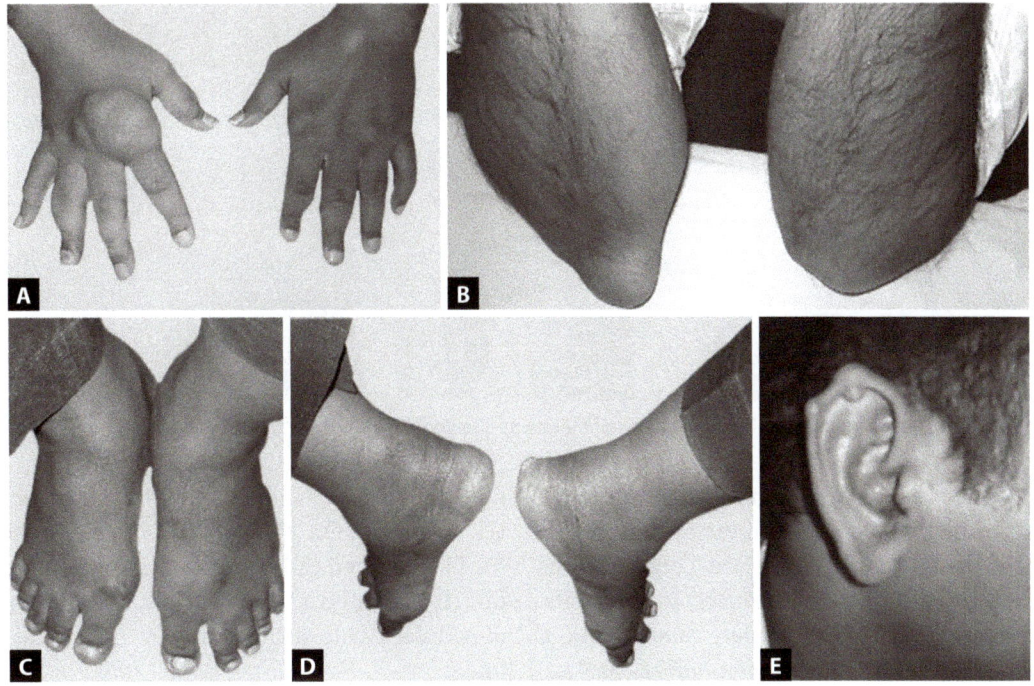

Figs. 10A to E: Man with chronic polyarticular gout: Showing bulging olecranon bursae, tophi over ear pinna, in both hands and the feet, joints are asymmetrically swollen.

Stage 3—Intercritical gout: In between attacks of gouty arthritis, the patient is asymptomatic but may still have urate crystals present in both previously affected and unaffected joints.

Stage 4—Chronic gout: Approximately 50% of patients who have had attacks of gout for a period of 10 years or more develop tophi, nodules in the skin and soft tissues containing precipitated uric acid crystals. *Tophi* and the associated inflammatory reaction to urate crystals can damage cartilage, subchondral bone, tendons, and skin, leading to cosmetic and functional deformities.

Chronic Gout

Diagnostic and Classification Criteria for Gout

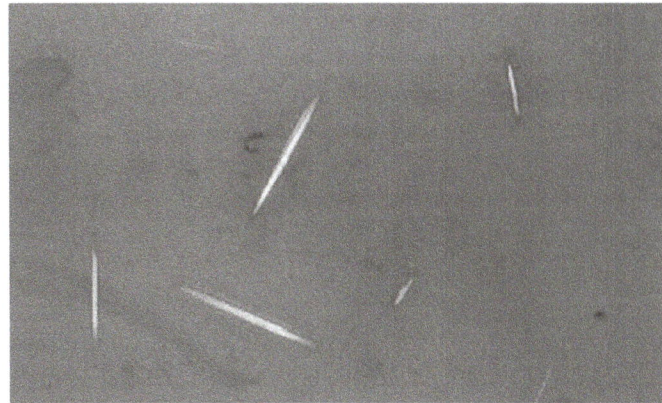

Fig. 11: Microscopy of monosodium urate crystals in polarized light. Urate crystals needle like, long and exhibit strong negative birefringence.

The key diagnostic features, reflected in the classification criteria, are recurrent attacks of acute monoarthritis of the first MTP or tarsal joints with maximal inflammation, producing redness over the involved joint, developing within one day, and the presence of tophus.

Laboratory Investigations

Synovial fluid examination: The most important procedure in establishing the diagnosis of acute gouty arthritis is the examination of synovial fluid under compensated polarized microscopy, urate crystals can be seen in the synovial fluids of 85% of acute gout patients. Urate crystals are slender and needle-shaped and have strong negative birefringence under polarized light. (Calcium pyrophosphate crystals are pleomorphic, are predominantly rhomboid-shaped, and have weakly positive birefringence.) In most joint fluids, urate crystals can be found inside neutrophils; however, in chronic gout, crystals may also be found free in the synovial fluid. Under polarized light, urate crystals appear yellow when parallel to the axis of the red compensator and blue when perpendicular to the axis **(Fig. 11)**.

Biochemical findings: Serum uric acid is usually elevated but is normal in about 10% of patients with acute gout. The creatinine and urea nitrogen will be elevated if secondary gout attributable to renal failure is responsible for the acute attack.

Radiographic Findings

- *Erosions*: These are caused by deposition of sodium biurate and are typically punched out in appearance.

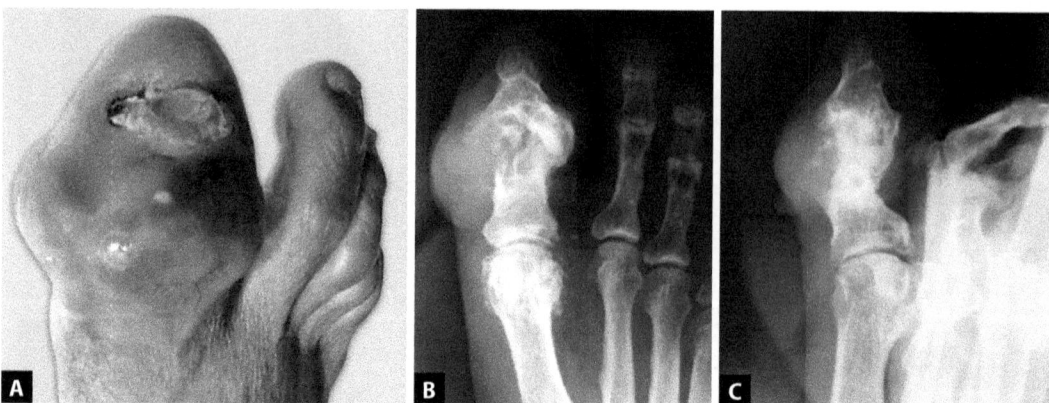

Figs. 12A to C: Most common site of gouty arthritis of metatarsophalyngeal joint of great toe showing typical gouty tophus.

They tend to appear near joint margins (**Figs. 12A to C**). As they enlarge, they tend to involve more of the cortex of the shaft rather than the articular surface. Large erosions extend to the articular cortex and diffusely in the shafts. Cartilage destruction is a relatively late manifestation. Usually much bony destruction is seen before cartilage loss supervenes. In the hand, gout tends to attack the distal and proximal interphalangeal joints, whereas rheumatoid arthritis affects the metacarpophalangeal and proximal interphalangeal joints.

- *Osteoporosis* is not seen except in advance cases which have been immobilized.
- *Tophi*: These are shown as soft-tissue swellings eccentric in distribution, in contradistinction to the fusiform soft-tissue swellings of rheumatoid arthritis. Eventually, both soft-tissue and intraosseous tophi may become calcified but this is uncommon.

In practice, the most frequent difficulty is in differentiating gout from rheumatoid arthritis. Important points are: the longer latent period of gout; its eccentric, often gross soft-tissue swellings; and tendency to attack distal interphalangeal joints. Osteoporosis is found much more frequently in rheumatoid arthritis. Rheumatoid erosions are not as sharply defined as those of gout. Calcified tophi are, of course, diagnostic of gout. In difficult cases, differentiation will be made by laboratory tests revealing a raised uric acid level in blood. Radiologic features are usually not seen until 6–12 years after initial attack. Radiologic features present in 50% of inflicted patients.

Computed tomography using advanced multi-slice CT scanning tophi were likely to be responsible for bone erosion in gout—an impression gained from XR review but not previously confirmed by using a multiplanar high-definition modality. Clearly, CT would have no role in the diagnosis of acute gout, prior to the development of bone erosions or tophi, as it does not provide imaging of synovitis, tenosynovitis, or osteitis.

MRI scanning can also be used to image tophi, and the information this modality reveals about the inflammatory nature of these lesions cannot be appreciated from XR or CT scanning. On MRI, tophi typically exhibit low signal on T1-weighted (T1W) images and medium to high signal on T2-weighted (T2W) images, indicating the presence of cellular tissue surrounding or infiltrating the crystalline mass.

Ultrasound (US) provides a different "sonar" picture of tophi, which may appear as hypoechoic, hyperechoic, or mixed echogenicity nodules. US detection of tophi could be helpful in diagnosing gout, especially when these lesions are not detectable clinically.

Both ultrasound and MRI scanning can also image the inflammatory aspect of gouty arthropathy, including synovitis, tenosynovitis, and edematous soft tissue inflammation. Regions of thickened soft tissue that have moderate US echogenicity and that might represent diffuse infiltration with MSU crystals have been described. Evidence of increased vascularization within the synovial membrane can be obtained on power Doppler images and contrast-enhanced MRI scans.

Differential Diagnosis of Gout

Infection: Cellulitis, septic bursitis, an infected bunion or septic arthritis must all be excluded. If necessary, perform an immediate joint aspiration for synovial fluid analysis. One should remember that crystals and sepsis may coexist, so always send fluid for both culture and crystal analysis.

Pseudogout: CPPD crystal deposition may cause an acute arthritis indistinguishable from gout-except that if tends to affect large rather than small joints and is somewhat more common in women than in men. Articular calcification may show on X-ray. Demonstrating the crystals in synovial fluid establishes the diagnosis.

Reiter's disease: It may present with acute pain and swelling of a knee or ankle, but the history is more protracted and the response to anti-inflammatory drugs less dramatic.

Rheumatoid arthritis (RA): Polyarticular gout affecting the fingers may be mistaken for RA, and elbow tophi for rheumatoid nodules. In difficult cases, biopsy will establish the diagnosis. RA and gout seldom occur together.

Management of Gout

Patient education is important that the patient realize that gout is a chronic disease and that certain lifestyle modifications, such as maintenance of an ideal weight and moderation of alcohol intake, are important. A purine-restricted diet may be of benefit in some patients, but only small changes in serum uric acid can be attained. Other factors worth emphasizing are ingestion of at least 2 L/day of fluids to help prevent renal stones and avoidance of alcohol and low-dose aspirin, which aggravate hyperuricemia.

Drugs used in Gout

The goals of therapy are to prevent renal parenchymal damage and nephrolithiasis and to suppress articular flares. Drug strategy in chronic gout is determined by the pattern of 24-hour urate excretion and the severity of disease.

For acute gout: (1) Anti-inflammatory and analgesics: nonsteroidal anti-inflammatory drugs (NSAIDs) and corticosteroids. (2) Drugs inhibiting leukocyte migration into joint: Colchicine.

For chronic gout: (1) Inhibits uric acid synthesis: Allopurinol, febuxostat and rasburicase. (2) Increase uric acid excretion (Uricosuric): Probenecid, sulfinpyrazone and benzbromarone **(Flowchart 2)**.

NSAIDs: Nonsteroidal anti-inflammatory drugs are superior to colchicine in terms of speed of onset of action but are relatively contraindicated in some patients, particularly those with renal insufficiency, hypertension, peptic ulceration or congestive heart failure. Despite having been used for centuries, *colchicine is now usually reserved for those patients in whom NSAIDs are contraindicated*. Among the various NSAIDs, indomethacin has been the most widely used but most other NSAIDs, if they are used in appropriate doses, have been shown to be effective in the treatment of an acute attack of gout. The newer COX-2 selective inhibitors, celecoxib and rofecoxib, have not yet been assessed in the management of an intense inflammatory arthritis such as occurs in gout, but it is likely that they would be effective if given in appropriate anti-inflammatory dosage.

Indomethacin: Patients will often notice that the pain has begun to ease within 2 hours of taking the first dose. Generally, 50 mg four times a day is an average and effective dose schedule, although mild attacks may respond to lower doses. This dose may be doubled with benefit in particularly severe cases. The dose should be maintained for 2 days or until the severe pain settles, and then reduced to three times a day. Provided the attack continues to settle, the dose is further reduced to 25 mg three times a day and continued for 1–2 days after the acute inflammation has settled completely.

Other NSAIDs: The doses of the several other NSAIDs used to treat gout tend to be toward the upper limit of, or above, the usual therapeutic range. In most cases, a higher initial dose has been advocated and, as with indomethacin, the dose is generally reduced as the inflammation resolves.

Some of the dose schedules are as follows:
- Ibuprofen 800 mg every 8 hours reducing to 400 mg every 8 hours.
- Diclofenac 50 mg every 8 hours reducing to 25 mg every 8 hours
- Naproxen 750 mg initially, then 250 mg every 8 hours
- Piroxicam 40 mg daily for 5 days
- Sulindac 200 mg initially, then 100 mg every 6 hours.

Several of the NSAIDs available in suppository or injectable form may be useful in patients unable to take oral medications.

Colchicine: Colchicine is one of the oldest available therapies for acute gout. Plant extracts containing colchicine were used for joint pain in the sixth century. *Colchicine is considered second-line therapy* because it has a narrow therapeutic window and a high rate of side effects, particularly at higher doses. It has antimitotic effects, arresting cell division in G1 by interfering with microtubule and spindle formation. It may alter neutrophil motility. It decreases the crystal-induced secretion of chemotactic factors and superoxide anions by activated neutrophils. It also limits neutrophil adhesion to endothelium by modulating the expression of endothelial adhesion molecules.

Higher concentrations inhibit IL-1β processing and release from neutrophils. The absorption is rapid and variable. There is significant enterohepatic circulation. It is metabolized by CYP3A4 oxidative demethylation. Its t½ is 9 hours but it can be detected in leukocytes and urine for at least 9 days. Nausea, vomiting, diarrhea, and abdominal pain are the most common untoward effects and the earliest signs of impending colchicine toxicity. Drug administration should be discontinued as soon as these symptoms occur. Acute intoxication causes hemorrhagic gastropathy. Intravenous

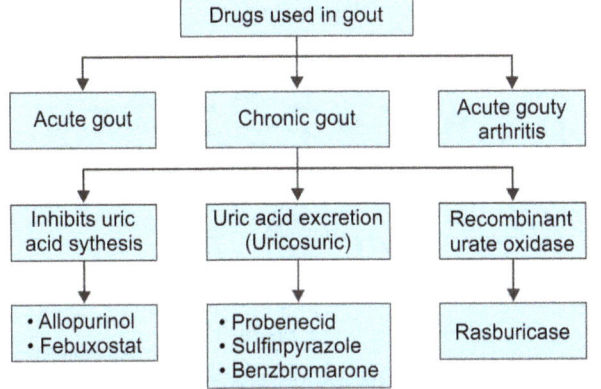

Flowchart 2: Classification of drugs used in gout.

colchicine was previously used to treat acute gouty arthritis; however, this route obviates early GI side effects that can be a harbinger of serious systemic toxicity.

Other serious side effects of colchicine therapy include myelosuppression, leukopenia, granulocytopenia, thrombopenia, aplastic anemia, and rhabdomyolysis. Life-threatening toxicities are associated with administration of concomitant therapy with P-glycoprotein or CYP3A4 inhibitors. It is contraindicated in patients with hepatic or renal impairment.

Colchicine is the drug of choice in acute attack to be administered within few hours. It is given in a dose of 0.6 mg/h until pain relives or diarrhea develops or 0.6 mg 2 tablets (1.2 mg) at first sign of gout and 0.6 mg PO after 1 hour. The intravenous dose for acute gouty arthritis is 1–2 mg given slowly through an established venous line over 10 minutes, and two additional doses of 1 mg each may be given at 6 hour intervals, but the total dose should never exceed 4 mg. A minimum of 3 days should elapse between courses to avoid cumulative toxicity. The off-label indication is in the prevention of recurrent gout. It is also useful for the prevention of attacks of familial Mediterranean fever and amyloidosis.

Corticosteroids: Corticosteroids are potent anti-inflammatory drugs. "Intra-articular administration of corticosteroids is a particularly effective means of terminating an attack of gout". Resolution is typically complete within 12–24 hours. This form of treatment is of particular value in some patients with monoarticular gout associated with renal impairment and other conditions where the use of full doses of other drugs may be relatively contraindicated. These are useful in resistant cases and patients not tolerating/not responding to NSAIDs/colchicine. A good response without rebound has been reported with either oral prednisone 30–50 mg/day tapering over 7–9 days or intra-articular triamcinolone acetonide (20–40 mg) or methylprednisolone (25–50 mg).

Allopurinol: Allopurinol is a hypoxanthine analog. It is the *first choice drug in chronic gout*. It is a substrate as well as inhibitor of xanthine oxidase, which is responsible for uric acid synthesis. Allopurinol itself is a short-acting (t½ 2 hours) competitive inhibitor but its major metabolite alloxanthine is a long-acting (t½ 24 hours) noncompetitive inhibitor of xanthine oxidase. This leads to decreased plasma concentration of uric acid and increased plasma concentration of xanthine and hypoxanthine which have more solubility and higher renal clearance. So crystallization in tissues and urine does not occur.

There is some feedback inhibition of de novo purine synthesis and reutilization of metabolically derived purine also occurs. 80% of orally given dose is absorbed. It is not bound to plasma proteins. It inhibits its own metabolism. One-third is excreted unchanged and the rest as alloxanthine. In chronic gout start with 100 mg OD gradually increase to maintenance dose of 300 mg/day. Maximum dose is 600 mg/day.

Liberal fluid intake is advocated during allopurinol therapy. It can be used in both over producers and under excretors of uric acid. It should not be started during an acute attack. During the initial months of treatment, acute attacks may precipitate probably due to fluctuating plasma urate levels favoring intermittent solubilization and recrystallization in joints; cover with NSAIDs/colchicine may be provided. It can be used in secondary hyperuricemia due to cancer chemotherapy/radiotherapy/thiazides or other drugs. It is used in the treatment of kala-azar as it inhibits the metabolism of purine in Leishmania. Allopurinol inhibits the metabolism of 6-mercaptopurine, azathioprine, warfarin and theophylline. It prolongs t½ of probenecid. It increases incidence of skin rash when ampicillin is used along with this. Iron treatment is not recommended along with allopurinol.

It is contraindicated in hypersensitive patients, during pregnancy and lactation. It should be used cautiously in the elderly, children and in kidney or liver disease. Adverse effects are uncommon. Hypersensitivity reactions are common. Steven-Johnson syndrome is rare. Gastric irritation, headache, nausea, and dizziness are infrequent.

Febuxostat: Febuxostat is a novel non-purine inhibitor of xanthine oxidase (**Fig. 13**). It is rapidly absorbed. Food decreases absorption. $Mg(OH)_2$ and $Al(OH)_3$ delay absorption. It is highly plasma protein bound. It is extensively metabolized by CYPs and conjugation. Its t½ is 5–8 hours and is eliminated by both hepatic and renal pathways. The most common adverse reactions are liver function abnormalities, nausea, joint pain, and rash. There is increased incidence of MI and stroke. It inhibits the metabolism of mercaptopurine, theophylline and azathioprine. Interactions between febuxostat and CYP inhibitors are likely. It is approved for hyperuric patients with gout attacks but not for asymptomatic hyperuricemia. It is available in 40 and 80 mg tablets.

Rasburicase: Rasburicase is a recombinant urate oxidase that catalyzes the enzymatic oxidation of uric acid into the soluble and inactive metabolite allantoin (**Fig. 14**). It is indicated for the initial management of elevated plasma uric

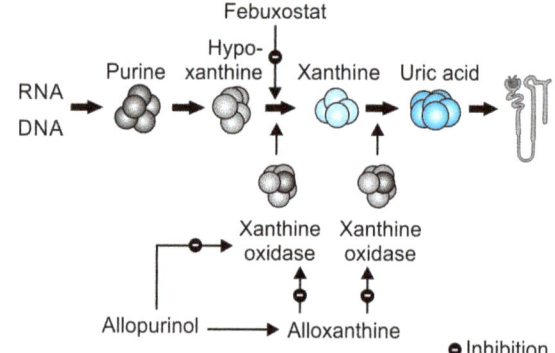

Fig. 13: Mechanism of action of febuxostat.

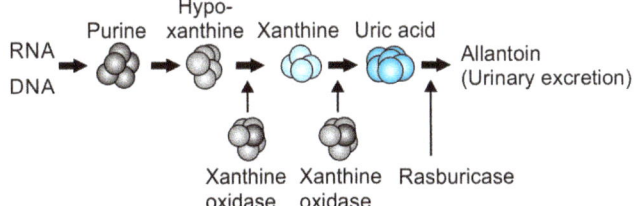

Fig. 14: Mechanism of action of rasburicase. Oxidazes uric acid to soluble and easily excreted metabolite allantoin.

acid levels in pediatric patients who are receiving anticancer therapy expected to result in tumor lysis and hyperuricemia. The therapeutic efficacy may be hampered by antibodies.

It causes hemolysis in G6PD deficient patients, methemoglobinemia, acute renal failure and anaphylaxis. The recommended dose is 0.15 mg/kg or 0.2 mg/kg as a single daily dose for 5 days.

Probenecid: Probenecid is a highly lipid soluble benzoic acid derivative. It inhibits the transport of organic acids across the epithelial barriers. It inhibits the reabsorption of uric acid by organic anion transporter URAT-1. This action is blunted by the coadministration of salicylates. It inhibits the tubular secretion of methotrexate, penicillin, cephalosporins and metabolites of clofibrate, naproxen, ketoprofen and indomethacin, thereby increases their plasma concentrations. It inhibits monoamine transport to CSF. It inhibits biliary secretion of rifampicin. It is absorbed completely. Its t½ is dose dependent. 95% of the drug is bound to albumin. The drug is secreted actively by the proximal tubule. Reabsorption occurs unless the urine is alkaline. It is well tolerated. It produces GI irritation. *It is ineffective in renal failure patients.* Hypersensitivity reactions can occur. Overdosage results in CNS stimulation, convulsion and death from respiratory failure. Probenecid is used in under excretors and should not be used in gouty patients with nephrolithiasis or uric acid over producers. Liberal fluid intake should be maintained as it increases urinary urate levels which may result in renal stones. It is used as an adjuvant to prolong penicillin concentration to treat gonorrhea or neurosyphilis infections.

Sulfinpyrazone: Sulfinpyrazone is a pyrazolone derivative related to phenylbutazone. It inhibits renal tubular reabsorption of uric acid. It is well absorbed orally. 98% of the drug is protein bound. It is excreted in urine. It is used in chronic gout in a dose of 100–200 mg BD, maximum dose is 800 mg/day. It produces gastric irritation and hypersensitivity reactions.

Benzbromarone: Benzbromarone is a potent and reversible inhibitor of organic anion transporter in the proximal tubule thereby inhibits reabsorption of uric acid. It is metabolized to monobromine and dehalogenated derivatives which also have uricosuric activity. It is excreted primarily in bile. The uricosuric action is blunted by aspirin or sulfinpyrazone.

It is effective in a single daily dose of 40–80 mg. It is effective in patients with renal insufficiency and in patients who are allergic to probenecid and sulfinpyrazone. *Combination of allopurinol and benzbromarone is more effective.*

Surgical Treatment for Gouty Arthritis

Immobilization of the affected joint will lessen the degree of joint destruction, during an acute attack of gout. Excision of the gouty lesion and other surgical measures are necessary certain times. Deposits of urate crystals (creamy and semiliquid or chalky and inspissated) usually may compromise various structures by compression or infiltration and destruction. Nervous tissue is resistant to invasion, but compression of digital nerves causes sensory disturbances. Gouty bursitis with a bursa may become so distended by urate deposits that the overlying skin is thinned and penetrated; resulting in a draining sinus; or the tendon or the bone beneath the bursa may be invaded.

Gouty tophi might cause tendon rupture due to urate crystals deposition within a tendon. Thereby parenchymal degeneration leads to tendon destruction by replacing the tendon fibers with development of fusiform, nodular enlargement, which interferes with tendon motion and may predispose to tendon rupture. Invasion of a joint destroys articular cartilage and capsular structures. If destruction is mild, a painful degenerative arthritis supervenes.

Surgical stabilization of the joint in a functional position is indicated and if a large bony lesion lies adjacent to a point, removal of the focus may preserve joint function.

Joint aspiration and intra-articular injection of corticosteroid preparations may be indicated for patients with persisting chronic synovitis.

Ultrasound allows a "hands on" approach for the practicing clinician to assess tophi, erosions, and synovitis and may be particularly applicable in the longitudinal setting. It can also be used to guide aspiration of the joint or tophus to obtain material for crystal examination.

Surgical removal of large tophi is indicated if they become infected or interfere with joint function.

Indolent tophus ulcers: By breakdown of skin over a tophus produces a characteristic indolent ulcer with a base of urate crystals and little surrounding inflammatory reaction. With conservative treatment, the base eventually granulates, and the area epithelializes over with minimal scarring. Removal of the gouty deposit, with awaiting appearance of granulation, and applying a skin graft. Urates possess a bacteriostatic property thereby secondary infection of the gouty ulcer does not occur usually.

Severe joint destruction is usually followed by fibrous ankylosis, which is eventually converted into a bony ankylosis. *Total joint replacement arthroplasty* is the treatment modality for these types of cases.

Principles for surgery of gouty lesions:
1. Avoidance of local anesthesia, which might impair local blood supply
2. Incisions to be given parallel with course of blood vessels
3. Using sharp dissections
4. Making loose suturing to allow escape of liquefied deposits
5. Putting pressure dressings
6. Avoidance of prolonged splinting, which encourages ankylosis.

Minimization of postoperative acute attacks by medical therapy, colchicine (0.5 mg) is given for 3 days preoperatively and 1 week postoperatively. In addition, postoperatively, Probenecid (0.5–3.0 g) is given daily preoperatively and is continued indefinitely.

Orthopedic interventions consist mainly of prevention of joint destruction by immobilization and may be removal of large tophi that interfere with joint and tendon motion.

Prognosis

Prognosis of properly managed gout is excellent, and most patients have a normal life span. Chronic deforming arthritis and periarthritis can occur in long-standing untreated cases. Rare patients with severe tophaceous renal disease develop chronic renal failure.

■ PSEUDOGOUT

Calcium Pyrophosphate Dihydrate Crystal Deposition Disease

Definition

The hallmark of calcium pyrophosphate dihydrate deposition disease (CPPD) is the formation of CPPD crystals in articular hyaline and fibrocartilage. CPPD deposition comprises three overlapping conditions:
1. *Chondrocalcinosis*: Calcification of articular fibro- or hyaline cartilage
2. *Pyrophosphate arthropathy*: Structural abnormality of cartilage and bone (cartilage loss, osteophyte, cysts) associated with intra-articular CPPD deposition **(Fig. 15)**.
3. *Calcium pyrophosphate deposition disease (Pseudogout)*: The clinical syndrome of acute synovitis associated with intra-articular CPPD deposition.

Historical Milestones

In 1857, Adams was the first who described that articular cartilage calcification is a common phenomenon occurring either alone or in association with arthritis.

In 1903, Bennet reported that the autopsy of patients with polyarticular chondrocalcinosis owing to crystalline chalk containing tiny rhomboidal crystals.

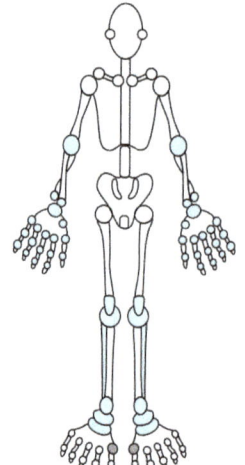

Fig. 15: Chronic arthropathy: Common sites of involvement of chronic pyrophosphate arthropathy.

In 1929, Tobler examined menisci from cadavers and found degenerative changes in 75% and calcification in 15% of menisci.

In 1958, Zitnan and Sitaj described the clinical and roentgenological features of what they called chondrocalcinosis articularis (familiaris).

In 1962, McCarty et al. identified previously unrecognized square rod-like, or rhomboid non-urate crystals, when examined with compensated polarized light microscopy, subsequently were identified as calcium pyrophosphate dihydrate by their X-ray diffraction powder pattern.

Clinical similarity to gout promoted the term *pseudogout* for this new "'crystal-induced arthropathy".

It was soon realized that chondrocalcinosis polyarticularis was also caused by CPPD.

Classification and Diagnostic Criteria

Calcium pyrophosphate dihydrate deposition disease can be subclassified as hereditary, secondary, chiefly associated with metabolic disease, or sporadic according to the presence or absence of recognized predisposing factors. A tentative classification is given in **Table 5**.

Epidemiology

Chondrocalcinosis: One of the common disorders associated with intra-articular crystal formation. Deposition of calcium pyrophosphate dihydrate (CPPD) crystals in synovial membranes (pseudogout), joint cartilage (chondrocalcinosis), ligaments and tendons. Usually >50 years of age; more common with increasing age; M=F.

Pathogenesis

Calcium pyrophosphate dihydrate crystal-associated arthropathy: CPPD is divided into: (1) Sporadic (Idiopathic); (2) Hereditary; and (3) Secondary types.

TABLE 5: Diagnostic criteria for calcium pyrophosphate deposition disease.

Criteria

I	Definitive identification of CPPD crystals obtained by joint aspiration or biopsy by X-ray or electron diffraction, infrared spectroscopy or chemical analysis
IIa	Identification of monoclinic or triclinic crystals showing no birefringence or a weakly positive elongation by compensated polarized light microscopy
IIb	Presence of typical calcifications of fibrocartilage and hyalin cartilage on X-rays
IIIa	Acute arthritis attacks especially in knees and wrists
IIIb	Subacute or chronic arthritis, with or without acute episodes

Categories

A	Definite diagnosis:	Criterion I, or IIa plus IIb
B	Probable diagnosis:	Criterion IIa or IIb
C	Possible diagnosis:	Criterion IIIa or IIIb in any combination

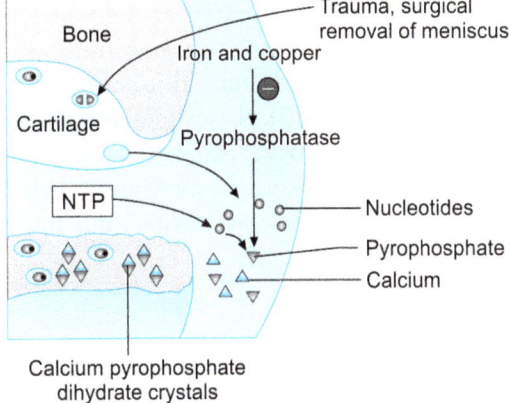

Fig. 16: A pathogenesis of pseudogout: CPPD deposition in knees after trauma and after surgical removal of the meniscus nucleotides released after injury to articular cartilage—act as substrates for nucleotide triphosphate pyrophosphohydrolase (NTP)—increase production of pyrophosphate Iron and copper- inhibit pyrophosphatase—decreased degradation of pyrophosphate.

The disease is caused by germline mutations in the pyrophosphate transport channel. The CPPD deposition in knees occurs after trauma and surgical removal of the meniscus. Nucleotides that are released after injury to articular cartilage act as substrate for nucleotide triphosphate pyrophosphohydrolase (NTP)—increased production of pyrophosphate. Iron and copper—inhibit pyrophosphatase—decreased degradation of pyrophosphate **(Fig. 16)**.

Hereditary: Crystals develop relatively early in life and are associated with severe osteoarthritis. Autosomal dominant form of the disease is caused by germline mutations in the *ANKH* gene. *ANKH* gene encodes a membrane pyrophosphate transporter that inhibits mineralization of several tissues including joints, articular cartilage and tendons.

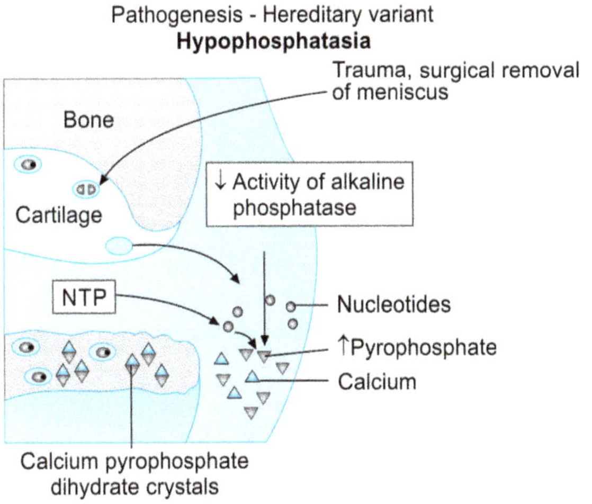

Fig. 17: Pathogenesis of pseudogout—hereditary variant: AD, *ANKH* gene—encode a membrane pyrophosphate transporter that inhibits mineralization of several tissues including joints, articular cartilage and tendons. Mutated ANKH elevates intracellular pyrophosphate and reduces extracellular pyrophosphate. Hypophosphatasia: activity of alkaline phosphatase (hydrolyzes pyrophosphate) in serum and tissue - deficient.

Mutated ANKH elevates intracellular pyrophosphate and reduces extracellular pyrophosphate. Hypophosphatasia (HPP) results from *ALPL* mutations leading to deficient activity of the tissue-non-specific alkaline phosphatase isozyme (TNAP) and thereby extracellular accumulation of inorganic pyrophosphate (PPi), a natural substrate of TNAP and potent inhibitor of mineralization **(Fig. 17)**.

Secondary: Diseases associated with CPPD include previous joint damage, hyperparathyroidism, hemochromatosis, hypophosphatasia, hypomagnesemia, gout, neuropathic arthropathy, hypothyroidism, ochronosis, osteoarthritis, Wilson disease and diabetes. Basis of crystal formation is altered activity of the matrix enzymes that produce and degrade pyrophosphate is suspected.

Pathology of Pseudogout

The inflammation present in pseudogout is usually milder than in gout. The basis for crystal formation in calcium pyrophosphate dihydrate arthropathy is not well-known. The current studies suggest that articular cartilage proteoglycans are normally inhibit the mineralization and are degraded by allowing crystallization around chondrocytes. As in gout, inflammation in pseudogout is caused by activation of the *inflammasome* in macrophages.

The CPPD crystals first develop in the articular cartilage, menisci, and intervertebral discs **(Fig. 18)**. The enlarged CPPD deposits may rupture and seed the joint. Once released into the joint-elicit an inflammatory infiltrate rich in neutrophils. Neutrophils produce damage through the release of oxygen metabolites and cytokines. Chronic reactions associated with macrophages and fibrosis. The CPPD crystals form chalky, white friable deposits. These

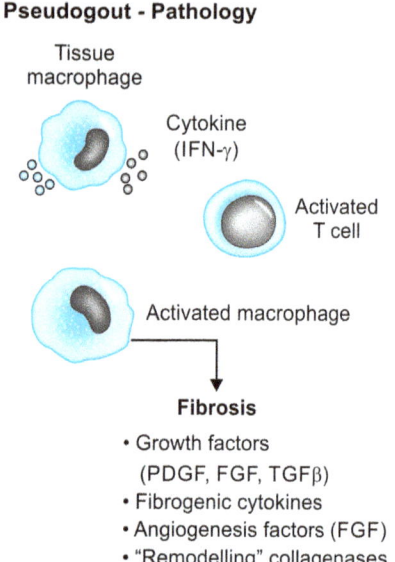

Fig. 18: Pathogenesis of pseudogout: Neutrophils: produce damage through the release of oxygen metabolites and cytokines. Chronic reactions associated with macrophages and fibrosis. Crystals form chalky white friable deposits.

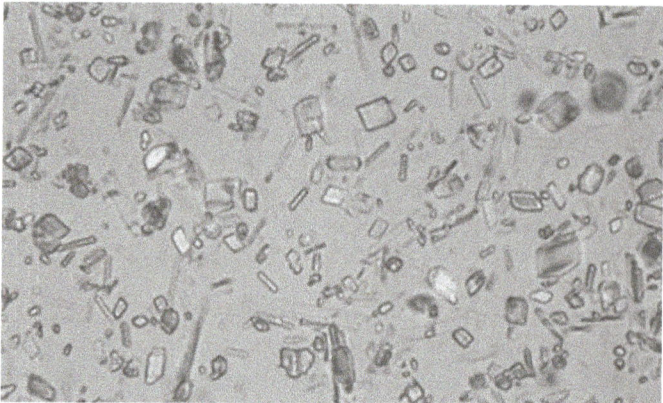

Fig. 19: Microscopy of CPPD crystals. Calcium pyrophosphate dehydrate crystals on rhomboid shaped rods, rectangle 1–2 μ (Coffin shaped) slightly smaller than urate crystals and show weak positive birefringence.

are seen histologically in stained preparations as oval blue-purple aggregates. Individual CPPD crystals are rhomboid-shaped, 0.5–5 μm in greatest dimension, slightly smaller than the urate crystals and show week positively birefringence.

Clinical Features

Most of the patients are women over the age of 60 years. CPPD is frequently asymptomatic. The incidence of CPPD arthropathy rises with increasing age; men and women are equally affected and in some cases the disease runs in families. CPPD deposition syndromes occur in the following clinical patterns:

Asymptomatic chondrocalcinosis: Radiographic finding of calcified cartilage in patients without any joint complaints. Calcification of the menisci is common in elderly people and is usually asymptomatic or is seen in association with osteoarthritis. Both are common in elderly people and X-rays may reveal chondrocalcinosis.

Acute synovitis ("pseudogout"): The classic presentation is the acute monoarthritis in the elderly patients. The knee is the most commonly involved joint. Any joint may be involved, including the first metatarsophalangeal joint ("pseudopodagra"). The patient, typically a middle-aged woman, complains of acute pain and swelling in one of the larger joints—usually the knee. The typical attack develops rapidly, with severe pain, stiffness, and swelling, maximum within 6–24 hours of onset. If untreated, the acute synovitis of pseudogout lasts for a few weeks and then subsides spontaneously. X-rays may show signs of chondrocalcinosis, and the diagnosis can be confirmed by finding positively birefringent crystals in the synovial fluid. Situations that may trigger acute pseudogout include direct trauma to joint, intercurrent medical illness (e.g., chest infection, myocardial infarction), surgery (especially parathyroidectomy), blood transfusion, parenteral fluid administration, institution of thyroxin replacement therapy and joint lavage.

Chronic pyrophosphate arthropathy: Usually an elderly woman, presents with polyarticular "osteoarthritis" affecting large joints (hips, knees) and unusual joints, such as the ankles, shoulders, elbows and wrists where osteoarthritis is seldom seen. There are the usual features of pain, stiffness, swelling, joint crepitus and loss of movement. It is often diagnosed as "generalized osteoarthritis", but the X-ray features are distinctive.

Investigations

Synovial fluid: Study of aspirated joint fluid is required to confirm the diagnosis with WBC count 3,000–15,000 with 70% or more neutrophils. CPPD crystals can be identified with compensated polarized microscopy showing rhomboid shaped crystals and exhibit weakly positive birefringence **(Fig. 19)**.

Radiographs show characteristic features of combination of intra-articular and periarticular calcification, and degenerative arthritis in distinctive site. Chondrocalcinosis appears as linear or punctate radiodensities within cartilage. Subchondral bone cysts and hook-like osteophytes of metacarpophalangeal joints may be observed. Calcification is usually seen in and around the knees, wrists, shoulders, hips, pubic symphysis and intervertebral disks and is often bilateral and symmetrical. In advanced cases joint destruction may be marked, with the formation of loose bodies.

Differential Diagnosis

The acute attack: Pseudogout must be distinguished from other acute inflammatory disorders.

Acute gout usually occurs in men, and typically in smaller joints or in the olecranon bursa. Joint aspiration

TABLE 6: Differentiating features of gout and pseudogout.

	Gout	Pseudogout
Joints affected	Small joints—first MTP, foot, ankle, knee	Large joints–knee
Initial attack	90% monoarticular	90% monoarticular
Distribution	Asymmetric, additional joints added with subsequent attacks	Usually monoarticular, more than three joints unusual
Pain	Intense	Moderate
Joint feature	Inflamed	Swollen
Onset	Hyperacute, within a few hours	Acute, with 6–24 hours
Biochemical	Hyperuricemia	Chondrocalcinosis
Tophi	Present in chronic gout	May develop tophi-like deposits
Provocants	• Disorders of urate metabolism • Diuretics • Ethanol • Cold	• Joint trauma • Systemic illness • Endocrine disorders
Crystals	Monosodium urate	Calcium pyrophosphate dehydrogenate
	Needle-shaped	Rhomboidal or rod-shaped
	Negatively birefringent	Positively birefringent
Cell count	Inflammatory, usually >50,000, mostly PMNs	Usually inflammatory, may be <50,000, mostly PMNs
Viscosity	Markedly decreased	Decreased, but variably
Treatment	NSAIDs	Joint aspiration and injection
	Analgesics	NSAIDs
	Colchicine	Early mobilization

(MTP: metatarsophalangeal)

and identification of the characteristic monosodium urate crystals with strong negative birefringence in synovial fluid. Simultaneous existence both gout and pseudogout may occur **(Table 6)**.

Post-traumatic hemarthrosis can be misleading; pseudogout is often precipitated by trauma. A clear history and aspiration of blood-stained fluid from joint will establish the diagnosis.

Septic arthritis shows prominent systemic science of infection, when present need for aspiration of synovial fluid with Gram stain and culture helpful for diagnosis.

Reiter's disease affects single large joint and with signs of conjunctivitis, urethritis and colitis.

Chronic CPPD Arthropathy

Chronic pyrophosphate arthropathy usually affects multiple joints and it has to be distinguished from other types of polyarticular arthritis:

Hydroxyapatite crystal deposition disease may produce synovitis or tendinitis. Crystals may be seen with electron microscopy but not with routine polarizing microscopy.

Osteoarthritis and joint calcification are both common in older people. The distinctive X-ray features, and especially the involvement of unusual joints (the elbow, wrist and ankle), point to a CPPD disorder rather than a simple concurrence of two common conditions.

Inflammatory polyarthritis usually involves the smaller joints as well, and systemic features of inflammation are more marked.

Metabolic disorders include hyperparathyroidism, hemochromatosis and alkaptonuria may be associated with calcification of articular cartilage and fibrocartilage as well as joint symptoms.

Hemochromatosis resulting from chronic iron overload, usually in men, shows clinical features of cirrhosis and diabetes, with a typical bronze pigmentation of the skin. About half of the patients develop joint symptoms (particularly in the hands and fingers); some also have chronic backache. X-rays reveal chondrocalcinosis and a destructive arthropathy, typically in the metacarpophalangeal joints. The plasma iron and iron-binding capacity are raised.

Alkaptonuria is characterized by the appearance of homogentisic acid in the urine, dark pigmentation of the connective tissues (*ochronosis*) and calcification of hyaline and fibrocartilage. The inborn error is an absence of homogentisic acid oxidase in the liver and kidney. X-rays reveal narrowing and calcification of the intervertebral disks at multiple levels, and spinal osteoporosis. At a later stage the large peripheral joints may show chondrocalcinosis and severe osteoarthritis.

Hyperparathyroidism is caused by solitary adenoma of thyroid gland with hypercalcemia, anorexia, nausea, abdominal pain, depression, fatigue and muscle weakness, polyuria, kidney stones or nephrocalcinosis with joint symptoms due to chondrocalcinosis (less than 10% present with bone disease with generalized osteoporosis).

Treatment

Pseudogout is treated same as that of acute gout: Rest with immobilization and high-dosage anti-inflammatory therapy. In elderly patients, *joint aspiration and intra-articular corticosteroid injection is the treatment of choice* as these patients are more vulnerable to the side effects of NSAIDs.

When it is associated with progressive joint degeneration the treatment is essentially that of advanced osteoarthritis with total replacement arthroplasty.

Prognosis

Pseudogout itself has no known effect on life expectancy; associated diseases carry their own prognosis. Chronic chondrocalcinosis appears to be irreversible and fortunately usually causes few symptoms and little disability. Patients with associated osteoarthritis may eventually require prosthetic joints, if symptoms and disability become chronic and severe.

Basic Calcium Phosphate Crystal Deposition Disease

Basic calcium phosphate (BCP) is a primary material of normal bone mineral, in the form of *calcium hydroxyapatite* crystals. Abnormal accumulation of basic calcium phosphates, largely carbonate substituted apatite, can occur in areas of tissue damage such as dystrophic calcification or hyperthyroid states like metastatic calcification and certain others **(Box 2)**. Minute deposits in joints and periarticular tissues can give rise to either an acute reaction (synovitis or tendinitis) or a chronic, destructive arthropathy.

Prolonged hyperphosphatemia, of whatever cause, may result in widespread metastatic calcification. The most common cause of BCP crystal deposition in and around joints is local tissue damage–strained or torn ligaments, tendon attrition and cartilage damage or degeneration.

Pathology

Apatite aggregates are commonly present in synovial fluid in an extremely destructive chronic arthropathy. In the elderly this occurs most often in the shoulders (Milwaukee shoulder) and in a similar process in hips, knees, and erosive osteoarthritis of fingers. Joint destruction is associated with damage to cartilage and supporting structures, leading to instability and deformity.

Progression tends to be indolent, and synovial fluid leukocyte counts are usually <2,000/L. Symptoms range from minimal to severe pain and disability that may lead to joint replacement surgery. Whether severely affected patients merely represent an extreme synovial tissue response to the apatite crystals that are so common in osteoarthritis is uncertain. Synovial lining cell or fibroblast cultures exposed to apatite (or CPPD) crystals can undergo mitosis and markedly increase the release of prostaglandin E2 and cytokines and also collagenases and neutral proteases, underscoring the destructive potential of abnormally stimulated synovial lining cells

Calcific deposit has a creamy consistency but in longstanding cases it is more like chalk. Crystal shedding into joints may give rise to synovitis. More rarely this is complicated by the development of a rapidly destructive, erosive arthritis. Bits of articular cartilage and bone or fragments of a meniscus may be found in the synovial cavity.

Clinical Features

Two clinical syndromes are associated with BCP crystal deposition:

Acute or subacute periarthritis: It is the most common form of BCP crystal deposition disorder affecting joints. Adults between 30 and 50 years, presents with complains of pain close to one of the larger joints—most commonly the shoulder or the knee. Symptoms may start suddenly, perhaps after minor trauma, or more gradual in onset and can easily localize the area of tenderness over periarticular structures. Both forms of the BCP crystals deposition disease are seen most commonly in rotator cuff lesions of the shoulder. Symptoms usually subside after a few weeks or months; sometimes they are aborted only when the calcific deposit is removed or the surrounding tissues are decompressed. In acute cases, operation may disclose a tense globule or creamy material.

Chronic destructive arthritis: Basic calcium phosphate crystals are sometimes found in association with a chronic erosive arthritis.

Milwaukee shoulder: Milwaukee shoulder syndrome or rapid destructive arthritis of the shoulder; it is a particular form of arthritis which affects mainly elderly patients, predominantly women, with limited pain and sometimes neuropathic joints, rotator cuff tear, joint instability, mildly inflammatory or non-inflammatory, blood-stained effusion, calcium apatite crystals deposition, and marked joint and bone destruction.

Differential Diagnosis

Acute calcific periarthritis: The differential diagnosis of acute calcific periarthritis should include gout, pseudogout and sepsis. The distribution of the lesions and the acute onset are often characteristic. X-rays showing the evolution of the calcific deposit are virtually pathognomonic. The diagnosis can be confirmed if material can be aspirated from the area.

Box 2: Conditions associated with BCP crystal deposition disease.

- Aging
- Osteoarthritis
- Hemorrhagic shoulder effusions in the elderly (Milwaukee shoulder)
- Destructive arthropathy
- Tendinitis, bursitis
- Tumoral calcinosis (sporadic cases)
- Disease-associated
  - Hyperparathyroidism
  - Milk-alkali syndrome
  - Renal failure/long-term dialysis
  - Connective tissue diseases (e.g., systemic sclerosis, idiopathic myositis, SLE)
  - Heterotopic calcification after neurologic catastrophes (e.g., stroke, spinal cord injury)
- Heredity
  - Bursitis, arthritis
  - Tumoral calcinosis
  - Fibrodysplasia ossificans progressiva

Chronic periarticular syndromes: The usual features are those of a tendinitis, and the only way of implicating crystal deposition in the diagnosis is through visualizing the deposit on the radiograph. Other causes of tendonitis, such as trauma, impingement, and inflammatory arthritis, are possible differential diagnoses.

Acute and chronic arthritis: It may mimic gout, pseudogout or other systemic inflammatory rheumatic disease has been attributed to BCP crystals. BCP crystals are often detected in osteoarthritic joints and appear to promote the degenerative process, as their presence is associated with more advanced radiographic change and larger joint effusions than in joints without BCP crystals. Erosive arthritis with recurrent episodes of pain and swelling involving the wrists and the finger joints has been associated with BCP crystal deposition.

Destructive arthropathies of the elderly: The main differential diagnoses include neuropathic or Charcot joints, chronic sepsis, advanced rheumatoid disease, osteonecrosis and CPPD deposition disease. Radiographic involvement of both sides of the joint helps differentiate this condition from osteonecrosis. The absence of any neurologic deficit distinguishes it from Charcot's arthropathy.

Investigations

Synovial fluid: Individual crystals from synovial fluid or tissue are very small and can be seen only by electron microscopy. Clumps of crystals may appear as 1- to 20-m shiny intra- or extracellular nonbirefringent globules or aggregates that stain purplish with Wright's stain and bright red with alizarin red S. Tetracycline binding is under investigation as a labeling alternative. Absolute identification depends on electron microscopy with energy-dispersive elemental analysis, X-ray diffraction, infrared spectroscopy, or Raman microspectroscopy, but they usually are not required in clinical diagnosis.

Radiographs: Intra- and/or periarticular calcifications with or without erosive, destructive, or hypertrophic changes may be seen on radiographs. They should be distinguished from the linear calcifications typical of CPPD deposition disease. In peri-arthritis, calcification may be seen in tendons or ligaments close to the joint, most commonly in the rotator cuff around the shoulder. "Loose bodies" may be seen in synovial joints with erosive arthritis show loss of the articular space, with little or no sclerosis or osteophyte formation, with severe destruction of subchondral bone and in advanced case unstable joints may dislocate.

Treatment

Asymptomatic deposits require no treatment. Acute periarthritis should be treated by rest and NSAIDs or oral colchicine for 2 weeks. Resistant cases may respond to local injection of corticosteroids (EDTA). Operative removal of the calcific deposit or "decompression" of the affected tendon or ligament indicated for persistent pain and tenderness. Erosive arthritis is treated like osteoarthritis. Rapidly progressive bone destruction needs early operation by synovectomy and soft-tissue repair for shoulder and usually total joint replacement for the hip.

■ OTHER CRYSTAL DEPOSITION DISORDERS

Clinical significance of other joint crystals: Calcium Oxalate Crystals and Synthetic Depot Corticosteroid Crystals have established pathogenic potential. Other crystalline material with possible pathogenic implications include Liquid Lipid crystals, Cholesterol crystals, other lipid crystals, Hematoidin crystals, immunoglobulins, Charcot-Leyden crystals, Protein Crystals (Immunoglobulin, Amyloid Crystal) and Foreign Bodies (bacteria, others).

Oxalate (CaOx) Crystal Deposition Disease

To date, oxalate crystals have only been described in the joints of patients with renal failure.

Primary oxalosis is a rare hereditary metabolic disorder with enhanced production of oxalic acid with enzyme defects, leading to hyperoxalemia and deposition of calcium oxalate crystals in tissues. Nephrocalcinosis, renal failure, and death usually occur before age 20. Acute and/or chronic CaOx arthritis and periarthritis may complicate primary oxalosis during later years of illness.

Secondary oxalosis is more common than the primary disorder and is one of the many metabolic abnormalities that complicate end-stage renal disease. In chronic renal disease, calcium oxalate deposits have long been recognized in visceral organs, blood vessels, bones, and cartilage and are now known to be one of the causes of arthritis in chronic renal failure.

Clinical Features

Acute CaOx arthritis features are similar to MSU, CPPD, or apatite. CaOx aggregates can be found in bone, articular cartilage, synovium, and periarticular tissues. From these sites, crystals may be shed, causing acute synovitis. Persistent aggregates of CaOx can, like apatite and CPPD, stimulate synovial cell proliferation and enzyme release, resulting in progressive articular destruction. Deposits have been documented in fingers, wrists, elbows, knees, ankles, and feet. Oxalates may also be found in intervertebral disks and contribute to disk destruction in dialysis patients.

Investigations

Synovial fluid: Definitive diagnosis is by crystal identification in joint fluid or by biopsy of joints, bones or other tissues. Synovial fluid crystals can be pleomorphic, but characteristically include at least some with *bipyramidal or envelope-like shapes*. CaOx-induced synovial effusions are usually noninflammatory, with <2,000 leukocytes/L, or mildly inflammatory. Neutrophils or mononuclear cells can predominate. CaOx crystals have a variable shape and variable birefringence to polarized light. The most easily recognized forms are bipyramidal, have strong birefringence, and stain with alizarin red S.

Radiographs may reveal chondrocalcinosis or soft tissue calcifications and radiographs are not helpful.

Treatment of CaOx Arthropathy

Treated with NSAIDs, colchicine, intra-articular glucocorticoids, and/or an increased frequency of dialysis has produced only slight improvement. In primary oxalosis, liver transplantation has induced a significant reduction in crystal deposits.

Lipid Crystals: Cholesterol, Lipid Liquid Crystals and Others

Cholesterol crystals are seen most commonly as a complication of joint effusions resulting from *RA or OA* and are also found in sites such as olecranon bursae. Cholesterol crystals are most often seen as broad plates with a notched corner. Needle-shaped crystals with negative elongation (which are not MSUM crystals) and also be seen in cholesterol-laden fluids. Cholesterol crystals may develop in rheumatoid nodules, in gouty tophi, and have been found in rheumatoid pericarditis. Recent hemarthrosis or trauma followed by joint inflammation is another clinical setting in which lipids might be considered.

Most patients present with monoarthritis. Most commonly knee joint is involved, but cases with wrist involvement and even polyarthritis. Lipid liquid crystals are readily identified under compensated polarized light as 2–20/Lim. *Maltese cross-like spherules* with the two blue parts of the cross lined up parallel to the axis of slow vibration of the compensator (positive elongation). Nonbirefringent droplets composed largely of neutral lipids are common after trauma, lymphatic obstruction, in pancreatic disease, and occasionally in type IV hyperlipoproteinemia. Needle-shaped crystals with negative elongation can precipitate in these droplets, especially during storage, and can be a source of confusion with urates. Crystalline lipids generally do not stain with fat stains as do neutral fat droplets.

Protein Crystals

Patients with *cryoglobulinemia* may have arthritis without synovial fluid crystals. In vessels, crystallized cryoglobulin or myeloma proteins can cause vascular obliteration. Cryoglobulin crystals have been emphasized as causes of both destructive arthritis and vasculopathy. A mouse model for IgG3 cryocrystal globulinemia has been reported with deposits in kidneys.

Immunoglobulin crystals are pleomorphic and may be over 60 cm in size. These can also appear as smaller squares, hexagons, rhomboids or rods, and be potentially confused with known pathogenic crystals. Because they are proteins, they will stain with methylene blue. Some crystals are negatively birefringent. Monoclonal antibodies can provide specific identification. Other protein crystals described in synovial fluid include *Charcot-Leyden crystals*, felt to be composed of lysophospholipase in eosinophil-laden fluids, hemoglobin, and hematoidin. Charcot-Leyden crystals have a characteristic spindle shape and are weakly birefringent, with positive or negative elongation. *Hematoidin crystals*, derived from the breakdown of hemoglobin, are rhomboids very similar to CPPD, except for their golden color on regular light microscopy.

Crystalline Foreign Bodies

Foreign bodies can cause acute or recurrent arthritis that is usually monoarticular. The penetrating injury may not be recalled. Most foreign bodies become embedded or sequestered in synovial tissue and so are not seen in synovial fluid (**Box 3**). *Arthroscopy or arthrotomy* may be required for diagnosis. *Plant thorns* can show dramatic packing of cells and cellulose that is accentuated with polarized light. Calcium carbonate from *sea urchin spines* is birefringent and irregular; *fiberglass* birefringent fibrils, or *polyethylene and methacrylate* in patients with replacement joints, have also been described in joints. *Aluminum crystals* have been reported in joints in systemic aluminum toxicity. Most foreign bodies are not radiopaque and magnetic resonance imaging (MRI) may help identify some of these.

Treatment

Nonsteroidal anti-inflammatory drugs are generally used when the clinical situation permits for oxalate-associated inflammation or to temporarily help with depot corticosteroid-induced bouts. Rarely, depot corticosteroid crystals have to be aspirated in unusually prolonged iatrogenic corticosteroid crystal-induced inflammation. Oxalate accumulation in hemodialysis patients may be slowed by avoiding the use of

---

Box 3: Crystal-like artifacts seen in synovial fluid wet preparations.

- Depot corticosteroid crystals
- Glass fragments
- Nail polish from sealed cover slip edges
- Wood fragments from sticks used in transport
- Starch from gloves
- Anticoagulant crystals—sodium oxalate, lithium, heparin
- Precipitates from storage—calcium phosphates, oxalates, hemoglobin, hematoidin, lipids, unidentified material
- Dust
- Lens paper fibrils

vitamin C, which is metabolized to oxalate. *Foreign bodies, of course, are best managed by removal.*

Lesch–Nyhan Syndrome

Lesch–Nyhan syndrome is a genetic disorder associated with three major clinical elements.
1. Overproduction of uric acid
2. Neurological disability
3. Behavioral problems.

The enzyme hypoxanthine-guanine phosphoribosyl transferase (HGPRTase) deficiency results in increased levels of phosphoribosyl pyrophosphate (PRPP) and decreased levels of IMP and GMP causing increased de novo purine synthesis. Thus, resulting in overproduction of uric acid.

Genetics

It is a rare X-linked recessive disorder associated with a virtually *complete deficiency of HGPRTase*. It mostly occurs in males. The prevalence of Lesch–Nyhan syndrome is approximately 1 in 380,000 individuals **(Fig. 20)**.

Clinical Features

Increased uric acid levels leading to gout like swelling in some of the joints. In some cases, kidney and bladder stones develop. Males with this disease have delayed motor development followed by abnormal movements and increased reflexes. A significant feature of this syndrome is self-destructive behavior including chewing of fingertips and lips. The behavioral problems include cognitive dysfunction, aggressive and impulsive behavior **(Figs. 21A and B)**.

Treatment

Treatment of Lesch–Nyhan syndrome is *symptomatic*. Gout can be treated with allopurinol to control excessive uric acid. Kidney stones may be treated with lithotripsy. There is no standard treatment for the neurological symptoms

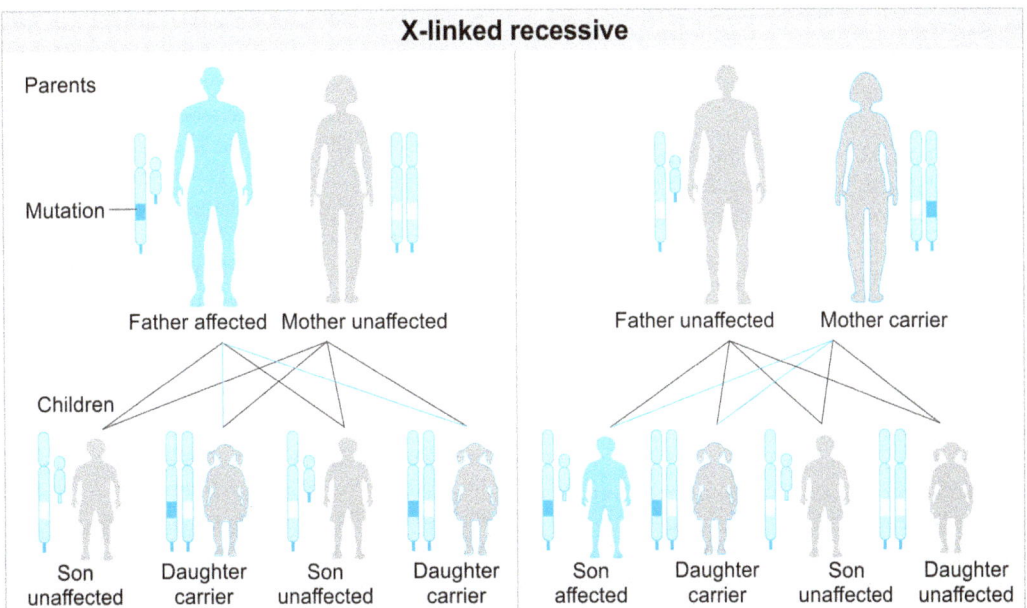

Fig. 20: The inheritance detects of Lesch-Nyhan syndrome. This X-linked recessive syndrome is solely for the male and the chance taken from the sons and daughters with either affected father and unaffected mother or unaffected father and carrier mother are showed.

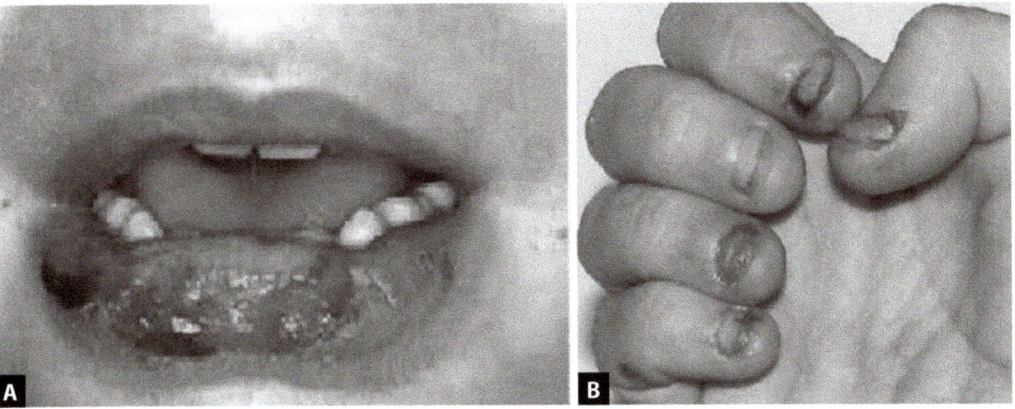

Figs. 21A and B: Self-destructive behavior of Lysch-Nyhan syndrome showing chewing of lips and finger tips.

of Lesch–Nyhan syndrome but some may be relieved with drugs such as carbidopa or levodopa, phenobarbital, etc.

■ FURTHER READING

1. Ames BN, Cathcart R, Schiviers E, Hochstein P. Uric acid provides an anti-oxidant defense in humans against oxidant and radicals. Proc Natl Acad Sci USA. 1981;78(11):6858-62
2. Brunton L, Chabner BA, Knollman B. Goodman and Gilman's The Pharmacological Basis of Therapeutics, 12th edition. New York: McGraw Hill; 2011.
3. Coe FL, Moran E, Kavalich AG. The contribution of dietary purine over-consumption to hyperuricosuria in calcium oxalate stone formers. J Chron Dis. 1976;29: 793-800.
4. Davis S, Park Y, Abuchowwski A, Davis F. Hypouricaemic effect of polyethyleneglycol modified urate oxidase. Lancet. 1981:1.
5. Dieppe PA, Alexander GJM, Jones HE, Doherty M, Scott DG, Manhire A, et al. Prophosphate arthropathy: a clinical and radiological study of 105 cases. Ann Rheum Dis. 1982;41(4):371-6.
6. Dieppe PA, Huskisson EC, Crocker P. Willoughby DA, Apatite deposition disease: a new arthopathy. Lance. 1976;1:266-9.
7. Dougados M, Benhanou L, Amor B. Charcot-Leyden crystals in synovial fluid. Arthritis Rheum. 1983;26:1416.
8. Fam AG. Gout in the elderly. Clinical presentation and treatment. Drugs Aging. 1998;13:229-43.
9. Halverson PB, McCarty DJ. Identification of hydroxyapatite crystals in synovial fluid. Arthritis Rheum. 1979;22:389-95.
10. Hochberg MC. Rheumatology, 3rd edition. Mosby: Elsevier; 2003.
11. Hoffman GS, Schumacher HR, Paul H, Cherian V, Reed R, Ramsay AG, et al. Calcium oxalate microcrystalline associated arthritis in end stage renal disease. Ann Intern Med. 1982;97:36-42.
12. Ishikawa K, Masuda I, Ohira T, Yokoyama M. A Histological study of calcium pyrophosphate dihydrate crystal-deposition disease. J Bone Joint Surg. 1989:71A:875-6.
13. KD Tripathi. Essentials of Medical Pharmacology, 7th edition. New Delhi: Jaypee Brothers Medical Publishers; 2013.
14. Kumar V, Abbas AK, Aster JC, Fausto N. Robbins and Cotran Pathologic Basis of Disease, 8th edition. New York: Saunders/Elsevier; 2010.
15. Lipkowitz MS, Leal-Pinto E, Rappoport JZ, Najfeld V, Abramson RG. Functional reconstitution, membrane targeting, genomic structure, and chromosomal localization of a human urate transporter. J Clin Investig. 2001;107:1103-15.
16. Longo DL, Kasper DL, Larry JJ, Anthony FS, Hauser SL. Harrison's Principles of Internal Medicine, 18th edition. New York: McGraw Hill; 2012.
17. Maldonado I, Prasad V, Reginato AJ. Oxalate crystal deposition disease. Curr Rheumatol Rep. 2002;4(3):257-64.
18. McCarty DJ, Gatter RA. Recurrent acute inflammation associated with focal apatite crystal deposition. Arthritis Rheum. 1966; 9:804-19.
19. McCarty DJ, Halverson PB, Carrera GF, Brewer BJ, Kozin F. 'Milwauke shoulder'- association of microspheroids containing hydroxyapatite crystals, active collagenase and neutral protease with rotator cuff defects. Arthritis Rheum. 1981;24(3):464-73.
20. McCarty DJ. Calcium pyrophosphate dihydrate crystal deposition disease - 1975. Arthritis Rheum. 1976;19(Suppl): 275-86.
21. McCarty DJ. Robert Adams' rheumatic arthritis of the shoulder: "Milwaukee Shoulder" revisited. J Rheumatol. 1989; 16:668-670.
22. McQueen FM, Doyle A, Dalbeth N. Imaging in gout - What can we learn from MRI, CT, DECT and US? Arthritis Res Ther. 2011;13:246.
23. Molloy ES, McCarthy GM. Basic calcium phosphate crystals: pathways to joint destruction. Curr Opinion Rheumatol. 2006;18:187.
24. Reiders MK, aagsma C, Jansen TL, van Roon EN, Delsing J, van de Laar MA, et al. A randomised controlled trial on the efficacy and tolerability with dose escalation of allopurinol 300–600 mg/day versus benzbromarone 100–200 mg/day in patients with gout. Ann Rheum Dis. 2009;68(6):892-7.
25. Resnick CS, Resnick D. Crystal deposition disease, Semin Arthritis Rheum. 1983;12: 390-403.
26. Richette P, Bardin T, Doherty M. An update on the epidemiology of calcium pyrophosphate dihydrate crystal deposition disease. Rheumatology (Oxford). 2009;48(7):711-5.
27. Robert K. Murray et al., Harper's Illustrated Biochemistry, 29th edition, Mc Graw Hill, Lange; 2012.
28. Rosenthal A, Mandel N. Identification of crystals in synovial fluids and joint tissues. Curr Rheumatol Rep. 2001;3:11-6.
29. Rundles RW, Metz EN, Silberman HR. Allopurinol in the treatment of gout. Ann Intern Med. 1966;64:229-58.
30. Stevens CR, Benboubetra M, Harrison R, Sahinoglu T, Smith EC, Blake DR. Localisation of xanthine oxidase to synovial endothelium. Ann Rheum Dis. 1991;50:760-2.
31. Thouverey C, Bechkoff G, Pikula S, Buchet R. Inorganic pyrophosphate as a regulator of hydroxyapatite or calcium pyrophosphate dihydrate mineral deposition by matrix vesicles. Osteoarthritis Cartilage. 2009;17(1):64-72.
32. Wortmann RL, Schumacher HR, Becker MA, Ryan LM. Crystal-Induced Arthropathies: Gout, Pseudogout and Apatite-Associated Syndromes. New York: Taylor and Francis; 2006.

17. Osteoarthritis: Etiology, Pathogenesis, and Management

Venus Khanna, Manju Agrawal, Alok Chandra Agrawal

■ INTRODUCTION

The term "Osteoarthritis" is derived from three Greek words, "osteo," which means "of the bone," "arthr," which means "joint," and "itis," which implies "inflammation". It is a progressive degenerative disorder of the joints caused by the destruction of the articular cartilage, marginal osteophytes, subchondral cyst, and sclerosis.

Incidence

As per the Framingham study, it is estimated that women (1%) are more commonly affected than men (0.7%) each year. Bilateral knee osteoarthritis (OA) is more common than unilateral disease, affecting 5% versus 2%, respectively.

Pathogenesis

The normal balance between chondrocyte synthesis, articular cartilage, and extracellular matrix formation and degeneration is destabilized due to repeated mechanical and biological factors. This leads to series of molecular, biochemical, morphological, and biochemical changes in the cells. It is characterized by softening of the cartilage, fibrillations and ulcerations, erosion of the articular cartilage, subchondral cysts, formation of osteophytes, subchondral sclerosis of the bone.

■ ARTICULAR CARTILAGE

Composition

In adults, the normal articular cartilage occupies 2% of the total volume. It consists of a specialized extracellular matrix that is regulated by the chondrocytes. The matrix predominantly contains type II collagen, proteoglycans such as aggrecan with hyaluronic acid (HA). The microfibrillar framework is formed by the type II, IX, X collagens entrapped in proteoglycan aggrecan. Type VI collagen forms an additional fibers meshwork in the pericellular matrix (between the matrix and the cell surface).

Proteoglycans consist of a "protein core" to which glycosaminoglycans chains (mainly keratan sulfate and chondroitin sulfate) are covalently attached. The physicochemical properties of the structure provide swelling pressure, hydration, and its ability to withstand compressible forces. The structure of the proteoglycan unit is depicted in **Figure 1**.

Articular cartilage is divided into four layers (**Fig. 2**), namely

1. *Superficial/Tangential zone (Lamina splendens)*: It consists primarily of collagen type IV, fibers parallel to the surface and closely packed, relatively acellular, has tightly bound smaller proteoglycan, namely decorin and biglycan. Orientation of fibrous cartilage tissue is vital for biomechanical integrity. When the deforming forces are against the orientation of its fibers, it can cause a break in collagen fibril and the first step to joint degeneration.

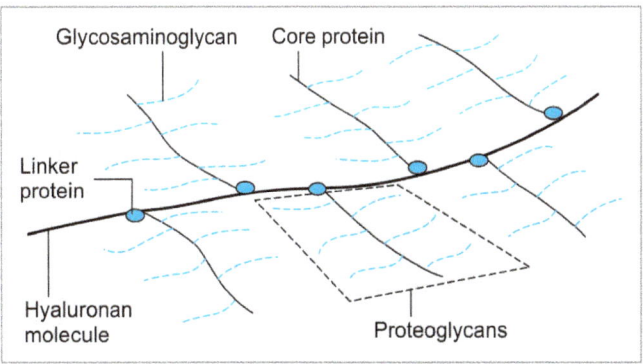

Fig. 1: Structure of proteoglycans.

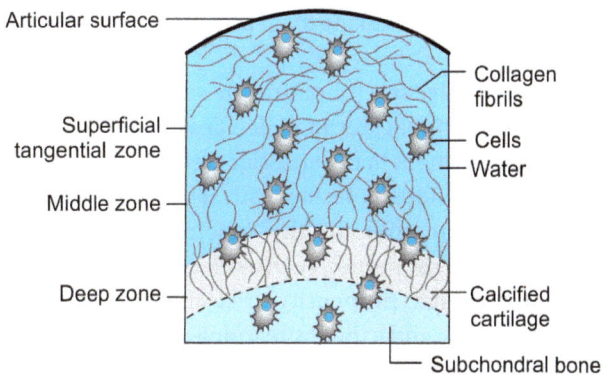

Fig. 2: Hyaline cartilage.

2. *Middle/Intermediate/Transition zone*: Collagen fibers form a coiled interlacing network, fibers are more widely spaced, and ground substance is abundant. Cells are numerous spheroidal and dispersed. When articular cartilage is subjected to physiologic compressive load for a period of 12 hours, the open fibrous network becomes obliterated and fibers are becoming oriented at right angles to the direction of loading.
3. *Deep/Basal/Radial zone*: This zone contains large amounts of aggrecan with few collagen fibrils. Cells are arranged in columnar fashion and show abundant rough endoplasmic reticulum, which is rich in glycogen. The calcification at the deep end of radial zone cartilage is called tidemark/mineralization front.
4. *Calcified zone*: Here cartilage consists mainly of type X collagen. Below this, layer is the subchondral bone. Overall, type II collagen is most common. The highest degree of metabolic activity takes place in zones II and III. The water content of articular cartilage constitutes approximately 75% of the wet weight and does not change with aging. Keratan sulfate is more intense in the deep zone matrix lying remote from the chondrocytes. Chondroitin sulfate stains most intensely in the deeper parts of zone III immediately about the cells.

Biomechanics of Articular Cartilage

Articular cartilage acts as a low-friction cushion between the joints which supports the load, enables motion, and weight transmission across the joint. Biomechanically, it is considered a permeable, porous, fiber-reinforced composite material with a high quantity of water as its interstitial fluid. These features give anisotropic (dependent on direction), viscoelastic (time-or rate-dependent), and non-linear (dependent on the magnitude of strain) mechanical advantage to the surface.

In response to load, the tensile properties from the high-water content, the non-linear properties of collagen fibril, are responsible for distributing compressible forces. These properties progressively decrease after 30 years due to the accumulation of advanced glycation end products (AGE). These end products cause biomechanical alteration in the articular cartilage by making them brittle and prone to tissue fractures.

The proteoglycans (chondroitin sulfate and keratan sulfate) chains with aggrecan molecules create a negatively charged environment in the articular cartilage. The complex interaction with these molecules with HA in the extracellular matrix is responsible for the electrokinetic and the physicochemical properties, such as electro-osmotic effects, streaming currents, propensity to swell under enormous osmotic pressure, and exhibit streaming potentials. Synovial fluid provides a high viscosity squeeze layer which acts as a joint lubricant and distributes the load.

Biomechanical Regulation of Cartilage Metabolism

The normal homeostasis between cartilage synthesis and breakdown is regulated by genetic (growth factors, cytokines), extracellular matrix composition, and environmental factors (mechanical stress). The mechanical stress on chondrocytes leads to activation of cyclic AMP, inositol trisphosphate through various intercellular and intracellular signaling pathways.

■ RISK FACTORS FOR OSTEOARTHRITIS

- *Abnormalities in joint biomechanical and biomaterial attributes, an endocrine disorder, and chemical injuries*: Mutations in the *COL2A1 gene* localized on chromosome 12 leading to alteration of type II collagen can cause a spectrum of disease, such as cartilage dysplasia, familial OA, severe form of OA with defective collagen. It usually appears after growth arrest. Osteoarthritis can also be caused by endocrine disorders, like acromegaly, which causes interference with cartilage metabolism or metabolic diseases such as ochronosis, hemochromatosis, or alkaptonuria abnormal build-up of the matrix in cartilage. Traumatic injury to the cartilage can lead to joint incongruity and predispose OA.
- *Abnormal loading of forces in joint*: Repeated mechanical trauma, abnormal loading over joints, and progressive wear can change the cartilage's structure, composition, and material properties. These changes associated with unstable joints (ligament or meniscal injury) can lead to secondary OA. Obesity itself can cause increased joint loading along with endocrine changes causing low-grade chronic inflammation. Lack of proper rehabilitation, specific neurological disorder, or even prolong immobilization due to casting can cause secondary disuse atrophy of the articular cartilages. This alteration in biomechanical properties halts cartilage proteoglycan aggrecan synthesis and increases metalloproteinases (MMPs), which itself can cause damage to the articular cartilage.

Various age-related changes can cause muscle weakness, altered impact loading, which fails to absorb impact during the various day-to-day activities. One of the most common causes of knee pain in patients with OA is quadriceps muscle weakness. Certain nutritional factors such as vitamin C and E deficiency have some evidence as risk factors for accelerated OA development.

■ CAUSES OF OSTEOARTHRITIS

The important causes of osteoarthritis are given in **Table 1**.

■ THE DEGENERATION OF ARTICULAR CARTILAGE IN OSTEOARTHRITIS

In vivo, cartilage swelling (hypertrophic reaction) occurs due to increased synthesis of the matrix with an increased

TABLE 1: Causes of osteoarthritis.

Primary	Secondary (Degenerative process that takes place in a previously unhealthy joint)
Unknown etiology in a previously healthy joint	• Trauma • Arthritis (such as rheumatoid arthritis, infectious arthritis, etc.) • Deformities (genu varum, genu valgum, recurvatum, flexion) • Instability (ACL/PCL/MCL/LCL injury) • Obesity • Osteochondritis dissecans disease • Meniscal cyst, discoid meniscus

(ACL: anterior cruciate ligament; LCL: lateral collateral ligament; PCL: posterior cruciate ligament; MCL: medial collateral ligament)

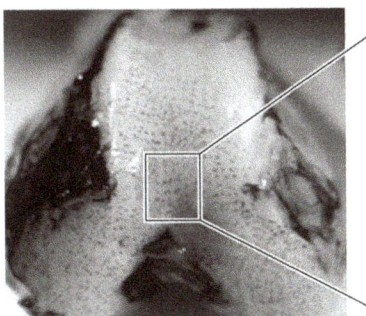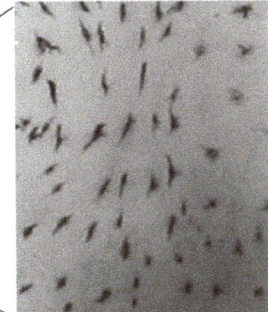

Fig. 3: Split-line pattern on rabbit femur.

aggrecan seen in articular cartilage degeneration. It is followed by increased matrix turnover and gradual depletion of matrix components leading to loss of collagen framework **(Fig. 3)**. This cycle of degeneration of articular cartilage may begin with the loss of articular cartilage in a particular area to gradually involve multiple compartments. This degeneration presents the fibrillations parallel to the articular surface which later denudes the articular cartilage, causing exposure to the subchondral bone. In patients with a fracture of the articular surface, damage to the joint stabilizers such as anterior cruciate ligament, meniscal injuries, and progressive degeneration of the articular cartilage leads to post-traumatic osteoarthritis. The medial compartment of the tibia is prone to such changes.

Proteinases of Osteoarthritis Cartilage

The regulation of matrix macromolecules such as aggrecan, type II collagen is highly regulated via MMPs. In osteoarthritis, there is increased expression of various MMPs with downregulation of ADAMTS-4 (a disintegrin and metalloproteinase with thrombospondin motifs) or ADAMTS-5. This causes excessive proteolysis.

Metalloproteinases such as 1, 8, 13, 14 are highly active in the articular cartilage and are mainly responsible for cleavage in articular cartilage and collagenases. MMP-13, as compared to other MMPs and collagenase, is primarily responsible for the separation of articular cartilage.

Aggrecanases and other MMPs cause break in aggrecan, which is also increased during OA.

The Causes and Regulation of Cartilage Matrix Degradation

A vicious cycle forms when the matrix degradation products stimulate further damage by activating chondrocyte and synovial cell receptors, e.g. In OA, there is increased production of fibronectin. The degradation products stimulate autocrine and paracrine roles for cytokine production such as interleukin (IL)-1, which causes further degradation. Fragments of type II collagen can when present in sufficient concentration, also induce matrix resorption. In OA, there is the increased expression on chondrocytes of the receptors for IL-1 and IL-1 itself, even more than in rheumatoid arthritis.

The pathologic changes in a cartilage matrix structure in OA are likely to cause fundamental disturbances in the normal balance between the cytokine and growth factor signaling, which leads to changing gene expression of signaling molecules, enzymes, and the matrix macromolecules. These MMPs are regulated extracellularly at the level of inhibition by tissue inhibitors of metalloproteinases (TIMPs) and intracellularly at transcriptional activation, translation, and extracellular proenzyme activation. Four such inhibitors have been described; namely, TIMP-1, -2, -3, and -4. These react with the active MMP in a 1:1 molar ratio. In OA, there is a deficiency of TIMP activity favoring excessive proteolysis. TIMP-3, which is the only TIMP that can bind to the extracellular matrix, can inhibit aggrecan degradation in hyaline cartilage. Its expression is upregulated in OA cartilage, whereas TIMP-1 and -4 are downregulated.

General Changes in Cartilage Matrix Protein Content and Gene Expression

The early damage to the more superficial matrix in early OA is accompanied by an increased content of biglycan and decorin and aggrecan in the mid and deep zones, no doubt to compensate for the increased loading on the chondrocytes and the damage to and loss of these molecules from the more superficial cartilage. This accompanies the marked increase in the synthesis of type II procollagen in these deeper sites, mainly type MB and some type IIA, which is usually observed only before chondroblast differentiation early in development. Overall there is a loss of type II collagen, starting in the more superficial cartilage. There is limited-expression and synthesis of type III collagen. Type VI content is, however, increased, and its filamentous structure is altered, presumably as a result of pericellular remodeling, which frequently results in an enlargement of the pericellular matrix. These changes are also reflected as a loss of mechanical properties of the pericellular matrix, which results in significant alterations in the biomechanical environment of the chondrocytes.

The Regulation of Cartilage Matrix Assembly in Osteoarthritis

Cytokines such as IL-1 can inhibit matrix synthesis, whereas IGF-1 can suppress this inhibition. IGF-1 and mRNA levels are increased in OA articular tissue. IGF-1 can decrease the degradation and inhibition of synthesis induced by IL-1. IL-1 stimulates IGF-1 release from chondrocytes. Despite the increase in IGF-1 in OA, OA chondrocytes are hyporesponsive to this growth factor. This may be because IGF-1 activity is excessively restricted by IGFBPs, which are also upregulated by cytokines such as IL-1. Proteases can also cleave these binding proteins, regulating their activity. Fibroblast growth factor-2 stimulates cell proliferation in articular chondrocytes but does not stimulate the synthesis of glycosaminoglycans.

Changes in the Chondrocyte Phenotype in Relationship to Cell Death—Matrix Degradation and Calcification in Osteoarthritis

Usually, hypertrophy is only seen in the growth plate when the extracellular collagen network is partially resorbed by MMP-13 and then calcified as cells die as a result of apoptosis. In OA, these events, including apoptosis, reappear in degenerate OA cartilage. Parathyroid hormone-related peptide (PTHrP), also produced by prehypertrophic cells in the growth plate and suppresses hypertrophy, is also upregulated in OA cartilage. The calcium-sensing receptor, expressed by hypertrophic cells, is upregulated with the onset of OA. These changes are initially observed in OA cartilage, mainly in the more superficial and mid zones where damage to collagen is most pronounced and may represent a chondrocyte response to a damaged extracellular matrix with the reversion to a more fetal phenotype. There is also a marked increase in the expression of type II collagen, which is also a feature of the shift to hypertrophy in the growth plate.

In the partially calcified OA cartilage delimited by the tidemark and bordered by the subchondral bone, there is a reactivation of endochondral ossification characterized by upregulation of type X collagen expression and duplication or replication of the tidemark, separating this zone from uncalcified cartilage. Vascular invasion from subchondral bone is reinitiated, resembling that seen in endochondral ossification. Moreover, osteophyte formation and the endochondral process are initiated peripheral to the articular cartilages, leading to bone spurs capped with articular cartilage. Thus, there is a significant shift in the physiology of the articular cartilage character. Hypertrophy is accompanied by calcification of the normally uncalcified extracellular matrix of articular cartilage. More than 90% of OA subjects show evidence for limited calcification of articular cartilages; there is also a high incidence of hydroxyapatite crystals in joint fluids.

Articular cartilage:
Normally:
- Spatial distribution of chondrocytes
- Avascular
- Sparsely cellular at its joint surface with increased cellularity toward subchondral bone
- *Site of calcification*: Tidemark/mineralization front

Osteoarthritis:
- Unevenness and fibrillation/fraying of the surface
- Cartilage is thin, fissured, with clefts or slits
- Chondrocytes proliferate adjacent to the fissures
- These cartilage clones/brood capsules represent various stages of the evolution of degenerative joint disease (DJD)
- Marked variation in cellularity and variation in the intensity of the proteoglycan matrix, which is identified by particular stains—Alcian blue, toluidine blue, and safranin O
- At the base, vascular penetration is noted from the underlying subchondral bone with duplicate and marked irregularity to the tidemark
- Eventually-cartilage is eburnated
- Mesenchymal proliferation ensues
- Enchondral ossification (near to growth plate)

THE REMODELING OF SUBCHONDRAL BONE IN OSTEOARTHRITIS

Pronounced changes in subchondral bone occur in OA and may even occur in sites remote from the affected joints. As suggested by bone scintigraphy, the degeneration of articular cartilage may be accompanied or possibly preceded by increased subchondral bone turnover. In the absence of MRI, it is not possible to be clear as to whether the bone changes preceded those in articular cartilages. Such bone changes are predictive of the progression of knee OA and generalized nodal OA. Studies in humans using histologic analyses and magnetic resonance imaging suggest that degenerative changes in articular cartilages are accompanied by local changes in subchondral bone that involve cyst formation and altered trabecular and osteoid thickness and bone formation and turnover.

The development of osteophytes so often seen peripherally in an OA joint involves the formation of a cap of new articular cartilage and new bone formation as part of an endochondral process.

SYNOVITIS AND INFLAMMATION IN OSTEOARTHRITIS

Osteoarthritis is not considered inflammatory arthritis, and the synovial fluid leukocyte count is characteristically less than 3,000 cells/mL. To the extent that acute synovial fluid leukocytic inflammation does occur in OA, it is often the result of secondary crystal-induced synovitis (either calcium apatite or calcium pyrophosphate dihydrate). However, low-grade inflammatory processes nevertheless occur in osteoarthritic synovial tissues that contribute to disease pathogenesis, and many of the clinical symptoms and signs seen in OA joints reflect synovial inflammation (e.g., joint swelling and effusion, stiffness, occasionally redness). Synovial histological changes include synovial hypertrophy and hyperplasia with an increased number of lining cells, often accompanied by infiltration of the subliming tissue with scattered foci of lymphocytes. Cartilage breakdown products derived from the articular surface due to mechanical or enzymatic destruction of the cartilage can provoke collagenase and other hydrolytic enzymes from synovial cells and macrophages.

Hyaluronic acid is also often increased in OA patients. Those with persistently elevated serum HA levels exhibit more rapid disease progression. HA levels also indirectly correlate with minimal joint space.

PAIN IN OSTEOARTHRITIS

Arthritis pain is the most common cause of pain in aged populations and arguably the most debilitating aspect of OA. Although knee pain increases with radiographic disease severity in most studies, it is apparent that the severity of abnormalities by routine radiography does not correlate with pain severity in the individual patient. MRI studies have indicated that in patients with knee OA, knee pain severity was associated with synovitis/effusion, meniscal tears, bone marrow lesions, and subchondral bone erosion.

Pain severity in persons with OA is not a simple phenomenon and can arise from several innervated tissues. The joints of the appendicular skeleton are innervated by the peripheral nervous system in every tissue except cartilage, where innervation is peripheral in the periosteum, synovium, capsule, ligaments, and subchondral bone. Here nociceptors monitor the environment. Neuroinnervation can determine disease onset. Limbs paralyzed by hemiplegia or poliomyelitis are often spared in the development of OA.

THERAPEUTIC TARGETS FOR THE MANAGEMENT OF OSTEOARTHRITIS

Cartilage is a principal target because of its paramount importance in joint articulation. Despite the tremendous impact of this disease, however, current therapies are palliative, and there are no disease-modifying OA drugs (DMOADs) approved for clinical use. Nonetheless, many promising molecular targets exist in the development of pharmacologic therapies for OA, and a valuable and comprehensive review of such therapeutic approaches has recently been published. To date, doxycycline is the only molecule that can regulate collagenase activities in vitro, control the progression of experimental OA, and be used without severe side effects in the treatment of knee OA.

IGF-1 is of obvious importance because of its potency and upregulation in OA, but there may be more potent growth factors or combinations that can be used to renew matrix assembly and control degradation. A combination of MMP inhibitors and enhanced stimulation of matrix synthesis may prove most effective. Pharmacologic stimulation of the vagus nerve cholinergic anti-inflammatory pathway offers new therapeutic opportunities.

Management of Osteoarthritis

Osteoarthritis, more aptly osteoarthrosis, is a noninflammatory degenerative state of joint principally striking weight-bearing joints such as hip, knee, and ankle, almost certainly due to normal wear and tear of articular cartilage, and is accountable for global disability and diminishing the quality of life of an individual.

CLINICAL EVALUATION

Degenerative OA of the knee is blameworthy for 83% of OA disability. Patient conventionally presents with knee arthralgia symptoms, which gets angry on weight-bearing and soothe on rest, swelling, morning stiffness less than 30 minutes, gait disturbance, deformity of joint, incapability to squat and sit cross leg, and trouble to execute the daily activity.

On examination, the patient has joint line tenderness, swollen knee due to synovial hypertrophy, varus or valgus deviation, variable degree of fixed flexion and external torsion of the tibia, and crepitus knee range movement and overall decreased range of motion.

Laboratory and Radiological Evaluation

- Hematology and biochemistry
- Complete blood counts with an erythrocyte sedimentation rate (ESR) and C-reactive protein (CRP)
- Serum calcium, alkaline phosphatase, and phosphorous
- Serum uric acid and RA factor
- Serum Vitamin D3
- *Radiology*:
  - X-ray—*semiquantitative assessment [Kellgren-Lawrence grading system **(Table 2)**]*
    - Weight-bearing anterior-posterior and lateral view of the bilateral knee.
    - Axial or skyline view for patellofemoral joints.
    - Typically show asymmetrical decreased joint space, subchondral sclerosis and cyst formation, osteophytes and malalignment due to varus or valgus, fixed flexion, and external tibial torsion deformities.

TABLE 2: Kellgren–Lawrence grading.

Grade	Radiologic findings
Grade 0	Normal
Grade 1	Doubtful narrowing of joint space with possible osteophytes
Grade 2	Joint space narrowing with osteophytes
Grade 3	Narrowing of joint space, osteophyte formation, and subchondral sclerosis
Grade 4	Large osteophytes, gross destruction of joint space, and definite deformity of bone ends

- *MRI—semiquantitative and quantitative assessment*
  - It provides semiquantitative assessment along with the status of articular cartilage, meniscus, collateral ligaments, bone marrow lesion (BML), and synovium with a grading system.
  - MRI is also helpful in quantitative assessment by measuring joint cartilage thickness and meniscus and joint effusion volume.

Synovial Fluid Analysis

Synovial fluid aspiration from the knee (minimum two examinations) revealing clear normal viscous fluid with leukocyte count not more than 2,000/mL favors the diagnosis of degenerative joint pathology.

CLASSIFICATION OF DEGENERATIVE KNEE OA

Depending on the anatomical region involved, it is classified into:
- Degenerative knee OA proper
- Chondromalacia patellae
- Patellar tendonitis
- Subpatellar fat pad inflammation
- Medial collateral ligament (MCL) inflammation
- Lateral collateral ligament (LCL) inflammation

DIAGNOSTIC CRITERIA

According to the Chinese Medical Association (CMA), knee osteoarthritis can be diagnosed in patients if they have criteria 1st plus any two criteria from 2nd, 3rd, 4th, and 5th as mentioned here:
1. Multiple episodes of knee pain within 1 month duration.
2. X-ray showing joint space reduction with sclerosis and cystic changes and osteophytes.
3. Middle age group >50 years.
4. Morning stiffness <30 minutes.
5. Crepitus on knee range of motion.

TREATMENT

The administration of OA knee requires commingled outlook from orthopedic doctors and physiotherapist. Treatment aims to restore the normal biomechanics and function of the knee through pain management and physiotherapy, which slow the progression of disease and deformity correction by osteotomy and arthroplasty. All approaches are directed to improve the quality of life of the individual.

Treatment armamentarium to doctors includes pharmacological, nonpharmacological, and surgical modalities depending upon the severity of the disease process.

Nonpharmacological Treatment

Patient education: Educating the patient about the disease process and explaining different treatment modalities significantly minimize the psychosocial burden and improve quality of life.

Lifestyle changes: Asking the patient to avoid stairs, cross-leg sitting, and squatting. Usage of commode lavatory should be encouraged.

Weight reduction: A patient with a high BMI should be advised for dietitian consultancy to provide patients with a low calorie and high protein diet. The patient should be encouraged for aerobic exercises.

Exercise therapy: Stretching and range of motion exercise, quadriceps and hamstring strengthening exercises, aerobic exercises, water-based exercises, and slow walking on level ground with electronic monitoring should be advised.

Walking aids: Usage of the stick in opposite sides for unilateral involvement and walker-assisted walking for bilateral disease. The application of elastic knee braces and foot orthoses also relieves pain, gives a soothing effect to patients, and improves function.

Others therapy: Short wave diathermy, ultrasound therapy, transcutaneous electric nerve stimulation, infrared treatment, and magnetic therapy. All these therapies relieve pain and somewhat improves the function of the knee.

Pharmacological Treatment

Paracetamol: They have antipyretic and analgesic effect. Dosage up to 4 g/day. They are no longer regarded as the first-line drug for the management of OA. Paracetamol is used in those patients showing renal and gastrointestinal adverse effects to nonsteroidal anti-inflammatory drugs (NSAIDs).

NSAIDs: These are the first-line drugs in the management of OA. They are used with caution in the elderly and contraindicated in the patient having renal compromise and a history of GI bleed and perforation. They cause gastrointestinal upset. Prolong usage is responsible for cardiovascular dysfunction. They are superior to paracetamol in relieving pain and improving joint function. NSAIDs are available in oral, parenteral, and topical formulations.

Selective COX-2 inhibitors such as etoricoxib and celecoxib are better tolerated in a patient with GI dysfunction.

Capsaicin: Capsaicin and diclofenac are available in gel form for topical usage and have shown results better than placebo.

Opioids and duloxetine: Opioid analgesics (tramadol) are first-line drugs in the patient who have a contraindication to the usage of NSAIDs. Adverse effects are dryness of the mouth, nausea, vomiting, and dizziness. Overdosage may cause respiratory depression. Pain in the OA knee is of heterogeneous origin, and chronicity of symptoms may lead to depression. Duloxetine is mainly used to fight the neuropathic component and depression when used as an adjunct to NSAIDs.

SYSADOs: They are called as symptomatic slow-acting drugs in osteoarthritis. They include glucosamine, chondroitin, diacerein and Avocado soy unsaponifiables. They are dietary adjuncts used with NSAIDs. Efficacy is controversial.

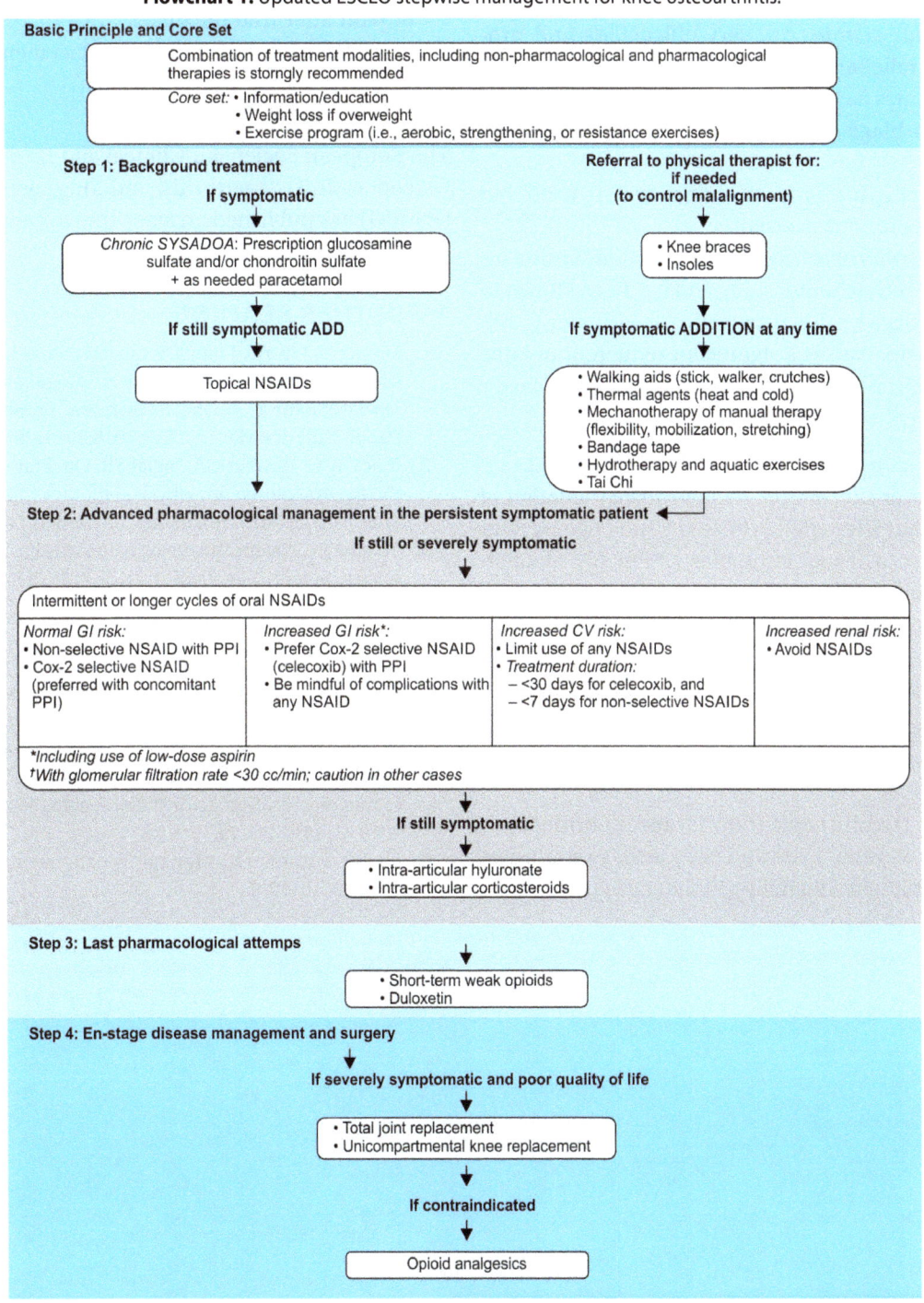

Flowchart 1: Updated ESCEO stepwise management for knee osteoarthritis.

(COX-2: cyclo-oxygenase-2; CS: chondroitin sulfate; CV: cardiovascular; GI: gastrointestinal; GS: glucosamine sulfate; IA: intra-articular; NSAID: nonsteroidal anti-inflammatory drug; PPI: proton pump inhibitor; SYSADOA: symptomatic slow-acting drugs in osteoarthritis; OA: osteoarthritis)

Vitamins: Antioxidant vitamins such as A, C, and E are under study. Vitamin D has a therapeutic effect by bone mineralization.

Traditional Chinese Medication (TCM) includes internal application pills such as Huoluo pills and Duhuojisheng pills. External application methods such as Chinese herbal fumigation, Chinese herbal iontophoresis, and Chinese herbal plaster. They inhibit the inflammatory pathway and delay cartilage destruction.

Intra-articular Injections

- *Intra-articular steroids* are very efficacious and provide instant relief and improvement in joint functions. However, studies have shown that frequent injection can accelerate cartilage destruction and the overall disease process.
- *Intra-articular hyaluronic acid* injections are used, but their benefits are controversial.
- *Intra-articular platelet-rich plasma (PRP)* is an autologous platelet concentrate under study and has been shown to improve cartilage health. Intra-articular PRP, along with hyaluronic acid, causes a significant reduction in knee pain and improved Western Ontario and McMaster Universities Arthritis Index (WOMAC) pain score.

Other therapy: Acupuncture therapy has a good effect on knee OA with fewer side effects. *Radiofrequency* ablation of genicular nerve has been tried in knee OA and ongoing pain management after total knee arthroplasty. Similarly, ablation of the infrapatellar branch of the saphenous nerve by injecting nitrous oxide called *cryoneurolysis* has been tried.

Surgical Treatment

A patient with Grade 4 OA changes and who has exhausted the conservative methods are candidates for surgical management.

- *Arthroscopy*: Arthroscopic joint lavage, debridement, and removal of osteophytes and torn cartilage, meniscus give relief to patient with mild-to-moderate OA.
- *Osteotomy*: High tibial osteotomy (HTO) and distal femoral osteotomy for varus and valgus correction are performed in young patients with minimal deformity and unicompartmental OA disease.
- *Fibular osteotomy* has been tried to have mild-to-moderate OA changes in the medial compartment with promising results.
- *Arthroplasty*: Unicompartmental knee replacement is reserved for unicompartmental involvement and minimal deformity. Progressive knee OA, fixed deformity, global disability in daily activity, and patient complaining of pain after trial of conservative treatment modalities are candidates for total knee replacement surgery.

TREATMENT GUIDELINES

The European Society for Clinical and Economic Aspects of Osteoporosis, Osteoarthritis, and Musculoskeletal Diseases (ESCEO) has published an algorithm for managing OA knee in 2014 **(Flowchart 1)**.

FURTHER READING

1. Huang D, Liu YQ, Liang LS, Lin XW, Song T, Zhuang ZG, et al. The Diagnosis and Therapy of Degenerative Knee Joint Disease: Expert Consensus from the Chinese Pain Medicine Panel. Pain Res Manag. 2018;2018:2010129.
2. MacKay C, Hawker GA, Jaglal SB. Qualitative study exploring the factors influencing physical therapy management of early knee osteoarthritis in Canada. BMJ Open. 2018;8(11):e023457.
3. Tanchev P. Osteoarthritis or osteoarthrosis: commentary on misuse of terms. Reconstruct Rev. 2017;7(1):178.
4. Vitaloni M, Botto-van Bemden A, Sciortino Contreras RM, Scotton D, Bibas M, Quintero M, et al. Global management of patients with knee osteoarthritis begins with quality of life assessment: a systematic review. BMC Musculoskelet Disord. 2019; 20(1):493.
5. Xia W, Cooper C, Li M, Xu L, Rizzoli R, Zhu M, et al. East meets West: current practices and policies in the management of musculoskeletal aging. Aging Clin Exp Res. 2019;31(10):1351-73.
6. Yu SP, Hunter DJ. Managing osteoarthritis. Aust Prescr. 2015;38(4):115-9.

Osteoporosis

SS Jha, Lalit Kishore

■ INTRODUCTION

In general term osteoporosis mean weakness of bone. It is a metabolic bone disease which mostly progresses silently. In this disease bone mass gradually reduced. Women are affected more commonly than men especially older age groups and postmenopausal women. Men can also be affected in their groups or in younger age with some underlying conditions associated with bone mineralization process. It commonly presents with generalized body pain or back pain or sometimes presents with fractures commonly vertebral and hip area. Bone loss starts as early as in 30–40 years age group, but in females it increases rapidly after menopause which reaches to equilibrium after about 10 years.

■ DEFINITION AND ITS EVOLUTION

Osteoporosis is commonly perceived as a modern disease, particularly in view of its apparently greater prevalence in the more prosperous societies of the world, but the contribution of bone fragility to fractures in the elderly has been known for at least 200 years. In 1822, Sir Astley Paston Cooper first reported the connection between fracture and "abnormal bones". In 1835, Jean Lobstein first coined the term osteoporosis, although that was probably osteogenesis imperfecta type I.

It is worth mentioning that in 1930s the "crush fracture syndrome" at clinical level was still being confused with osteomalacia. For almost a century, there were no further major specific mentions of osteoporosis. In 1941, a case was reported by Fuller Albright in which a fracture was seen in vertebra of a woman after she lost her ovarian function which he definitively identified it with osteoporosis and defined as "too little calcified bone".

In 2006, group of scientist gave the definition of osteoporosis as "a skeletal disorder characterized by compromised bone strength predisposing to an increased risk of fracture".

Osteoporosis was defined by World Health Organization (WHO) on the basis of bone mineral density (BMD). It is amount of bone mineral mass per volume of the bone (relating to density in terms of "physics sense"), but clinically it is measured by proxy according to optical density per square centimeter of bone surface upon imaging. It is measured by a procedure called densitometry. For measurement of BMD, dual energy X-ray absorptiometry (DEXA or DXA) scan is used which measures it in term of T-score. T-score is a statistical term which compares BMD to a reference mean of healthy 30-year-old adult. It means a T-score shows how much one individual's bone density is higher or lower than the bone density of a healthy 30-year-old adult. Z-score is the comparison of BMD to the age-matched normal. This is the number of standard deviations a patient's BMD differs from the average BMD of their age, sex, and ethnicity.

WHO definition: "Osteoporosis is defined as a BMD that falls 2.5 standard deviations (SD) below the mean for young healthy adults of the same sex also referred to as a T-score of -2.5". T-score between -1 and -2.5 comes in category of osteopenia, means low bone density. People having low T-score are also have chances of fractures.

■ EPIDEMIOLOGY

It is estimated that about 200 million women worldwide is affected by osteoporosis (about 10% women <60 years of age, 20% <70 years age, 40% <80 years age and about 66% <90 years of age). A source estimated in 2013 that about 50 million people in India are either osteoporotic or osteopenic. Several studies report different data about prevalence of osteoporosis in India ranging 8–62% affection in Indian women. In these studies, osteopenia has been prevalent in higher percentage ranging from 29 to 62% than osteoporosis. Urban/upper socioeconomic class as per expectation had better BMD than rural/slum/lower socioeconomic class. Similarly premenopausal women had lower osteopenia/osteoporosis than postmenopausal women.

■ CLASSIFICATION

Earlier days, diagnosis of osteoporosis was made on the basis of plane radiograph as newer diagnostic modalities such as DEXA scan, computed tomography (CT) scan, and magnetic resonance imaging (MRI) were not available. It was observed that osteoporosis changes trabecular pattern of proximal femur according to severity which can be seen in plane X-ray **(Fig. 1)**. In 1960, Manmohan Singh et al. described changes in trabecular pattern of proximal femur on plane anteroposterior radiograph for diagnosis of osteoporosis known as "Singh Index grading system" **(Figs. 2A to F)**.

- *Grade 6*: All the normal trabecular patterns are visible.
- *Grade 5*: The structure of principal tensile and principal compressive trabeculae is accentuated. Ward's triangle appears prominent.
- *Grade 4*: Principal tensile trabeculae are markedly reduced in number but can still be traced.
- *Grade 3*: There is a break in the continuity of the principal tensile trabeculae.
- *Grade 2*: Only the principal compressive trabeculae stand out prominently, the others have been more or less completely resorbed.
- *Grade 1*: All trabeculae are markedly reduced in number.

Singh index was a diagnostic classification. It was widely used in clinical practice for diagnosing osteoporosis and in research papers. However, when compared to DEXA in several studies, it was found unreliable and is therefore unsuitable for diagnosing osteoporosis.

In 1983, Riggs and Melton classified osteoporosis into four types.

Primary Osteoporosis

1. *Type I*: Postmenopausal
2. *Type II*: Senile
3. Idiopathic
4. Juvenile

Subsequently in 1990, Gallagher added secondary osteoporosis to the above classification and called it as type III **(Table 1)**.

In 1995, Nordin simplified the classification into:
- *Generalized*: Primary and secondary
- Localized

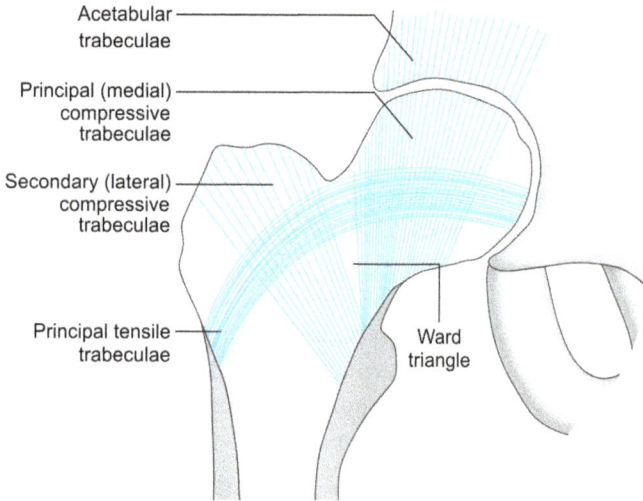

Fig. 1: Normal trabecular pattern of femur bone.

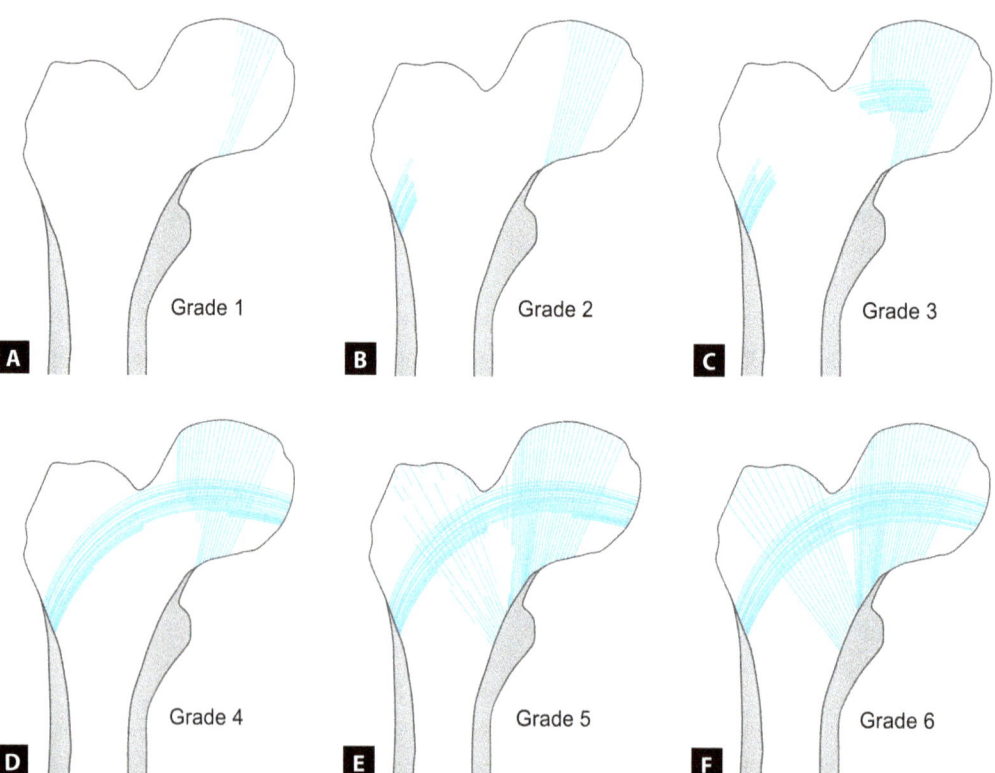

Figs. 2A to F: The basic trabecular patterns of the Singh index, from grade 6 (normal) to grade 1 (severe osteoporosis).

TABLE 1: Classification of osteoporosis by Gallagher.

Characteristic	Type I Postmenopausal	Type II Senile	Type III Secondary
Age (years)	55–70	75–90	Any age
Years past menopause	5–15	25–40	-
Sex ratio	20:1	2:1	1:1
Fracture site	Spine	Hip, spine, pelvis, humerus	Spine, hip, peripheral skeleton
Trabecular bone loss	+++	++	+++
Cortical bone loss	+	++	
Contributing factor			
Menopause	+++	++	++
Age	+	+++	++

TABLE 2: WHO classification of osteoporosis.

Classification	T-score
Normal	-1.0 or greater
Low bone mass (osteopenia)	Between -1.0 and -2.5
Osteoporosis	-2.5 and below
Severe osteoporosis	-2.5 and below + fragility fracture

Nowadays, criteria given by WHO is most useful because it is helpful in diagnosis, prevention and treatment **(Table 2)**. It is based on DEXA scan.

■ PATHODYNAMICS

Process of formation and destruction is continuously going on throughout the life at cellular level in bone tissues, so it is called dynamic tissue. It provides strength to the body and gives attachment for various muscle, tendons, ligaments and capsule. It also acts as reservoir for many minerals and ions mainly calcium and phosphorus, and helps in maintaining the normal homeostatic metabolic function of body. Skeletal tissue consists of two components:

1. *Cellular component*: It consists of osteocytes which are formed by osteoblast. It is of mesenchymal cell origin. Organic matrix is synthesized and secreted by these osteoblast cells which later becomes mineralized and developed into osteocyte. There is another cell present which is responsible for bone resorption called osteoclast. It also derived from same mesenchymal cells and is multinucleated cell.
2. *Extracellular component*: Alongside organic matrix there is solid mineral phase which consists of primarily type I collagen (90–95%). Noncollagenous portion is made up of different types of proteins. In between collagen fiber there are "holes" in which mineral phase is located which is made up of mainly calcium and phosphorus.

Modeling and Remodeling

Modeling and remodeling are the part of bone metabolism through which formation and destruction of bone cells occurs. Cells responsible for formation of bone cell are called osteoblasts while cell responsible for destruction is known as osteoclast. Both cells are derived from common precursors, mesenchymal stem cells. Osteoclast is formed by fusion of many cells thus are multinucleated. There are many factors that control cell proliferation and differentiation into either osteoblast or osteoclast.

Factors promoting osteoblast formation are: parathyroid hormone (PTH), vitamin D, insulin-like growth factor (IGF), bone morphogenetic proteins (BMPs).

Factors promoting osteoclast formation are: RANK ligand, macrophage colony stimulating factor (M-CSF), interleukin (IL)-1, IL-6.

They exert their effect by mainly two pathways. First is osteoprotegerin (OPG)/RANK/RANKL pathway in which RANK/RANKL activation causes osteoclastogenesis while OPG activation inhibits osteoclastogenesis. Second is Wnt/β-catenin Signaling System, in which Wnt activation promotes osteoblastogenesis.

Modeling: It occurs during normal growth process of skeletal tissue. Growth in bones occurs by growth in length (linear growth) and growth in width (new bone tissue apposition on outer cortex). At the end of skeletal maturation the amount of bone tissue present in bones is called peak bone mass. Up to 90% peak bone mass is achieved by the age of 18 years in females and 20 years in males. It keeps growing until around age of 30 years where bones have reached their maximum strength and density known as *peak bone mass*.

Remodeling: It is the process through which new bone tissues are deposited and old bone tissues are removed. It has mainly two functions.
1. To repair microdamage within skeleton
2. Calcium homeostasis by supplying calcium from bone tissue

Mechanism of bone remodeling: At cellular level it occurs via basic molecular unit (BMU) in which osteoblastic and osteoclastic activities are going simultaneously. Following **Figures 3A to F** explain the mechanism of remodeling.

Bone remodeling is regulated by large number of factors such as vitamin D, PTH, IGF-I, transforming growth factor (TGF)-β, PTHrP, interleukins, prostaglandins, tumor necrosis factor (TNF), sex hormones, IL-1, IL-6 and various cytokines.

In young age groups remodeling process is well balanced, that is the amount of bone resorbed is equally replaced by new bone tissue formation. So, total skeletal

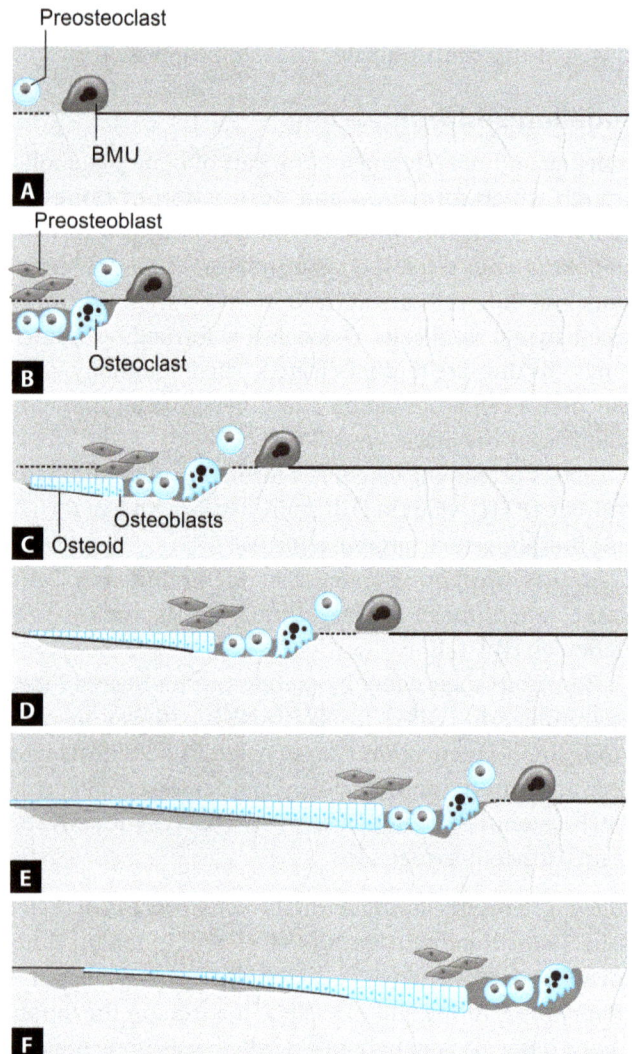

Figs. 3A to F: Mechanism of bone remodeling: (A) Origination of basic molecular unit (BMU): Lining cells contracts to expose collagen and attract preosteoclasts; (B) Osteoclasts fuse into multinucleated cells that resorbs cavity. Mononuclear cells continue resorption, and preosteoblasts are stimulated to proliferate; (C) Osteoblasts align at bottom of cavity and start forming osteoid (black); (D) Osteoblasts continue formation and mineralization. Previous osteoid starts to mineralize (horizontal lines); (E) Osteoblasts begin to flatten; (F) Osteoblasts turn into lining cells; bone remodeling at initial surface (left of drawing) is now complete but BMU is still advancing (to the right).

mass remains constant. But in later phase of life, mostly after 40 years, this formation and resorption process of bone become imbalanced and resorption takes place at greater pace than formation. This imbalance is more pronounced in postmenopausal women. So loss of bone tissue can be either due to decrease osteoblastic activity and/or increased resorptive activity.

Factors Responsible for Osteoporosis Developement

Lifestyle factors: Alcohol abuse, high salt intake, low calcium intake, inadequate physical activity, excessive thinness, vitamin D insufficiency, immobilization, prior fractures, excess vitamin A, smoking (active or passive).

Genetic factors: Cystic fibrosis, homocystinuria, osteogenesis imperfecta, Ehlers-Danlos syndrome, Gaucher's disease, glycogen storage diseases, hemochromatosis, hypophosphatasia, idiopathic hypercalciuria, Marfan's syndrome, Menkes' steely hair syndrome, Parental history of hip fracture, porphyria, Riley-Day syndrome.

Hypogonadal States

Androgen insensitivity, hyperprolactinemia, athletic amenorrhea, anorexia nervosa and bulimia, panhypopituitarism, premature menopause, premature ovarian failure, Turner's and Klinefelter's syndromes.

Endocrine Disorders

Adrenal insufficiency, Cushing's syndrome, central adiposity, diabetes mellitus (types I and II), hyperparathyroidism, thyrotoxicosis.

Gastrointestinal Disorders

Celiac disease, inflammatory bowel disease, primary biliary cirrhosis, gastric bypass, Malabsorption, gastrointestinal (GI) surgery, pancreatic disease.

Hematologic Disorders

Multiple myeloma, monoclonal gammopathies, sickle cell disease, hemophilia, leukemia and lymphomas, systemic mastocytosis, thalassemia.

Rheumatologic and Autoimmune Diseases

Ankylosing spondylitis, lupus, rheumatoid arthritis and other rheumatic and autoimmune diseases.

Central Nervous System Disorders

Epilepsy, Parkinson's disease, stroke, multiple sclerosis, spinal cord injury.

Miscellaneous Conditions and Diseases

AIDS/HIV, alcoholism, amyloidosis, chronic metabolic acidosis, chronic obstructive lung disease, congestive heart failure, depression, end-stage renal disease, hypercalciuria, idiopathic scoliosis, muscular dystrophy, post-transplant bone disease, sarcoidosis, weight loss.

Medications

Aluminum (in antacids), anticoagulants (heparin), anticonvulsants, aromatase inhibitors, barbiturates, cancer chemotherapeutic drugs, cyclosporine A and tacrolimus, Depomedroxyprogesterone (premenopausal contraception), glucocorticoids (≥5 mg/day prednisone or equivalent for ≥3 months), gonadotropin-releasing hormone antagonists and agonists, lithium, methotrexate, proton pump inhibitors, selective serotonin reuptake inhibitors, tamoxifen (premenopausal use), thiazolidinediones (such as pioglitazone and rosiglitazone), thyroid hormones (in excess), parenteral nutrition.

Role of Calcium, PTH, Vitamin D, and Estrogen

Inadequate calcium intake has detrimental effects on bones. Due to low intake serum level of calcium decreases and to maintain serum calcium parathyroid starts secreting parathormone which increases bone remodeling by increasing osteoclastic activity and thus calcium is released into systemic circulation from bone. PTH also increases GI absorption of calcium and decreases renal calcium loss through increasing hydroxylation of vitamin D. Vitamin D increases osteoblastic activity. Low vitamin D level also causes secondary hyperparathyroidism.

Estrogen affects bone remodeling directly. It increases life span of osteoblasts while its deficiency causes increase activity and life span of osteoclast. Low estrogen state tilt Osteoprotegerin/RANK/RANKL system into RANKL side which promotes osteoclastogenesis.

Investigations

Osteoporosis can be suspected in elderly persons presented with fractures or back pain or sometimes generalized body pain. So detail history and physical examination should be taken such as age, sex, height, weight, history of previous fractures, and about other medical conditions known to affect bone strength.

Laboratory Investigations

First-line laboratory investigation is complete blood count, TSH, renal function test, serum calcium, serum phosphate, serum alkaline phosphatase, 24-hour urine calcium, liver function test (LFT), etc.

Second-line investigation which often not needed is focused on finding the cause of secondary osteoporosis.

- Level of hormones which regulates calcium homeostasis such as PTH, calcitonin, vitamin D, cortisol
- *Markers of bone formation*: Serum total alkaline phosphatase, bone specific alkaline phosphatase, osteocalcin, type I procollagen extension peptides.
- *Markers of bone resorption*: Plasma tartrate-resistant acid phosphatase, urine hydroxyproline, pyridinoline cross links, assays for the N- or C-telopeptide cross-linking domains of type I collagen.
- Bone biopsy in some specific situations such as multiple myeloma, osteoporosis in younger age group individuals.

Radiological Investigations

- *Conventional radiography*: Common sites for radiography are spine, hip and wrist region. It gives qualitative picture of bone density.
- *Bone density measurements*: Earlier days it was very difficult to measure bone density. X-rays were taken along with pieces of aluminum or ivory, and then density of bone was compared to density of these materials. It gave rough estimation of bone density. In 1963, single-photon absorptiometry (SPA) was invented by Cameron and Sorenson. They used radioactive material iodine (I-125) or americium (Am-241). Gamma rays were passed through limbs and bone density was calculated by differential photons attenuation by soft tissues and bones. Later in 1965 came the addition of a dual energy source for measuring bone density at axial sites called dual-photon absorptiometry (DPA) which used gadolinium-153. Both these methods were much costly, used harmful radioactive material, time taking process and limited to peripheral sites, so not much used. Later single energy X-ray absorptiometry (SXA) and dual energy X-ray absorptiometry (DXA) came which used X-rays so were cheaper and very less harmful. DXA was more informative than SXA, so later was not much used. Other methods to measure BMD are quantitative computed tomography (QCT), quantitative ultrasonography (QUS), single-photon emission computed tomography (SPECT) and MRI.

Dual-energy X-ray absorptiometry: It measures bone density very accurately, even 1–2% loss of bone can be detected while X-ray cannot detect until up to 30% loss in bone mass occurred. Common sites for measurement of BMD are spine, wrist and hip.

DXA was first introduced by Hologic Inc. in 1987. In this technique two different X-ray energy (30–50 KeV and >70 KeV) are passed through two planes of bones and mineral content of that area is calculated. Since it is a two dimensional measurement, depth or height of bone cannot be estimated by it so it may give false high bone density report in individuals having extra bone growth like bone spurs or osteoarthritis patients who have osteophytes while slim people may have false low bone density report.

Quantitative computed tomography: It is more sensitive and accurate method than DXA. True density of mineral inside bone can be measured. It measures density in even bony trabeculae. Bone density is measured in terms of g/cm^3. It is not influenced by size or extra growth in bones, but individuals are exposed with more harmful radiographic radiation than DXA and it is also more costly, thus less used.

Quantitative ultrasonography: It is a convenient and low cost method, mostly used as screening tool. It is not as accurate as DXA but it has no radiation exposure. Its clinical use is limited to only heels to measure BMD.

Single-photon emission computed tomography (SPECT): It is more sensitive and specific than planar technique.

It is a CT-like bone imaging technique and it localizes lesions more accurately. SPECT is a simple, effective, painless and noninvasive examination in diagnosing painful vertebrae of osteoporotic vertebral compression fracture, and the SPECT showed the great potential for replacing MRI in the case of patients who cannot be diagnosed by MRI due to the implanted metal in body. SPECT scanning is helpful in localizing metabolically active bone disease. It is largely used for malignant lesions.

Magnetic resonance imaging: It is safe and it has no radiation exposure but it is costly so not used for measuring BMD. It is mainly useful in identifying stress fractures, in differentiating chronic and acute fracture, identifying metabolic bone disease.

- *Bone scan (Bone scintigraphy)*: It uses small amounts of radioactive material to diagnose and assess the severity of a variety of bone diseases and conditions. It visualizes metabolically active sites of bone formation or sites of bones in remodeling phase which cannot be assessed by other imaging method (such as CT, MRI), so it provides functional imaging.

In the field of nuclear medicine imaging for skeletal metabolism, first name was a Nobel Prize winner Hungarian Radiochemist George Charles de Hevesy who used phosphorus-32 as radioactive material in 1930s. Charles Pecher, a Belgian nuclear medicine scientist, worked on radioactive calcium and strontium in 1940s. In later decades other radioactive molecule such as fluorine-18 and isotopes of strontium also studied and found useful. In 1971 came technetium-99m (99mTc) labeled phosphates, diphosphonates or similar agents which revolutionized the bone scan technique.

Radioactive compound used most commonly in modern era are:
- Methylenediphosphonate (MDP),
- Hydroxymethylenediphosphonate (HMDP)
- Hydroxyethylenediphosphonate (HDP)
- 2,3-dicarboxypropane-1,1-diphosphonate (DPD)

These compounds adsorbs onto the crystalline hydroxyapatite mineral of bone. During remodeling process, bone mineralization occurs at osteoblasts, representing sites of bone growth, where MDP (and other diphosphates) bind to the hydroxyapatite crystals in proportion to local blood flow and osteoblastic activity and are therefore markers of bone turnover and bone perfusion. For doing bone scan, radioactive dye (Tc99-MDP) is injected into veins. After about 4–6 hours about 50–60% of these compounds became fixed to skeletal tissues and then scanned by gamma camera. It gives exact localization of picture of active metabolically bone growth sites where vascularization is increased and increased osteoblastic activity. It can detect metabolically active sites of bone at very early stage even weeks or months before they appear in conventional X-rays. It is most commonly used for oncology, metabolic bone diseases, rheumatology, bone and joint infections and trauma and various other skeletal diseases.

■ TREATMENT

Treating osteoporosis involves treating and preventing fractures, using medication to strengthen bones as well as treatment of underlying disease. Prevention of development of osteoporosis should be also considered in high risk groups and older population especially females.

First osteoporosis should be treated medically and if fractures occur then according to fracture type, surgical option should be considered.

Treatment of Osteoporotic Fractures

Osteoporotic bones are weak, fragile, have less trabeculations, may have cortical thinning, so can be easily fractured with trivial trauma. Metaphyseal region is most common site for osteoporotic fractures. Common sites for osteoporosis related fractures are hip, spine and forearm while other uncommon sites are upper end humerus, around knee and skull.

Surgical fixation in these types of fractures is not easy as it differs from normal healthy bone and have different biomechanical problems like
- Fractures are usually unstable and communited
- As it mostly occurs in metaphyseal area so have very short length available in epiphyseal area for fixation
- Healing is delayed as bone formation mechanism is abnormal
- Screw purchasing capacity is reduced in osteoporotic bone
- Early implant-bone fatigue which leads to implant loosening and loss of fixation

Osteoporotic fractures can be subdivided into two subgroups: (1) long bone fractures and (2) flat bone fractures.

Long Bone Fractures

Depending on site, quality of bone, type of fracture, intensity of trauma, managements can be done by either conservatively or surgically. In upper limbs, low trauma fractures commonly treated with casting or splinting, but in lower limb fractures usually surgical management is needed to allow early mobilization. Different types of surgical fixation fractures are plating, nailing, external fixator, arthroplasty with or without augmentation.

Plate fixation: Cortical thinning is the main issue in osteoporotic fracture fixation by plates as holding power of screws is reduced by 50% by 1 mm cortical thinning. So implant failure is rare in this type of surgical fixation as bony failure occurs earlier than implant failure. Conventional plates has higher incidence of screw pull out in osteoporotic bone than locking plates. Conventional plates exert compressive force between plate and bone through screw. Force around screw increases preload on bones that may cause screw pull out in already thinned out cortex with less holding power. Whereas loads are transferred across fracture site in locking plates by plate and screw construct to screws in bones. However, locking plates still has some limitations and complications. Locking plate constructs are sometime very rigid that may leads to nonunion. So longer plates with fewer screws are used spreading over a longer working distance from the fracture to increase flexibility and bending resistance. The current concept about locking plate fixation is "far cortical locking" and "near cortical slots" with unicortical fixation in distal cortex. This type of screw placement has better pull out strength.

Intramedullary nailing: It is usually used in diaphyseal fractures. Its use in osteoporotic bone was limited, however with newer designed nails with better instrumentation and technique osteoporotic fractures can be treated with nailing. Nailing is done in medullary canal which is close to mechanical axis of bone so nails give greater resistance to bending forces. Patient can be mobilized early and early weight bearing can be allowed with nailing. Weakest point of nailing is where interlocking screw are placed that is in metaphyseal area. Here screw nail construct is more loaded because of wider canal and small gap between nail surface and bone inner cortex. Newer generation nails are locked in multiplane or have helical blade like device which has larger surface area which causes distribution of loads over larger area of bone and screw nail constructs are less loaded. So there are fewer chances of failure of internal fixation. Thus, IM nails have biologic and biomechanical advantages over plates in osteoporotic fracture fixation.

Augmentation techniques: Bone grafts—it can be taken from the patient (autograft) or can be used from donor bone (allograft). Bone grafts provides scaffold for new bone growth, fills void space and helps in stabilize implants. For filling larger space as in tumor surgery or large defects in bone, allograft is used. Autograft is most commonly taken from iliac crest as a cancellous bone graft or from fibula as fibular strut graft. Commonly used sites are upper end of humerus, upper end of tibia, femoral neck. Use of fresh frozen allograft in geriatric osteoporotic bone fractures gives comparable results to nongeriatric patients.

Bone graft substitute: Bone grafts have limitation of availability and quantity, so bone graft substitute were developed. While bone grafts possess osteoinductive and osteogenic property bone graft substitute only provide osteoconductive property that is it only provides scaffold for bone growth. Commonly used bone graft substitute materials are calcium sulfate, calcium phosphate or polymethylmethacrylate (PMMA).

Calcium sulfate: It is moldable, self-setting and biologically inert material. It dissolves in 6–8 weeks so causing early loss of augmenting effect and early implant loosening.

Calcium phosphate: It comes in form of synthetic tricalcium phosphate, beta tricalcium phosphate, and coralline hydroxyapatite. It comes in block, granules, or cement. They provide good structural support and osteoconductive effect as these are highly porous. They have clear benefits in osteoporotic fracture management when used for screw augmentation or in filling voids.

PMMA: It comes in form of cements. It is used primarily in arthroplasty, fixation of prosthetic implants, osteoporotic vertebral fractures (vertebroplasty) and neoplastic lesions. It can also be used in newer implants where it can be injected through cannulated or perforated screw into bones.

These bone graft substitute has only osteoconductive effect, it provides support for bone growth and supports and stabilize implant but do not induce bone growth or not enhance healing potential of osteoporotic bones. So others molecules are needed which not only provide structural support but also helps in bone growth or induces osteoblast cells. Platelet rich plasma and bone morphogenic proteins (BMP) are found very effective in osteoinductive effects in fracture healing in osteoporotic bones.

Primary arthroplasty: Intra-articular fractures in osteoporotic bone are difficult to manage due to poor subchondral bone quality and impacted articular surface. Anatomic reduction is difficult to achieve in these case and if achieved, it is difficult to maintain after starting of weight bearing and beginning range of motion exercises. Conservative treatment often gives poor results. In order to allow early mobilization and weight bearing the concept of primary arthroplasty has been adopted.

Flat Bone Fractures

Vertebral compression fractures (VCF) are most common among flat bones. Other sites are skull, facial bones, and ribs. Diagnosis of osteoporosis is self-established if VCF occurs without any history of trauma. VCF occurs mostly spontaneously or with subtle trauma during daily routine activities such as lifting objects, bending, twisting or sudden sitting. Most common areas involved are mid-thoracic or thoracolumbar spine. Most of patients experiencing an osteoporotic VCF remain asymptomatic or minimally symptomatic. Some patients may complain of sudden onset acute back pain. These pain usually resolved by symptomatic treatment with analgesic, rest and braces. It should be differentiated from chronic back pain.

German Society for Orthopedics and Trauma (DGOU) has developed a classification system [osteoporotic fracture (OF)

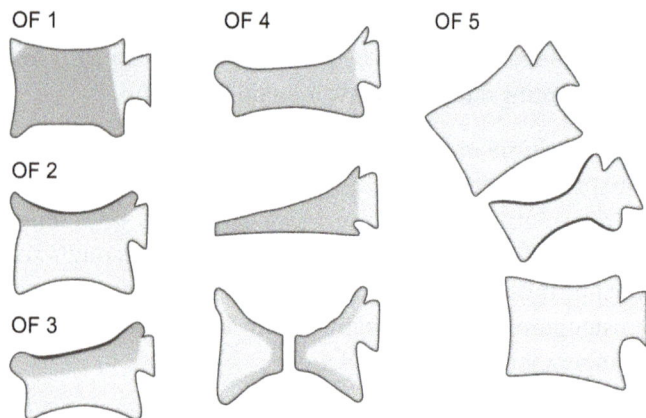

Fig. 4: Schematic representation of the 5 osteoporotic fracture (OF) subtypes (OF 1–5).

classification] for osteoporotic thoracolumbar fractures into five types **(Fig. 4)**:
1. *OF 1*: No vertebral deformation (vertebral body edema in MRI-STIR only). This is rare type. X-rays and CT scan show normal vertebral architecture. This is stable fracture.
2. *OF 2*: End plate deformation with no or only minor involvement of the posterior wall (<1/5). This is also stable fracture type.
3. *OF 3*: Posterior wall involvement (>1/5) with deformation. Only one endplate is affected, with both anterior and posterior wall involved (incomplete burst fracture). It can be unstable and may collapse later.
4. *OF 4*: Loss of integrity of the vertebral frame structure, or vertebral body collapse, or pincer-type fracture. This subgroup consists of three fracture types. In case of a loss of integrity of the vertebral frame structure both endplates and the posterior wall are involved (complete burst fracture). A vertebral body collapse is typically seen as a final consequence of a failed conservative treatment and can impose as a plain vertebral body. Pincer-type fractures involve both endplates and may lead to severe deformity of the vertebral body. These are unstable fractures and intravertebral vacuum clefts are often visible.
5. *OF 5*: Injuries with distraction or rotation. It is rare but unstable fracture type. The injury includes not only the anterior column but also the posterior bony and ligamentous complex. OF 5 injuries can be caused either by a trauma directly or by ongoing sintering and collapsing of an OF 4.

Based on this OF classification, a scoring system was developed to guide the option of nonsurgical versus surgical management **(Table 3)**.

A score of less than 6 points advocate nonsurgical management, more than 6 points recommend surgical management while point 6 is gray zone depends on surgeon decision. Decision should be taken by surgeon on individual patient basis considering all factors.

Medical managements include analgesics drugs, nonsteroidal anti-inflammatory drugs (NSAIDs), muscle relaxants, activity modification, spinal braces, neuropathic pain agents, different modes of physiotherapy such as short wave diathermy, ultrasonic therapy, TENS, different forms of dry heat and lastly medication for osteoporosis. Acute pain of VCF usually diminishes when fracture heals in about 3 months. But sometimes pain persists due to deformity developed from vertebral compression. Surgical management option should be considered when conservative methods fail to give relief in pain or neurological signs and symptoms develop. Commonly used surgical methods for VCF are vertebroplasty and kyphoplasty. In vertebroplasty bone cement (PMMA) is injected through cannulated syringe into compressed vertebral body while in kyphoplasty, first fractures is reduced by balloon pump inflation inside fractured vertebral body followed by cement injection. These surgical methods provide quick pain relief. Depending on the type and severity of vertebral fracture other surgical procedures like posterior stabilization, posterior instrumentation, with or without anterior reconstruction can be done.

TABLE 3: Osteoporotic fracture (OF) classification-based scoring system.

Parameter	Grades	Point
Fracture classification type (OF 1–5)	1-5	2–10
Bone mineral density	T-score < -3	1
Ongoing fracture process	Yes : No	1 : -1
Pain (under analgesia)	VAS ≥ 4 : <4	1 : -1
Neurological deficit	Yes	2
Mobilization (under analgesia)	No : Yes	1 : -1
Health status	ASA > 3 : dementia : BMI <20 kg/m²: nursing case: anticoagulation	Each 1 : Maximum

(ASA: American Society of Anesthesiologists risk classification; BMI: body mass index; VAS: visual analog scale for pain)

Medical Management

Medical management of osteoporosis start with proper diagnosis and suspicion on individuals with risk factors as this disease is not only a preventable disease but also can be treated.

The principles of management are:
- Prevention and control of risk factors
- Management of menopause and hormone replacement therapy
- Drug therapy
- Musculoskeletal and psychological rehabilitation

Prevention and Control of Risk Factors

Risk group for osteoporotic fracture should be identified from population. BMD can be used for diagnosis of osteoporosis but it will be little help in prevention of development of osteoporotic fractures as risk of developing fractures is not only depends upon only weakness of but bone but it varies markedly with age, sex, ethnicity, habitat, local environment. So besides T-scores we need another tool for fracture risk assessment. Several tools are available for risk assessment. Most commonly used one is FRAX tool.

FRAX is a computer-based algorithm that calculates the 10-year probability of a major fracture. It is calculated from parameters like age, sex, BMI, prior fragility fracture, parental history of hip fracture, addictions such as tobacco, smoking, alcohol, long-term steroid use, BMD of femoral neck and another causes of secondary osteoporosis. But it is not a perfect tool as it could not tell about risk of fall and it has not any term to include multiple fractures or recent or old fractures.

The aim is to provide safety and all fall prevention in risk group individuals. Proper care should be given to older age group individuals in family. Bathroom, corridors, stairs should be well lighted and should be kept dry. Sedatives should be avoided in nights. Walking sticks should be given for proper walking. Daily exercise should be started from early age of life. Exercise increases BMD and muscle strength so regular exercise routine should be included in daily life. Sunlight exposure to body is also important. Healthy nutrition should be taken specially calcium and vitamin D rich foods. Addictions such as tobacco, smoking, alcohol should be discouraged as it directly affects bone mass. Long term use of certain drugs like steroids, anticancer drugs, anticonvulsant should be avoided.

Exercise: Daily exercise should be started from early age of life. As peak bone mass is attained during adolescent age, so exercise starting at younger age helps individuals to attain higher peak bone mass. Mechanical loading plays an important role in maintaining bone mass and skeletal integrity. The osteocyte network senses and transduces strain to the effector cells, osteoclasts and osteoblasts, to decrease bone resorption and enhance bone formation at sites where more strength is required to counter stress. Resistant exercise produces stress on bone so helps in stimulation of bone growth at desired area. Exercise increases BMD and muscle strength so regular exercise routine (at least 5 hours per week) should be included in daily life.

Nutrition: Nutrition is a modifiable pathogenic factor for osteoporosis.

Calcium: Proper and adequate calcium and mineral intake is necessary in all age group persons especially in children and younger age group when new bone are forming to achieve higher peak bone mass. Good dietary source of calcium are milk and dairy products, green vegetables, sardines, finger millet, fruits like orange, etc. Milk and dairy products have more benefits as they have some antiosteoclastic activity and they increase insulin-like growth factors. Current recommendations from the American Association of Clinical Endocrinologists (AACE) for daily calcium intake are as follows:

- *Age 0-6 months*: 200 mg/day
- *Age 6-12 months*: 260 mg/day
- *Age 1-3 years*: 700 mg/day
- *Age 4-8 years*: 1,000 mg/day
- *Age 9-18 years*: 1,300 mg /day
- *Age 19-50 years*: 1,000 mg/day
- *Age 50 years and older*: 1,200 mg/day
- *Pregnant and breastfeeding women age 18 years and younger*: 1,300 mg/day
- *Pregnant and breastfeeding women age 19 years and older*: 1,000 mg/day

Dietary calcium has no side effects but increased risks of renal stone formation are reported with supplemental calcium.

Vitamin D: It plays a significant role in calcium metabolism. It increases calcium absorption from gastrointestinal tract and reabsorption from renal tubules. It has negative feedback level on PTH so it decreases osteoclastic activity. It is also needed for proper muscle functioning and maintain body balance. It also helps in maintain blood pressure and decreases susceptibility to fall by decreasing body swaying. It is synthesized in body under skin by sunlight exposure from cholesterol. Dietary sources of vitamin D are nonvegetable products and some dairy products like butter. Recommended daily dose of vitamin D is 600 IU/day in both sexes and its dose should increase to 800 IU/day in individuals more than 70 years age. Requirement of vitamin D is increased in pregnant and lactating mother.

Management of Menopause and Hormone Replacement Therapy

Hormone replacement therapy (HRT) consists of giving estrogen with or without progesterone. Earlier before 1990 it is the mainstay of therapy for prevention of osteoporosis. Maximum bone loss occurs during early years of menopause so maximum benefit can be taken by early starting of estrogen. It has proven role in decreasing fracture risk of both vertebral and nonvertebral fractures. Even after stopping of HRT, fracture protection is continued but bone loss starts as same rate as during pretreatment level of menopause. There are various types of estrogen available in the market such as estradiol, estrone, ethinyl estradiol, mestranol, etc. Progestins are available in form of medroxyprogesterone acetate, norethindrone acetate, norethindrone, micronized progesterone, etc.

Mode of action:
- Decrease bone loss by directly acting via estrogen receptors on bone

- Decreasing RANKL production and increasing osteoprotegerin production by osteoblasts causing increase rate of bone synthesis
- May also directly inhibit osteoclast causing decreases the rate of resorption
- It can decrease renal calcium loss and increase GI absorption indirectly.

Side effects: Return of menstrual bleeding can occur in initial days. In many clinical trials combined therapy of estrogen and progestin showed increased risk of CHD, stroke, venous thromboembolism, breast malignancy and dementia while estrogen only therapy showed no increased risk for CHD or breast cancer. It is contraindicated in renal and liver disease patients, thromboembolic disease. Blood pressure should be controlled before starting of therapy. Risk of breast cancer is increased by progestin only pills.

Drug Therapy

Calcitonin: It was first discovered by Coop and colleagues in the course of investigations to identify hormones that regulate serum levels of calcium. It decreases blood calcium level by inhibiting bone resorption and increasing renal calcium excretion. It decreases osteoclast activity by direct action on the osteoclast calcitonin receptor by inducing contraction and inhibits osteoclast motility. It is also able to interfere with osteoclast differentiation from precursor cells.

It has some effect on CNS producing central analgesia, so may be useful in acute vertebral fracture. Its analgesic action may be due to production of endogenous opioid, because elevated levels in plasma endorphin levels are found in calcitonin treated patients. So it can be used in pain related to bone metabolic disorders like Paget's disease and malignancy.

This analgesic effect of calcitonin can be used in lumbar canal stenosis (LCS) pain. LCS can cause back and leg pain due to the compression of neuronal structures and intraspinal vascular by narrowed spinal canal. Some studies suggested that calcitonin therapy can be used as a conservative treatment in selected cases of lumbar spinal stenosis. Meta-analysis and systematic reviews of studies on use of calcitonin in LCS concluded that calcitonin is not an effective analgesic and does not significantly improve walking distance in LSS patients, thus it is no better than placebo or paracetamol regardless of mode of administration or outcome assessed.

Mainly two form of calcitonin is available, salmon calcitonin and human calcitonin. Human calcitonin is 40–50 times less potent than salmon calcitonin but also less antigenic. It can be given by nasal or parenteral route. The absorption of the nasal dose is delayed compared with the parenteral route. Common side effects are facial flushing and nausea but seen much less with nasal spray form. With long-term use resistance may develop in few patients due to neutralizing antibodies formation.

With its long-term use marginal increase in BMD was observed but significant decrease in fracture risk was found. In recent years, concerns have been raised about association of calcitonin use and cancer particularly prostate cancer. The European Medicines Agency (EMA) and US Food and Drug Administration (FDA) prohibited its use in indication of osteoporosis. However, further studies do not support the role of calcitonin as an oncogen or tumor-accelerating agent. So it has limited role in prevention of osteoporosis.

Selective estrogen receptor modulators (SERMs): This group of drugs acts by stimulating some of the receptors of estrogen, but it has selective action depending on the organ system, it can acts as either antagonist or agonist. In this group three drugs are available: Tamoxifen, Raloxifen and Bazedoxifene.

Tamoxifen: It is the first medicine in this group made by chemist Dora Richardson in 1962. Initially it was used as antagonist to estrogen so as side effects osteoporosis was expected but when clinically found that it increased BMD, then further research on this group of drugs started and concept of SERMs came. It acts on bone tissue as oestrogen agonist thus inhibiting osteoclasts so can be used in prevention of osteoporosis. Its main indication is in treatment of breast cancer. Other indications are treatment of infertility and prevention or treatment of gynecomastia. Most common side effects are nausea, hot flashes, vaginal dryness, loss of sexual desire. Its prolong use increases the risk of DVT, stroke, pulmonary embolism, uterine cancers. So this drug was discontinued.

Raloxifene: It is developed by Eli Lilly in 1997. It is a second generation benzothiophene-derived SERM, produces beneficial effects on bone without harmful effects on breast and uterus.

Mechanism of action—there are two different isoforms of estrogen receptors: (1) ERα (predominantly activating) and (2) ERβ (predominantly inhibiting). ERβ inhibits the action of ERα by forming a heterodimer. Both type of action (agonist and antagonist) by a single compound can be explained by these mechanisms:
- Differential ER expression in a given target tissue
- Differential ER conformation on ligand binding
- Differential binding to the coregulator proteins

So relative levels of expression of these two isoforms will decide the effect on that tissue. It also reduces osteoclastic resorption by decreasing the production of IL-6 and TNFα, and increasing the production of TGF-$β_3$.

In various studies it shows beneficial effects on bone. It increases BMD, decreases vertebral fracture risk (insignificant effect on nonvertebral fracture risk), reduces bone turn over markers and improves bone quality with increase mineralization of bones. It reduces the risk of breast cancer and cataract. It lowers LDL cholesterol while increases HDL cholesterol. Common side effects are hot flushes, leg cramps and peripheral edema. It is not associated with risk of uterine cancer as seen in tamoxifen. So this drug is indicated in prevention and treatment of postmenopausal osteoporosis.

Bazedoxifene: This drug has raloxifene like profile but approved only in Europe and available only in Spain and Germany. It also increases BMD, reduces risk of both vertebral and nonvertebral fractures, and has beneficial effect on lipid metabolism. Common side effects are hot flushes, leg cramps, and thromboembolic events.

Bisphosphonates: These are pyrophosphate analog. Earlier their use were limited to industries mainly oil and textile industry. They were used as water softeners, antiscaling and anticorrosive agents for their property of inhibiting calcium carbonate precipitation. Fleisch and his colleagues showed that a pyrophosphate like substance present in urine and serum had ability to prevent calcification by binding to newly forming crystals of hydroxyapatite. Thus work started on pyrophosphates and like molecules in relation to prevent calcification. In the 1990s their actual mechanism of action was demonstrated with the initial launch of alendronate.

Mechanism of action—bisphosphonate has two phosphonate group attached to single carbon atom. It is very stable compound resistant to any enzymatic or chemical hydrolysis. Its carbon atom has two side chains attached which produces different range of activity among bisphosphonates.

On the basis of presence of nitrogen atoms it is divided into two groups:
1. Nitrogen-containing bisphosphonates are alendronate, risedronate, pamidronate, Neridronate, Olpadronate, ibandronate, and zoledronate.
2. Non-nitrogen containing bisphosphonates are Etidronate, Clodronate and Tiludronate.

Both groups have different mechanism of action.

Non-nitrogen containing bisphosphonates produces toxic analogs of ATP that cause cell death thus inhibiting osteoclastic activity.

Nitrogen-containing bisphosphonates inhibit the farnesyl pyrophosphate synthase step in the mevalonate pathway, so the isoprenylation of guanosine triphosphate binding proteins is modified **(Flowchart 1)**.

Thus, it inhibits osteoclast precursor cells differentiation, prevents attachment to osteoclast to bone and starts apoptosis of osteoclast. Potency for inhibiting farnesyl pyrophosphate synthase from increasing to decreasing order is zoledronate, risedronate, ibandronate, alendronate. It also causes marked decrease in vascular endothelial growth factor and reduces angiogenesis, thus reduce healing capacity.

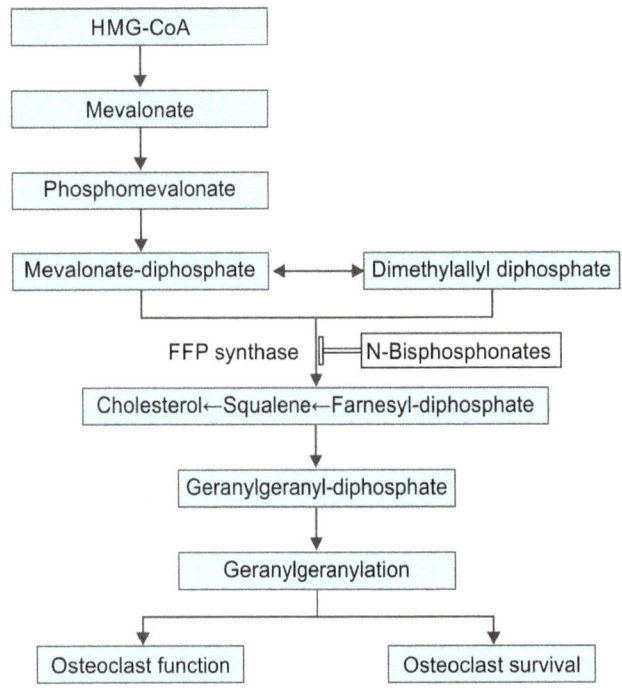

Flowchart 1: Mechanism of action of bisphosphonates.

The affinity to bind bones is different for different bisphosphonates. Decreasing order from highest to lowest binding affinity are zoledronate, alendronate, ibandronate, risedronate, etidronate and clodronate.

Pharmacology—bisphosphonates can be given intravenously or orally. Risedronate, alendronate, tiludronate and etidronate are given orally and pamidronate and zoledronic acid are given intravenously while ibandronate and clodronate can be given by both routes. Food, calcium, iron, coffee, tea, etc., can interfere with drug absorption in GIT. About half of them is excreted in urine and remaining half of them is deposited in bones and can remain there for several years even after discontinuation of drug. It is deposited more on that bone site where bone metabolism is high.

Effects on bone—its effect on bones is related to its relative mineral binding capacity. Drugs with high mineral binding affinity have greater effect on reducing bone turn over and having prolonged effect. Its effect is continued even after treatment is stopped. It decreases number of bone remodeling sites and osteoclastic bone resorptive activity. With oral therapy, markers of bone resorption decreases to 50% in 1 month and up to 70% after 3 months below baseline and stabilizes after 6–12 months of therapy. It increases BMD mainly in first 2 years. It decreases risk of both vertebral and nonvertebral fractures. Alendronate decreases risk of both vertebral and nonvertebral fractures by 50% and multiple vertebral fractures by 90% after 3 years of use while risedronate decreases risk of vertebral fracture 41–49% and nonvertebral fractures by 33–39%. Ibandronate decreases risk of vertebral fractures by 50–60% while it has no significant effect on risk of nonvertebral fracture. Zoledronic acid decreases risk of vertebral fractures by 70% and nonvertebral fractures by 25%.

Among commonly used bisphosphonates, alendronate and risedronate are used daily or weekly, ibandronate used monthly and zoledronic acid used yearly.

Adverse effects of bisphosphonates:

GIT: Esophageal irritation, ulceration, nausea, dysphasia, and heartburn, are well known side effects mainly seen with oral drugs. These side effects can be minimized by taking drugs in empty stomach with plenty of waters, remain upright for about 30 minutes after taking drug without further eating.

Acute phase response: Mild to moderate inflammatory symptoms, such as fever, myalgia, arthralgias, and headache can be developed by intravenous administration but these are respond well to symptomatic treatment and many times self-limiting.

Hypocalcemia: It reduces serum calcium by inhibiting osteoclastic bone resorption but it is clinically insignificant as long as baseline serum calcium is normal.

Skeletal effects: Sometimes joint pain, muscle pain or severe bone pain can be experienced even after many days or months of taking drugs but it subsided after discontinuation.

Ocular inflammations: Nonspecific conjunctivitis, uveitis, iritis, episcleritis and scleritis can be developed by nitrogen containing compounds especially pamidronate but it responds well to corticosteroid treatment.

Atypical femoral fractures (AFF): Odvina and colleagues in 2005 first reported these types of fractures. For the diagnosis of femoral fractures to be atypical there are following major and minor criteria:

Major features:

- The fracture is associated with minimal or no trauma, as in a fall from a standing height or lower
- The fracture line originates at the lateral cortex and is substantially transverse in its orientation, although it may become oblique as it progresses medially across the femur
- Complete fractures extend through both cortices and may be associated with a medial spike; incomplete fractures involve only the lateral cortex
- The fracture is noncomminuted or minimally comminuted
- Localized periosteal or endosteal thickening of the lateral cortex is present at the fracture site ("beaking" or "flaring")

Minor features:

- Generalized increase in cortical thickness of the femoral diaphysis
- Unilateral or bilateral prodromal symptoms such as dull or aching pain in the groin or thigh
- Bilateral incomplete or complete femoral diaphyseal fractures
- Delayed fracture healing
- Comorbid conditions (e.g., vitamin D deficiency, rheumatoid arthritis, hypophosphatemia)
- Use of pharmaceutical agents (e.g., bisphosphonates, glucocorticoids, proton pump inhibitors)

At least four of five major features must be present for diagnosis of AFFs while minor feature is not necessary although commonly present.

Pathogenesis of bisphosphonate-related AFFs: Long-term bisphosphonate therapy sometime oversuppresses bone remodeling leading to impair ability to heal microcracks in bone by itself and bone fragility increased. It accumulates at the site of high metabolic region where bone remodeling is going on or at microfracture site that may lead to changes in bone mineralization (increased mineralization and reduced heterogeneity of mineralization), decrease or alter collagen cross linking or bone matrix production. It also may have reduced vascularity and antiangiogenic effects. Other possible risk factors for developing AFFs are obesity, early menopause, decreased neck shaft angle of femur, increased bowing, younger age (<70 years) and inadequate response of parathyroid hormone to hypocalcemia.

For prevention of AFFs, assessment for continuing or discontinuing bisphosphonate therapy after 3–5 years is needed **(Flowchart 2)**.

These fractures usually treated by IM nailing, but thorough investigation is needed regarding osteoporosis. **Flowchart 3** shows the treatment pathway for these types of fractures.

Atrial fibrillation: In some cases increased incidence of atrial fibrillation was reported. It has not any apparent risk of thromboembolic complications.

Nephrotoxicity: Bisphosphonates are excreted via kidney so, may accumulate in patients with diminished renal function, and toxicity may occur. Intravenous bisphosphonates are more nephrotoxic than oral drugs. It is both dose-dependent and infusion time-dependent. Intravenous bisphosphonates, zolendronate and pamidronate, may produce toxic acute tubular necrosis and collapsing focal segmental glomerulosclerosis, respectively. So these drugs are not used in renal disease patients.

Osteonecrosis of the jaw: It is a rare complication mostly reported in cancer patients who were treated with high doses of bisphosphonates. It was first described by Marx and Stern in 2002. Patients may be considered to have bisphosphonate-related osteonecrosis of the jaw (BRONJ) if all of the following three characteristics are present:

Flowchart 2: Possible pathway for prevention of bisphosphonate-related atypical femoral fractures (AFFs).

```
                    Assessment (3 to 5 years)
        ┌───────────────────┼───────────────────┐
  T score < –2.5    –2.5 < T score < –2.0 and    T score > –2.0
  • Continue         existing vertebral fracture  • Discontinue therapy
    bisphosphonate   • Continue bisphonate
    therapy            therapy
        └───────────────────┤
                            ▼
                  Role for surveillance
                  Physiological risk factors:
                  • Inadequate response of
                    parathyroid hormone
                    hypocalcemia
                  • Obesity
                  • Early menopause
                  • Younger age (<70 years)
                  Machanical risk factors:
                  • Varus neck-shaft angle and
                    narrow center-edge angle
```

Flowchart 3: Management of atypical femoral fractures (AFFs).

```
        Atypical femoral fracture diagnosed
        • Discontinue bishophonate
        • Check calcium and vitamin D levels +/– supplement
        • Consider teriparatide
              ┌──────────────┴──────────────┐
        Incomplete fracture            Complete fracture
         ┌──────┴──────┐                     │
   Pain present:   Asymptomatic:       Intramedullary nailing
   • Intramedullary • MRI surveillance
     nailing       • Minimal weight-bearing until
                     MRI shows no bone edema
```

1. Current or previous treatment with a bisphosphonate
2. Exposed bone in the maxillofacial region that has persisted for more than 8 weeks
3. No history of radiation therapy to the jaws

Oral bisphosphonates therapy has lower risk of BRONJ than IV BPs. Longer duration of treatment more than 3 years is associated with higher risk of developing BRONJ. Dentoalveolar surgery including dental extractions is considered important risk factors. Any dentoalveolar surgery combining with IV bisphosphonate therapy has 7 times higher risk of developing BRONJ. Its management is done by pain control, any secondary infection should be treated by antibiotics and debridement of exposed bone should be done.

Denosumab: It is a human monoclonal antibody mimicking IgG2 immunoglobulin. It was developed in the process of reducing skeletal tumor burden in cancer patients. It inhibits osteoclast induced bone resorption.

Mechanism of action—it acts on OPG/RANK/RANKL pathway in calcium metabolism. RANK (receptor activator of nuclear factor-kappa B) receptor is expressed on osteoclast precursor cells called preosteoclast (**Fig. 5**). It is activated by binding to RANKL (the RANK-Ligand) which is expressed on the surface of osteoblasts, bone stromal cells and activated T cells. Osteoclastogenesis is activated by RANKL–RANK interaction by converting preosteoclast into osteoclast and increasing osteoclast survival. Osteoprotegerin (OPG) is an anti-inflammatory protein, which is derived from the osteoblasts binds to RANKL and inhibits RANKL–RANK interaction thus inhibiting osteoclastogenesis. Denosumab acts by mimicking OPG, binds to RANKL and thus inhibits osteoclast differentiation, activation and survival.

It is given by parenteral route as SC injection. Its dose is 60 mg half yearly. It is absorbed via lymphatic system and has plasma half-life of 25–38 days. It is metabolized by reticuloendothelial system. It is minimally excreted by renal filtration. It does not incorporate in bones.

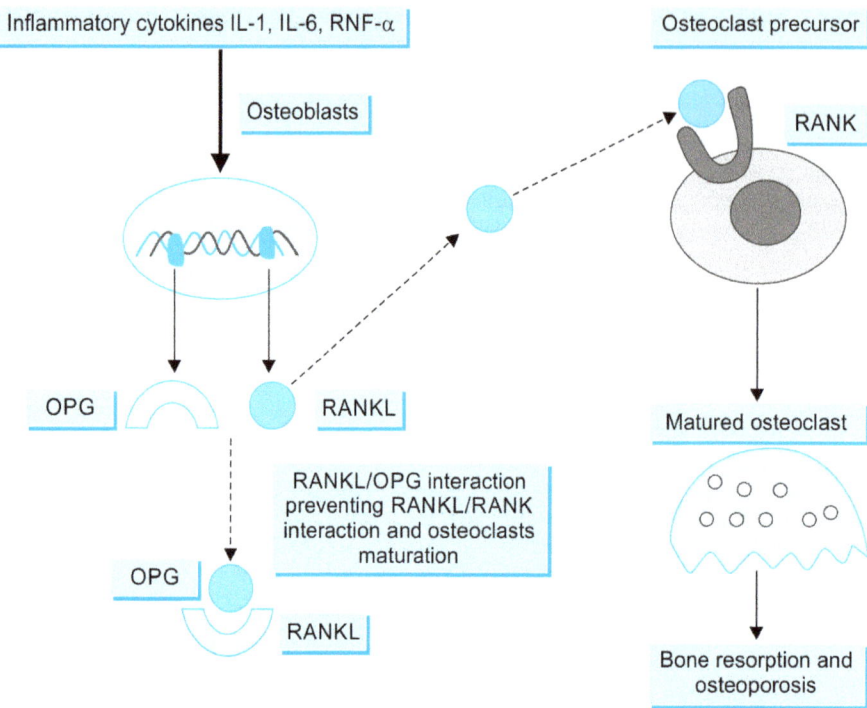

Fig. 5: Relationship between RANK (receptor activator of nuclear factor-kappa B), RANKL (the RANK-Ligand), and osteoprotegerin (OPG) in bone metabolism.

It reduces incidence of both vertebral and nonvertebral fractures and increases BMD. Bone mass is increased in both trabecular and cortical compartments by denosumab therapy. It significantly increases BMD in lumbar spine and hip by 9.2% and 6% respectively after 3 years of therapy and reaches to 18.4% and 8.3% respectively after 8 years of continuous therapy.

As it does not bind to bone its effect is shot lived after stopping of treatment. BMD comes to initial level within 1 year of discontinuation of treatment. In some recent studies rebound phenomenon is seen as few cases of increased vertebral fractures are observed within months of stopping denosumab therapy.

Side effects—common side effects are arthralgia (25%), nasopharyngitis, back pain, headache, extremity pain, upper respiratory infection, constipation, urinary tract infection, shoulder pain, Sore throat, rash, and asymptomatic hypocalcemia. It is contraindicated in hypocalcemia. Others side effects are rash, eczema, dermatitis, cataract, etc. Osteonecrosis of jaw and severe hypophosphatemia is also reported in few cases.

Besides its proven role in prevention of postmenopausal osteoporosis, its other uses are unresectable giant cell tumor of bone, breast cancer, nonmetastatic prostate cancer, and bone metastasis induce skeletal events such as pathologic fractures, spinal cord compression, intractable pain, etc.

Strontium ranelate: It is a newer drug. It is a combination of strontium chloride ($SrCl_2$, $6H_2O$) and sodium ranelate. Strontium has atomic number 38 and is placed just beneath calcium in group II in atomic table so it has some similarity with calcium. It has dual mode of action as it acts on both osteoblast and osteoclast cells, so promoted as a "dual action bone agent (DABA)".

Mechanism of action—due to its similarity to calcium molecule the body takes up strontium in place of calcium in bones. The exact cellular mechanism by which it affects osteoclast and osteoblast is unknown but stimulation of calcium sensing receptor on osteoclast and osteocyte is a contributing factor.

Its effects on bone are mediated by various ways:

It increases BMD by increasing cortical thickness, increasing bone diameter, trabecular thickness and bone volume.
- It inhibits osteoclast proliferation and differentiation, thus decrease bone resorption
- It increases osteoblastic proliferation, differentiation and its survival as indicated by increased DNA synthesis in osteoblast
- It promotes the differentiation and survival of osteocytes
- It promotes collagen synthesis, proteoglycan synthesis and cartilage matrix formation
- It stimulates the synthesis of PG by human chondrocytes possibly by IGF-I stimulation

It reduces risk of both vertebral and nonvertebral fractures. It increases BMD in lumbar spine and proximal femur by 12.7% and 8.6% respectively after 3 years of treatment, however BMD measurement by DEXA was not accurate because strontium has higher atomic no. (38)

than calcium (20), so it strongly attenuate X-rays giving higher BMD value. It can replace 1 out of 10 calcium atoms preferentially in newly formed bones.

It is given orally in dose of 2 g per day. Food and milk reduce its absorption from GIT. Its most side effects are mild and transient. Myocardial infarction, venous thromboembolism and pulmonary embolism are serious side effects of strontium ranelate. Other side effects are disturbed consciousness, seizures, mental impairment, memory loss, GIT disturbance, deranged LFT, Stevens-Johnson syndrome, toxic-epidermal necrosis, and rashes. It is contraindicated in renal diseases.

Teriparatide: It is a human recombinant peptide which exerts its action by mimicking parathyroid hormone. Parathyroid hormone has resorptive effects on bones. Continuous increased level of this hormone causes bone loss and weakening of bones but it was found that when it was given intermittently by exogenous administration, it increased bone mass at both cortical and cancellous area and increased osteoblastic activities. Teriparatide is a recombinant peptide which has an identical sequence to the 34 N-terminal amino acids (the biologically active region) of the 84-amino acid human parathyroid hormone.

Mechanism of action—PTH is an endogenous hormone which causes renal and GIT calcium absorption and release of calcium from bone by bone resorption. There is the PTH/PTH-related protein (PTHrP) receptor present on osteoblasts and renal tubular cells, to which PTH binds and this binding starts a cascade that activates protein kinase 1-cyclic AMP, protein kinase C, and phospholipase C. This cascade finally leads to increases the number of active osteoblasts and decreases osteoblast apoptosis. Teriparatide binds with these receptors with same affinity and exerts same physiological effect as PTH. It causes increase bone mass in both cortical and cancellous area, increase bone strength and causes increase in markers of both bone formation and resorption. Markers of bone formation appears early than bone resorption. So there is an "anabolic window" period where bone formation precedes bone resorption. So its intermittent dosing causes anabolic effects on bones. It decreases risk of fractures in both vertebral and non-vertebral area. It increases BMD more in spinal area than hip.

Its recommended dose is 20 µg per day by subcutaneous route. Its half-life is 1 hour and almost clears from body after 3 hours. Its bioavailability is 95%. It is excreted in urine.

Side effects—injection-site pain and swelling, nausea, headaches, leg cramps, and dizziness are common side effects Allergic reaction and transient hypercalcemia are less common side effects. It increases risk of osteosarcoma so contraindicated on patients with high risk factors for osteo-sarcoma such as Paget's disease, unexplained elevations in alkaline phosphatase, open epiphyses (children), or prior radiation therapy. It should not be used for long terms (>2 years).

Sodium fluoride: It increases BMD by increasing osteoblastic activity, its proliferation and function. It is deposited in bone. In several studies, BMD was increased significantly but there was no change in fracture reduction. In addition, nonvertebral fracture rates were increased with sodium fluoride treatment groups, raised concern about impaired bone quality and reduced bone strength. It may be due to the initial bone formed in response to sodium fluoride is partly woven in texture, but such bone is gradually replaced by apparently lamellar bone. Much of the added bone is incompletely mineralized, and its effect on bone strength is uncertain. It is more useful in combination therapy. When used with HRT, it increases BMD synergistically that is increased bone density by either agent alone and reduces fracture much more when given with calcium and vitamin D.

The usual dose is 50–75 mg/day. Gastrointestinal symptoms and painful lower extremity syndrome are common side effects of this drug. Currently its use is restricted to treatment of dental caries.

Newer Drugs

Cathepsin K inhibitors: Odanacatib, Balicatib.

This group of drugs acts on osteoclastic pathway of bone resorption. Various enzymes are secreted by osteoclast for bone matrix resorption and Cathepsin K is among one of these enzymes. It is a lysosomal cysteine proteinase which has high collagenase activity. It dissolves hydroxyapatite crystals from bone. These drugs block this enzyme and thus bone resorptive activity is reduced. It increases BMD by decreasing bone loss rather increasing bone formation. It causes sustained suppression of bone resorption biomarkers. It showed significant reduction of fracture risk in both vertebral and nonvertebral area in a 5-year long study. Its effects are reversed after treatment discontinuation.

Its adverse effects are increased risk of stroke, atrial fibrillation, atypical fractures, etc. Balicatib causes plaque-like skin thickening (morphea) in few cases. These group of drugs are still under development and further studies are needed for established use.

Anti-sclerostin antibodies: Romosozumab, Blosozumab, BPS804.

These group of drugs are humanized monoclonal antibody that binds a protein sclerostin. This protein is secreted by osteoclast which interferes with Wnt signaling pathway in bone remodeling process. Wnt signaling promotes osteoblastogenesis by stimulating differentiation of pluripotent mesenchymal stem cell toward the osteoblast lineage and osteoblast survival by inhibiting its apoptosis. Wnt proteins binds with LDL receptor-related protein 5 (LRP5)/6 and frizzled receptors (Frz) and forms a complex

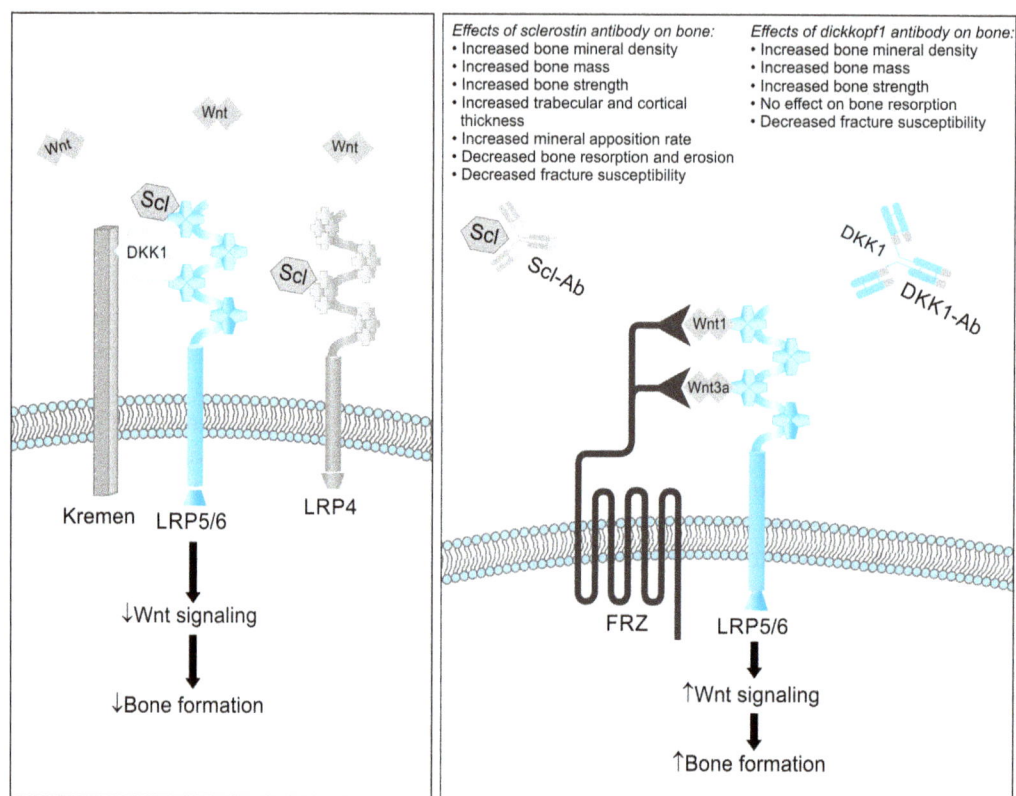

Fig. 6: Wnt pathway, sclerostin, and DKK1; effects of monoclonal antibodies on bone. (DKK1: dickkopf-related protein 1; DKK1-Ab: dickkopf-1 antibody; FRZ: frizzled; LRP: lipoprotein receptor-related protein; Scl: sclerostin; Scl-Ab: sclerostin antibody)

which starts a cascade to upregulate osteoblastogenesis and bone formation. Sclerostin and Dickkopf (DKK) blocks binding to wnt proteins with LDL receptor-related protein and thus complex with frizzled receptors cannot be formed and Wnt pathway is down regulated. Antibody against these proteins (Sclerostin and Dickkopf) blocks their action and allows wnt proteins to bind their receptors and thus increases differentiation, function and survival of osteoblasts and bone formation increased. **Figure 6** explains the action of antisclerostin antibodies.

In clinical trials BMD was found profoundly increased during 1st year (16.9%) but it decreased during subsequent year and returned to baseline. Bone formation markers which were increased previously and bone resorption markers which were decreased also came to lower than baseline values. This phenomenon may be occurred due to other pathway existence or compensatory increase in other signaling molecules.

Common side effects are deranged LFT and injection site complication. Stroke and cardiovascular complications are rare. Clinical researches are still going on this drug. Currently, it is not recommended for osteoporosis prevention or treatment.

Combination therapy: Compounds with different mode of action such as antiresorptive and bone forming or with same mechanism may have synergistic effect in combination therapy. Calcium and vitamin D are used in combination with most of drugs. Sodium fluoride and HRT has synergistic effect on bone formation. Bisphosphonates and teriparatide combination therapy did not show favorable results as BMD was not increased more than the individual therapy with single drug. Combinations of teriparatide and denosumab showed good results. Teriparatide does not adequately prevent bone loss after denosumab therapy whereas denosumab stabilizes and further increases BMD when used after teriparatide or combination therapy. Combination denosumab/teriparatide therapy followed by denosumab alone results in the largest 4-year increases in hip and wrist BMD. Estrogen in combination with SERMs had small additive effect.

So treatment of osteoporosis should be planned according to patient profile.

Musculoskeletal and Psychological Rehabilitation

Osteoporosis should be treated not only drugs. Preventive aspects of this disease should also be explained to the patient. Modification of lifestyle and good nutrition intake can modify many factors of osteoporosis. Patients can be taught about how they can keep their body healthy with regular exercise, walking, yoga and proper nutrition. Consultation with psychologist is also important as they can create positive energy in depressed patients and can taught awareness about bone health. Physiotherapist consultation is also important for proper exercise regime and physical rehabilitation of patients with established osteoporosis or with complications.

COPD, asthma and osteoporosis: Chronic obstructive pulmonary disease (COPD) is a chronic inflammatory airway disease associated with various systemic comorbidities. Osteoporosis is among the major systemic comorbidities of COPD. Osteoporosis associated with respiratory diseases is grossly underevaluated and undertreated. Treatment is mainly focused on symptomatic relief due to respiratory problems but various mechanism in COPD causes osteoporosis leading to fractures in these patients.

Various factors leading to development of osteoporosis in COPD and asthma patients are:
- Systemic inflammation
- Vitamin D deficiency
- Smoking
- Anemia
- Hypercapnia and hypoxia
- Hypogonadism
- Reduced BMI and reduced physical activity
- Use of corticosteroid
- *Systemic inflammation*: In COPD patients there is chronic inflammation in lung tissues. Mucosa, submucosa and glandular tissue are infiltrated by inflammatory cells, leading to increased mucous content, epithelial hyperplasia, and airway wall thickening, and ultimately terminal bronchioles become narrowed, obliterated or destructed **(Flowchart 4)**. This chronic inflammations leads to increase in CRP and various inflammatory markers such as TNFα, IL-1, and IL-6. These cytokines induces osteoclast leading to osteoporosis. In addition, other pathways are also involved. Osteoporotic patients having lower BMD showed higher serum levels of RANK ligand and a higher ratio of RANK ligand/osteoprotegerin compared with those with normal BMD. Higher RANKL promotes osteoclast induced bone resorption. In COPD patients, Wnt/β-catenin pathway is also downregulated, thus contributing in osteoporosis.
- *Vitamin D deficiency*: Vitamin D deficiency and insufficiency is defined as 25D levels below 20 and 20–30 ng/mL, respectively. Vitamin D is very well-known factor in calcium homeostasis. In COPD patients, there is high prevalence of vitamin D deficiency, particularly in advance stages of this disease, lower levels of 25D is found. Various factors that have been implicated for the deficiency of vitamin D in COPD patients include poor diet, less exposure to sunlight because of decreased physical activity, accelerated skin ageing, renal dysfunction, depression, and treatment with corticosteroids. Vitamin D deficiency causes decrease calcium absorption from GIT and kidney and causes secondary hyperparathyroidism that ultimately leads to osteoporosis.
- *Smoking*: It is an important risk factor for development of COPD as well as osteoporosis. Ward and Klesges demonstrated that tobacco smoking had a cumulative, dose-dependent independent effect on bone mass. Smoking induces osteoporosis by several potential mechanisms:
  - Altered metabolism of calciotropic hormone
  - Dysregulation in the production, metabolism, and binding of estradiol
  - Altered metabolism of adrenal cortical hormone
  - Effects on the RANK–RANKL–OPG system

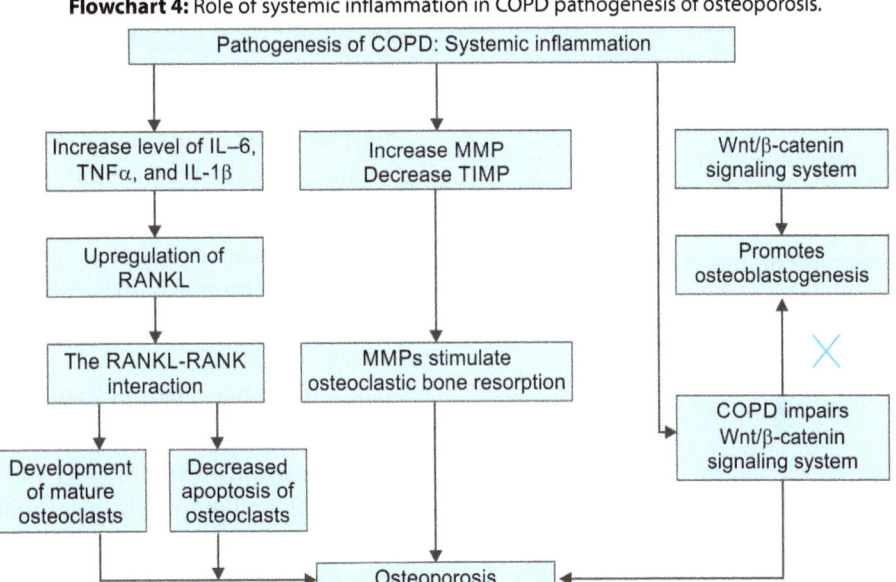

Flowchart 4: Role of systemic inflammation in COPD pathogenesis of osteoporosis.

(COPD: chronic obstructive pulmonary disease; IL: interleukin; TNF: tumor necrosis factor; RANK: receptor activator of nuclear factor-kappa B; RANKL: RANK-Ligand; MMP: matrix metalloproteinase; TIMP: tissue inhibitors of matrix metalloproteinases)

- Effects on collagen metabolism and bone angiogenesis
- Increased free radicals and oxidative stress
- *Anemia*: It is common in COPD patients, and its prevalence varies from 7.5 to 34%. Anemia is associated with low BMD and higher bone loss especially in cortical bone. In a study it was demonstrated that presence of anemia among postmenopausal women was an independent predictor of low BMD of the spine, after adjusting for BMI and other confounders. The exact pathophysiology behind anemia and osteoporosis development is not well understood but in some experiments it was suggested that anemia-associated hypoxia may be the cause of development of osteoporosis.
- *Hypercapnia and hypoxia*: Hypercapnia is a state of CO_2 retention in the body. In a study it was found that COPD patients with hypercapnia had lower BMD, low arterial pH, and a higher serum cross-linked telopeptide of type I collagen (a bone resorption marker) than COPD patients with eucapnia. Osteoclasts are directly stimulated by carbon dioxide as they have receptor for CO_2. Also CO_2 stimulates the carbonic anhydrase II within the osteoclasts, leading to activation of osteoclastic-mediated bone resorption.

  Hypoxia has also a role in the development of osteoporosis. Hypoxia stimulates osteoclast and inhibits osteoblast leading to osteoporosis. Hypoxia inhibits osteoblast formation by reducing the expression of RUNX2, a key transcription factor required for stem cell selection toward osteoblastic lineage and osteoblast differentiation **(Fig. 7)**.
- *Hypogonadism*: Sex steroids are important for muscle strength and bone mass. It maintains skeletal integrity by increasing bone formation and decreasing bone resorption. The reported prevalence of hypogonadism in men with COPD varies from 22 to 69%. Estradiol has also direct effect on increasing bone mass as described earlier.
- *Reduced BMI and reduced physical activity*: Physical inactivity cause muscle wasting and generalized weakness. Mechanical loading and physical stress are important for bone growth, maintaining bone mass and its integrity. Exercise increases BMD and physical inactivity leads to bone loss.

COPD patients generally have low BMI. They are physically less active due to breathing problem. Less physical activity causes muscle wasting, decrease BMI, less mechanical loading on bone that ultimately leads to osteoporosis.

- *Use of corticosteroid*: Steroids are commonly used medication for COPD and asthma either in inhaled form or in systemic form. Weakness in bones is a well-known side effect of steroid use. Glucocorticosteroids (GCSs) use is the common cause of iatrogenic and secondary osteoporosis and it was found to be a predictor of the increased risk of fractures, independent of previous history of fractures and BMD. More than 10% of patients who receive long-term GC treatment are diagnosed with a fracture, and 30–40% have radiographic evidence of vertebral fractures. GCs exerts its effect more on trabecular bone than cortical bone, so risk of vertebral fractures are increased more than long bone. If fractures occur at long bone it usually occurs at metaphyseal area where trabecular bone area is more **(Figs. 8A and B)**. It can lead to osteoporotic fracture within 6 months of use and risk of fracture remains present up to 1 year after discontinuation of its therapy, indicating that its effects are reversible. After stopping treatment BMD begins to rise and fracture risk declines. Children can also be affected with prolong steroid use which can cause decrease in bone strength, decrease growth and may develop fractures.

Mechanism of steroid-induced osteoporosis: Corticosteroids affect all three major cells involved in bone homeostasis, tilting the balance in favor of bone resorption and increasing the risk of fractures **(Flowchart 5)**. Steroid-induced fractures are unique in many senses.

- Fracture can occur with normal BMD, where as in osteoporotic patients, fractures occur after decrease in BMD.
- The number of osteoclasts is usually maintained in the normal range after long-term steroid therapy whereas numbers of osteoblast cells are decreased.
- Loss of bone strength occurs even before the loss of BMD.

Steroid-induced osteoporosis occurs in two phases. First phase is of rapid bone loss phase which is osteoclast induced. Second phase is of decreased bone formation which is due to osteoblast inhibition.

Pathophysiology behind development of this type of osteoporosis are:

- It decreases the levels of OPG and enhance expression of RANKL and monocyte/macrophage-colony stimulating factor (M-CSF), similar to RANKL, that stimulates osteoclastogenesis
- It inhibits Wnt/β-catenin pathway leading to inhibition of osteoblast proliferation, differentiation and maturation

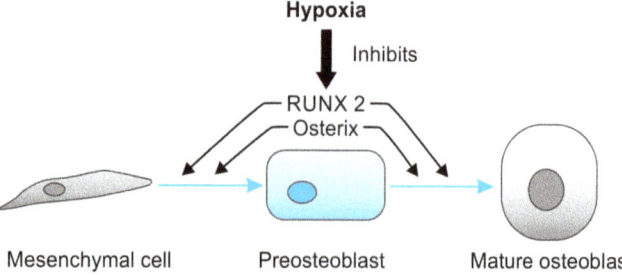

Fig. 7: Effect of hypoxia on osteoblast.

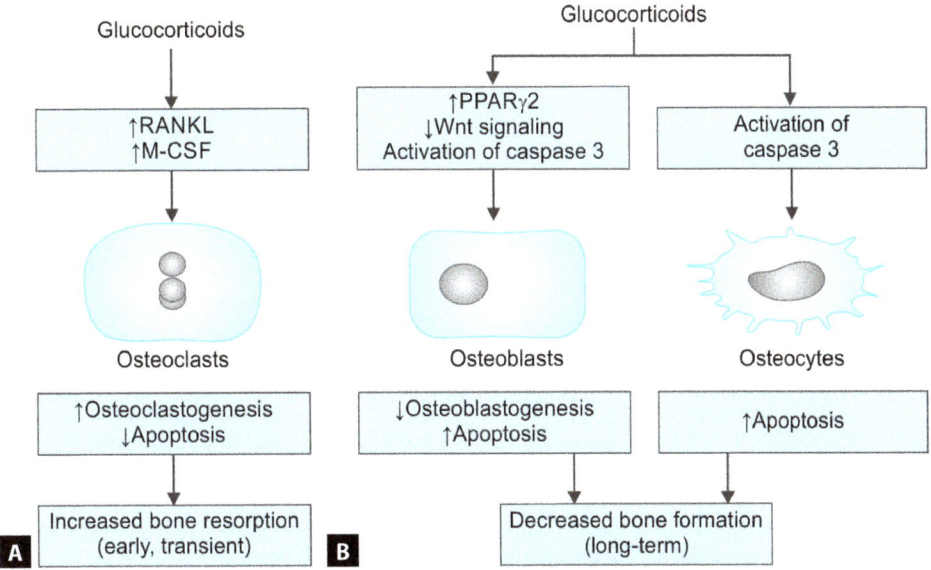

Figs. 8A and B: Direct effects of glucocorticoids on bone cells.

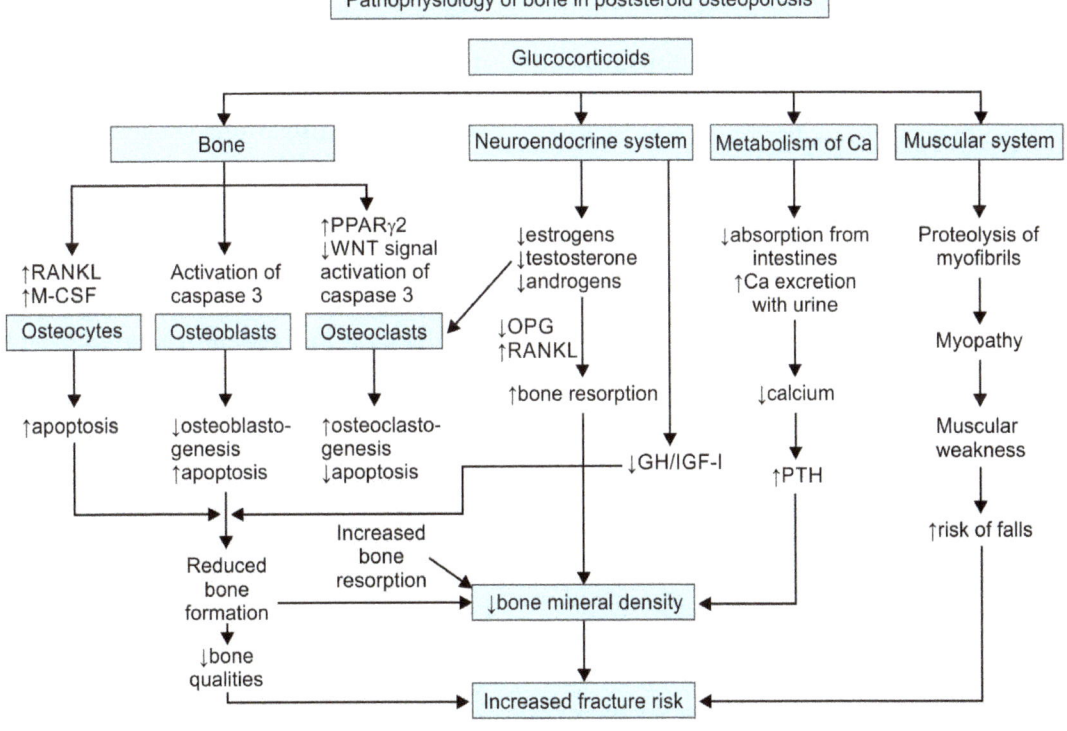

Flowchart 5: Overview of mechanism of steroid-induced osteoporosis.

- Osteocytes cells have ability to detect microdamages and repair the damage. Steroids adversely affect this ability leading to increase susceptibility to fractures. Osteocyte also enhances VEGF level via hypoxia-inducible factor-α (HIF-α), which causes angiogenesis. Steroids promote apoptosis of osteocyte causing bones harder, less vascular and more brittle. Also VEGF production is reduced causing reduce bone hydration and decrease bone strength
- It decreases sex hormones and growth hormones which has direct effect on bone formation
- It also affects calcium homeostasis by decreasing intestinal calcium absorption and increasing urinary calcium excretion.

Management of Osteoporosis due to COPD and Asthma

Chronic obstructive pulmonary disease is a lifestyle related disorder, change in lifestyle is necessary for prevention of osteoporosis. Patients should remain physically active and do daily exercises. Proper nutrition is necessary especially calcium, iron, vitamin D rich foods. These patients should

Flowchart 6: Schematic diagram summarizing the risk factor assessment, diagnosis and treatment for osteoporosis in chronic obstructive pulmonary disease (COPD).

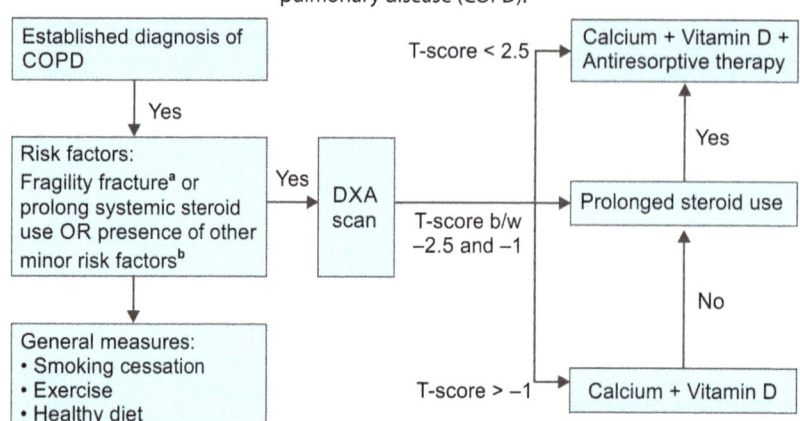

a = Fragility fracture is defined as a fracture of the hip or spine; prolonged systemic steroid use duration is defined as 3 months.
b = Risk factors include: BMI < 21, active smoking, daily significant alcohol intake, age > 65 years, menopause, rib fracture, inactivity, FEV1 < 50%, parental hip fracture.

avoid going to dusty environment. They should stop or minimize tobacco and alcohol intake **(Flowchart 6)**. Smoking is a major factor for causing osteoporosis so smoking must be stopped. Patients should be discouraged for taking more steroids.

If patients have history of fragility fracture or taking steroids more than 3 months in a year then pharmacological interventions is needed. Other criteria for medical treatment for osteoporosis include low BMI (<21 kg/m^2), active smoking, significant alcohol use, age above 65, rib fracture, physical inactivity, menopause, FEV1 <50% and parental hip fracture. Pharmacological interventions consist of calcium and vitamin D supplementation, Bisphosphonates, SERMs, teriparatide, denosumab, and newer drugs such as romosozumab/odanacatib.

Management of Steroid-induced Osteoporosis

Management starts with detailed history of steroid use about its doses, duration patterns. Patients should be asked for any alcohol, tobacco, or smoking habit. An evaluation for risk of fracture should be done about malnutrition, significant weight loss or low body weight, hypogonadism, secondary hyperparathyroidism, thyroid disease or family history of hip fracture. Thorough physical examination should also be done about weight, height, bony tenderness or any deformity. Clinical fracture risk assessment should be performed within 6 month of starting treatment with long term steroids. Fracture risk can be estimated using FRAX tool. Adjustments for steroid use should be done in final calculation of fracture risk (the risk of major osteoporotic fracture calculated with the FRAX tool should be increased by 1.15, and the risk of hip fracture by 1.2, if the prednisone dose is 7.5 mg/day).

American College of Rheumatology (ACR) gave following guidelines for the Prevention and Treatment of glucocorticoid-induced osteoporosis in 2017. The important recommendations of ACR are:

- **All adults taking prednisone at a dose of ≥2.5 mg/day for ≥3 months:** Optimize calcium intake (1,000–1,200 mg/day) and **vitamin D intake** (600–800 IU/day) and **lifestyle modifications** (balanced diet, maintaining weight in the recommended range, smoking cessation, regular weight-bearing or resistance training exercise, limiting alcohol intake to 1–2 alcoholic beverages/day) **over no treatment or over any of these treatments alone.**
- **Adults with low risk of fractures:** Optimize calcium and vitamin D intake and lifestyle modifications over treatment with bisphosphonates, teriparatide, or denosumab.
- **Adults with moderate or high risk of fractures:**
  - Treat with an oral bisphosphonate over calcium and vitamin D alone.
  - Treat with an oral bisphosphonate over IV bisphosphonates, teriparatide, denosumab, or raloxifene.
- **Children ages 4–17 years treated with GCs for ≥3 months:** Optimize calcium intake (1,000 mg/day) and vitamin D intake (600 IU/day) plus lifestyle modifications.
- **Children ages 4–17 years with an osteoporotic fracture who are continuing treatment with GCs at a dose of ≥0.1 mg/kg/day for ≥3 months:** Treat with an oral bisphosphonate (IV bisphosphonate if oral treatment contraindicated) plus calcium and vitamin D.

Recommendations for follow-up treatment for prevention of glucocorticoid-induced osteoporosis:
- **Adults age ≥40 years continuing GC treatment who have had a fracture that occurred after ≥18 months of treatment with an oral bisphosphonate or who have had a significant loss of bone mineral**

density (≥10%/year): Treat with another class of OP medication (teriparatide or denosumab; or, consider IV bisphosphonate if treatment failure is judged to be due to poor absorption or poor medication adherence) with calcium and vitamin D over calcium and vitamin D alone or over calcium and vitamin D and continued oral bisphosphonate.

- **Adults age ≥40 years who have completed 5 years of oral bisphosphonate treatment and who continue GC treatment and are assessed to be at moderate-to-high risk of fracture:** Continue active treatment [with an oral bisphosphonate beyond 5 years or switch to IV bisphosphonate (if concern with regard to adherence or absorption) or switch to an OP treatment in another class] over calcium and vitamin D alone.
- **Adults age ≥40 years taking an OP medication in addition to calcium and vitamin D who discontinue GC treatment and are assessed to be at low risk of fracture:** Discontinue the OP medication but continue calcium and vitamin D over continuing the OP medication.
- **Adults age ≥40 years taking an OP medication in addition to calcium and vitamin D who discontinue GC treatment and are assessed to be at moderate-to-high risk of fracture:** Complete the treatment with the OP medication over discontinuing the OP medication.

FURTHER READING

1. Abrahamsen B. Bisphosphonate adverse effects, lessons from large databases. Curr Opin Rheumatol. 2010;22:404-9.
2. Alexanderson P, Riis BJ, Christiansen C. Monofluorophosphate combined with hormone replacement therapy induces a synergistic effect on bone mass by dissociating bone turn over and resorption in postmenopausal women: a randomised study. J Clin Endocrinol Metab. 1999;84: 3013-20.
3. Ammendolia C, Stuber K, de Bruin LK, Furlan AD, Kennedy CA, Rampersaud YR, et al. Nonoperative treatment of lumbar spinal stenosis with neurogenic claudication a systematic review. Spine. 2012;37(10): E609-E616.
4. Athanasios AD, Toulis KA, Polyzos SA, Anastasilakis CD, Mkras P. Long-term treatment of osteoporosis: safety and efficacy appraisal of denosumab. Ther Clin Risk Manag. 2012;8:295-306.
5. Bagger YZ, Tanko LB, Alexandersen P, Hansen HB, Mollgaard A, Ravn P, et al. Two to three years of hormone replacement treatment in healthy women have long-term preventive effects on bone mass and osteoporotic fractures: the PERF study. Bone. 2004;34:728-35.
6. Balasubramanian V, Naing S. Hypogonadism in chronic obstructive pulmonary disease: incidence and effects. Curr Opin Pulm Med. 2012;18(2):112-7.
7. Baron R, Tsouderos Y. In vitro effects of S12911-2 on osteoclast function and bone marrow macrophage differentiation. Eur J Pharmacol. 2002;450(1):11-7.
8. Baud'huin M, Duplomb L, Teletchea S, Lamoureux F, Ruiz-Velasco C, Maillasson M, et al. Osteoprotegerin: multiple partners for multiple functions. Cytokine Growth Factor Rev. 2013;24(5):401-9.
9. Bischoff-Ferrari HA, Dawson-Hughes B, Willett WC, Staehelin HB, Bazemore MG, Zee RY, et al. Effect of Vitamin D on falls: a meta-analysis. JAMA. 2004;291(16):1999-2006.
10. Black DM, Cummings SR, Karpf DB, Cauley JA, Thompson DE, Nevitt MC, et al. Randomised trial of effect of alendronate on risk of fracture in women with existing vertebral fractures. Lancet. 1996;348:1535-41.
11. Blake GM, Fogelman I. Long-term effect of strontiumranelate treatment on BMD. J Bone Miner Res 2005;20:1901-4.
12. Blattert TR, Schnake KJ, Gonschorek O, Gercek E, Hartmann F, Katscher S, et al. Nonsurgical and Surgical Management of Osteoporotic Vertebral Body Fractures: Recommendations of the Spine Section of the German Society for Orthopaedics and Trauma (DGOU). Global Spine J. 2018;8(2 Suppl):50S-55S.
13. Blick SK, Dhillon S, Keam SJ. Teriparatide: a review of its use in osteoporosis. Drugs 2008;68:2709-37.
14. Bone HG, Hosking D, Devogelaer JP, Tucci JR, Emkey RD, Tonino RP, et al. Ten years' experience with alendronate for osteoporosis in postmenopausal women. N Engl J Med. 2004;350:1189-99.
15. Brenner A, Koshy J, Morey J, Lin C, DiPoce J. The Bone Scan. Semin Nuc Med. 2012; 42(1):11-26.
16. Buckley L, Guyatt G, Fink HA, Cannon M, Grossman J, Hansen KE, et al. 2017 American College of Rheumatology Guideline for the Prevention and Treatment of Glucocorticoid-Induced Osteoporosis. Arthritis Rheumatol. 2017;69(8):1521-37.
17. Cadogan J, Eastell R, Jones N, Barker M. Milk intake and bone mineral acquisition in adolescent girls: randomised control intervention trial. BMJ. 1997;315:1255-60.
18. Cakarer S, Selvi F, Keskin C. Bisphosphonates and Bone. In: Al-Aubaidi Z (Ed). Orthopedic Surgery. New York: InTech; 2010.
19. Cameron JR, Mazess RB, Sorenson JA. Precision and accuracy of bone mineral determination by direct photon absorptiometry. Invest Radiol. 1968;3:141.
20. Cameron JR, Sorenson J. Measurement of bone mineral in vivo: an improved method. Science. 1963;11:230-2.
21. Canalis E, Mazziotti G, Giustina A, Bilezikian J. Glucocorticoid-induced osteoporosis: pathophysiology and therapy. Osteoporos Int. 2007;18(10):1319-28.
22. Carlson S. A glance at the history of nuclear medicine. Acta Oncologica. 2009;34(8):1095-102.
23. Chesnut III CH, Skag A, Christiansen C, Recker R, Stakkestad JA, Hoiseth A, et al. Ibandronate: a comparison of oral daily dosing versus intermittent dosing in postmenopausal osteoporosis. J Bone Miner Res. 2004;19:1241-9.
24. Chhibber G, Roy R, Eunice M, Srivastava M, Ammini AC. Prevalence of osteoporosis among elderly women living in Delhi and rural Haryana. IJEM. 2007;11(1):11-4.
25. Compston J. Management of glucocorticoid-induced osteoporosis. Nat Rev Rheumatol. 2010;6:82-8.
26. Coop DH, Camenon EC, Chenwy BA, Davidson GF, Henze G. Evidence for calcitonin—a new hormone from the parathyroid that lowers blood calcium. Endocrinology. 1962;70:638-49.
27. Cornell CN, Lane JM, Poynton AR. Orthopedic management of vertebral and long bone fractures in patients with osteoporosis. Clin Geriatr Med. 2003;19:433-55.
28. Cummings SR, Eckert S, Krueger KA, Grady D, Powles TJ, Cauley JA, et al. The effect of raloxifene on risk of breast cancer in postmenopausal women: results from the MORE randomized trial. JAMA. 1999;281:2189-97.

29. Eskola A, Pohjolainen T, Alaranta H, Soini J, Tallroth K, Slatis P. Calcitonin treatment in lumbar spinal stenosis: a randomized, placebo-controlled, double-blind, cross-over study with one-year follow-up. Calcif Tissue Int. 1992;50:400-3.
30. Hanley DA, Adachi JD, Bell A, Brown V. Denosumab: mechanism of action and clinical outcomes. Int J Clin Pract. 2012; 66(12):1139-46.
31. Hanley DA. The investigation of osteoporosis. J SOGC. 1995;17:1211-4.
32. Harris ST, Watts NB, Genant HK, McKeever CD, Hangartner T, Keller M, et al. Effects of risedronate treatment on vertebral and nonvertebral fractures in women with postmenopausal osteoporosis: a randomized controlled trial. Vertebral Efficacy With Risedronate Therapy (VERT) Study Group. JAMA. 1999;282:1344-52.
33. Harris ST, Watts NB, Li Z, Chines AA, Hanley DA, Brown JP. Two-year efficacy and tolerability of risedronate once a week for the treatment of women with postmenopausal osteoporosis. Curr Med Res Opin. 2004;20: 757-64.
34. Harvey HA, Kimura M, Hajba A. Toremifene: an evaluation of its safety profile. Breast (Edinburgh, Scotland). 2006; 15(2):142-57.
35. Hinds RM, Garner MR, Tran WH, Lazaro LE, Dines JS, Lorich DG. Geriatric proximal humeral fracture patients show similar clinical outcomes to non-geriatric patients after osteosynthesis with endosteal fibular strut allograft augmentation. J Shoulder Elbow Surg. 2015;24(6):889-96.
36. Hunter DJ, Sambrook PN. Bone loss. Epidemiology of bone loss. Arthritis Res Ther. 2000;2:441-5.
37. Ishibashi H, Crittenden DB, Miyauchi A, Libanati C, Maddox J, Fan M, et al. Romosozumab increases bone mineral density in postmenopausal Japanese women with osteoporosis: a phase 2 study. Bone. 2017;103:209-15.
38. Jameson JL, Fauci AS, Kasper DL, Hauser SL, Longo DL, Loscalzo J. Harrison's Principles of Internal Medicine, 19th edition. New York: McGraw-Hill Education/Medical; 2017. pp. 2488-504.
39. Jilka RL, Noble B, Weinstein RS. Osteocyte apoptosis. Bone. 2013;54(2):264-71.
40. Jordan VC. Tamoxifen (ICI46, 474) as a targeted therapy to treat and prevent breast cancer. British Journal of Pharmacology. 2006;147(Suppl 1):S269-76.
41. Mithal A, Kaur P. Osteoporosis in Asia: a call to action. Curr Osteoporos Rep. 2012;10(4):245-7.
42. Nordin B, Chatterton B, Need A, Horowitz M. The definition, diagnosis and classification of osteoporosis. Physical Med Rehab Clin North Am. 1995;6(3):395-414.
43. Nordin BE. The definition and diagnosis of osteoporosis. Calcif Tissue Int. 1987; 40(2):57-8.
44. Odvina C, Zerwekh J, Rao D, Maalouf N, Gottschalk F, Pak C. Severely suppressed bone turnover: a potential complication of alendronate therapy. J Clin Endocrinol Metab. 2005;90:1294-301.
45. Ohnaka K, Tanabe M, Kawate H, Nawata H, Takayanagi R. Glucocorticoid suppresses the canonical Wnt signal in cultured human osteoblasts. Biochem Biophys Res Commun. 2005;329(1):177-81.
46. Osterhoff G, Morgan EF, Shefelbine SJ, Karim L, Mcnamara LM, Augat P. Bone mechanical properties and changes with osteoporosis. Injury. 2016;47:S11-20.
47. Saha S, Burke C, Desai A, Vijayanathan S, Gnanasegaran G. SPECT-CT: applications in musculoskeletal radiology. Br J Radiol. 2013;86(1031):20120519.
48. Salamat MR, Rostampour N, Zofaghari J, Hoseyni-Panah H, Javdan M. Comparison of Singh index accuracy and dual energy X-ray absorptiometry bone mineral density measurement for evaluating osteoporosis. Iran J Radiat Res. 2010;8(2):123-8.
49. Sarkar M, Bhardwaj R, Madabhavi I, Khatana J. Osteoporosis in chronic obstructive pulmonary disease. Clin Med Insights Circ Respir Pulm Med. 2015;9:5-21.
50. Sawyer A. Current Clinical Practice: Bone Densitometry in Growing Patients: Guidelines for Clinical Practice. Totowa, New Jersey: Humana Press; 2010. pp. 41-57.
51. Schnake KJ, Blattert TR, Hahn P, Franck A, Hartmann F, Ullrich B, et al. Classification of Osteoporotic Thoracolumbar Spine Fractures: Recommendations of the Spine Section of the German Society for Orthopaedics and Trauma (DGOU). Global Spine J. 2018;8(2S):46S-49S.
52. Schousboe JT, Shepherd JA, Bilezikian JP, Baim S. Executive summary of the 2013 International Society for Clinical Densitometry Position Development Conference on bone densitometry. J Clin Densitom. 2013;16(4):455-66.
53. Seeman E, Delmas PD. Bone quality-the material and structural basis of bone strength and fragility. N Engl J Med. 2006;354:2250-61.
54. Sewerynek E. Current indications for prevention and therapy of steroid-induced osteoporosis in men and women. Endokrynologia Polska. 2011;62(Suppl 2):1-8.
55. Shane E, Burr D, Abrahamsen B, Adler RA, Brown TD, Cheung AM, et al. Atypical subtrochanteric and diaphyseal femoral fractures: second report of a task force of the American Society for Bone and Mineral Research. J Bone Miner Res. 2014;29:1-23.
56. Simman R, Hoffmann A, Bohinc RJ, Peterson WC, Russ AJ. Role of platelet-rich plasma in acceleration of bone fracture healing. Ann Plast Surg. 2008;61:337-44.
57. Singh M, Nagrath AR and Maini PS. Change in trabecular pattern of the upper end of the femur as an index to osteoporosis. J Bone Jt Surg. 1970;52-A:457-67.
58. Stefanick ML. Risk-benefit profiles of raloxifene for women. N Engl J Med. 2006;355:190-2.
59. Subramanian G, McAfee JG. A New Complex of 99mTc for Skeletal Imaging. Radiology. 1971;99(1):192-6.
60. Tabatabaei-Malazy O, Salari P, Khashayar P, Larijani B. New horizons in treatment of osteoporosis. Daru. 2017;25:2.
61. Thomas T. Intermittent parathyroid hormone therapy to increase bone formation. Joint Bone Spine. 2006;73:262-9.
62. UPTODATE. Parathyroid hormone therapy for osteoporosis. [online] Available from: www.uptodate.com. [Last accessed May, 2021].
63. World Health Organization. Assessment of fracture risk and its application to screening for postmenopausal osteoporosis. Geneva: WHO; 1994.

18.2 Osteomalacia

SS Jha, Rahul Ranjan

DEFINITION

The word *osteomalacia* means soft bone (osteo = bone, malacia = softening). Osteomalacia is a condition of defective mineralization (deposition of hydroxyapatite) of existing bone during the remodeling process and occurs ubiquitously in bones of adults or adolescents (closed growth plates) resulting in reduction of bone stiffness.

CAUSES

The most common cause of osteomalacia is vitamin D deficiency. The other causes of osteomalacia are enlisted in **Table 1**.

RISK FACTORS

- Older people living in long-term care setting who do not get adequate exposure to sunlight or people with restricted mobility who are unable or lack the confidence to venture outside.
- *Dark skin pigmentation*: In developed countries, the prevalence of vitamin D deficiency is several hundred-fold higher in dark-skinned immigrants compared to native population. There has been steady increase in the prevalence of osteomalacia in the developed countries due to increase in the proportion of dark-skinned populations due to immigrants.
- *Resident of high northern or Southern latitudes (more than approximately 34°)*: They have seasonal lack of the ultraviolet-B (UV-B) spectrum of sunlight that causes seasonal vitamin D deficiency (also known as "Vitamin D winter").
- Other risk factors are diet low in calcium, cultural full body clothing, use of sunscreen with protection factor 15 or more, renal disease, malabsorption in the intestines as a result of conditions such as lactose intolerance, celiac disease or inflammatory bowel disease.

PATHOGENESIS

Regardless of the specific etiology, the basic pathophysiological abnormality in all the osteomalacic syndromes is the diminution of the level of calcium, phosphate, or both, in the plasma and extracellular fluid.

Vitamin D deficiency produces the simplest and most specific form of osteomalacia, and in this condition the metabolic abnormality is most clearly defined. In the absence of an adequate intake of vitamin D or failure of sunlight to convert the 7-dehydrocholesterol in the skin to calciferol, insufficient 1,25-dihydroxy vitamin D is produced, with the result that there is decreased absorption of calcium across the intestinal barrier and decreased transport of calcium in (and out) of the bone. Of the ingested calcium, only a small amount is absorbed and the rest is excreted in the feces. The body pool of calcium depleted, and the patient became hypocalcemic and hypocalciuric.

When hypocalcemia reaches a significant level, a negative feedback response causes hyperplasia of the parathyroid glands and elaboration of parathormone in excess. This hormone increases the serum level of calcium by direct and indirect mobilization of calcium and phosphate from the bone, by increasing the absorption of calcium in the gut, and by increasing the reabsorption of calcium in the renal tubules. In addition, parathormone acts on the renal tubules to reduce reabsorption of phosphate, thus causing phosphaturia, which, if sustained, results in hypophosphatemia. Bone resorption is excessive, but bone formation is also increased in an abortive attempt at

TABLE 1: Causes of osteomalacia.

Vitamin D deficiency	- Inadequate oral intake - Inadequate exposure to sunlight - Intestinal malabsorption
Abnormal vitamin D metabolism	- Liver disease - Renal disease - Medication
Hypophosphatemia	- Low oral phosphate intake - Excess renal phosphate loss
Inhibition of mineralization	- Bisphosphonates - Aluminum - Fluoride
Hypophosphatasia (inherited autosomal disorders)	

compensation. The pattern seen in the bone therefore is one of markedly increased resorption and formation, but overall, there is a state of negative balance, with insufficient calcium and phosphate available for the mineralization of the newly formed bone.

Bony Abnormalities

The gross, microscopic, and biochemical changes which occur in the bones of patients with rickets or osteomalacia can be related more directly to the altered physiology. Grossly the bones are smaller and lighter in weight than normal bone, and are deformed. When analyzed, they are found to contain considerably less calcium and phosphate than normal. Although recent evidence has suggested an abnormality in collagen crosslinking, it is postulated that collagen in synthesized at a normal rate but that diminished levels of calcium or phosphate, or both, decrease appetite crystal deposition in and on the collagen fibrils, so that the volume of mineralized bone decreased without significant decline in osteoid.

Other changes which occur are related to alterations in vitamin D and parathormone metabolism. The decreased level of 1,25-dihydroxy vitamin D probably decreases the exchange of calcium between bone and extracellular fluid, an effect which favor retention of mineral within the skeleton. The chronic hypocalcemia, however, causes an increase in circulating parathormone, parathyroid hyperplasia, and secondary hyperparathyroidism which increase bone destruction and decrease renal tubular reabsorption of phosphate. Thus, findings of a mild-to-moderate osteitis fibrosa may be superimposed on the histological changes of osteomalacia in long-standing rachitic or osteomalacic syndromes.

Above-mentioned chemical abnormalities are clearly reflected by the histological picture. Microscopic examination shows that both the cortical and medullary bones are affected by the osteomalacic process. The cortex shows increased porosity and diminished density, and this pattern is reflected histologically by thinned cortices containing large channels and irregular Haversian system. Trabecular bone is also thinned and appears more porous than normal, while the total number of trabeculae are diminished. The trabeculae show a characteristic feature, the presence of "osteoid seams". However, this is not a pathognomonic feature of osteomalacia. These trabeculae are composed of thin strips of mineralized bone surrounded by a layer of unmineralized osteoid presumably synthesized by the cells in preparation for nucleation and mineralization. However, because of the deficit of calcium and phosphate, mineralization of osteoid does not occur. Osteoid seams are the cardinal feature of the bone changes in osteomalacia and are important both in the diagnosis and in the evaluation of treatment. The width and number (total count) of the osteoid seams provide a good index of the severity of the process. In addition to the osteoid seams, the bones of patients with long-standing osteomalacic syndromes, show histological evidence of secondary hyperparathyroidism. Osteoclastic resorption, formation of new bone, marrow fibrosis, and occasionally small "brown tumor" may be observed.

Osteoid seams are generally found in relation to a single trabecula of bone, but occasionally in one or more bones, there is a large segment of the cortex or medullary bone which consists almost entirely of osteoid, with very little mineralization present. When this region is large enough, it produces a characteristic ribbon-like linear radiolucency visible on the radiograph. Such lesions, called Looser's lines, umbauzonen, or Milkman's pseudofracture, are virtually diagnostic of the osteomalacic syndrome.

■ CLINICAL PRESENTATION

The clinical diagnosis of osteomalacia in an adult is often subtle and is considerably more difficult to establish than that of rickets in a child. Part of this difficulty lies in the relatively mild changes in this syndrome, but the diagnosis is also obscured by the historical confusion surrounding the nature of the osteomalacic process. The first case was reported by an Arabian physician, the entity has been described as a lesion of obscure etiology, variously named mollities ossium, malacosteon, or hunger or war osteopathy. In the early 18th century, the syndrome was recognized by obstetricians, since most of the cases occurred during pregnancy, and severe narrowing of the pelvis outlet was defined as a characteristic deformity, "Kilian's pelvis".

The clinical findings in osteomalacia are often subtle, and the patient with mild or moderate disease may be totally asymptomatic for years. With moderately severe or advanced disease, poorly localized pain and tenderness are common and occurs in multiple sites, most often the spine, pelvis, and proximal part of the extremities. Muscular weakness and hypotonia may be present and result in mild-to-moderate decrease in functional capacity, a waddling gait, or, in severe cases, inability to walk.

Patient with osteomalacia may suffer from Milkman's syndrome, a roentgenographic entity in which the patient shows multiple spontaneous ribbon-like pseudofractures of the long and flat bones without displacement or callus formation. A Milkman's pseudofracture (Looser's line or umbauzonen) occasionally becomes the site of a true fracture, presumably as a result of torsional, tensile, or shearing stress on the weakened area in the bone.

Occasionally, an acute fracture is the initial complaint leading to the diagnosis of the primary disease. The most common features are in the neck of the femur, pubic ramus, spine, or ribs, and may produce severe debility. Considerable shortening of trunk may occur when the spine is extensively involved.

Roentgenographic Features of Osteomalacia

The roentgenographic changes associated with osteomalacia clearly reflect the physiological and pathological changes, particularly those in the shafts of the long bones. The lack of calcium, phosphate, or both available for mineralization of the skeleton, and the specific alterations in the bones, presumably in response to the deficiency of these elements, are readily translated into the characteristic and almost pathognomonic radiographic appearance.

Roentgenogram of the long and flat bones shows a generalized decrease in density affecting both the cortical and medullary areas. The cortices appear thinned and the loss of trabeculae and its number. Small bones are generally less severely affected and may appears relatively normal. The most commonly and severely affected are the vertebrae.

In addition to the reduction in the amount of bone, there is often a distinct difference in the quality, which may be helpful in distinguishing the osteomalacia from other form of osteopenia such as osteoporosis. The cortices are not only thinned, but their outline is fuzzy and indistinct, and endosteal margin tends to merge with the medullary bone. The trabeculae in the medulla are reduced in the amount, lacking the pencil-line sharpness characteristic of normal or osteoporotic bone, and appear fuzzy, coarse, and irregular in outline. Occasionally, patients with long-standing osteomalacia show findings of secondary hyperparathyroidism, characterized by erosions of the phalangeal cortices and tufts and of distal ends of the clavicles.

As already described, one of the unusual and pathognomonic features of the osteomalacic syndromes is the presence of Milkman's pseudo fractures (umbauzonen or Looser's lines). The characteristic locations of these symmetrical, transverse, ribbon-like zones of decreased density are: the concave side of the long bones, medial side of the neck of the femur, the pubic rami, the ribs, clavicles, and axillary borders of the scapula. Although pathogenesis of these defects is largely unknown, their proximity to the sites of vessels in the bones has suggested that they are vascular in origin, probably the result of pressure on the softened bone or of the increased local blood supply.

Occasionally, one may see radiolucencies suggestive of pseudofractures in hyperparathyroidism, fibrous dysplasia, Paget's disease, or neurofibromatosis, but they are more likely to be true stress fractures, which may progress in a relatively short time to fracture with displacement or show evidence of healing and callus formation. The pseudofracture of osteomalacia occasionally become complete fractures with displacement, particularly when the part is subjected to significant trauma, but this occurrence is unusual and one rarely sees radiographic evidence of callus formation.

In patients with long-standing osteomalacia, multiple pathological and often "silent" fractures can result in significant deformities and disabilities. Compression fractures of the vertebral segments may alter the normal spinal curves or cause gibbus formation. Coxa vara may result from fracture in the neck and proximal part of the shaft of the femur. Pelvis fractures may so distort the shape and symmetry of the innominate bones that the obstetrical dimensions are grossly disturbed. Occasionally, areas of increased bone density are seen in patients with classic osteomalacia.

EVALUATION OF BIOCHEMICAL PARAMETERS

The diagnosis of osteomalacia may be suspected on the basis of history and physical examination and may be supported by suitable roentgenograms. Proof of the diagnosis and, perhaps more important, determination of the etiology must depend on the laboratory evaluation. The diagnosis of the disease process is done on the basis of the aberrations of the calcium and phosphate contents in the blood, urine, and feces. It should be performed in the patient suspected of osteomalacic syndrome.

Calcium

The calcium content of the serum in patients with osteomalacia is generally normal or slightly to moderately decreased. The serum calcium rarely falls below 7.5–8 mg/100 mL and may be as high as 10 mg/100 mL. Despite the fact that in most patients, osteomalacia is caused by a decrease in the body's pool of calcium, the serum calcium is maintained at relatively high level, probably on the basis of increased activity of the parathyroid gland in response to the chronic calcium deficit. Urinary calcium is almost invariably decreased, the finding that is highly significant. The usual finding in the patient is a fairly marked decreased in the 24 hours output of calcium with values ranging between 80 and 150 mg per 24 hours. On a dietary intake of 750–1,000 mg of calcium per day, urinary excretion of under 200 mg of calcium per 24 hours is significant. Fecal calcium is usually increased, but the level depends considerably on the dietary intake. It is not unusual in patients receiving 1 g of calcium per day in their diet to excrete almost all of it in the feces, or, at times, even slightly more than the amount ingested. This is particularly common in the patients with renal osteodystrophy.

Inorganic Phosphate

The levels of inorganic phosphate in the patients of osteomalacia are considerably decreased due to action of parathyroid hormone (PTH). The exception is renal osteodystrophy, in which filtration of phosphate through the glomerulus is inadequate and as a result the serum values rise considerably above normal.

The decreased reabsorption of phosphate by renal tubules, or, expressed in another way, the increase phosphate clearance is an integral part of the pathogenesis of the osteomalacia. Some patients with relatively high serum phosphate level excrete large amounts of phosphate in the urine, far exceeding the expected normal values of 300–1,000 mg/day in adults.

Vitamin D Level

The most specific screening test for vitamin D deficiency is a serum 25(OH)D level. The level of serum 25(OH) D of <37 nmol/L is associated with increased PTH level and lower bone density.

Serum Alkaline Phosphatase

Due to increased bone turnover under impact of PTH level, serum ALP increases in the patient of osteomalacia.

PREVENTION AND TREATMENT

Like nutritional rickets, osteomalacia is fully preventable disease. The global consensus recommends, 800 IU of vitamin D daily lifelong in risk groups, including individuals with dark skin, full body clothing, limited sun exposure either due to geographic location, limited outdoor activity or restricted mobility, low socioeconomic background and poor diet (Harrison). Individuals at risk should also meet daily minimum requirement of sufficient calcium intake as shown in **Table 2**.

Diet

Encouraging a diet rich in vitamin D and calcium will help to maintain nutritional level required for effective mineralization of the bones. Discussing dietary requirements and highlighting foods that are rich in calcium and vitamin D will help raise awareness of important food sources. Referral to a dietitian can also be helpful in assessing and planning nutritional support, especially where people have specific dietary requirement.

Exposure to Sunlight

Where possible, people should be encouraged to go outside and expose their arms and face to the sun to increase vitamin D level. Approximately, 15 minutes exposure will increase levels, although care should be taken not to allow the skin to burn in strong sunshine.

TABLE 2: Global consensus definition of vitamin D deficiency and dietary calcium intake.

	Serum 25(OH)D levels	Daily calcium intake
Deficient	>50 nmol/L	>500 mg
Insufficient	30–50 nmol/L	300–500 mg
Sufficient	<30 nmol/L	<300 mg

Exercise

As stiffness and weakness increase with advanced osteomalacia, it can become difficult to perform a variety of activities. It helps in the strengthening of the muscles and bones, although high impact and intensive exercise should be avoided until Looser's zones or fracture have healed. As mobility become more difficult with advanced osteomalacia it is important to assess the risk of falling because it may increase with reduced muscle strength and increased pain and stiffness.

Treatment of Vitamin D Deficiency

Treatment of vitamin D deficiency should be directed at the underlying disorder, if possible, and should also be tailored to the severity of the condition. Recommendation is to give 50,000 IU weekly for 3–12 weeks followed by maintenance therapy of 800 IU daily. Higher dose may be required if patient is taking medication such as phenytoin or barbiturate which accelerate the metabolism of vitamin D.

If patient is having intestinal malabsorption, repletion can be performed with IM vitamin D (250,000 IU biannually).

Normocalcemia is usually observed within 1 week of therapy, although increase in PTH and ALP level may persist for 3–6 months. The most efficacious method to monitor treatment and resolution of vitamin D deficiency are serum and urinary calcium measurements.

The safety margin of vitamin D is large, and its toxicity is usually observed only in patient taking dose in the range of 40,000 IU daily.

FURTHER READING

1. Albright F, Reifenstein EC. The Parathyroid Glands and Metabolic Bone Disease. Baltimore: Williams and Wilkins; 1948.
2. Arnaud C, Rasmusen H, Fischer J. Role of parathyroids in phosphaturia of vitamin D deficiency. J Clin Investig. 1964;43(6):1256.
3. Arnaud CD, Tenenhouse AM, Rasmussen H. Parathyroid Hormone. Annual Rev Physiol. 1996;29:349-72.
4. Arnstein AR, Frame B, Frost HM. Recent progress in osteomalacia and rickets. Annals of Internal Medicine. 1967;67(6):1296-330.
5. Arthritis Research UK (2013). Osteomalacia. [online] Available from: www.arthritisresearchuk.org/arthritisinformation/conditions/osteomalacia.aspx. [Last accessed May, 2021].
6. Barnes MJ, Constable BJ, Morton LF, Kodicek E. Bone Collagen Metabolism in Vitamin D Deficiency. Biochem J. 1973;132:13-5.
7. Bartlett A. A Case of Mollities Osteum. Boston Med Surg J. 1840;22:205-6.
8. Beal VA. Calcium and phosphorus in infancy. J Am Diet Assoc. 1968;53:450-9.
9. Caffey J, Silverman FN. Pediatric X-ray diagnosis. New York: Year Book Medical Publishers; 1967.
10. Cashman KD, Dowling KG. Vitamin D deficiency in Europe: pandemic? Am J Clin Nutr. 2016;103(4):1033-44.

11. Chalmers J, Conacher WD, Gardner DL, Scorr PJ. Osteomalacia: a common disease in elderly women. J. Bone and Joint Surg. 1967;49-B:403-23.
12. Cousins RJ, Deluca HF. Vitamin D and Bone. In: Bourne GFF (Eds). The Biochemistry and Physiology of Bone. New York: Academic Press; 1971. pp. 281-335.
13. Dodds GS, Cameron HC. Studies on experimental rickets in rats: IV. The relation of rickets to growth, with special reference to the bones. Am J Pathol. 1943;19(1):169.
14. Feist JH. The biologic basis of radiologic findings in bone disease. Recognition and interpretation of abnormal bone architecture. Radiol Clin North Am. 1970;8(2):183-206.
15. Fourman P, Royer P. Calcium Metabolism and the Bone, 2nd edition. Philadelphia: FA Davis Co.; 1968.
16. Fraser D. Hypophosphatasia. Am J Med. 1975;22:730-46.
17. Frost HM. The bone dynamics in osteoporosis and osteomalacia. Springfield: Charles C. Thomas Publisher; 1966.
18. Goldsmith RS. Laboratory aids in the diagnosis of metabolic bone disease. Orthop Clin North Am. 1972;3:545-60.
19. Harris WH, Heaney RP. Skeletal renewal and metabolic bone disease. N Engl J Med. 1969;280(4):193-202.
20. Hodkjnson HM. Fracture of the Femur as a Presentation of Osteomalacia. Geront Clin. 1971;13:189-91.
21. Jaffe HL. Metabolic, Degenerative, and Inflammatory Diseases of Bones and Joints, Philadelphia: Lea and Febiger; 1972. pp. 381.
22. Jaworski ZF. Pathophysiology, diagnosis and treatment of osteomalacia. Orthop Clin North Am. 1972;3:623-52.
23. Kilian HF. Spondylolysteses gravissimae pelvangustiae cause nuper detecta. Commentatio Anatomica Obstetricia. Bonnae: Lit. C. Georgii; 1854.
24. Kirkwood JR, Ozonoff MB, Steinbach HL. Epiphyseal displacement after metaphyseal fracture in renal osteodystrophy. Am J Roentgenol. 1972;115(3):547-54.
25. Lafferty FW, Herndon CH, Pearson OH. Skeletal dynamics in vitamin D resistant rickets. Dynamic Studies on Metabolic Bone Disease. Pearson OH, Joplin K (Eds). Oxford: Blackwell Scientific Publications; 1964. pp. 163.
26. Le May M, Blunt JW. A factor determining the location of pseudo fractures in osteomalacia. J Clin Investig. 1949;28(3):521-5.
27. Longo DL, Fauci AS, Kasper DL, Hauser SL, Jameson J, Loscalzo J. Harrison's Principles of Internal Medicine, 18th edition. New York: McGraw-Hill; 2012.
28. Looser E. Uber pathologische von Infraktionen und Callusbildungen bei Rachits und Osteomalcie und Knochenerkrankungen. Zbl Chir. 1920;47:1470-4.
29. Morgan B. Osteomalacia, renal osteodystrophy, and osteoporosis. Springfield: Charles C. Thomas Publisher; 1973.
30. Munns CF, Shaw N, Kiely M, Specker BL, Thacher TD, Ozono K, et al. Global consensus recommendations on prevention and management of nutritional rickets. J Clin Endocrinol Metab. 2016;101(2):394-415.

18.3 Paget's Disease of Bone

SS Jha, Rahul Ranjan

DEFINITION

Paget's disease of bone (PDB) or osteitis deformans is a metabolic bone disease characterized by abnormal and excessive bone remodeling. This results in bone expansion and trabecular disorganization and hence compromises the strength and quality of the affected.

EPIDEMIOLOGY

- The prevalence of PDB is highest in England, the United States, Australia and New Zealand, especially in patients of age more than 55 years.
- It is rarely seen in Indian subcontinent, Scandinavian countries, Japan, China, the Middle East and black African.
- The peak incidence is in the age of 70–80 years and rarely seen in the age before 40 years. However, the prevalence double every decade after the age of 50 years.
- The overall prevalence 8% in men and 5% in female after the age of 80 years.
- The isolated raised in plasma alkaline phosphatase level of more than 150 U/L is known as "biochemical Paget's disease". Its prevalence is almost equal to radiographic Paget's disease which is significantly lower than the scintigraphy Paget's disease.
- Probably due to change in the environmental trigger and/or in change of ethnic make-up of the geographic population, fall in the prevalence and clinical severity is reported in the population of developed countries in the last three decades.
- PDB is called monostotic, if affect one bone and polyostotic if multiple bones are involved. Later is more common.
- The pelvic bone is the most commonly involved site (in approximately 50% of case). Other commonly involved bones are the spine, femur, skull and sternum.

ETIOPATHOGENESIS

Normal bones are strong and hard due to balance between the osteoclastic activity and osteoblastic activity. However, in PDB, enhanced activity of osteoclastic is observed both in the form of bigger and more active osteoclasts. The osteoblasts response to this by depositing new bone at an increased rate, resulting the structure of formed bone abnormal and fragile.

Although, the exact cause of PDB is unclear, there are evidences indicating both genetic and environmental influence.

Genetic Factors

- There are several genetic bone disorders with clinical, radiological and histological features are similar to the classic form of PDB. These differentials are familial expansile osteolysis (FEO), expansile skeletal hyperphosphatasia (ESH), idiopathic hyperphosphatasia (also known as juvenile PDB), inclusion body myopathy along with early onset PDB, early onset PDB and frontotemporal dementia.
- The most important associated gene is *SQSTM1/p-62* (*sequestosome 1 encoder*), located on chromosome 5q35. Random mutation (*P392L*) of this gene is detected in more than 30% of PDB family member. This mutation reduces the ability to sequester cytoplasm proteins, altering nuclear factor κB (NF-κB), resulting in increased osteoclastogenesis.
- Another associated gene is *TNFRSF11A* (*encoder of the RANK*) located on chromosome 18q21-22. The mutation causing loss in the *TNFRSF11B gene*, encoding the osteoprotegerin (OPG), could also lead to an activating effect in the signalization of NF-κB.
- Interaction between *TNFRSF11B* gene allelic variants with *SQSTM1* mutation, cause the severity of the disorder.

Environmental Factors

- *Paramyxovirus infection*: In a biological hybridization studies as well as immunohistochemistry suggest that infection of osteoclast by this virus cause PDB.
- *Measles*: This virus nucleocapsid affects gene expression and the *SQSTM1* mutation both contribute to the increased osteoclastic activity in PDB.
- High prevalence of vitamin D deficiency has been seen in the patients with PDB. This is probably because osteoclast

precursors have a high responsiveness and sensitivity to 1, 25 $(OH)_2D_3$, resulting in increased expression of coactivators of vitamin D receptors in PDB.

PATHOPHYSIOLOGY

Paget's disease of bone evolves through various stages of activity followed by a quiescent phase.

- *Initial phase*: This phase shows intense resorption of normal bone by multinucleated giant cells of osteoclast. This osteolytic front progress approximately 1 cm yearly.
- *Second phase*: It is a phase of osteoblastic response to initial excessive ostoclastic activity, which leads to an excessive and disorganized new bone formation. This abnormal bony tissue have increased vascularity and pronounced connective tissue reaction which resembles woven bone. This hypervascularity of the Pagetic bone and adjacent cutaneous vasodilation lead to an increase in regional blood flow, manifested clinically by rise in overlying skin temperature.
- *Quiescent phase*: After a variable period of time, there is decrease in osteoclastic activity. The abnormal bone and some of the immature woven bone may be replaced by normal-appearing lamellar bone. The resulted bone is heavier and ivory hard because of their incapacity to form Haversian systems or to center about blood vessel. Osteoblastic activity may eventually decline too and the disease became quiescent. In this stage, sclerotic bone is observed and there is no evidence of resorption and increased cellular activity.

CLINICAL FEATURES

The PDB has spectrum of symptoms which is highly variable and depends on the sites affected, the type and magnitude of the complications, and the metabolic activity. Most (70%) of the patients are asymptomatic and are diagnosed incidentally.

- The most common symptom is the *bone pain*. It is present in 40–45% of the patients. It is usually deep, precisely located and persists when the patient is at rest, constant, exacerbated both at night and by weight overload. Pain is also due to Pagetic injury, complications caused by the breakdown of bone structure, leading to degenerative arthritis, nerve compression or sarcomatous degeneration.
- *Deformities* are the second most common symptom. Its prevalence ranging from 12 to 36%. The common sites affecting are the femur and tibia, causing anterolateral bending of femur and anterior bending of tibia. These deformities can lead to changes in gait and mechanical stress, increases the likelihood of joint degeneration.
- Pagetic bones are brittle and may *fracture* even spontaneously, particularly the femur, the tibia, the humerus, and the forearm. The acute fractures are typically transverse and mend rapidly. Sometimes, the chronic *fissure fractures* may occur along convex surfaces of the long bones and are frequently asymptomatic, but when painful may represent a complete fracture. This fissure fracture is a unique feature of PDB but the differential diagnosis are the fractures occurring hyperparathyroidism and osteomalacia.
- Spine involvement may be responsible for "*vascular steal*", causing pain, dysesthesias or paralysis. This is due to diversion of blood to the adjacent cutaneous circulation because of vasodilatation.

COMPLICATIONS

- *Osteoarthritis*: Most often affecting the knee and hip joints. This is due to alteration of bone biomechanics that causes bone and cartilage degeneration.
- *Deformities and fractures*: This is due to abnormal bone formation, and associated with high morbidity due to pain.
- Cranial bone involvement causes hearing loss, headache, dizziness and rarely vascular dementia and hydrocephalus.
- Jaw bone involvement cause periodontal disease and dental malocclusion.
- *Malignant transformation*: Like osteosarcoma, and giant cell tumor (<1%) and is seen in case of polyostotic PDB. This is to be suspected in case of increased bone pain, swelling, and more rarely pathological fracture.
- *Hypercalcemia*: It is often associated with prolonged immobilization or dehydration.

RADIOGRAPHIC FINDINGS

Different phases of PDB give different radiographic picture and still remain the mainstay of diagnosis.

- *Resorption of bone trabeculae* that appears on radiograph as an osteolytic advancing front. It is typically seen in skull at which site it is termed *osteoporosis circumscripta* and begins in frontal and occipital regions.
- In tubular bones, osteolysis begins in the subchondral regions of the epiphysis and subsequently extends in the metaphysic and diaphysis. Exception to this is tibia in which osteolytic front is diaphysis.
- "*Blade of grass*" or "*flame*": Advancement of the osteolytic front to the diaphysis of the bone forms a wedge-shaped radiolucent area, which is clearly demarcated from the adjacent bone. This gives a characteristic appearance of "blade of grass" or "flame".
- *Bone sclerosis* may be seen both in active and inactive staged of the disease. In the long bones, the flame-shaped osteolytic advancing edge proceeding toward the shaft is replaced, in the epiphysis and metaphysic, by focal radiodensity. Besides, coarsened trabeculae, cortical thickening and enlargement of bone are prominent.

BIOCHEMICAL MARKERS

The role of the biochemical markers of bone turnover helps in objective assessment of both disease activity and the response to treatment. Among many markers, the main is the elevation of total alkaline phosphatase (total ALP).

- *Total ALP*: It reflects the spreading of osseous involvement, with exception of *osteoporosis circumscripta*, in which there is higher bone ALP than other skeletal segments. Serum ALP has a sensitivity of 78% and a specificity of almost 100%. The mean increase in serum ALP is more pronounced in polyostotic disease. Serum ALP may be normal in 20% cases of monostotic disease.
- *Osteocalcin*: It is considered a specific marker for bone formation. It is found normal in approximately 40% of cases, limiting its clinical significance. Also there occurs a transient elevation with the treatment of bisphosphonate.
- *C-terminal (CTX) crosslinking telopeptide of type I collagen*: It is the most sensitive bone resorption marker both for assessing disease activity and for monitoring efficacy of therapy.
- *Procollagen type I-N-propeptides*: Helpful in monitoring of efficacy of treatment as its level decrease more rapidly than total ALP after treatment with bisphosphonates. A significant reduction after treatment would be >40%.

TREATMENT

The primary aim of the treatment is to relief pain and to reduce the rate of bone remodeling. Restoration of typical bone turnover balances the rate of bone deposition, reducing bone hypervascularization, and slowing progression of the disease.

Indications of pharmacotherapy are:
- All symptomatic patients
- Asymptomatic patients, planned for surgery at an active Pagetic site in order to reduce the risk of bleeding (including blood loss during surgery)
- Those with hypercalcemia
- The cases involving locations liable to present complications

Pharmacological Agents

The osteoclast cells play the pivot role in the development and progression of PDB. Hence the drugs targeting, suppression of osteoclast over activity will help in modification of disease course.

Calcitonin

It acts directly on calcitonin receptor located on the osteoclast, and hence inhibits its activity. Due to its short duration of action, partial response, and acquired resistance, is rarely used nowaday. It is only indicated in the patient who is not tolerating the bisphosphonate. Recurrence is common after discontinuation of medicine. Its common side effects are flushing, nausea and vomiting.

Bisphosphonates

It is the most widely used agent. Mechanism of action is by blocking osteoclastic bone resorption. Nitrogenous bisphosphonates (alendronate, risedronate, pamidronate and zoledronic acid) are drugs of choice.

- *Etidronate*: It is a non-nitrogenous bisphosphonate recommended in the dose of 5 mg/kg per day (mean dose 400 mg/day) for 6 months. Main concerns of its use are high relapse rate after discontinuation and resistance after repeated course of treatment.
- *Tiludronate*: It is also a non-nitrogenous class of bisphosphonate recommended in the dose of 400 mg/day for 3 months. It normalizes ALP in 35% of the patient. It is more effective than etidronate and does not cause bone demineralization.
- *Alendronate*: It is nitrogenous bisphosphonate recommended in the dose of 40 mg daily for 6 months. It is generally well-tolerated drug, effective in normalizing serum ALP. It is to be avoided in the patient with creatinine clearance below 35 mL/min. Alendronate and pamidronate have similar efficacy in achieving biochemical remission.
- *Risedronate*: It is nitrogenous bisphosphonate recommended in the dose of 30 mg daily for 2 months but should be avoided in the patient with a creatinine clearance of less than 30 mL/min. 73% of the patients treated with risedronate achieve normalization of serum ALP. Relapse rate after discontinuation of medication is 3%.
- *Pamidronate*: It is well-tolerated drug and can be used in the patient with creatinine clearance of less than 30 mL/min. It is given intravenously in 30 mg doses daily for 3 days. Main drawback is the development of resistance, which may influence the effectiveness of retreatment. It normalizes serum ALP in 60–80% of the patients treated with pamidronate.
- *Ibandronate*: It is effective in the dose of 2 mg intravenous doses. It has been seen that more than 80% and more than 50% patient treated with ibandronate have normal serum CTX and ALP.
- *Zolendronate*: It is the most potent bisphosphonate approved for the treatment of PDB. It is given in a single IV dose of 5 mg. It is not preferred in the case with clearance below 35 mL/min. Sustained remission is observed in most of the patients, lasting up to 2 years. The effective response being considered normalization of ALP which is seen in approximately 90% of cases.

MONITORING OF DISEASE ACTIVITY

- Alkaline phosphatase level is directly related to disease activity. Normal ALP is associated with biochemical remission, histological evidence of normal bone turnover, and its elevated level is related to the increase disease activity. The measurement of ALP level should be conducted after first 3–6 months of treatment, in order to evaluate the initial response, followed by two annual measurements as a marker of bone activity.

- Remission is considered to be achieved when normal level of ALP are attained and partial remission when there is decrease in level greater than 75% after 3–6 months of treatment. Retreatment should be resumed when ALP level begin to rise again, or when there is a 25% increase compared to post-treatment levels.

Results from the PRISM study showed that most treatment approaches have limited impact on quality of life, pain and hearing loss, and highlighted the need for further studies to examine whether the effects of bisphosphonates on the bone remodeling can actually translate into a clinical improvement and lower risk of complications in the individual affected. Most of the study conducted so far have a short period of follow-up. So long-term study is required to draw a conclusion.

FURTHER READING

1. Altman RD. Paget's disease of bone: rheumatologic complications. Bone. 1999; 24(5):47S-8S.
2. Bandeira F, Griz L, Caldas G, Macedo G, Marinho C, Moutelik M, et al. A single center experience of 103 cases. Paget's disease of bone in Brazil. Proceedings of the International Symposium on Paget's disease of bone/fibrous dysplasia: advances and challenges. 2006. Bethesda, Maryland: The Paget's Foundation, National Institute of Health; 2006. p. 53.
3. Bone HG. Nonmalignant complications of Paget's disease. J Bone Miner Res. 2006; 21:64-8.
4. Chambers TJ, Magnus CJ. Calcitonin alters behaviour of isolated osteoclasts. J Pathol. 1982;136(1):27-39.
5. Colina M, La Corte R, De Leonardis F, Trotta F. Paget's disease of bone: a review. Rheumatology International. 2008;28(11): 1069-75.
6. Daroszewska A, Ralston SH. Mechanisms of disease: genetics of Paget's disease of bone and related disorders. Nat Clin Pract Rheumatol. 2006;2:270-7.
7. Davie M, Davies M, Francis R, Fraser W, Hosking D. Paget's disease of bone: a review of 889 patients. Bone. 1999;24(5):11S-2S.
8. Devogelaer JP, Bergmann P, Body JJ, Boutsen Y, Goemaere S, Kaufman JM, et al. Management of patients with Paget's disease: a consensus document of the Belgian Bone Club. Osteoporos Int. 2008;19(8):1109-17.
9. Douglas DL, Duckworth T, Russell RG, Kanis JA, Preston CJ, Preston FE, et al. Effect of dichloromethylene diphosphonate in Paget's disease of bone and in hypercalcaemia due to primary hyperparathyroidism or malignant disease. Lancet. 1980;1:10:43-7.
10. Doyle T, Gunn J, Anderson G, Gill M, Cundy T. Paget's disease in New Zealand: evidence for declining prevalence. Bone. 2002;31(5):616-9.
11. Eyres KS, Marshall P, McCloskey E. Spontaneous fractures in a patient treated with low doses of etidronic acid (disodium etidronate). Drug Saf. 1992;7(2):162.
12. Falchetti A, Di Stefano M, Marini F, Del Monte F, Mavilia C, Strigoli D, et al. Two novel mutations at exon 8 of the sequestosome (SQSTM1) gene in an Italian series of patients affected by Paget's disease of bone (PDB). J Bone Miner Res. 2004;19(6):1013-7.
13. Gallacher SJ, Boyce BF, Patel U, Jenkins A, Ralston SH, Boyle IT. Clinical experience with pamidronate in the treatment of Paget's disease of bone. Ann Rheum Dis. 1991;50(12):930-3.
14. Gennari L, Di Stefano M, Merlotti D, Giordano N, Martini G, Tamone C, et al. Prevalence of Paget's disease of bone in Italy. J Bone Miner Res. 2005;20(10):1845-50.
15. Griz L, Caldas G, Bandeira C, Assunção V, Bandeira F. Paget's disease of bone. Arq Bras Endocrinol Metab. 2006; 50(4):814-22.
16. Griz L, Colares V, Bandeira F. Treatment of Paget's disease of bone: importance of the zoledronic acid. Arq Bras Endocrinol Metabol. 2006;50(5):845-51.
17. Griz L, Fontan D, Mesquita P, Lazaretti-Castro M, Borba VZ, Borges JL, et al. Diagnosis and management of Paget's disease of bone. Arq Bras Endocrinol Metabol. 2014;58(6): 587-99.
18. Hosking D, Lyles K, Brown JP. Long-term control of bone turnover in Paget's disease with zoledronic acid and risedronate. J Bone Miner Res. 2007;22(1):142.
19. Janssens K, Van Hul W. Molecular genetics of too much bone. Hum Mol Genet. 2002;11(20):2385-93.
20. Kurihara N, Zhou H, Dempster D, Windle J, Brown J, Roodman D. Measles virus nucleocapsid gene expression and the SQTM1 mutation both contribute to the increased osteoclast activity in Paget's disease. J Bone Miner Res. 2010;25(Suppl 1): S11.
21. Langston AL, Campbell MK, Fraser WD, MacLennan GS, Selby PL, Ralston SH, et al. Randomized trial of intensive bisphosphonate treatment versus symptomatic management in Paget's disease of bone. J Bone Miner Res. 2010;25(1):20-31.
22. Merlotti D, Gianfrancesco F, Gennari L, Rendina D, Stefano M, Mossetti G, et al. TNFRSF11A gene allelic variants are associated with Paget's disease of bone and interact with sqstm1 mutations to cause the severity of the disorder. J Bone Miner Res. 2010;25(Suppl 1):S11.
23. Poór G, Donáth J, Fornet B, Cooper C. Epidemiology of Paget's disease in Europe: the prevalence is decreasing. J Bone Miner Res. 2006;21(10):1545-9.
24. Reginster JY, Colson F, Morlock G. Evaluation of the efficacy and safety of oral tiludronate in Paget's disease of bone: a double-blind, multiple-dosage, placebo-controlled study. Arthritis Rheum. 1992;35(8):967.
25. Reid IR, Miller P, Lyles K, Fraser W, Brown JP, Saidi Y, et al. Comparison of a single infusion of zoledronic acid with risedronate for Paget's disease. N Engl J Med. 2005;353: 898-908.
26. Reid IR, Nicholson GC, Weinstein RS. Biochemical and radiologic improvement in Paget's disease of bone treated with alendronate: a randomized, placebo-controlled trial. Am J Med. 1996;101(4):341.
27. Reid IR. Pharmacotherapy of Paget's disease of bone. Expert Opin Pharmacother. 2012;13(5):637-46.
28. Seitz S, Priemel M, Zustin J, Beil FT, Semler J, Minne H, et al. Paget's disease of bone: histologic analysis of 754 patients. J Bone Miner Res. 2009;24(1):62-9.
29. Seton M, Moses AM, Bode RK, Schwartz C. Paget's disease of bone: the skeletal distribution, complications and quality of life as perceived by patients. Bone. 2011;48:281.
30. Sharma H, Mehdi S, MacDuff E, Reece A, Jane M, Reid R. Paget sarcoma of the spine: Scottish Bone Tumor Registry experience. Spine (Phila Pa 1976). 2006;31:1344-50.

Childhood Rheumatic Disease and Tubercular Infection in Orthopedic Rheumatology

- **Juvenile Idiopathic Arthritis**
  Utkarsh Bansal, Manish Khanna
- **Mycobacterial Infections of Bone and Joints**
  Gyaneshwar Tonk, Sujit Kumar

19. Juvenile Idiopathic Arthritis

Utkarsh Bansal, Manish Khanna

INTRODUCTION

Juvenile idiopathic arthritis (JIA), the most common rheumatic pediatric disease, is one of the commonest chronic pediatric illnesses. The incidence varies from 1 to 20 per 100,000 children per year, with prevalence of 10–140 per 100,000. The wide variability reflects the population and environmental differences. The International League of Associations for Rheumatology (ILAR) used the term JIA to include all subtypes of chronic juvenile arthritis in its classification. JIA can lead to long-term morbidity and severe disability in a number of cases. JIA is defined as the presence of inflammation of at least one joint for a minimum duration of 6 weeks, with onset prior to the age of 16 years and exclusion of other causes of arthritis.

ILAR classification of JIA includes the following:
- Systemic JIA
- Oligoarthritis
- Polyarthritis
- Psoriatic arthritis
- Enthesitis-related arthritis
- Undifferentiated arthritis

ETIOPATHOGENESIS

The etiology is not well understood, but the immunogenetic susceptibility and environmental triggers are necessary for the development of the disease. JIA is associated with multiple genes making it a complex genetic trait. Environmental triggers may include viral and bacterial infections, joint trauma, enhanced host response to infections, and deranged sex hormones.

There is an alteration of both cell-mediated and humoral immunity in this autoimmune disease. Immunological derangements lead to inflammatory synovitis, which on further advanced stage lead to pannus formation and the progressive erosion of articular cartilage.

HISTORY

Arthritis is defined by intra-articular swelling or the presence of two or more of the following signs: Tenderness or pain on movement, limitation in range of movement, and warmth. For the diagnosis, arthritis must be present for at least 6 weeks. The onset of the disease can be insidious or abrupt and often includes morning stiffness or a *gelling phenomenon* (stiffness after long periods of inactivity) and arthralgia with easy fatigability occurring during the day. A morning limp that improves over the day may be the manifestation of a young child.

There can be a history of school absences, and children will have reduced ability to participate in physical activity that may manifest the disease severity or acute flares.

Systemic JIA is characterized by fever, arthritis, and visceral involvement. The spiking high-grade fever (≥39°C) is a characteristic, which occurs once or twice at about the same time every day, for at least 2 weeks in duration with temperature rapidly returning to normal. The predictable fever pattern differentiates it from infections, malignancy, or Kawasaki disease.

Fever is usually accompanied by an evanescent (nonfixed) erythematous rash. The salmon-colored rash is linear or circular, on the trunk and proximal extremities. Superficial trauma evoking the rash (*Koebner phenomenon*) is a cutaneous hypersensitivity. Classically, the rash is nonpruritic and migratory.

Psoriatic arthritis may present with typical psoriasis and arthritis or arthritis with subtle dermatological manifestations like pitting of nails. Dactylitis is a characteristic feature.

Enthesitis-related arthritis presents as postexercise and evening pain. There is a history of back pain that improves with activity. Children suffering from this condition cannot lie in the bed all morning due to back pain.

PHYSICAL EXAMINATION

Juvenile idiopathic arthritis is essentially a clinical diagnosis. A complete physical examination provides criteria for diagnosis. JIA can be diagnosed in a child younger than 16 years presenting with arthritis persisting for at least 6 weeks in at least one joint, with other causes of arthritis excluded.

On examination, there should be arthritis or the presence of two or more of the following signs: Tenderness or pain on motion, limitation of joint motion, warmth, or erythema of the joint. The temporomandibular joint (TMJ), hips, and small joints in the spine when affected by synovitis rather than swelling demonstrates loss of motion and pain. The physical findings reflect the extent of joint involvement.

In synovitis, the child tends to keep the joint in a position of maximum. Generally, limbs are held in flexion, while the limitation in range of motion is rarely seen.

An early sign of synovitis is guarding. The fingers are swollen in synovitis with a painful range of motion. In the lower limb, a doughy synovium may be palpable over the knee joint and a soft, boggy swelling may be palpated in the popliteal fossa. The hip is kept in flexion, abduction, and external rotation with a painful range of motion.

The presence of cutaneous erythema is rare finding and should alert to search for an alternate diagnosis.

Systemic-onset Juvenile Idiopathic Arthritis (SoJIA)

Spiking fever with twice-daily peaks which may be accompanied or followed by arthritis few days to months later.

Physical examination findings include the following:
- Ill child
- Evanescent, salmon-colored, erythematous, macular rash, predominantly on the trunk and the proximal extremities
- Myalgia
- Arthralgia
- Hepatosplenomegaly
- Lymphadenopathy, especially the axillary lymph nodes
- Serositis
- Pericarditis or pleuritis may present with chest pain or shortness of breath
- Friction rub may occur in pericarditis
- Myocarditis may lead to heart failure presenting with basilar rales, and hepatomegaly.

Oligoarticular Juvenile Idiopathic Arthritis

- Arthritis affecting four or fewer joints in first 6 months of disease onset, often only single joint.
- Those who never develop the disease in more than four joints are having *persistent oligoarticular JIA* while those who develop in more than four joints after 6 months are suffering from *extended oligoarticular JIA*.
- Typically affects the large weight-bearing joints of the lower extremity. Isolated upper extremity involvement is rare.
- Usually present with swelling in the joint rather than pain.
- Well looking child, though walking with a limp.
- Leg-length discrepancy can occur because of chronic inflammation-related hyperemia in asymmetrical arthritis cases, leading to overgrowth of the limb.
- Extensor muscle atrophy (vastus lateralis, quadriceps in knee arthritis) may occur.

Atypical features include small joint involvement in the hands, which suggests development of polyarticular JIA or psoriatic arthritis. Dactylitis or sausage digit (tenosynovitis of a finger or toe) is usually seen in psoriatic arthritis or enthesitis-related arthritis. Isolated hip joint involvement is seldom a presenting sign and is suggestive of a nonrheumatic cause or enthesitis-related arthritis.

One out of five children with oligoarticular and polyarticular JIA may have asymptomatic anterior uveitis, and thus screening by an ophthalmologic slit-lamp examination is necessary. Antinuclear antibody (ANA) positivity confers increased risk of anterior uveitis.

Polyarticular Juvenile Idiopathic Arthritis

- Five or more joints are affected in the first 6 months after the onset of the disease.
- Joints of both upper and lower extremity are affected, especially the weight-bearing joints.
- Rheumatoid nodules, on the extensor surfaces of the spine, elbows, and ankles, are sometimes present. Presence is associated with a severe course and rheumatoid factor (RF)-positive cases.
- Small joints in the hands are symmetrically involved.

Two forms of presentation may be there:
1. *Rheumatoid factor negative*: About 20–30% of patients having a symmetrical involvement of joints and a benign course of the disease.
2. *Rheumatoid factor positive*: The presentation resembles characteristic adult rheumatoid arthritis. There is a typical symmetrical small joints involvement. Rheumatoid nodules may be present. Extra-articular manifestations are very rare. Micrognathia is seen in chronic TMJ disease.

Psoriatic Arthritis

Usually, a mild disease in children and in majority the onset of arthritis precedes that of psoriasis. Characteristics include the following:
- Asymmetrical arthritis
- Distal interphalangeal joint involvement
- Dactylitis
- Nail pitting (minimum of 2 pits in 1 or more nails) and onycholysis.

Enthesitis-related Arthritis

Enthesitis is tenderness at the insertion of tendon, ligament, joint capsule, or fascia to the bone.

Pain and tenderness at the enthesis is the usual presentation, but sometimes swelling may also be seen.

In children, the peripheral joint involvement (dactylitis) precedes the axial involvement (e.g., sacroiliitis).

Diagnostic criteria include the presence of both arthritis and enthesitis, or arthritis or enthesitis with at least two of the following:
- Onset of arthritis in a male >6 years old. Sacroiliac joint tenderness or inflammatory lumbosacral pain, or both.
- Positive human leukocyte antigen B27 (HLA-B27) antigen.
- Acute symptomatic anterior uveitis.
- History of the presence of ankylosing spondylitis, enthesitis-related arthritis, inflammatory bowel disease with sacroiliitis, reactive arthritis, or acute anterior uveitis in a first-degree relative.

Enthesitis can be present with both oligoarticular and polyarticular JIA cases, but spondyloarthropathy is differentiated from the fact that it develops into a predominant enthesitis.

Undifferentiated Arthritis

This diagnosis is made when the manifestations fulfill the criteria for no category or for more than one category.

Polyarticular RF-negative JIA with either enthesitis-related JIA or psoriatic JIA, usually falls in the second category.

■ DIAGNOSTIC CONSIDERATIONS

Many conditions may mimic JIA as they may present with arthritis or arthritis-like symptoms. Leukemia is the most important differential diagnosis of JIA.

Differential Diagnoses
- Systemic lupus erythematosus (SLE)
- Polyarteritis nodosa
- Scleroderma
- Juvenile dermatomyositis
- Behçet syndrome
- Sjögren syndrome
- Kawasaki disease
- Pediatric sarcoidosis
- Infectious mononucleosis
- Reactive arthritis
- Septic arthritis
- Lyme disease
- Gout
- Trauma
- Scurvy
- Rickets
- Benign bone tumors
- Acute lymphoblastic leukemia
- Lymphoma
- Hemophilia

■ INVESTIGATIONS

Inflammatory Markers

Erythrocyte sedimentation rate (ESR) or C-reactive protein (CRP) levels are elevated in children with systemic and polyarticular JIA, but rarely in oligoarticular disease. These inflammatory markers can serve to monitor disease activity.

Leukocytosis, thrombocytosis, increased complement, decreased albumin, and microcytic anemia are the other markers of inflammation.

Complete Blood Count and Metabolic Panel

The degree of systemic and articular inflammation is reflected by leukocytosis, thrombocytosis, and microcytic anemia. Due to the migration of activated lymphocytes migrate out of the circulation into synovium, lymphopenia may be present. However, the presence of neutropenia, particularly with lymphocytosis or thrombocytopenia, should raise a suspicion of acute lymphocytic leukemia.

A complete hemogram, liver, and kidney function tests should be done before starting treatment with immunosuppressant drugs.

Antinuclear Antibody Testing

About half to three-fourth of the children with oligoarticular or polyarticular JIA will have high ANA titers but rarely in children with systemic JIA. However, in case of a positive ANA test, SLE should be ruled out.

Children with a positive ANA test are at increased risk of chronic anterior uveitis. In a child where the onset of arthritis is below 6 years of age and who is also ANA seropositive should be screened for development of uveitis every 3–4 months by slit-lamp examination.

Other Laboratory Tests

Rheumatoid factor is positive in about 5–15% cases of polyarticular JIA and indicates a severe course. Anticyclic citrullinated peptide antibody (anti-CCP antibody) also indicates aggressive disease. In systemic JIA, often the total protein and albumin levels are low, while fibrinogen, ferritin, and D-dimer levels may be elevated.

Sarcoidosis may be differentiated from JIA by an elevated angiotensin-converting enzyme (ACE) level, while acute rheumatic fever or post-streptococcal arthritis can be diagnosed by an elevated anti-streptolysin O (ASO) and anti-DNase B levels.

Urinalysis should be performed to rule out infection that may act as a trigger for JIA or transient postinfectious arthritis.

Macrophage-activating syndrome [MAS, also referred to as *secondary hemophagocytic syndrome or hemophagocytic lympho-histiocytosis (HLH)*], is rare but a fatal complication in patients with systemic onset JIA, indicated by:

- Falling ESR
- Leukopenia
- Low platelets
- Elevated liver enzymes
- Increased triglycerides
- Increased ferritin
- Increased lactate dehydrogenase
- Low fibrinogen
- Low albumin
- Erratic high spiking fevers
- Splenomegaly
- Hepatomegaly
- Lymphadenopathy
- Purpura and mucosal bleeding
- Encephalopathy

Radiography

The radiographic changes in JIA include:
- Soft tissue swelling
- Periarticular osteopenia and/or osteoporosis
- Periosteal new bone apposition around affected joints
- Loss of joint-space
- Subchondral erosions
- Bony erosions
- Intra-articular bony ankylosis
- Periostitis
- Growth disturbances (epiphyseal overgrowth or ballooning)
- Epiphyseal compression fracture
- Joint subluxation
- Synovial cysts
- Ankylosis in the cervical spine progressing to atlantoaxial subluxation

The inability of direct visualization of synovium, articular cartilage, and other noncalcified structures in a joint by conventional radiography limits its utility.

Computed Tomography and Magnetic Resonance Imaging

Though computed tomography (CT) scan is the best modality to analyze bone deformities, but in the assessment of JIA magnetic resonance imaging (MRI) has proved to be more beneficial.

Magnetic resonance imaging is the most sensitive radiologic indicator of early pathological changes and disease activity. It can demonstrate synovial hypertrophy, soft tissue swelling, and the status of articular cartilage. Contrast-enhanced sequences detect cartilaginous erosions.

It is difficult to differentiate synovitis and a joint effusion on T2-weighted (T2W) images as they show similar hyperintensity. So, gadolinium-enhanced T1-weighted (T1W) MRIs are needed to diagnose active synovitis.

Ultrasonography

Basic findings in JIA include:
- Synovial inflammation is visualized around the articular cartilage as an area of mixed echogenicity.
- Synovial vasculature is depicted with Doppler flow studies.
- The serial measurements of effusion volumes and synovial thickness can help to assess disease progression.

Ultrasound is helpful to evaluate the joints, which cannot be clinically examined easily. It has further advantages that it there is no need of sedation, no risk of radiation and can be therapeutically useful to guide injections to the joint space.

Others

Bone scan, arthrocentesis, biopsy, etc., may be required in certain cases.

■ TREATMENT AND MANAGEMENT

Approach Considerations

For remission, the criteria of the American College of Rheumatology (ACR) are as follows:
- No joint pain
- No morning stiffness
- No fatigue
- No synovitis
- No damage progression
- No elevation of the ESR and CRP levels

In 2011, the following five treatment groups for the treatment of JIA were included in the ACR recommendations:
1. History of arthritis in four or fewer joints
2. History of arthritis in five or more joints
3. Active sacroiliac arthritis
4. Systemic arthritis without active arthritis
5. Systemic arthritis with active arthritis

The management depends upon disease activity, severity, and the presence or absence of poorprognostic features **(Flowchart 1)**.

History of Arthritis in Four or Fewer Joints (Table 1)

Nonsteroidal anti-inflammatory drugs (NSAIDs) monotherapy may be adequate for patients without any joint contracture and low disease activity with no poor prognostic features. The response usually comes within 2 months. NSAIDs are a useful adjunctive treatment as needed in other patients.

In cases with medium to high disease activity, or low diseases activity with poor prognostic features glucocorticoid intra-articular injections (triamcinolone) can be used. It usually provides a clinical relief for about 4 months. In patients not responding to NSAID monotherapy even after 2 months, should be switched to this therapy.

Flowchart 1: Medical management of JIA based on ACR 2011 recommendations.

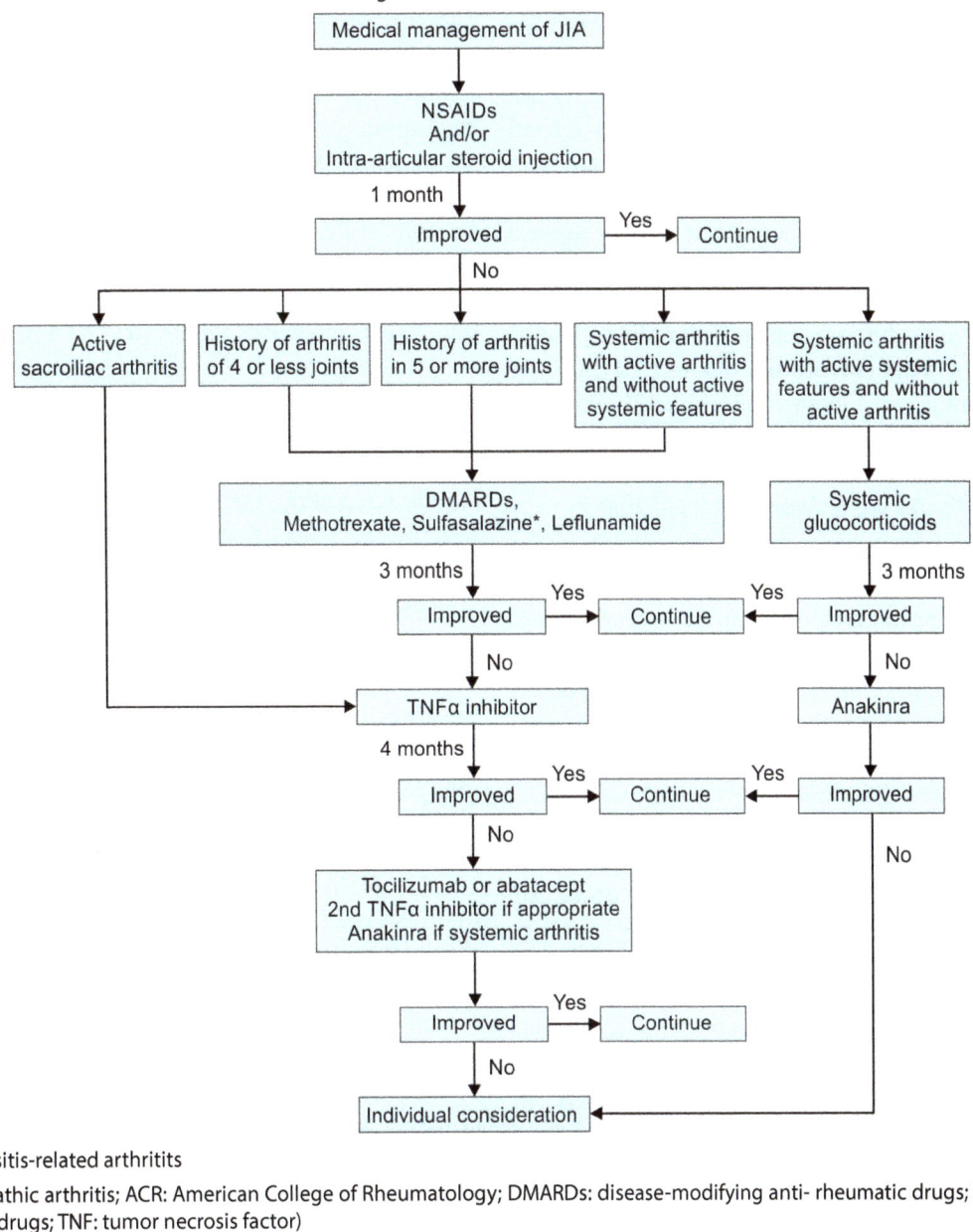

*Preferred if enthesitis-related arthritits

(JIA: juvenile idiopathic arthritis; ACR: American College of Rheumatology; DMARDs: disease-modifying anti-rheumatic drugs; NSAIDs: nonsteroidal anti-inflammatory drugs; TNF: tumor necrosis factor)

TABLE 1: Features of poor prognosis and disease activity for a history of arthritis of four or fewer joints according to ACR 2011.

Features of Poor Prognosis (Must satisfy 1)

Arthritis of the hip or cervical spine

Arthritis of the ankle or wrist AND marked or prolonged inflammatory marker elevation

Radiographic damage (erosions or joint space narrowing by radiograph)

Disease Activity Levels

Low disease activity (Must satisfy all)	Moderate disease activity (Does not satisfy criteria for low or high activity)	High disease activity (Must satisfy at least 3)
One or fewer active joints	One or more features greater than low disease activity level AND fewer than three features of high disease activity	Two or more active joints
ESR or CRP level normal		ESR or CRP > twice upper limit of normal
Physician global assessment of overall disease activity <3 of 10		Physician global assessment of overall disease activity ≥7 of 10
Patient/parent global assessment of overall well-being <2 of 10		Patient/parent global assessment of overall well-being ≥4 of 10

(ACR: American College of Rheumatology; ESR: erythrocyte sedimentation rate; CRP: C-reactive protein)

Patients not responding to NSAIDs and/or glucocorticoid intra-articular injections should be treated with methotrexate with other therapies as an adjunct. Methotrexate is the initial treatment of choice for patients with high disease activity and poor prognosis features. In patients with enthesitis-related JIA, NSAIDs, or joint injections failure warrants therapy with sulfasalazine rather than methotrexate.

Patients who continue to have moderate to high-disease activity with poor prognostic features after even 3 months or high disease activity after even 6 months of methotrexate therapy should be given tumor necrosis factor-alpha (TNFα) inhibitor treatment. In patients of enthesitis-related JIA TNFα inhibitor treatment is recommended over methotrexate or sulfasalazine.

Patients who continue to have moderate to high-disease activity with poor prognostic features after even 3 months or high-disease activity after even 6 months of methotrexate or leflunomide therapy, should be escalated to TNFα inhibitor treatment.

Patients who show features of moderate to high-disease activity even after 4 months of TNFα inhibitor treatment can be switched to a non-TNFα inhibitor biologic (tocilizumab or abatacept) rather than to a second TNFα inhibitor. A second TNFα inhibitor may be appropriate for patients with good initial response to their first TNFα inhibitor.

Rituximab may be used in cases who fail to respond to the above treatment and in RF-positive polyarticular JIA cases it may be more appropriate (**Flowchart 1**).

History of Arthritis in Five or More Joints (Table 2)

This group includes children with RF-negative and RF-positive polyarthritis, extended oligoarthritis, psoriatic arthritis, enthesitis-related arthritis, and undifferentiated arthritis..

First-line NSAIDs monotherapy may be tried for 1 month in patients with low disease activity, or 1–2 months in those with moderate disease activity but without poor prognostic features. Patients uncontrolled should be escalated to methotrexate therapy. Latest recommendations suggest the use NSAIDs only as an adjunct not as monotherapy.

For patients with moderate disease activity and poor prognostic features and those with high-disease activity should be initiated with methotrexate. Using subcutaneous methotrexate is conditionally recommended over oral methotrexate. NSAIDs and/or glucocorticoid intra-articular injections are adjunct therapies in all stages of treatment.

Leflunomide or sulfasalazine can be tried as an alternative to methotrexate in cases of side effects, but recommendations prefer methotrexate over leflunomide or sulfasalazine.

Active Sacroiliac Arthritis (Table 3)

Patients with active sacroiliitis mostly within the ILAR categories of enthesitis-related arthritis, psoriatic arthritis, and undifferentiated arthritis but may include patients from any of the ILAR JIA categories.

Initial monotherapy with NSAIDs is recommended. In those who have a failure of an adequate trial of NSAIDs therapy and continue to have high disease activity with features of poor prognosis, TNFα inhibitor treatment is recommended.

Using sulfasalazine for patients who have contraindications to TNFα inhibitor or have failed more than one TNFα inhibitor is recommended. In ACR 2019 guidelines, methotrexate monotherapy is not recommended based on data from adult spondyloarthritis suggesting lack of effectiveness. Intra-articular glucocorticoid injection of the sacroiliac joints as an adjunct therapy is recommended.

Systemic Arthritis with Active Systemic Features and without Active Arthritis (Table 4)

Nonsteroidal anti-inflammatory drug monotherapy is recommended in patients who have fever and less severe

TABLE 2: Features of poor prognosis and disease activity for a history of arthritis of five or more joints according to ACR 2011.

Features of Poor Prognosis (Must Satisfy 1)

Arthritis of the hip or cervical spine

Positive rheumatoid factor or anticyclic citrullinated peptide antibodies

Radiographic damage (erosions or joint space narrowing by radiograph)

Disease Activity Levels

Low disease activity *(Must satisfy all)*	Moderate disease activity *(Does not satisfy criteria for low or high activity)*	High disease activity *(Must satisfy at least three)*
Four or fewer active joints	One or more features greater than low disease activity level AND fewer than three features of high disease activity	Eight or more active joints
ESR or CRP level normal		ESR or CRP level > twice upper limit of normal
Physician global assessment of overall disease activity <4 of 10		Physician global assessment of overall disease activity ≥7 of 10
Patient/parent global assessment of overall well-being <2 of 10		Patient/parent global assessment of overall well-being ≥5 of 10

(ACR: American College of Rheumatology; ESR: erythrocyte sedimentation rate; CRP: C-reactive protein)

TABLE 3: Features of poor prognosis and disease activity for active sacroiliac arthritis according to ACR 2011.

Features of Poor Prognosis

Radiographic damage of any joint (erosions or joint space narrowing by radiograph)

Disease Activity Levels

Low disease activity (Must satisfy all)	Moderate disease activity (Does not satisfy criteria for low or high activity)	High disease activity (Must satisfy at least two)
Normal back flexion	One or more features greater than low disease activity level AND fewer than two features of high disease activity	ESR or CRP > twice upper limit of normal
ESR or CRP level normal		Physician global assessment of overall disease activity ≥7 of 10
Physician global assessment of overall disease activity <4 of 10		Patient/parent global assessment of overall well-being ≥4 of 10
Patient/parent global assessment of overall well-being <2 of 10		

(ACR: American College of Rheumatology; ESR: erythrocyte sedimentation rate; CRP: C-reactive protein)

TABLE 4: Features of poor prognosis and disease activity for systemic arthritis with active systemic features (and without active arthritis) according to ACR 2011.

Features of Poor Prognosis

Six months duration of significant active systemic disease, defined by: Fever, elevated inflammatory markers, or requirement for treatment with systemic glucocorticoids

Disease Activity Levels **(2 levels)**

Active fever AND physician global assessment of overall disease activity <7 of 10

Active fever AND systemic features of high disease activity (e.g., significant serositis) that result in physician global assessment of overall disease activity ≥7 of 10

TABLE 5: Features of poor prognosis and disease activity for active sacroiliac arthritis according to ACR 2011.

Features of Poor Prognosis (Must satisfy 1)

Arthritis of the hip

Radiographic damage (erosions or joint space narrowing by radiograph)

Disease Activity Levels

Low disease activity (Must satisfy all)	Moderate disease activity (Does not satisfy criteria for low or high activity)	High disease activity (Must satisfy at least 3)
Four or fewer active joints	One or more features greater than low disease activity level AND fewer than three features of high disease activity	Eight or more active joints
ESR or CRP level normal		ESR or CRP level > twice upper limit of normal
Physician global assessment of overall disease activity <4 of 10		Physician global assessment of overall disease activity ≥7 of 10
Patient/parent global assessment of overall well-being <2 of 10		Patient/parent global assessment of overall well-being ≥5 of 10

(ACR: American College of Rheumatology; ESR: erythrocyte sedimentation rate; CRP: C-reactive protein)

disease and without poor prognostic feature for 2 weeks. For nonresponders, treatment is escalated to systemic glucocorticoids, with as needed adjunct NSAIDs.

Systemic glucocorticoids are the initial treatment for children with high systemic disease activity or/and poor prognostic features.

Anakinra (human interleukin 1 receptor antagonist protein) is used in patients who have persistent fever despite systemic steroid therapy and may be used as first-line therapy in those with poor prognostic features.

Systemic Arthritis with Active Arthritis and without Active Systemic Features (Table 5)

Nonsteroidal anti-inflammatory drug monotherapy, with intra-articular joint injections as needed, is the initial treatment for patients with low disease activity and no poor prognostic features. Treatment should be tried for 1 month, but if disease activity persists methotrexate should be started.

Methotrexate is given for a period of 3 months, and if the disease activity remains at moderate to severe level the treatment should be escalated to anakinra or a TNFα inhibitor.

Patients having moderate to severe disease activity even after 4 months TNFα inhibitor treatment, can be switched to abatacept.

In September 2013, ACR updated the guidelines for the treatment of systemic JIA defining three primary clinical phenotypes. The case should meet the ILAR criteria for systemic JIA at disease onset. The features of poor prognosis and levels of disease activity specified in the 2011 ACR JIA recommendations were not applied. The decision thresholds of active joint count (AJC; ≤4 or >4) and physician global assessment (MD global; <5 or ≥5) were chosen.

1. *Systemic JIA with active systemic features and varying degrees of synovitis*: Active systemic features are the presence of any combination of the following: Fever, evanescent rash, lymphadenopathy, hepatomegaly, splenomegaly, or serositis.

   As an initial treatment, for patients with:
   - MD global <5 and AJC = 0: NSAIDs monotherapy
   - MD global <5 and AJC 1–4: NSAIDs or anakinra
   - MD global <5 and AJC > 4: NSAIDs or systemic glucocorticoids or anakinra
   - MD global >5 and AJC irrespective: Systemic glucocorticoids or anakinra

   For patients with continued disease activity:
   - Following NSAID monotherapy for 1 month:
     – MD global <5 and AJC = 0: Anakinra
     – MD global <5 and AJC >0: Systemic glucocorticoids or anakinra
     – MD global >5 and AJC irrespective: Systemic glucocorticoids or anakinra or canakinumab (interleukin-1 β blocker) or tocilizumab (interleukin-6 blocker)
   - Following systemic glucocorticoids monotherapy for 2 weeks:
     – MD global <5 and AJC = 0/MD global >5 and AJC irrespective: anakinra or canakinumab or tocilizumab
     – MD global <5 and AJC > 0: Anakinra or canakinumab or methotrexate or leflunomide or tocilizumab
   - Following anakinra for 1 month:
     – MD global irrespective and AJC = 0–4: Canakinumab or methotrexate or leflunomide or tocilizumab
     – MD global irrespective and AJC > 4: Canakinumab or methotrexate or leflunomide or tocilizumab or TNFα inhibitor

2. *Systemic JIA without active systemic features but with active synovitis*:

   As an initial treatment, for patients with:
   - AJC = 0–4: NSAIDs monotherapy or intra-articular glucocorticoids injection
   - AJC > 4: NSAIDs or methotrexate or leflunomide

   For patients with continued disease activity:
   - Following NSAID monotherapy for 1 month:
     – AJC = 0–4: Methotrexate or leflunomide
     – AJC > 4: Anakinra or methotrexate or leflunomide
   - Following initial intra-articular glucocorticoids injection:
     – AJC = 0–4: Methotrexate or leflunomide
     – AJC > 4: Anakinra or methotrexate or leflunomide
   - Following methotrexate or leflunomide for 3 months:
     – AJC > 0: Abatacept or anakinra or tocilizumab or TNFα inhibitor
   - Following anakinra for 1 month:
     – AJC > 0: Abatacept or methotrexate or leflunomide or tocilizumab or TNFα inhibitor

3. *Systemic JIA with features concerning for MAS*: Macrophage activating syndrome treatment includes anakinra, a calcineurin inhibitor, or systemic glucocorticoids monotherapy for up to 2 weeks. They may be used in combination too.

Hospital Admission

Hospitalization is required for patients presenting with:
- Persisting fevers of unknown origin
- Severe exacerbation of disease
- Loss of ability to walk
- Pericarditis in children with systemic JIA

Exercise and Other Nonpharmacologic Therapy

Exercise has a significant role in maintaining the range of motion of the joints and its integrity by providing better shock absorption. Exercise also improves muscular strength. Muscle-strengthening program, stretching of deformities, range-of-motion activity, endurance development, and recreational exercises should be advised like hydrotherapy. Joint contractures developed may be helped by splinting or serial casting.

The leg-length discrepancy occurs due to the neovascularization of growth plates of an affected knee. This may be difficult to detect in knee flexion contracture. The problem becomes evident with contracture correction, and then the length discrepancy can be treated with a shoe lift on the contralateral side.

Surgical Treatment

The need for surgical procedures in cases of JIA has comparatively decreased due to increased advancement in medical therapy.

Synovectomy

Synovectomy is a sparsely needed procedure, because it yields poor outcomes in the long-term. It may be performed in cases where the involvement is confined to a single joint or few joint with active, proliferative synovitis. Even after arthroscopic debridement, recurrence is a rule, if the disease process is not controlled.

Osteotomy and Arthrodesis

In patients with severe joint destruction or deformity, osteotomy, and arthrodesis may be the terminal procedures.

Arthrodesis is better than arthroplasty for children with disease involving the wrist, fingers, and the ankle.

Total Hip and Total Knee Replacements

Replacements can provide a good outcome in children who have a debilitating disease and are functionally disabled. The limitation with this procedure is that it cannot be performed until epiphyseal closure, which indicates that bone growth has been completed.

Treatment of uveitis: Uveitis is the most common extra-articular manifestation of JIA. The patients of uveitis are mainly young girls with positive levels of ANA in their blood who are frequently asymptomatic so ophthalmic screening every 3 months is important.

Uncontrolled uveitis can lead to complications such as synechiae, cataracts, and glaucoma in 25–50% and vision loss in 10–20% of children. Thus, early detection and treatment can prevent these complications. The topical treatment includes topical corticosteroids and mydriatic agents.

For systemic treatment for uveitis, using subcutaneous methotrexate is recommended over oral methotrexate. In cases severe active chronic uveitis and sight-threatening complications, starting methotrexate and a monoclonal antibody TNFα inhibitor immediately is recommended over methotrexate monotherapy.

Diet and Activity

There is no special dietary recommendation for patients of JIA. As JIA is associated with decreased osteoblast activity, which may lead to osteopenia, calcium-rich food is advised. Calcium and vitamin D supplementation can be done in poor dietary intake. Diet may also be compromised due to TMJ involvement.

Bed rest is normally not advised in patients of JIA, in fact for better long-term prognosis patient should be encouraged to be as active as possible. As the patients may encounter an increased pain during routine physical activities they must be advised to limit their activities, especially strenuous activities, accordingly. An exercise program, with emphasis on joint protection, stretching exercises, pain modalities, and focusing on domiciliary exercises, is important to keep the patients active.

Long-term Monitoring

Patients of JIA are followed with complete hemogram, liver, and kidney function tests. The patients on long-term daily NSAIDs therapy should have urinalysis twice yearly.

On initiation of methotrexate therapy, these tests should be performed after the first month of treatment and similarly in case of any increase in dose, tests are repeated a month later. When the patient is on a stable dose with normal previous reports, the investigations can be done every 3–4 months.

Patients on TNFα inhibitors, require investigations every 3–6 months. Initial screening for latent tuberculosis should be done before starting a biologic agent but repeat testing is only required, if there is some increased risk of TB in the child.

■ PROGNOSIS

The course of JIA is usually unpredictable. Disease type and course may help to provide some estimate of prognosis. Persistent oligoarticular JIA has a better prognosis with majority achieving remission. But extended oligoarticular disease has a poorer prognosis. The risk of development of chronic uveitis is highest in children with arthritis onset at a younger age, female sex, and ANA positivity. Polyarticular JIA has a prolonged course requiring early treatment. Risk factors for poor prognosis are RF positivity, rheumatoid nodules, anti-CCP antibodies presence, young age, more joints involved and involvement of hip and wrist. Systemic JIA has the poorest outcome and predictors of poor prognosis are fever of more than 3-month duration, polyarticular arthritis and raised inflammatory markers for more than 6 months.

Ophthalmic complications include posterior synechiae, cataracts, glaucoma, and blindness. Orthopedic complications are leg length discrepancy and flexion contractures. Psychosocial and psychological complications may develop due to the chronic nature of the disease.

■ MEDICATION

An integrated approach of pharmacological and nonpharmacological therapy is required for treatment of JIA patients.

Nonsteroidal Anti-inflammatory Drugs

Nonsteroidal anti-inflammatory drugs act inhibiting the activity of cyclooxygenase (COX) enzyme, which blocks the prostaglandin synthesis leading to decreasing the symptoms of pain and swelling. NSAIDs include naproxen, ibuprofen, and diclofenac, which can be used for the treatment of all subtypes of JIA.

Aspirin is avoided due to its side effects like gastritis and hepatotoxicity. Celecoxib, a selective inhibitor of COX-2 is more useful in treating patients with bleeding diathesis.

A particular NSAID may not be useful in every JIA patient so the choice of NSAID varies from case to case depending upon patient response. In the active systemic JIA cases with fever and pericarditis, indomethacin is preferred over other drugs.

Naproxen: 15 mg/kg/day PO divided bid (maximum dose 500 mg bid)
Ibuprofen: 40 mg/kg/day PO divided tid (maximum dose 800 mg tid)
Diclofenac: 3 mg/kg/day PO divided tid (maximum dose 50 mg tid)
Celecoxib: <25 kg 50 mg bid, >25 kg 100 mg bid
Indomethacin: 1–2 mg/kg/day PO divided tid (maximum dose 50 mg tid)

Disease-modifying Antirheumatic Drugs

These drugs prevent the disease progression process, which leads to the destruction of joint and functional loss. NSAIDs are needed for relief of pain and swelling until the action of disease-modifying antirheumatic drugs (DMARDs) take place. Methotrexate remains the drug of choice in most cases except enthesitis-related JIA where sulfasalazine may be preferred. Methotrexate therapy requires folic acid supplementation and monitoring of complete blood counts and liver function. Sulfasalazine can cause gastrointestinal disturbances, pancytopenia and rashes. Leflunomide is rarely used due to serious hepatic, hematologic, respiratory and dermatologic adverse effects.

Methotrexate: 0.5–1 mg/kg PO or SC weekly (maximum dose 25 mg/week)
Sulfasalazine: Initial 12.5 mg/kg PO daily; increase by 10 mg/kg/day
Maintenance: 40–50 mg/kg divided bid (maximum dose 2 g/day)
Leflunomide: 10–20 mg PO daily

Corticosteroids

Corticosteroids are used to buy time until the action of DMARDs take place. Bridging therapy with a limited course of oral glucocorticoids (<3 months) during initiation or escalation of therapy in patients with high or moderate disease activity is recommended in cases with moderate to high-disease activity. But the long term use carries the risk of unacceptable side effects, thus only short courses or low doses should be used. Intra-articular steroid injections are useful as monotherapy in oligoarticular JIA and as an adjunct therapy in other categories. Triamcinolone hexacetonide is a long-lasting preparation that provides a prolonged response and is preferred over Triamcinolone acetonide.

Intra-articular triamcinolone: 1 mg/kg for large joints (knees and hips) and 0.5 mg/kg for smaller joints (ankles, wrists, and elbows)
Prednisolone: 1 mg/kg PO daily (maximum dose 60 mg) for first week, depending on response can be tapered, continued at same dose or increased to 2 mg/kg PO daily (maximum dose 100 mg)
Methyl Prednisolone: Pulse therapy 30 mg/kg IV for 3 days (maximum dose 1 g), depending on the response can be repeated

Immunomodulators (Biologics)

The proinflammatory cytokines, TNFα, and interleukin (IL)-1 play an important role in the pathogenesis of JIA. The drugs acting as inhibitors of these cytokines thus effect the disease progression. The biologic agents have a role in the prevention of joint erosion. The TNFα inhibitor are adalimumab, etanercept, infliximab, golimumab. Non-TNFα inhibitor are abatacept (CTLA-4Ig), tocilizumab (anti-IL-6 receptor), rituximab (anti-CD20), Canakinumab (anti-IL-1β monoclonal antibody), and anakinra (anti-IL-1 receptor).

The biological, according to consensus statements, should be used only after a poor response to DMARDs. But they should not be used as a monotherapy but in combination with DMARDs. Treatment with biologics should be done under expert supervision with complete baseline investigations to monitor toxicity.

Side effects like autoantibodies production, infections, antinuclear antibodies and drug-induced lupus can occur. Rarely demyelinating disorders and bone marrow suppression can occur. Contraindications for administration of TNFα inhibitor include infections, recent malignancies, congestive heart failure and demyelinating disorders. Chest radiography and Mantoux test should be essentially done before starting biologics to detect the presence of latent tuberculosis.

Etanercept: 0.8 mg/kg SC weekly or 0.4 mg/kg SC twice weekly (maximum dose 50 mg/week)
Infliximab: 3–10 mg/kg IV q4–8 wk
Adalimumab: <30 kg: 20 mg SC every other week, >30 kg: 40 mg SC every other week
Golimumab: 80 mg/m^2 IV infusion over 30 minutes at weeks 0 and 4, and every 8 weeks thereafter
Abatacept: <75 kg: 10 mg/kg/dose IV q4 wk, 75–100 kg: 750 mg/dose IV q4 wk, >100 kg: 1,000 mg/dose IV q4 wk
Rituximab: 750 mg/m^2 IV 2 wk × 2 (maximum dose 1,000 mg)
Anakinra: 1–2 mg/kg SC daily (maximum dose 100 mg/day)
Canakinumab: 15–40 kg: 2 mg/kg/dose SC q8 wk, >40 kg: 150 mg SC q8 wk
Tocilizumab: <30 kg: 12 mg/kg/dose q2 wk, >30 kg: 8 mg/kg/dose q2 wk (maximum dose 800 mg)

CONCLUSION

- JIA is the most common type of arthritis and the most common rheumatic disease, affecting children.
- JIA is essentially a clinical diagnosis without any diagnostic laboratory tests. A complete physical examination provides criteria for diagnosis.
- ACR criteria of JRA is used in clinical diagnosis.
- ESR and CRP are elevated in systemic onset JIA and serves to monitor disease activity.
- MRI is a more sensitive indicator of early pathological changes and disease activity.
- NSAIDs, intra-articular triamcinolone injection, methotrexate, anti-TNF-alpha agents, anti-interleukin-1 agents are various treatment modalities available and administered based on age, severity of disease, and prognosis.

- Physiotherapy and exercise have a significant role in preserving the joint range of movements and the muscle strength.
- Need for surgical intervention in JIA has largely reduced due to advancement in medical therapy. Surgical procedures like synovectomy, osteotomy, and arthrodesis, and hip and knee replacement may be performed in few cases.
- The risk of development of chronic uveitis is highest in children with arthritis onset at a younger age, female sex, and ANA positivity. They are predominantly asymptomatic, making routine screening essential as a part of the treatment regimen.
- Risk factors for poor prognosis are RF positivity, rheumatoid nodules, anti-CCP antibodies presence, young age, more joints involved and involvement of the hip and wrist. Thus, persistent oligoarticular JIA has a better prognosis.

FURTHER READING

1. American College of Rheumatology, Subcommittee on Rheumatoid Arthritis Guidelines. Guidelines for the management of rheumatoid arthritis: 2002 Update. Arthritis Rheum. 2002;46(2):328-46.
2. Angeles-Han ST, Ringold S, Beukelmann T, Lovell D, Cuello CA, Becker ML, et al. 2019 American College of Rheumatology/Arthritis Foundation guideline for the screening, monitoring, and treatment of juvenile idiopathic arthritis–associated uveitis. Arthritis Care Res. 2019;71:703-16.
3. Beukelman T, Patkar NM, Saag KG, Tolleson-Rinehart S, Cron RQ, DeWitt EM, et al. 2011 American College of Rheumatology recommendations for the treatment of juvenile idiopathic arthritis: initiation and safety monitoring of therapeutic agents for the treatment of arthritis and systemic features. Arthritis Care Res (Hoboken). 2011;63(4):465-82.
4. Cassidy J, Kivlin J, Lindsley C, Nocton J. Ophthalmologic examinations in children with juvenile rheumatoid arthritis. Pediatrics. 2006;117(5):1843-5.
5. Dabov G, Perez EA. Miscellaneous nontraumatic disorders: rheumatoid arthritis. In: Canale ST (Ed.). Campbell's Operative Orthopaedics, 10th edition. St Louis, Mo: Mosby; 2003.
6. DeWitt EM, Kimura Y, Beukelman T, Nigrovic PA, Onel K, Prahalad S, et al. Juvenile Idiopathic Arthritis Disease-specific Research Committee of Childhood Arthritis Rheumatology and Research Alliance. Consensus treatment plans for new-onset systemic juvenile idiopathic arthritis. Arthritis Care Res (Hoboken). 2012;64(7):1001-10.
7. Gerss J, Roth J, Holzinger D, Ruperto N, Wittkowski H, Frosch M, et al. Phagocyte-specific S100 proteins and high-sensitivity C reactive protein as biomarkers for a risk-adapted treatment to maintain remission in juvenile idiopathic arthritis: a comparative study. Ann Rheum Dis. 2012;71(12):1991-7.
8. Gylys-Morin VM. MR imaging of pediatric musculoskeletal inflammatory and infectious disorders. Magn Reson Imaging Clin N Am. 1998;6(3):537-59.
9. Hanson V, Kornreich HK, Bernstein B, King KK, Singsen BH. Three subtypes of juvenile rheumatoid arthritis: correlations of age at onset, sex, and serologic factors. Arthritis Rheum. 1977;20(Suppl 2):184-6.
10. Helmick CG, Felson DT, Lawrence RC, Gabriel S, Hirsch R, Kwoh CK, et al. Estimates of the prevalence of arthritis and other rheumatic conditions in the United States. Part I. Arthritis Rheum. 2008;58(1):15-25.
11. Ho ACH, Wong SN, Leung LCK, Chan WKY, Chong PCY, Tse NKC, et al. Biological disease-modifying antirheumatic drugs in juvenile idiopathic arthritis of polyarticular course, enthesitis-related arthritis, and psoriatic arthritis: a consensus statement. Hong Kong Med J. 2020;26:56-65.
12. Ilowite NT. Current treatment of juvenile rheumatoid arthritis. Pediatrics. 2002; 109(1):109-15.
13. Johnson K, Gardner-Medwin J. Childhood arthritis: classification and radiology. Clin Radiol. 2002;57(1):47-58.
14. Lamer S, Sebag GH. MRI and ultrasound in children with juvenile chronic arthritis. Eur J Radiol. 2000;33(2):85-93.
15. Lovell DJ. Juvenile idiopathic arthritis: Clinical features. In: Kippel JH, Stone JH, Crofford LJ, White PH (Eds). Primer on the Rheumatic Diseases. 13th edition. New York: Springer Science; 2008.
16. McHugh K, Gupta R, Murray K. Imaging in juvenile chronic arthritis. Imaging. 1999;11:91-7.
17. Mulhall KJ, Saleh KJ, Thompson CA, Severson EP, Palmer DH. Results of bilateral combined hip and knee arthroplasty in very young patients with juvenile rheumatoid arthritis. Arch Orthop Trauma Surg. 2008;128(3):249-54.
18. Ostring GT, Singh-Grewal D. Juvenile idiopathic arthritis in the new world of biologics. J Paediatr Child Health. 2013; 49(9):E405-12.
19. Petty RE, Southwood TR, Manners P, Baum J, Glass DN, Goldenberg J, et al: International League of Associations for Rheumatology (ILAR) classification of juvenile idiopathic arthritis: Second revision, Edmonton, 2001. J Rheumatol. 2004;31:390-2.
20. Prakken B, Albani S, Martini A. Arthritis 3: Juvenile idiopathic arthritis. Lancet. 2011; 377:2138-46.
21. Prince FHM, Otten MH, van Suijlekom-Smit WA. Diagnosis and management of juvenile idiopathic arthritis. BMJ. 2011;342:95-102.
22. Ravelli A, Grom A, Behrens E, Cron RQ. Macrophage activation syndrome as part of systemic juvenile idtiopathic arthritis: diagnosis, genetics, pathophysiology and treatment. Genes Immun. 2012;13:289-98.
23. Ringold S, Angeles-Han ST, Beukelman T, Lovell D, Cuello CA, Becker ML, et al. 2019 American College of Rheumatology/Arthritis Foundation Guideline for the Treatment of Juvenile Idiopathic Arthritis: Therapeutic approaches for non-systemic polyarthritis, sacroiliitis, and enthesitis. Arthritis Care Res (Hoboken). 2019;71(6):717-34.
24. Ringold S, Weiss PF, Beukelman T, DeWitt EM, Ilowite NT, Kimura Y, et al. 2013 update of the 2011 American College of Rheumatology recommendations for the treatment of juvenile idiopathic arthritis: recommendations for the medical therapy of children with systemic juvenile idiopathic arthritis and tuberculosis screening among children receiving biologic medications. Arthritis Rheum. 2013;65:2499-512.
25. Sandborg CI, Wallace CA. Position statement of the American College of Rheumatology regarding referral of children

and adolescents to pediatric rheumatologists. Executive Committee of the American College of Rheumatology Pediatric Section. Arthritis Care Res. 1999;12(1):48-51.
26. Scott DL, Wolfe F, Huizinga TW. Rheumatoid arthritis. Lancet. 2010;376:1094-106.
27. Sikora KA, Grom AA. Update on the pathogenesis and treatment of systemic idiopathic arthritis. Curr Opin Pediatr. 2011;23:640-6.
28. Sullivan DB, Cassidy JT, Petty RE. Pathogenic implications of age of onset in juvenile rheumatoid arthritis. Arthritis Rheum. 1975;18(3):251-5.
29. Wittkowski H, Frosch M, Wulffraat N, Goldbach-Mansky R, Kallinich T, Kuemmerle-Deschner J, et al. S100A12 is a novel molecular marker differentiating systemic-onset juvenile idiopathic arthritis from other causes of fever of unknown origin. Arthritis Rheum. 2008;58(12):3924-31.
30. Wu EY, Rabinovich CE. Juvenile idiopathic arthritis. In: Kliegman R, St Geme J (Eds). Nelson Textbook of Pediatrics, 21st edition. Philadelphia: Elsevier; 2020. pp. 1258-68.
31. Yun AG, Martin S, Zurakowski D, Scott R. Bipolar hemi-arthroplasty in juvenile rheumatoid arthritis: long-term survivorship and outcomes. J Arthroplasty. 2002;17(8): 978-86.

Mycobacterial Infections of Bone and Joints

Gyaneshwar Tonk, Sujit Kumar

INTRODUCTION

Mycobacterial infections of bone and joints are quite challenging problems in orthopedics. Even after lots of recent advances in orthopedics these are difficult to manage. Development of multidrug resistant (MDR) and extensively drug resistant (XDR) tuberculosis along with spread of human immunodeficiency virus (HIV) infections has caused extensive damage to disease control and eradication in developing countries. Treatment is further complicated by the toxicities due to antitubercular drugs, immunocompromised host status, lesser penetration of drugs into the bones and various complicated surgical procedures required to eradicate the bony infection.

Mycobacterium can affect almost every organ system of the human body though the lung is the most commonly affected. Tuberculosis of bones and joints are relatively rare extrapulmonary complications of mycobacterial infection. In various studies, the incidence of osteoarticular tuberculosis (TB) is only 1–3% of all cases and about 10% of extrapulmonary TB (EPTB) cases. Among half of this population is having spinal involvement and rest are having extraspinal osteoarticular involvement.

Mycobacterium tuberculosis is the most common cause of tubercular osteomyelitis and arthritis. Nontuberculous mycobacterial (NTM) infections of bone and joints are extremely rare, although their incidence has increased in recent years. Various predisposing factors for NTM infections are puncture wounds, previous injuries, orthopedics surgeries such as knee and hip arthroplasty, etc. Some literature has reported *M. bovis* skeletal infections after intravesical Bacillus-Calmette-Guérin (BCG) therapy. Tuberculous tenosynovitis and arthritis occur primarily through hematogenous spread and infrequently through contiguous spread or by direct inoculation. Mycobacterial spondylitis and arthritis are usually diagnosed later and can be extensively destructive.

INCIDENCE

As per the World Health Organization (WHO) 2018 data global estimate is that worldwide 10.0 million people developed TB disease in 2017. Among these 5.8 million men, 3.2 million women and 1.0 million were children. These were cases in all countries and age groups but overall 90% were adults (age >15 years), 9% were people living with HIV (72% in Africa) and two-thirds were in eight countries. As per this data, India was the country with highest burden of tuberculosis (27%) followed by China (9%), Indonesia (8%), Philippines (6%), Pakistan (5%), Nigeria (4%), Bangladesh (4%) and South Africa (3%). These and 22 other countries in WHO's list of 30 high TB burden countries accounted for 87% of the World's cases. Only 6% of global cases were in the WHO European Region (3%) and WHO's region of America (3%).

MICROBIOLOGY

Mycobacterium is an obligate aerobe. It is a facultative intracellular organism of the macrophages and grows very slowly. Tubercular bacilli do not have peptidoglycan teichoic acids in their cell wall, hence they do not stain violet-like gram-positive or gram-negative bacilli. As cell walls of *Mycobacterium* species are impermeable to certain dyes and stains, they are classified as acid-fast bacilli (AFB). Out of these, one of the very popular stains is Ziehl–Neelsen stain.

Approximately, 10,000 AFB/mL are needed to detect in sputum with a 100X microscope (100 times magnification). Suspicion of MTB is raised even when one AFB is seen per slide film.

Oxygen tension is very low in bone and joint lesions (as also seen in other extrapulmonary TB sites) which results in a scary number of bacilli in the affected area as these are essentially slow metabolizing and dormant.

The metabolism of *Mycobacterium* requires a neutral or near neutral pH. The nature of pus in bone and joint tuberculosis is alkaline therefore this is an unfavorable environment for multiplication of the bacilli. This is the reason why less numbers of *Mycobacterium* are detected in the bone and joint tubercular abscess cavities.

NATURAL HISTORY OF DISEASE

Musculoskeletal TB is always a secondary lesion. Primary focus is present somewhere else, most commonly in lungs or gastrointestinal system. Sometimes the primary site is detected in the lymph nodes also. *Mycobacterium* disseminates through the bloodstream to reach bone or synovial tissue. Dissemination can occur either from a recent primary focus or sometimes from old lesions where bacilli remained for years.

Before Onset of Chemotherapy

In children, disease developed in three stages within the duration of 3–5 years.

1. *The first stage (i.e., stage of onset)* lesion occurred in the synovial membrane nearer to its insertion on bone, i.e., the juxta-articular region of the bone. Bony lesions had a zone of destruction surrounded by a zone of diffuse calcification. Bony lesions last for a few weeks to months as compared to lesions of synovial membrane where lesions may be confined for months or even years.
2. *Second stage (i.e., stage of destruction)*: This is followed by stage of onset. In this stage disease progresses until there is involvement and destruction of the whole joint including articular cartilage. Radiologically this destruction appears as diminution of joint space. Extensive synovial tissue might fill the joint, pus in the joint distends capsule and ligaments which are progressively destroyed. This might lead to joint deformities and abscess which subsequently became permanent in association with muscle contracture. Pathologic dislocation, spread of abscess in the form of cold abscess, secondary pyogenic infection and sometimes may ultimately cause death of the patient.
3. *Stage III (i.e., stage of repair)* may occur spontaneously after 2–3 years of development, the patient's general condition improves and disease declines progressively. Abscess reabsorbs, healing of sinuses and radiologic calcification occurs. Final outcome is either bony fusion or fibrous ankylosis.

Stages of disease were less obvious in adults. Abscess formation was more common and earlier. Deformities were minor as compared to the children because there were no growth problems. Stage of repair was hardly ever reached and bony fusion never occurred spontaneously.

After Introduction of Chemotherapy

Chemotherapy helps to arrest the destructive process at the stage it has reached and heals the disease. It has no osteogenic, chondrogenic or fibrogenic power.

After adding antitubercular agents in treatment of mycobacterial infections the final outcome of disease may be resolved either with no morbidity or with minimal morbidity. The disease is healed with residual deformity and walled off lesions with calcification of caseous tissue. Sometimes the antitubercular agents are not effective and lead to a chronic low grade granulomatous lesion, cold or miliary spread of disease.

PATHOGENESIS

Human immune response to mycobacterial infection has been very effective. Because of good immune response only about 5% of infected persons develop clinically evident primary disease and further only 5% of infected ones develop clinically evident post primary disorder later on in life. Skeletal TB is a reflection of inherent poor protective response of one's immune system at the time of infection.

Mycobacterium tuberculosis has developed multiple molecular mechanisms which allow them to evade the immune system. By these they also avoid their destruction and eventually propagate to effect clinical disease if not intervened. On inhalation, *Mycobacterium* adheres to the complement Fc receptor and mannose receptor of the macrophages. Once inside, it disturbs the expression of many proteins which are responsible for pH regulation and urease production. Urease prevents acidification of the phagosome. They also produce catalase, thioredoxin and superoxide dismutase, to decrease the reactive oxygen species which are produced by phagocytic cells. Cellular immunity becomes essential in clearing mycobacterial infections once they are established in the intracellular space.

After the phagocytosis of bacteria, their cell wall is broken down and lipid is dispersed inside the cytoplasm of mononuclear cells. Thus transforming these mononuclear cells into epithelioid cells, which are characteristic features of tuberculosis infection. Multiple epithelioid cells fuse to form Langhans giant cells. The main function of these Langhans cells is to digest and remove necrosed tissue. About the end of the first week, lymphocytes appear and aggregate around the peripheral part of the lesion in the form of a ring. This mass formed by reactive cells constitutes a nodule known as the tubercle. During the 2nd week, the tubercles grow by expansion and coalesce to form a granuloma. Coagulation necrosis of protein content of the tubercle bacilli in the center of the tubercle is known as caseous necrosis. Presence of caseous necrosis is diagnostic of tuberculosis. The caseous material usually softens and liquefies these tubercles, and hence such tubercles are also known as soft tubercles. However, in certain cases under the influence of treatment tubercles may not show central caseation and they are called hard tubercles.

Marked exudation reaction is a common feature of tubercular infection. Following infection, marked hyperemia occurs and causes severe osteoporosis. Further weight-bearing, muscular compression, and traction forces lead to compression, collapse or deformation of the bones. Due to ischemia of the juxta-articular vessels and segmental intervertebral arteries, adjacent articular cartilage and intervening disks are degenerated and separate to become sequestrum. Although vertebral end plates work as a barrier but once invaded disk destruction progresses rapidly and disk is degenerated. Behavior of the tubercular lesion very much depends upon the virulence of the tubercular bacilli, resistance and immune status of the host and the stage of the tubercular lesion. This also depends upon the use of antitubercular drugs and at what stage of the disease these drugs are given.

Two types of tubercular lesions are detected in bones and joints. The first one may be caseous exudate type characterized by marked caseation and more bone destruction. While the second one is granular type, which is less destructive. It is insidious in onset and here abscess formation is rare.

CLINICAL FINDINGS

The spine is the most commonly affected site in bone and joint tuberculosis. Almost 50% of osteoarticular TB cases show vertebral involvement. This is followed by affection of large joints of the human body such as hip and knees. Other commonly involved joints in the sequence are sacroiliac joints, shoulder, elbow, ankle, carpal and tarsal joints.

Constitutional symptoms though not commonly present may include malaise, evening rise, low-grade fever, night sweats, anorexia, weight loss, and anemia. They are conspicuously absent in patients with good nutrition, elderly, and immunocompromised. Other complaints include stiffness of joints, pain in the affected regions and swelling. Swelling may be present at the local sites or at a distance as a part of cold abscess. Night cries may also be present where patients wake up during night due to pain.

Bony involvement is associated with increase in localized temperature, swelling and tenderness while the articular involvement is associated with soft tissue swelling/effusion, superficial or deep tenderness and restriction of movements and muscle atrophy.

In patients with spinal disease, there is stiffness, back pain, swelling, tenderness (deep or rotatory), neurologic deficit and deformity (kyphosis/scoliosis/both).

Swelling and tenderness over synovial bursa and tendon sheath are seen though less frequently. Regional lymphadenopathy is commonly present and sinuses are frequently observed.

Tubercular sinuses may have traditional appearance like a flat-ulcerated base with irregular and bluish edges. Small quantity of pus drains from it. But when the sinus becomes old and secondarily infected with bacteria, it looks like a pyogenic sinus. Now, the edges become thick and prominent without any special color. Here pus is thick and profuse.

Tubercular arthritis is usually monoarticular and manifests with chronic indolent localized involvement. Although not common, tuberculosis may involve multiple sites at a time, it is known as multifocal tuberculosis. Rarely, it may cause prosthetic joint infections as well.

Some patients with osteoarticular tuberculosis also have concomitant active pulmonary infection. Sometimes, they may also be associated with healed pulmonary lesions. Hence presence or absence of pulmonary symptoms or radiographic abnormalities should not exclude the diagnosis.

Foot and ankle tuberculosis is seen in only 5% of osteoarticular cases, lesions are typically cystic with well-defined borders. Subperiosteal scalloping is an important finding which is seen in one or both sides of the joints (kissing lesions). Diagnosis can be made by fine needle aspiration, which is a good alternative to open biopsy and surgical intervention is the best approach to arrest the local spread of the disease.

Although upper extremity tuberculosis is not common but it may involve shoulder and other joints. Shoulder disease is usually present in adults, and it is a dry type also known as caries sicca. The usual deformity is adduction because patient tends to keep the limb in adducted position due to pain. Arthrodesis is a preferred method to treat the pain and have functional position of the limb. Elbow is the other joint affected in sequence of incidence, here excisional arthroplasty is preferred over arthrodesis. Although tuberculosis of the wrist is rare, intercarpal joints may be affected and gross swelling is present due to caseation and synovial hypertrophy. Sometimes it is due to subluxation of carpal bones and involvement of flexor tendon sheaths. Diagnosis is usually early because wrist is rather a superficial joint.

Splinting is helpful in the early stage but in later stage arthrodesis is a preferred method.

Sometimes, there can be atypical presentations of osteoarticular tuberculosis such as Poncet's disease (polyarthritis with active visceral or disseminated tuberculosis) and BCG-associated rheumatic syndrome where there is granulomatous bony lesion after vaccination or bladder cancer therapy.

DIAGNOSIS

Diagnosis of the mycobacterial infection is of utmost importance as the treatment in this disease is totally different from the other pyogenic infection. The diagnosis of musculoskeletal tuberculosis may be definite or probable. Sometimes it is difficult to make a definitive diagnosis because isolation of bacteria from the lesion is not always possible. Culture of *M. tuberculosis*, if successful may provide susceptibility of the organism to the drug, which is very important in identifying antitubercular drugs for the management part. Drug resistance can also be identified by this. Other nonspecific laboratory tests are only of limited value in diagnosing tuberculosis. Abnormally high ESR and CRP are nonspecific for diagnosing mycobacterial infection. By other noninvasive tests such as purified protein derivative (PPD) test and IFN- gamma release assay (IGRA) may be helpful in suspecting the diseases but latent infection cannot be differentiated with active infection by these tests. PPD test and IGRA does not exclude the diagnosis of tuberculosis.

Radiological investigations are very helpful in diagnosing musculoskeletal tubercular infections, though they are neither confirmatory nor differentiate between infections due to typical or atypical mycobacteria.

Once suspension is made on the basis of history, laboratory tests, and radiology, further invasive diagnostic tests are used to confirm the diagnosis of musculoskeletal mycobacterial infections.

Synovial fluid aspiration is one of the best investigations of choice for diagnosing tuberculous synovitis and tubercular arthritis. Although it may not provide firm evidence of diagnosis, AFB staining and culture should be performed at the same time from the synovial fluid samples.

Best diagnostic method is percutaneous or open biopsy from the bone, synovium, cartilage and nearby abscess material. Microscopic visualization of severely infected tissue sometimes fails to deduct causative organisms, thus culture is the gold standard to confirm the diagnosis.

To establish the microbiologic diagnosis of nontuberculous mycobacterial (NTM) disease is very important due to heterogeneity of this group of organisms and the differences of susceptibility to antimicrobial drugs. NTM evolved multiple sites other than bone also hence sample collect may be the other sites such as blood, urine, sputum and limb notes as an adjunct the bone specimens.

Polymerase chain reaction may be used to identify pathogens without knowing the drug susceptibility in patients which are suspected cases of mycobacterial infection but are culture negative. Polymerase chain reaction (PCR) cannot differentiate between infection and contaminating organisms hence contamination of specimens should be excluded before final result of the test is declared.

Molecular probes that assess the presence of genes which confer resistance to specific antibiotics have the capacity to identify resistant isolates. The gene Xpert nucleic acid amplification assay for rifampicin (RIF) resistance in *M. tuberculosis* is one most commonly used assay of this type. WHO has endorsed GeneXpert test as a rapid diagnostic tool for diagnosing pulmonary and extrapulmonary tuberculosis.

Tuberculin Skin Test

The Mantoux test is a common skin test and used widely. The technique used presently was described by Charles Mantoux, a French physician in 1912. Tuberculin is commercially available in 1, 2 and 5 tuberculin unit (TU) PPD (RT23 equivalent) forms. Tuberculin test detects whether someone has developed immune response to the mycobacterium or not. In this test 0.1 mL tuberculin PPD is injected intradermally by a 26 G needle in the volar surface of the forearm of the individual and the response is read after 48–72 hours. Ballpoint or palpatory method is commonly used to read the results.

Although the interpretation is difficult and controversial, in healthy individuals with normal immune response the test is marked positive if the induration is more than or equal to 15 mm. Redness is not counted in the final interpretation of results. False positive results are seen in BCG-vaccinated individuals and NTM infected patients while false negative results are observed in immunocompromised persons and cases of recent mycobacterium infections.

Interferon Gamma Release Assays

Interferon gamma release assays (IGRAs) indicate cellular immune response to *M. tuberculosis*. They are surrogate markers of MTB infection. They should not be used as a sole method of diagnosing tuberculosis as they cannot distinguish between latent and active infections. The negative test rules out the probability of both active and latent infections. As IGRAs are not affected by BCG vaccination status, they can be useful for evaluation of latent tuberculous infection in BCG vaccinated individuals particularly in nations where BCG vaccination is a common practice during infancy. Commercially available IGRA tests are QuantiFERON TB Gold and T-Spot TB test.

QuantiFERON Test (QFT) is an interferon gamma release assay which is a registered trademark. This is an enzyme-linked immunosorbent assay (ELISA) based, whole blood test which uses peptides from three TB antigens (ESAT-6, CFP-10 and TB 7.7) in an in tube format. The result is considered positive for MTB infection if the IFN-gamma response to TB antigens above the test cut-off. It is a rapid test and the results are available within 24 hours. The disadvantage of the test is that the sample should be processed within 12 hours of the collection while white blood cells are still viable.

Enzyme-linked Immunosorbent Assay

These serological tests used for tuberculosis have low diagnostic values due to poor specificity and sensitivity. In late 1980s, this test was developed in France using highly purified A-60 antigen extract from Mycobacteria. As A-60 extract is common from *M. tuberculosis, M. leprae, M. bovis and M. avium*, hence it cannot be used specifically for diagnosing *M. tuberculosis infections.* By using ELISA, both IgG and IgM can be tested separately. IgG presents early in the disease while IgM appears late hence timing and response is important. These tests have the advantage of being quick, technologically easy and require minimum training hence can be useful tools for diagnosing tuberculosis in low- and middle-income countries.

Bacteriology

Presence of AFB in body fluids or tissues is the gold standard in confirmation of tuberculosis, and hence every effort should be made to prove the bacteriological diagnosis in clinically suspected TB patients. Clinicians must preferably collect at least two or even three samples for bacteriological examination. Most commonly used bacteriological method is Ziehl–Neelsen staining which can detect AFB, if the sample has greater than 10,000 bacilli per milliliter. Mycobacterial culture like in Löwenstein–Jensen medium and radiometric (Bactec 12B liquid medium) and nonradiometric (Bactec MGIT 960 system) can be used in paucibacillary samples. It also plays an important role in detecting drug resistance. Based on results of bacteriological methods, MDR- and XDR-TB are defined. Absolute concentration method and proportion method are the main drug susceptibility testing methods (DST).

Imaging

The first radiological investigation in a suspected TB patient is the X-ray of anteroposterior and lateral views of the part and posteroanterior view of the chest. It is wise to have an identical X-ray with a contralateral region (by the same exposure) to detect the earliest abnormal signs of the disease. Usually it takes about 2–5 months for the radiographic features to appear in TB patients.

The earliest sign seen is the localized osteoporosis. In cases of tubercular tenovaginitis and arthritis, the classical radiological triad is juxta-articular osteoporosis, peripheral osseous erosion, and gradual narrowing of the intra-articular space. Unlike rheumatoid arthritis, the joint space in early TB is well preserved. Rarely, there may be enlargement of epiphysis due to hyperemia adjacent to the growth plate. Gradually, the margins of the articular surface become less defined and there may be the appearance of areas of bony destruction. With period of time collapse of bone, subluxation/dislocation and deformity of joint appears.

In the center of the tuberculous cavity, there is presence of an irregular soft, feathery, coke such as sequestrum. Subperiosteal new bone formation is a late feature seen after formation of sinus or supervening secondary infection. Irregular calcified plaques in the wall of abscess are most definitive sign of long-standing tuberculosis.

Depending upon the primary location and degree of involvement radiological findings vary considerably in the hip, as noted by Shanmugasundaram **(Fig. 1)**. A lesion in the acetabular roof "wandering acetabulum" may result in subluxation. True pathologic dislocation may occur as well. Protrusio may be associated with lesions in the acetabular floor. Coxa magna may be confused with Perthes disease in pediatric patients. Significant joint space narrowing without an osseous focus ("atrophic") may be difficult to differentiate from rheumatoid arthritis. Destruction on both sides of the joint may result in irregularity of the femoral head and incongruity ("mortar and pestle").

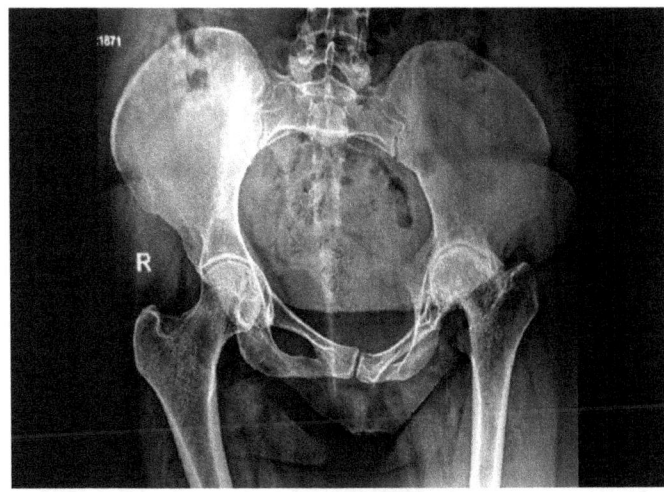

Fig. 1: X-ray of tubercular arthritis left hip.

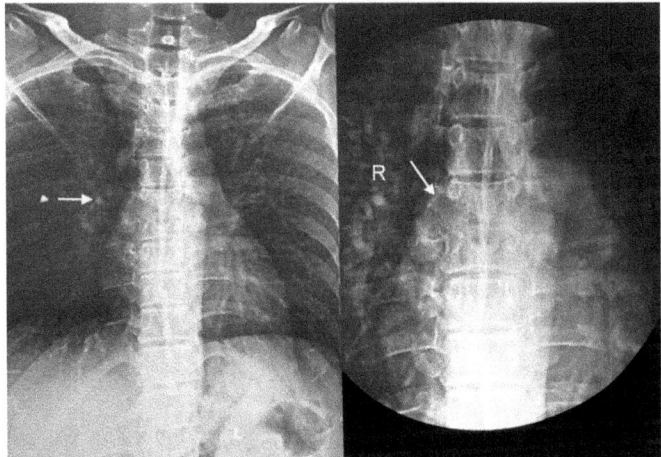

Fig. 2: X-rays of tubercular spine of dorsal region in anteroposterior view.

Tubercular spondylitis can be difficult to detect in the early stage due to relative preservation of the intervertebral disk space. Reduction in vertebral height is usually seen with irregularity of anterior-superior end plate being an early and subtle sign, due to subligamentous extension, there is irregularity of anterior vertebral margin. Paraspinal collection can develop which can be remarkably large **(Fig. 2)**.

MRI and CT

Magnetic resonance imaging (MRI) and computed tomography (CT) are helpful in further defining the disease. CT scan is helpful in detecting small bony erosions and cavities. Dystrophic calcification in soft tissue and encroachment of vertebral canal can be diagnosed by using CT scan. CT-guided needle biopsy is also an important method for obtaining tissue for histopathological and microbiological diagnosis. CT myelography is an imaging examination that is used for detecting mechanical block.

MRI is the investigation of choice to detect both the extent and severity of damage **(Fig. 3)**. It is useful in appreciating the nature of soft tissue mass. With the help of MRI fibrous

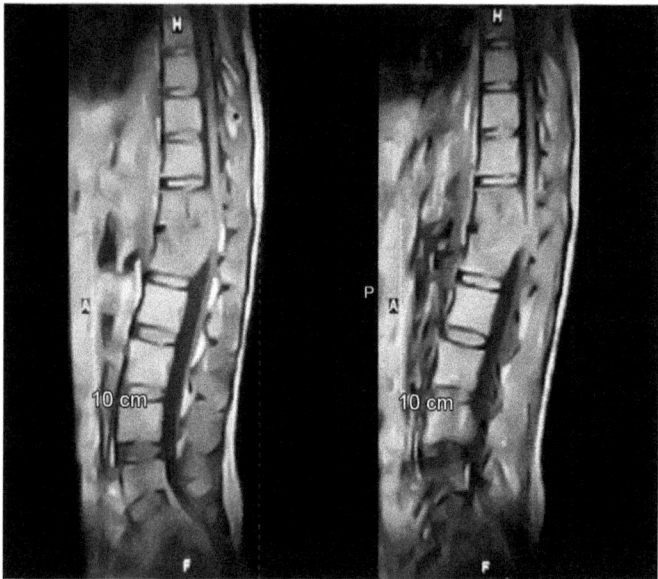

Fig. 3: MRI of tubercular spine of dorsolumbar region.

tissue, granulation, thick exudate or mixed lesion can be differentiated. Presence of rice bodies—another clue to mycobacterium infection may also be identified by using MRI scan. MRI of spine can detect involvement of vertebral canal, compression over dural sheath, localized abscess, generalized granuloma, shrinkage and edema of cord, myelomalacia and syrinx formation.

PET Scan

Positron emission tomography (PET) scan is a commonly used investigative modality for workup of malignant tumors. By this, we may know the metabolic activity of various tissues, increased uptake is detected in the areas of more metabolic activity. PET-CT images provide the metabolic map of the whole body. Thus, we can detect the lesions in the areas which are not reachable by the conventional imaging methods. This is not a specific test for tuberculosis because it is difficult to differentiate between infective, inflammatory and malignant lesions. But this can be very well used to know the activity of the lesion and guide about the active site of biopsy. We can also use this technique for treatment follow-up especially in MDR and XDR tuberculosis. By this, the disease extent can be well-defined and occult lesions can be detected. The limitation of this method is that it is nonspecific and expensive. Hence, it cannot be used in each and every case or for screening purpose.

Synovial Fluid Examination and Synovial Biopsy

Joint fluid examination from the affected joint is a standard routine investigation to differentiate the infective, inflammatory and traumatic lesions of the joints. Direct visualization of AFB or culture from the synovial fluid aspirate may provide a definitive diagnosis of tuberculosis.

In tuberculosis synovial fluid is nonhemorrhagic, it is turbid, and white blood cell (WBC) count is moderately increased. It is positive in 20–40% of cases.

The confirmation of diagnosis of tuberculous arthritis can be done by synovial biopsy, with positive results in 80% of cases. It shows typical granulomas, lymphocytic infiltration, and giant cells with caseation. These are characteristic of tubercular arthritis.

Polymerase Chain Reaction

Rapid and early diagnosis of skeletal tuberculosis, PCR has shown promising results. Nucleic acid sequence specific to *M. tuberculosis* can be identified in the clinical specimen by using an amplification system. This offers better efficacy and greater speed than AFB smear or culture. If sputum contains very small number of organisms, the traditional methods takes a long time to give results and sensitivity is also low, where diagnosis depends on tissue examination rather than microorganism detection in body fluids, DNA detection may be useful. PCR is also useful in certain circumstances where tissue has been sent for histopathological examination but culture could not be sent, and the specimen has already been mounted in formalin or other substances from where culture is not possible.

Because this methodology can detect *M. tuberculosis* in tissue samples even though the tissues have been preserved in formalin or other substances that preclude the possibility of culture.

Xpert MTB/RIF

Xpert MTB/RIF has been endorsed by WHO since 2010 as a rapid diagnostic tool for diagnosis of pulmonary and extrapulmonary TB. This is a nucleic acid amplification-based test (NAAT) and is performed from the sputum or abscess of the clinically suspected patient. This is a cartridge based test. The sputum or abscess sample is mixed with the reagent provided with the assay and a cartridge is placed in the GeneXpert machine. This assay quickly detects the possibility of drug resistance and help in making the diagnosis of MDR and XDR cases. Although this does not replace the need of AFB microscopy, culture and growth based drug susceptibility results. It is an addition for genotyping and early detection of cases.

■ TREATMENT OF SKELETAL TUBERCULOSIS

Various terminologies have been used by WHO and different authors in their descriptions. Some important terms and their definitions commonly used in tuberculosis are:

New case is a patient who has never had a treatment for TB, or has been anti-TB treatment for less than 4 weeks.

Drug resistant TB refers to cases of TB caused by an isolate of *M. tuberculosis* that is resistant to one of the first line anti-TB drugs: Isoniazid, Rifampin, Pyrazinamide, Ethambutol or Streptomycin.

Multidrug resistant TB refers to an isolate of *M. tuberculosis* that is resistant to at least isoniazid and rifampin, and possibly additional agents.

Extensively drug resistant TB is defined as TB which is resistant to any fluoroquinolone, and at least one of the three injectable second-line drugs (Capreomycin, Kanamycin and Amikacin), in addition to isoniazid and rifampin.

Total drug resistant TB refers to an isolate of *M. tuberculosis* resistant to all locally tested medications. However, the published studies initially describing TDR-TB did not include susceptibility testing for less frequently used agents with activity against TB, such as Cycloserine, Terizidone, Clofazimine, Linezolid or Carbapenems.

Primary drug resistance is said to occur in a patient who has never received anti-TB therapy.

Secondary drug resistance is defined as development of resistance during or following chemotherapy in patients who have previously had drug-susceptible TB.

Relapse is a patient who has been declared cured or treatment completed for any form of TB in the past, but who reports back to the health service and is found to be sputum positive or culture positive.

Treatment failure is a patient who, while on treatment remained sputum smear-positive or became sputum smear-positive at the end of the 5 months or more, after commencing the treatment difficult to define for OATB.

Treatment defaulter is a patient who had previously been recorded as defaulted from treatment or has discontinued treatment for a full 2 months in between and returns to the health service with smear positive sputum.

MANAGEMENT PRINCIPLES

General Approaches

The first priority, in treatment of any suspected case of TB, is to establish the diagnosis. In endemic regions, previously used concept of a therapeutic trial using the principle of treating based on clinical and radiographic features rather than confirming bacteriologically is not recommended by WHO nowadays, although it is still used in countries where disease load is high. This is due to lack of resources and manpower which limits every patient for microbial diagnosis. The probability of identifying the organism on a smear is 10–30% and cultures usually take up to 8 weeks, and are positive only in 30–60% of cases.

The initial management of osteoarticular tuberculosis consists of early and effective antitubercular therapy, assessing the clinical response and early identification of complications. This may merit additional intervention at any point of time and determination of duration of therapy.

Antitubercular drugs have been grouped into first-line and second-line agents. First-line agents include Isoniazid, Rifampicin, Pyrazinamide, Ethambutol, and second-line agents include Streptomycin, Capreomycin, Kanamycin, Ethionamide, Cycloserine, and Para-aminosalicylic acid and Thiacetazone. List of various antitubercular drugs along with dosing and adverse effects have been listed in **Table 1**.

Different regimens are in current practice which can be tailored by the physicians depending upon the clinicoradiological picture of the disease and drug sensitivity testing. Standard WHO or Tuli's regimen may be used to avoid any confusion **(Table 2)**.

According to WHO, treatment is divided into two phases: (1) Intensive phase, and (2) Continuation phase **(Table 2)**.

TABLE 1: Various antitubercular drugs with doses and common adverse reactions.

Drugs	Daily adult dose and administration	Minimum inhibitory concentration (μg/mL) for human mycobacteria	Main drug toxicity
Streptomycin (Sm) C	20 mg/kg maximum 1 (in children and elderly twice a week	1–2	Vestibular damage, deafness, fever, rashes, contact dermatitis, nephrotoxicity
Isoniazid (INH)*C	300–400 mg in single/two divided doses	0.1–0.2	Peripheral neuropathy, behavior disorder, convulsions, hepatitis, hypersensitivity osteomalacia life
Ethambutol (ETB) S	15–25 mg/kg in single/two divided doses	1–3	Retrobulbar neuritis with loss of vision, warned by diminution of visual field acuity, and color blindness
Rifampicin (RCN) C	450–600 mg/kg in single/two divided doses	0.25–1.0	Pinkish staining of urine, sweat and saliva, liver damage, bowel upset, rashes "flu-like" symptoms (purpura rarely)
Pyrazinamide C	40 mg/kg in single/two divided doses	10–20	Hepatotoxicity, gouty arthritis (hyperuricemic arthralgia)
Fluoroquinolones C	400–600 mg/kg	1–2	GI upset, rashes, transient liver disturbances

Contd...

Contd...

Drugs	Daily adult dose and administration	Minimum inhibitory concentration (μg/mL) for human mycobacteria	Main drug toxicity
Para-amino salicylic acid (PAS) S	12 g in single/two divided doses	1–4	GI disturbances, rashes, fever, lymphadenopathy, hepatotoxic, drowsiness
Thioacetazone** S	150 mg single dose	1	Anorexia, nausea, vomiting liver damage, marrow depression
Ethionamide/ Prothionamide S	1 g single dose	10–20	GI upset, abnormal liver tests, peripheral neuritis, convulsions
Cycloserine S	1 g single dose	5–10	Brain damage, mental disturbances, epilepsy
Capreomycin C (inj)	15 mg/kg single dose	2–3	Nephrotoxicity, others such as streptomycin, 8th nerve damage
Kanamycin C (inj)	15 mg/kg single dose (maximum 1 g/day)	8–16	Auditory toxicity, nephrotoxicity
Clofazimine C	100–200 mg/day	1–5	GI upset, headache, red discoloration
Amikacin (inj) C	15 mg/kg/day	4–8	Ototoxicity, nephrotoxicity
Minocyclines S	100–200 mg/day		GI disturbances, rashes, vestibular and hearing disturbances
Rifabutin	150–500 mg		Orange-brown staining of urine, saliva and cramps
Linezolid	600–1,000 mg/day		GI upset, vision disturbance
Ciprofloxacin	500–1,000 mg as two divided doses		GI upset, headache, insomnia
Clarithromycin	500 mg as 2 divided doses		GI upset, hepatotoxicity
Coamoxiclav	2 g twice a day		GI upset
Myser	250 mg twice a day		Hepatotoxicity, nephrotoxicity

*INH must form a part of any multidrug therapy.
**Thioacetazone is contraindicated in HIV-positive patients because of risk of severe skin reactions
(C: bactericidal; S: bacteriostatic; GI: gastrointestinal)
Source: Tuli SM. Tuberculosis of the skeletal system: bones, joints, spine and bursal sheaths, 5th edition. New Delhi: Jaypee Brothers Medical Publishers; 2016.

The medical therapy in intensive phase of drug-susceptible tuberculosis consists of a combination of drugs including rifampin (RIF), isoniazid (INH), pyrazinamide (PZA), and ethambutol (EMB) administered over a period of 2 months. Out of these, INH and RIF possess the most potent early antibacterial effect, and should be included in the regimen, whenever possible. Antitubercular agents achieve sufficient levels within nonsclerotic bone to perform bactericidal action against *M. tuberculosis*. After the intensive phase, patients with drug-sensitive disease should be continued for an additional 4–10 more months with INH and RIF depending on clinical and radiographic outcome. During the continuation phase of therapy, RIF remains especially important in eradicating the quiescent tubercular bacilli.

Chemotherapy is approximately 90% effective in eradicating the infection, provided that the appropriate drugs are administered in appropriate doses for appropriate duration. Since drugs have to be taken for a longer duration patient's compliance is always an issue and should be ensured. In the DOTS (directly observed treatment, short-course) program, compliance is tried to be ensured by local healthcare workers to document the ingestion of each dose of medication. The old policy of alternate day therapy has been changed to daily dosing in fixed dose combinations as per body weight. Although WHO recommends therapy of 6 months extendable to 9 months for extrapulmonary tuberculosis, the conventional duration of therapy is usually

TABLE 2: DOTS Regimen (WHO 2010).

Treatment group	Type of patient	Regimen	
		Intensive phase (IP)	Continuation phase (CP)
New (Category I)	• New sputum smear positive • New sputum smear negative • New extrapulmonary • New others	2H3R3Z3E3	4H3R3
Previously treated (Category II)	• Smear positive relapse • Smear positive failure • Smear positive treatment after default • Others	2H3R3Z3E3S3 1H3R3Z3E3	5H3R3E3

12 months, except for those with spinal disease, where it may be extended up to 18 months. The final duration of antimicrobial therapy depends upon the clinicoradiological healing of the disease.

Inadequate treatment without following standard protocol, improper documentation, and poor compliance results in the drug resistance of the organisms. Empirical treatment without confirming the diagnosis or starting ATT without biological diagnosis also contributes to the emergence of resistance. In different studies, multidrug resistance has been observed 1–3% while resistance to single drug has been reported approximately 13%. Treatment of recurrence and relapse is expensive and eradication of disease is difficult. According to WHO, the treatment of relapse involves 5 agents in the first phase, and 3 agents during the second phase.

In tuberculous arthritis, the goal is to achieve healing of the disease in such a way to obtain or maintain a normal or near normal range of motion. Chemotherapy is started in all the patients having active disease. During the early stages of disease, rest is advised, and weight bearing should not be allowed. Active and passive range of motion exercises (active and active-assisted) are started when symptoms allow. Casting and splinting helps to prevent deformity. Traction may be used to restore or improve motion before splinting or bracing.

Weightbearing within a splint is allowed when adequate alignment and movements are achieved, and the disease has been effectively controlled by multidrug therapy.

For patients coming in the later stages of disease, the joint is held in a functional position, as ankylosis is expected. In cases of tuberculous arthritis where medical therapy fails, debridement is required to improve the functional outcome. Patients with significant loss of motion and decreased joint space due to articular cartilage destruction may also be benefited by surgical debridement. For the joints where ankylosis may not be well-tolerated like in hip and elbow joints, excisional arthroplasty and arthrodesis might be considered. Optimally, total joint arthroplasty after tuberculosis arthritis should be delayed until patients show no evidence of recurrent disease after completion of therapy. Recent days though controversial arthroplasty is considered by many authors under cover of ATT once the clinical response is achieved even within 6–12 weeks. Corrective reposition osteotomy should be considered to those joints which are ankylosed in a suboptimal position. Prophylactic chemotherapy for several weeks to months may allow earlier implantation, and chemotherapy can often salvage a prosthetic joint when reactivation of infection has been observed.

The surgical management of prosthetic joint infection related to *M. tuberculosis* is debatable. Large effusions to be drained, and the devitalized tissue should be debrided. Implants and hardware may be retained in some periprosthetic infections after thorough debridement as *M. tuberculosis* does not form biofilms to the extent that *Staphylococcus* and other typical bacterial species do. Complicated infections characterized by hardware loosening, exposed hardware and formation of a significant involucrum are indications of hardware removal. For this single stage treatment, i.e., debridement removal and reinsertion of implant in one go or two stage treatment debridement and removal of implant followed by reinsertion of a new one may be used. It is not proven whether two stage hardware management strategy offers any advantage compared with a one stage exchange in such cases.

In tuberculous spondylitis, major focus is healing of the disease with prevention of kyphotic and scoliotic deformities. Treatment begins with chemotherapy and the measures to improve the general condition of the patient. For initial few months, bed rest is advised along with medical management. Healing of the disease is monitored by ESR and X-rays at 3-month intervals and MRI at 6 months interval. If disease is in control and patient is improving clinicoradiologically, patient is mobilized in spinal braces for next 18–24 months. Results are encouraging with outpatient treatment with chemotherapy and bracing along with surgical debridement. Results improve with the use of braces and orthoses. Many patients of uncomplicated tuberculosis can be treated without operative treatment, requirement of surgical debridement remains on the clinical condition of the patient and experience of the surgeon. In ambulatory patients, resection of infected bone and placement of bone graft confers no major advantage over medical therapy alone although in some cases, it can prevent deformity later on. The duration of chemotherapy remains controversial and has been tailored by different authors. Traditionally, 18 months of chemotherapy has been recommended. Recently, WHO and Parthasarathy et al. have suggested that the duration of therapy may be reduced to 9 months.

The role of surgery varies throughout different regions of the world, and both the indications for surgery and the specific procedures recommended remain somewhat controversial. To an extent, recommendations of surgery are based on the resources available locally, and the presence of surgeons with specialized training. Tuli's middle path regimen is a good guide in decision making of the surgical choice. Although the procedures are technically demanding, and intensive medical management is required during the perioperative period.

The philosophy of surgical treatment varies from routine decompression and arthrodesis (Hong Kong and others), to the "middle path" developed by Tuli in India, to chemotherapy alone when the resources for spinal surgery are unavailable. In the Tuli's "middle path" regimen surgical methods are recommended only for the treatment of the complications of disease. These may be increased in size of a paravertebral abscess despite adequate chemotherapy, lack of clinical response after 3–6 months of chemotherapy in neurologically normal individuals, lack of neurologic recovery or progression of neurologic deficits after 3–4 weeks of chemotherapy, involvement of the posterior elements and mechanical instability, recurrence of disease, or in cases of doubtful diagnosis.

Overall, requirement of surgery is in approximately 5% of uncomplicated cases, and 60% of those with neurologic deficits.

According to Jain et al., the indications for surgery may include certain clinical factors, few radiological factors and some patient related factors. Clinically, painful spasm and nerve root compression, recurrent paraplegia, and massive retropharyngeal abscess causing difficulty in respiration or swallowing, treatment factors such as persistent or progressive deficit even after an adequate course of conservative treatment. Imaging factors including paravertebral involvement scoliosis or severe kyphosis on plain X-rays, global destruction on CT scan and extradural compression on MRI (circumferential cord compression due to granulation tissue) will require surgery. While 80% of patients might have some localized kyphosis, only 3–5% progress to kyphosis greater than 60°. Progression may occur during the active phase or in healed disease. Risk factors for progression of kyphosis may include age, involvement of dorsal spine, greater initial loss of vertebral height, multiple levels of involvement. Prophylactic stabilization may be required in radiologically "at risk" factors, which include dislocation of the facets, retropulsion of diseased fragments, lateral translation of a vertebra, and toppling of a vertebra which may be later on responsible for increase in kyphotic deformity. In pediatric patients usually the deformity increases with increase in age but sometimes if anterior growth plate escapes infection kyphosis might not increase. Paraplegia in healed disease with kyphotic deformity is always a challenge and full of possibilities of complications. Upadhyay et al. reported that progression of kyphosis does not occur in children while Rajasekaran observed an increase in kyphosis of more than 20° in 22%.

As the disease is usually anterior, the procedure most commonly used is anterior decompression and arthrodesis, as popularized in Hong Kong. While decompressing from the anterior side structural graft is required to support the anterior column of the spine to resist the progression of kyphosis. This approach may be technically difficult in the presence of severe kyphosis. A lateral extrapleural approach may enhance visualization at the apex.

Graft complications are more common when multiple vertebrae are involved. And the frequent graft complications include subsidence, fracture of the graft, resorption, and loss of position. Progression of deformity may also be observed despite a successful anterior arthrodesis, although the frequency and magnitude vary within the literature.

Along with anterior decompression and fusion other approaches may be a posterior spinal fusion, an anterior and posterior spinal fusion, a posterior spinal fusion followed by an anterior spinal fusion (in same sitting or staged), costotransversectomy, and a lateral extrapleural approach. Both anterior and posterior arthrodesis is recommended to treat the instability associated with circumferential disease and for those with greater than 3 levels of involvement. This approach may be the only method which can be reliable in preventing the progression of kyphosis. Costotransversectomy facilitates evacuation of an abscess, but the exposure is not sufficient for decompression and bone grafting. In this procedure, the medial portion of the rib and the underlying transverse process are removed, and an extrapleural dissection leads to drainage of the abscess. The lateral extrapleural approach provides better exposure. This includes removal of the 8–10 cm medial portion of the rib, part of the transverse process and the pedicle to allow greater access to the vertebral body and spinal cord. Classically, 2 to 3 levels are exposed to facilitate debridement and bone grafting. The intercostal nerve is used as a guide to the foramen and spinal cord at each level.

A non-instrumented posterior spinal fusion may be performed through the same approach. Laminectomy may be indicated in the rare case in which isolated involvement of the posterior elements is observed. Bone graft may be selected from the rib, iliac crest, and fibula. The limited information is available for the use of allografts in anterior fusion of the spine. Fusion with the help of instrumentation may be used in the presence of mycobacterial infection, although posterior instrumentation has been used most frequently as compared to anterior instrumentation and fusion.

Cervical spinal involvement is relatively less common, and patients typically present with stiffness, pain and torticollis. Symptoms due to large abscesses may be hoarseness, stridor, and dysphagia. Swelling due to cervical lymphadenopathy and cold abscess, sinuses, and neurologic involvement are commonly observed. Atlantoaxial involvement may result in instability at this joint. Noncontiguous involvement may be seen, and involvement of more than two vertebrae is not uncommon in the mid-cervical spine. If the lateral radiograph shows widening of the retropharyngeal space the presence of an abscess should be suspected. MRI may demonstrate collection of pus and granulation tissue causing compression of thecal sac and the structures anterior to the cervical vertebrae **(Fig. 4)**.

Approaches for decompression include the transoral or an anterior approach along the anterior border of the sternomastoid muscle. Arthrodesis may be accomplished either anteriorly or posteriorly.

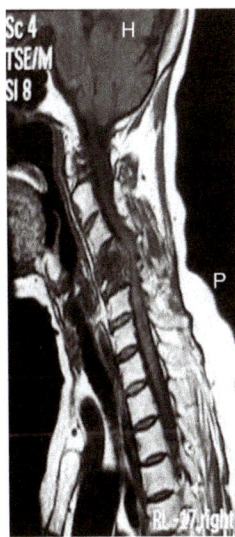

Fig. 4: MRI of tubercular spondylitis of cervical spine.

The lumbar spine is also involved though less frequently than the dorsal, or dorsolumbar spine. Patients often present with back pain and radiculopathy, and the neurologic involvement is uncommon though bladder and bowel dysfunction may be observed.

Kyphotic deformities are initially less prominent due to the natural lordotic curve of this region, later on if the disease involves more vertebrae and the patient remains ambulatory then it may become more prominent. Chemotherapy is effective, and the indications for surgery remain unclear. Compensatory lordosis in the upper lumbar and thoracic spine may also be observed.

Nontuberculous Mycobacteria

Nontuberculous mycobacterium (NTM) is usually seen in immunocompromised individuals. For the treatment of skeletal NTM infections, at least 6 months antitubercular treatment as guided by culture and sensitivity reports should be taken. However like in typical *Mycobacterium tuberculosis* patients the exact duration of treatment cannot be clearly demarcated and the duration of treatment depends upon the various factors such as virulence of the infecting species, disease burden, efficacy of the available drugs and the degree of immunosuppression to the host. Completeness of surgical debridement (when undertaken), and the clinical response also affect the decision making regarding the duration of therapy. Treatment durations of 12 months or longer may be required for severe infections. In the case of more resistant pathogens, such as *Mycobacterium abscessus*, use of combination intravenous antibiotics over a prolonged period may be required. Drug toxicity may also force the clinician to change the decisions about the therapy and the duration. NTM are intrinsically more resistant to antimycobacterial therapy compared with *M. tuberculosis*.

Thorough surgical debridement is often necessary for clinical cure. Sometimes even with thorough debridement

TABLE 3: Various drugs used in different species of NTM mycobacterial infections.

Species	Drug regimen
Mycobacterium avium complex	Rifampicin plus (azithromycin or clarithromycin) plus EMB
Mycobacterium kansasii	Rifampicin plus isoniazid plus EMB
Mycobacterium marinum	Rifampicin plus EMB plus (azithromycin or clarithromycin)
Mycobacterium abscessus	Clarithromycin or azithromycin plus amikacin plus (cefoxitin or imipenem)
Mycobacterium fortuitum	Amikacin plus trimethoprim/sulfamethoxazole plus quinolone
Mycobacterium chelonae	(Clarithromycin or azithromycin) plus tobramycin plus imipenem

and appropriate medical therapy, infection may recur and necessitate repeated debridement for control. NTM infection in presence of implants and prosthesis is difficult to treat and the hardware removal is recommended for control of infection whenever possible. Many chemotherapeutic agents active against NTM are thermostable and can be incorporated into cement. These include aminoglycosides, macrolides, carbapenem, some cephalosporins, and quinolones. Higher doses of these antimicrobial agents are required to be mixed with cement as higher minimal inhibitory concentration (MIC) may be necessary to achieve target drug concentration in the local tissues to hit the bacteria. However, the higher antibiotic doses may affect the stability of the cement leading to breakage of cement, and the risk of systemic toxicity, particularly with aminoglycosides. Different drugs may be used for different NTB species **(Table 3)** though these should be selected as per culture reports.

Because of the potential toxicity and the drug interactions, a careful understanding of comorbidities and other medications is necessary. For patients receiving immunomodulatory therapy, a strong suggestion is to stop the immunosuppressant drugs such as TNF-alpha, etc., if possible or substitute them with less immunosuppressive alternatives.

In Case of Drug Toxicity

A number of adverse drug reactions are described in the literature following use of antitubercular drugs as we are using multidrug therapy, it is sometimes difficult to single out the drug responsible for reaction. The commonly practiced techniques are the challenge and rechallenge methods where we withdraw a drug from the treatment and introduce another. If the reaction goes away it is considered because of the same drug, otherwise because of another one, the same process is repeated with another drug and so on till the responsible drug is pointed out. Rechallenge is started with a smaller dose with stepwise increase till the therapeutic dose is achieved. The step-up should be even more gradual, if the initial reaction is severe. Rechallenge should not be attempted in uncooperative patients or in cases where close watch is not possible. Individual tablets are better for challenge and rechallenge techniques rather than combination of drugs. Treatment may be continued by replacing the offending drug with a suitable alternative, or with a reduced number of drugs if none is suitable. Sometimes a new regimen should be considered if none drug of the regimen is found suitable. Hepatotoxicity is a common complication by many antitubercular drugs especially such as Isoniazid, rifampicin and pyrazinamide. Repeated liver function tests are advisable to detect these complications early. Baseline liver function tests are advisable before starting ATT. If no other cause of hepatitis is detected drug-induced hepatitis should be considered and the drug should be stopped. Symptoms aggravated if the exposure of the drugs is prolonged. Once the drug is stopped the symptoms start regressing and the elevated markers drop down. If hepatitis resolves the same regimen may also be continued but with caution. In case hepatitis is severe it is safer to avoid pyrazinamide and sometimes also rifampicin, in such cases an alternate regimen with initial phase of 2 months daily isoniazid, ethambutol and streptomycin followed by a 10-month continuation phase of isoniazid plus ethambutol may be used. A severely ill tuberculosis patient with drug-induced hepatitis may die without antitubercular treatment. In this case the patient may be treated with the two least hepatotoxic drugs, namely streptomycin and ethambutol instead of interrupting TB treatment. Isoniazid may be cautiously reintroduced after the hepatitis has resolved.

Treatment of Multidrug Resistant Tuberculosis

A mean delay of 6–8 months before the diagnosis of spinal tuberculosis is made is commonly observed, particularly in endemic countries. Drug resistant spinal tuberculosis is suspected when the patient is not responding to ATT for a minimum period of 5–6 months which leads to a further delay in diagnosing drug resistant cases of spinal tuberculosis.

Ideally all patients of spinal tuberculosis should be treated after obtaining drug sensitivity reports at the first instance. However, in a high disease load country it is not always possible and patients are often treated on clinicoimaging findings and patients are investigated for drug resistance only when failure of treatment is suspected, known as presumptive drug resistance. It is not uncommon to find a patient having failure of treatment where no bacteriological growth is detected, i.e., culture negative. In such patients if adequate clinical suspicion is present and histological examination is suggestive of tubercular pathology, they can be labeled as clinically drug resistant cases and may be treated as multidrug resistant tuberculosis.

A complete drug-o-gram, containing all particulars of the drugs their dose and duration, should be prepared for all the drug resistant tuberculosis patients. This helps to know which drugs have never been used for the treatment in the past for the particular patient. In each patient, all efforts should be made to obtain bacteriological culture and to have a subsequent drug sensitivity report, which would serve as a guide for subsequent ATT. The tissue sample may be obtained through percutaneous aspiration or through surgical debridement. Surgical debridement has an additional advantage of reducing the bacterial load of the lesion. Monitoring MDR-TB regimen with monthly culture rather than sputum microscopy alone is said to provide the best option for detecting a failing regimen in time for corrective action.

As per WHO (2011) guidelines for multidrug resistant pulmonary tuberculosis, a minimum four second-line antitubercular drugs based on individual drug sensitivity for 8 months of intensive phase and with a total duration of 20 months are recommended. The common practice of adding a one new drug to a failing regimen should be avoided. Second-line antitubercular drugs are highly toxic, hence an experienced physician should always be part of the treating team in MDR cases, this is particularly needed for early detection and treatment of drug toxicities. The second-line drugs are best given in once a day dosing.

The major challenges in treatment of drug resistant cases are the length of therapy, the high cost of the second-line drugs and the extensive side effects caused by these drugs. Based on the results on Bangladesh regimen and The STEAM trial, the WHO announced new guidelines in mid-2018 **(Table 4)**.

Generally MDR/RR-TB patients are on longer regimens. All three Group A agents and at least one group B agent should be included to ensure that treatment starts with at least four antitubercular agents. If only one or two Group A agents are used both Group B agents should be included. If the regimen cannot be composed with agents from Groups A and B alone, Group C agents should be added to complete it.

TABLE 4: Drugs for MDR-TB recommended by WHO (2018).

Group A	Group B	Group C
Levofloxacin (Lfx) or Moxifloxacin (Mfx)	Clofazimine (Cfz)	Ethambutol (E)
Bedaquiline (Bdq)	Cycloserine (Cs) Or Terizidone (Trd)	Delamanid (Dlm)
Linezolid (Lzd)		Pyrazinamide (Z)
		Imipenem-Cilastatin (Ipm-C n) or Meropenem (Mpm)
		Amikacin (Am) (or Streptomycin)
		Ethionamide (Eto) or Prothionamide (Pto)
		p-aminosalicylic acid (PAS)

Patients with resistance to additional antitubercular drugs should be advised individualized ATT as per their drug sensitivity results. WHO currently recommends individual tailor made regimens for each patient of drug-resistant tuberculosis as per their individual DST results.

A common mistake commonly practiced across the globe is to preserve the best drugs according to sensitivity for future use. The best way of achieving the cure is to hit the lesion hard by exposing it to the most sensitive drug at the first instance.

CONCLUSION

- Tuberculosis of bones and joints are relatively rare extrapulmonary complications of mycobacterial infection. And the most common cause of tubercular osteomyelitis and arthritis is *Mycobacterium tuberculosis*.
- Among cases of osteoarticular tuberculosis, spine is the most commonly affected site with predominant vertebral involvement followed by large joints such as hip and knee.
- The gold standard to confirm the diagnosis of tuberculous arthritis is synovial biopsy, with positive results in 80% of cases.
- Mantoux test, ELISA, rapidly advancing IGRA test, culture and sensitivity are widely used in diagnosing TB and deciding the drug susceptibility of the bacterium.
- *Radiological investigations*: X-ray, CT scan, PET scan, and MRI scan have been widely used to locate and learn the extent of the disease spread.
- Xpert MTB/RIF has been endorsed by WHO since 2010 as a rapid diagnostic tool for diagnosis of pulmonary and extra- pulmonary TB.
- The first step in the management of osteoarticular tuberculosis consists of early detection and effective antitubercular therapy. Assessment of complications might be ensued by the periodical follow-up. Analysis of the treatment response is must to decide the duration of the therapy.
- Chemotherapy is almost effective in 90% of cases for eradicating the infection, provided that the appropriate agents are prescribed in appropriate doses for appropriate duration and the patient's compliance is ensured.
- The duration of antimicrobial therapy depends upon the clinicoradiological healing of the disease, usually lasting from 12 to 18 months for spinal disease.
- In tuberculous arthritis, the aim is to achieve or maintain a normal or near normal range of motion. That is possible with adequate rest, chemotherapy, weight bearing with splinting or traction or casting to prevent deformity. For late presenters, aim is to allow fibrous ankylosis in functional position with concurrent pain management.
- In tuberculous spondylitis, major focus in management is to prevent or treat kyphotic deformities achieved with bed rest, braces, chemotherapy and serial ESR and routine radiological assessment.
- In case of toxicity, cautious rechallenge is the only and best way to identify the offending drug or drugs and prevent further toxicity.
- Individualized ATT as per their DST results is the right policy to be adopted in patients with resistance to additional antitubercular drugs. The best way of achieving the cure in MDR/XDR cases is to hit the lesion hard by exposing it to the most sensitive drug at the first instance.

FURTHER READING

1. Ankrah AO, van der Werf TS, de Vries EF, Dierckx RA, Sathekge MM, Glaudemans AW. PET/CT imaging of *Mycobacterium tuberculosis* infection. Clin Transl Imaging. 2016;4:131-44.
2. Babhulkar SS, Pande S. Tuberculosis of the hip. Clin Orthop Rel Res. 2002;398:93-9.
3. Bastian I, Colebunders R. Treatment and prevention of multidrug resistant tuberculosis. Drugs. 1999;58:633-61.
4. Bennett JE, Dolin R, Blaser MJ. Mandell, Douglas, and Bennett's Principles and Practice of Infectious Diseases, 8th edition. Philadelphia: Elsevier/Saunders; 2015.
5. Boachie-Adjei O, Squillante RG. Tuberculosis of the spine. Orthop Clin North Am. 1996;27:95-103.
6. Catanzaro A, Daley C. A summary of the Third Global Interferon-γ Release Assay Symposium. Infect Control Hosp Epidemiol. 2013;34:619-24.
7. CDC. Availability of an assay for detecting *Mycobacterium Tuberculosis*, including rifampin resistant strains, and considerations for Its Use—United States, 2013. MMWR. 2013;62(41).
8. Chakravorty S, Tyagi JS. Novel multipurpose methodology for detection of mycobacteria in pulmonary and extrapulmonary specimens by smear microscopy, culture, and PCR. J Clin Microbiol. 2005;43:2697-702.
9. Chan PC, Chang LY, Wu YC, Lu CY, Kuo HS, Lee CY, et al. Age-specific cutoffs for the tuberculin skin test to detect latent tuberculosis in BCG-vaccinated children. Int J Tuberc Lung Dis. 2008;12:1401-6.
10. Citak M, Argenson JN, Masri B, Kendoff D, Springer B, Alt V, et al. Spacers. J Arthroplasty. 2014;29(2 Suppl):93-9.
11. Colmenero JD, Jimenez-Mejias ME, Reguera JM, PalominoNicas J, Ruiz-Mesa JD, Marquez-Rivas J, et al. Tuberculous vertebral osteomyelitis in the new millennium: still a diagnostic and therapeutic challenge. Eur J Clin Microbiol Infect Dis. 2004;23:477-83.
12. Colmenero JD, Jimenez-Mejias ME, Sanchez-Lora FJ, Palomino Nicas J, Martos F, GarciadelasHeras J, et al. Pyogenic, tuberculous, and brucellar vertebral osteomyelitis: a descriptive and comparative study of 219 cases. Ann Rheum Dis. 1997;56: 709-15.
13. Colmenero JD, Morata P, Ruiz-Mesa JD, Bautista D, Bermudez P, Bravo MJ, et al. Multiplex real-time polymerase chain reaction: a practical approach for rapid diagnosis of tuberculous and brucellar vertebral osteomyelitis. Spine. 2010;35: E1392-6.
14. Cottle L, Riordan T. Infectious spondylodiscitis. J Infect. 2008;56:401-12.

15. Crespo M, Pigrau C, Flores X, Almirante B, Falco F, Vidal A, et al. Tuberculous trochanteric bursitis: report of 5 cases and literature review. Scand J Infect Dis. 2004;36:552-8.
16. Daniel TM. Antibody and antigen detection for the immunodiagnosis of tuberculosis: why not? What more is needed? Where do we stand today? J Infect Dis 1988;158:678-80.
17. Detjen AK, Keil T, Roll S, Hauer B, Mauch H, Magdorf K. Interferon-gamma release assays improve the diagnosis of tuberculosis and nontuberculous mycobacterial disease in children in a country with a low incidence of tuberculosis. Clin Infect Dis. 2007;45:322-8.
18. Dionisios V, Kazakos C, Tilkeridis C, Dermon A, Petrou H, Galanis V. Polymerase chain reaction for the detection of *Mycobacterium tuberculosis* in synovial fluid, tissue samples, bone marrow aspirate and peripheral blood. Acta Orthop Belg. 2003;69(5):366-9.
19. Eskola A, Santavirta S, Konttinen YT, Tallroth K, Lindholm ST. Arthroplasty for old tuberculosis of the knee. J Bone Joint Surg. 1988;70b:767-9.
20. Fang D, Leong JCY, Fang HSY. Tuberculosis of the upper cervical spine. J Bone Joint Surg. 1983;65b:47-50.
21. Ge Z, Wang Z, Wei M. Measurement of the concentration of three antituberculosis drugs in the focus of spinal tuberculosis. Eur Spine J. 2008;17(11):1482-7.
22. Glickman MS, Jacobs WR Jr. Microbial pathogenesis of *Mycobacterium tuberculosis*: dawn of a discipline. Cell. 2001; 104(4):477-85.
23. Good RC, Snide DE. Isolation of nontuberculous mycobacteria in the United States. J Infect Dis. 1982;146:829-33.
24. Guven O, Kumano K, Yalcin S, Karahan M, Tsuji S. A single stage posterior approach and rigid fixation for preventing kyphosis in the treatment of spinal tuberculosis. Spine. 1994;19:1039-43.
25. Hodgson AR, Skinsnes OK, Leong CY. The pathogenesis of Pott's paraplegia. J Bone Joint Surg. 1967;49a:1147-56.
26. Hogan JI, Hurtado RM, Nelson SB. Mycobacterial musculoskeletal infections. Thorac Surg Clin. 2019;29:85-94.
27. Hsu LCS, Cheng CC, Leong JCY. Pott's paraplegia of late onset: the causes of compression and results after anterior decompression. J Bone Joint Surg. 1988;70B: 534-8.
28. Hsu LCS, Leong JCY. Tuberculosis of the lower cervical spine (C2 to C7). A report on 40 cases. J Bone Joint Surg. 1984;66b:1-5.
29. Iademarco MF, Castro KG. Epidemiology of tuberculosis. Semin Respir Infect. 2003;18:225-40.
30. Jain AK, Kumar S, Tuli SM. Tuberculosis of spine (C1–D4). Spinal Cord. 1999;37:362-9.
31. Jarzembowski JA, Young MB. Nontuberculous mycobacterial infections. Arch Pathol. 2008;132:1330-4.
32. Jenkins DHR, Hodgson AR, Yau AMC, Dwyer AP, O'Mahoney G. Stabilization of the spine in the surgical treatment of severe spinal tuberculosis in children. Clin Orthop Rel Res. 1975;110:69-80.
33. Johansen IS, Nielsen SL, Hove M. Characteristics and clinical outcome of bone and joint tuberculosis from 1994 to 2011: a retrospective register based study in Denmark. Clin Infect Dis. 2015;61(4): 554-62.
34. Malaviya AN, Kotwal PP. Arthritis associated with tuberculosis. Best Pract Res Clin Rheumatol. 2003;17:319-43.
35. Narang S. Tuberculosis of the entheses. Int Orthop. 2012;36:2373-8.
36. Nikaido T, Ishibashi K, Otani K, Yabuki S, Konno S, Mori S, et al. *Mycobacterium bovis* BCG vertebral osteomyelitis after intravesical BCG therapy, diagnosed by PCR-based genomic deletion analysis. J Clin Microbiol. 2007;45:4085-7.
37. Perkins MD, Roscigno G, Zumla A. Progress towards improved tuberculosis diagnostics for developing countries. Lancet. 2006;367:942-3.
38. Rajasekaran S, Shanmugasundaram TK. Prediction of the angle of gibbus deformity in tuberculosis of the spine. J Bone Joint Surg. 1987;69a:503-9.
39. Rajasekaran S, Soundarapandian S. Progression of kyphosis in tuberculosis of the spine treated by anterior arthrodesis. J Bone Joint Surg. 1989;71a:1314-23.
40. Rajasekaran S. The natural history of post-tubercular kyphosis in children: radiological signs which predict late increase in deformity. J Bone Joint Surg. 2001;3b:954-62.
41. Rajasekaran S. The problem of deformity in spinal tuberculosis. Clin Orthop Rel Res. 2002;398:85-92.
42. WHO treatment guidelines for drug resistant tuberculosis (2010 update). Geneva: WHO; 2010.
43. WHO treatment guidelines for drug resistant tuberculosis (2018 update). Geneva: WHO; 2018.
44. WHO treatment guidelines for drug-resistant tuberculosis (2016 update). Geneva: WHO; 2016.

SECTION 6

Orthopedic Rheumatological Variants

- **Hand Radiograph: A Marker of Systemic Arthritis and Various Systemic Diseases**
  Kushal Singh

- **Various Arthritic Joint Disorders**
  Madhan Jeyaraman, Rakesh Kumar, Anil Gowtham Manivannan

- **Tendinopathies**
  Madhan Jeyaraman, Naveen Jeyaraman, Ravi VR

- **Periarthritis Shoulder**
  Krishna Subramanyam

- **Myofascial Pain Syndrome**
  SS Jha, Lalit Kishore

- **Fibromyalgia**
  SS Jha, Lalit Kishore

21. Hand Radiograph: A Marker of Systemic Arthritis and Various Systemic Diseases

Kushal Singh

INTRODUCTION

Hand being one of the most complex yet fine instruments to carry out simple day-to-day task to complex one. Apart from being a mechanical tool to express yourself, they can be really helpful in making diagnosis of various forms of arthritis. Being a radiologist we can say that a simple looking hand radiograph can give insight about multiple systemic diseases. We will be discussing the various forms of arthritis and few common diseases where a hand radiograph can be really helpful.

TECHNICAL ASPECTS

Evaluation of articular disease (actually all kind of bony pathologies) should begin with conventional radiography. My mentor always used to tell me "never ever report musculoskeletal magnetic resonance imaging (MRI) without reviewing radiographs." Symptomatic joints should be evaluated in at least two projections. Posteroanterior and anteroposterior oblique (also known as Nørgaard view) should be used if only two radiographs are being taken. Posteroanterior view provides information about mineralization and soft tissue component while Nørgaard view shows us early erosive changes. Nørgaard view is best to look for the radial aspect of base of proximal phalanges, triquetrum and pisiform which are earliest to get involved in any form of inflammatory arthropathy. Computed tomography (CT) has limited role in evaluation of joints of hand and wrist. The details given by a technically sound hand radiograph is far superior to CT. Other imaging modalities such as MRI, bone scan of hand should be done in specific clinical situations.

APPROACH TO HAND RADIOGRAPH

In any screening series of arthritis hand radiographs are probably the most informative one. Like elsewhere, a systematic approach should be used and we must observe the changes occurring in a specific joint and the pattern of these changes within the hand and wrist joints. Like other joints, a hand radiograph should be evaluated for mineralization, calcification/bone formation, joint space narrowing, erosion and subluxation/dislocation. Often ignored, soft tissue must be evaluated carefully.

- *Mineralization*: It is evaluated by observing the shaft of metacarpal of 2nd and 3rd digit. Normally, sum of cortical thickness should be equal or more than 50% of shaft thickness.

  Imaging pearls: Except rheumatoid arthritis, normal mineralization is typically seen in all arthropathies. Diffuse osteoporosis is associated only with rheumatoid arthritis (advanced disease).

  Diffuse osteoporosis, if seen in other arthropathies should be attributed to medication or aging, not to primary disease itself.

  Presence of juxta-articular osteoporosis is nonspecific finding and helps us only to establish that something is wrong.

- *Calcification*: Abnormal calcification can be seen in soft tissue, cartilage or of tendons and bursae.

  Imaging pearls: Urate crystals, seen in gout are not radiopaque. However when get deposited in soft tissue, they are associated with calcium deposition to variable degree, making it denser to soft tissue. Urate deposition in cartilage is never associated with calcium precipitation, so cartilage calcification is never seen in gout per se, unless associated with some other crystal deposition disease.

  Other than idiopathic calcium pyrophosphate dihydrate (CPPD), only two conditions are associated with true cartilage deposition of CPPD crystals, they are hyperparathyroidism and hemochromatosis. Hydroxyapatite crystals deposit in synovial joint and tendons, causing bursitis and tendinitis. In hand, it is associated with erosive arthropathy. Shoulder joint and greater trochanter are being the most common location for hydroxyapatite arthropathy.

  Various systemic diseases such as scleroderma, dermatomyositis and renal osetodystrophy are also associated with soft tissue hydroxyapatite deposition.

- *Joint space*: Except osteoarthritis, rest all other arthropathies show uniform narrowing of joint space.

List includes inflammatory arthropathies that erode the cartilage and all other arthropathies such as crystalline arthropathy, Wilson's disease and acromegaly, associated with deposition of extra substance within cartilage. Nonuniform joint space narrowing is seen in osteoarthritis and erosive osteoarthritis.

Imaging pearls: Gout can cause significant erosive changes around the joint while maintaining the joint space. Though pigmented villonodular synovitis (PVNS) rarely involves the hand, joint space is usually maintained.

- *Erosion*: They can be classified based on severity and location. As expected, aggressive erosions have no evidence of sclerotic border or reparative bone. Nonaggressive erosions or healing phase of aggressive lesions show a sclerotic margin with or without reparative bone. Locations of erosion within a joint can help us to narrow down differentials.

  Imaging pearls: "Bare area" of bone is first to get involved in inflammatory arthritis making disruption of white cortical line as first radiological sign. These early erosions are best seen at metacarpal head and radial aspect of base of proximal phalanges. In due course, diseases do not respect the cartilage barrier and involve more of joint space. In inflammatory arthropathies marginal erosions are seen, while in erosive arthritis they are seen centrally, giving classically described "mouse ear" and "gull wing" deformity respectively. Nonaggressive erosions are most commonly seen in gout arthropathy, which is caused by adjacent tophus.

- *Bone production*: New bone formation can be seen as reparative response or secondary to periostitis or enthesitis.

  Imaging pearls: New bone can be seen along shaft or at metaphysis adjacent to erosion. This pattern is classically described with psoriatic and Reiter's arthritis. In addition, bone formation can be seen at tendinous/ligamentous insertion. Both of the above-mentioned findings are not seen in rheumatoid arthritis. Bony ankylosis is seen in only those arthropathies which are associated with aggressive cartilage destruction, such as inflammatory arthropathies. In rheumatoid arthritis, "key point to remember" bony ankylosis is seen only in carpal joints. Bony ankylosis is also seen in erosive osteoarthritis because of inflammatory component associated with it. Obviously, it would not be seen in crystalline arthropathies. Subchondral bone formation and bony osteophytes which are seen as reparative response, typically seen in osteoarthritis (considered as hallmark) and crystalline arthropathies.

- *Distribution*: Distributions of radiographic changes within the joint are helpful in narrowing the differentials.

  Imaging pearls: Rheumatoid arthritis spares distal interphalangeal joint, which is classically involved in osteoarthritis. Random pattern of involvement is seen gouty arthritis. In wrist, erosive osteoarthritis involves only first carpometacarpal joint. If osteoarthritis of wrist present in some other location, possibility of post-traumatic osteoarthritis to be considered first. Radiocarpal compartment is involved in calcium pyrophosphate deposition (CPPD) arthropathy which extends to involve lunate-capitate joint. In wrist, gout has predilection for carpometacarpal joint.

Now we will be discussing hand radiograph in various forms of arthritis.

- *Rheumatoid arthritis*: It is a chronic autoimmune systemic arthropathy predominantly involving synovial joints and characterized by periarticular erosions. Symptoms typically first develop in hand and wrists in symmetric pattern and proximal distribution. Joints typically involved are distal radioulnar joint, radiocarpal, mid carpal and metacarpophalangeal joint. It is characterized by soft tissue swelling followed by joint space narrowing and periarticular demineralization. Periarticular erosions are seen in bare area of joints. Later, due to flexion and extension contractures, joint subluxation occurs, typically ulnar. Gross deformity and bony fusion seen in end stage disease **(Figs. 1 and 2)**.

- *Psoriatic arthritis*: It is a common seronegative spondyloarthropathy which is characterized by inflammatory arthritis, enthesitis, and periostitis. It has predilection for distal joints of hand **(Fig. 3)**. Erosion occurs at margin of joints giving a classic pattern which is classically described as "Pencil in Cup" appearance. New bone formation, which is usually bilateral and asymmetrical and associated with soft tissue swelling, giving the "sausage digit" appearance.

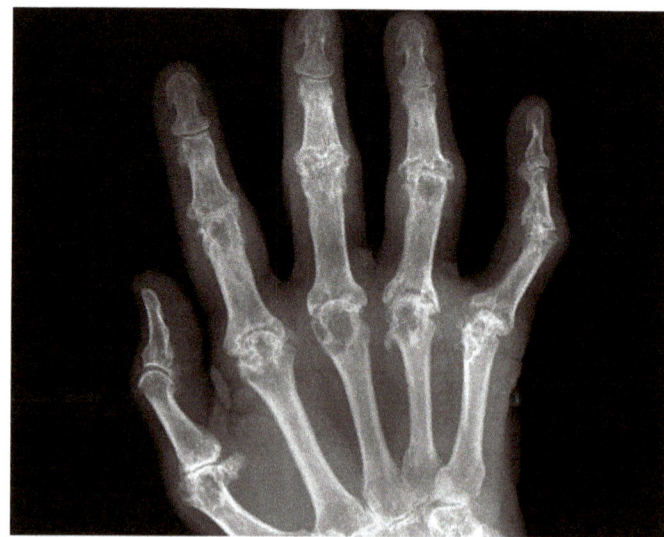

Fig. 1: Rheumatoid arthritis. This case shows arthropathy, predominantly involving the proximal joints along with ulnar subluxation at 5th metacarpophalangeal joint. Marginal erosions and periarticular osteopenia is also noted.

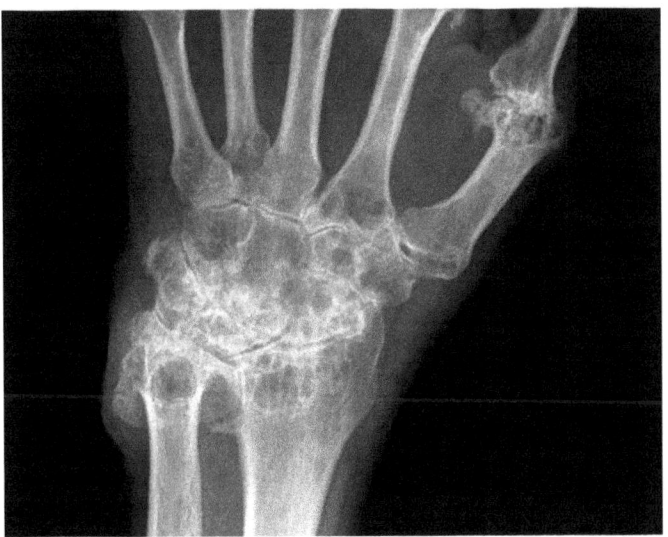

Fig. 2: Rheumatoid arthritis. This case shows bony fusion of carpal bones along with symmetric joint space narrowing. In addition, changes at radioulnar joint are also noted.

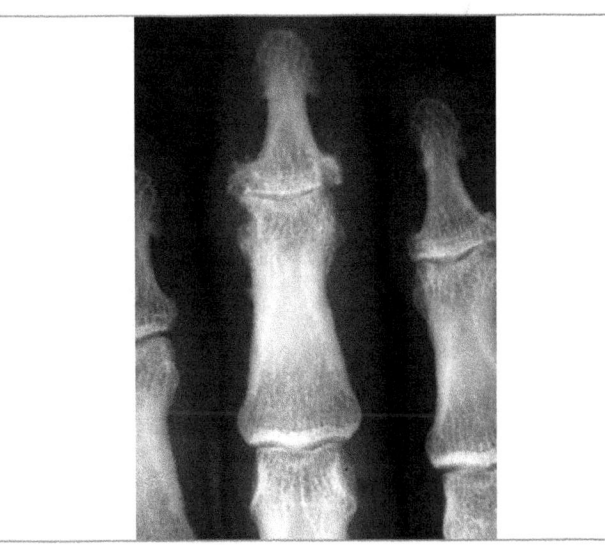

Fig. 3: Psoriatic arthritis. This case shows erosion and new bone formation involving distal interphalangeal joint of middle finger. Mild soft tissue swelling is also seen.

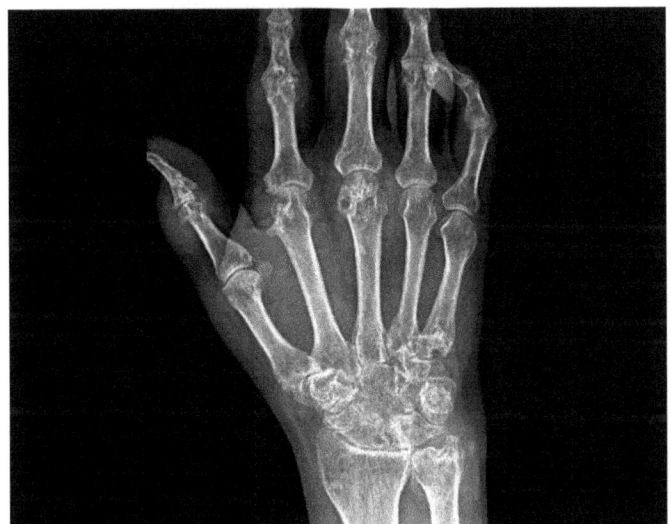

Fig. 4: Gout arthropathy. This case shows eccentric bone erosions with overhanging edges, involving the 2nd metacarpophalangeal joint. Mild soft tissue swelling is also seen.

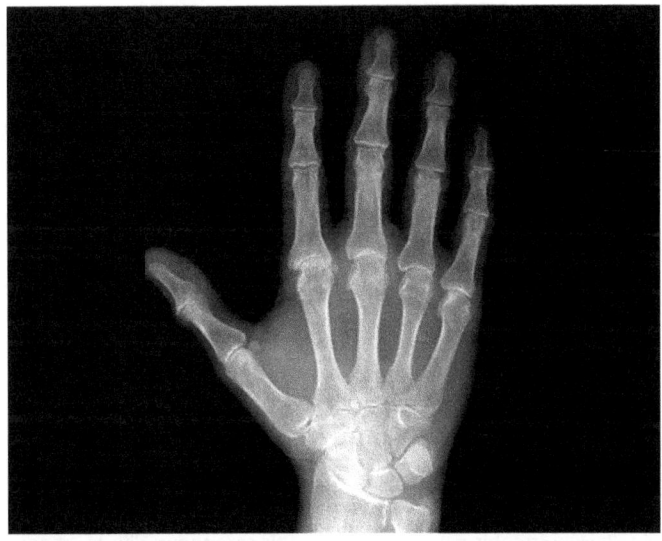

Fig. 5: Hemochromatic arthropathy. This case shows reduced joint space, overhanging "hooked osteophytes" with degenerative changes involving the metacarpophalangeal joint.
Courtesy: Dr Jan Frank Gerstenmaier, Radiopaedia.org, rID: 25057.

- *Gouty arthritis*: It is characterized is monosodium urate crystal deposition in and around the joint. Erosion margins are typically thin and sclerotic with a typically overhanging edge, giving the rat bite appearance **(Fig. 4)**. Erosions can be intra-articular, periarticular or can be seen distinct from the joint.
- *Hemochromatic arthritis*: This arthropathy is believed to have both degenerative and inflammatory component. It is caused by pathological deposition of iron in synovium. It has predilection for metacarpophalangeal joint (typically second) and characterized by symmetric uniform joint space narrowing. Hook like osteophyte, usually along the radial aspect of metacarpal head along with chondrocalcinosis are seen **(Fig. 5)**. Apart from its definite role in various arthropathies, hand radiograph is really helpful in diagnosing various systemic disorders. We will be discussing few of them which are seen in routine clinical practice.
  - *Hyperparathyroidism*: It occurs due to overproduction of parathyroid hormone. It is characterized by increased bone turnover and result in elevated serum alkaline phosphatase and calcium level. Accordingly bone osteopenia and demineralization is seen in hand radiographs. Classically it is along the radial aspect of middle phalanx of index and middle finger **(Fig. 6)**. In addition, cortical irregularity, acro-osteolysis and rarely browns (lytic lesion) tumor can be seen.

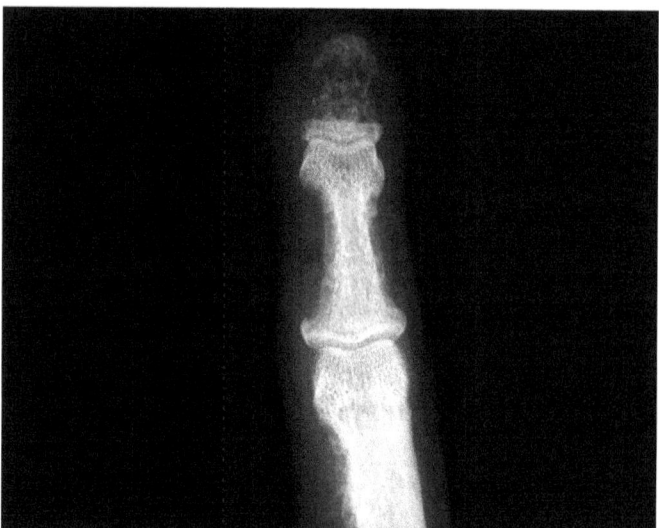

Fig. 6: Hyperparathyroidism. This case shows subperiosteal bone resorption, predominantly along the radial aspect of middle finger. Acro-osteolysis also noted.

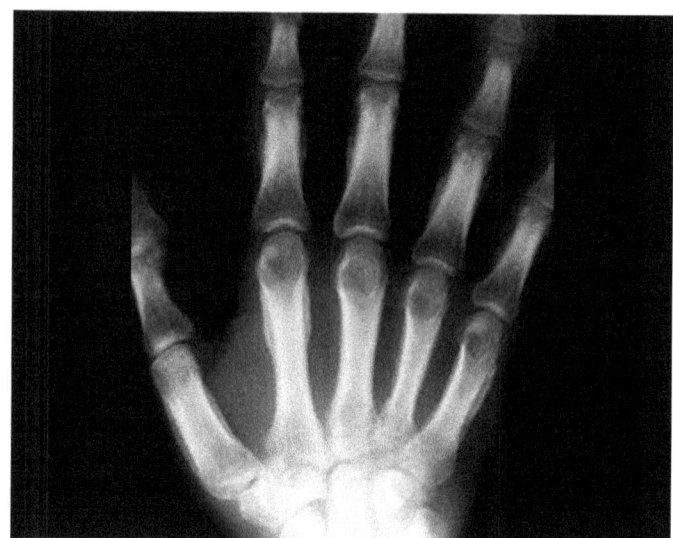

Fig. 7: Thyroid acropachy. This case showing thick benign smooth periosteal reaction involving diaphysis of metacarpals and phalanges.

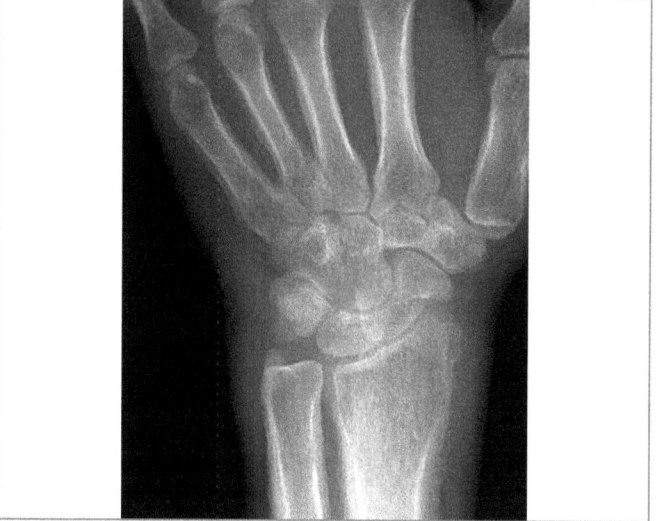

Fig. 8: Hypertrophic osteoarthropathy. This case shows diffuse smooth periosteal reaction involving the metacarpals and distal radius and ulna. Epiphysis is typically spared.

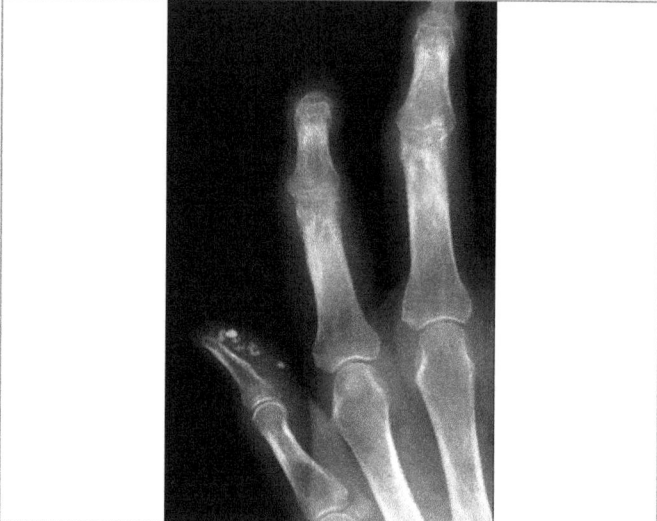

Fig. 9: Scleroderma. This case shows cutaneous calcification with acro-osteolysis. Periarticular osteopenia and early erosions are seen at interphalangeal joints.

- *Thyroid acropachy*: It is characterized by thickening of extremities and seen as one of manifestations of autoimmune thyroiditis. It is almost always seen in patients with ophthalmopathy and more common in patients with history of radioiodine treatment and smokers. Condition is usually bilateral, symmetric, and painless and involves the diaphysis of bones of hand. Solid periosteal reaction (classically described as feathery) along with clubbing and soft tissue swelling are seen **(Fig. 7)**.
- *Hypertrophic osteoarthropathy*: It is considered as paraneoplastic syndrome. It can be seen in plethora of conditions, most common being the pulmonary etiology. It is characterized by long bone metaphyseal and diaphyseal smooth periosteal reaction **(Fig. 8)**. The idiopathic form, pachydermo-periostosis is characterized by triad of skin thickening, clubbing and smooth periostosis. Epiphyseal involvement distinguishes idiopathic from the secondary form where epiphysis is usually spared.
- *Scleroderma*: It is multisystem connective tissue disorder. Triad of articular erosions, acro-osteolysis and subcutaneous calcinosis is highly suggestive of this condition. Periarticular osteopenia is also seen **(Fig. 9)**. Acro-osteolysis is thought to be secondary to pressure caused by dense sclerotic tissue.
- *Dermatomyositis*: It is an autoimmune inflammatory arthropathy with significant female predilection. It is characterized by swelling of distal joints of hand and arthritis. Cutaneous calcification and rarely acro-osteolysis can be seen. Cutaneous calcifications are more diffuse in nature compared to scleroderma.

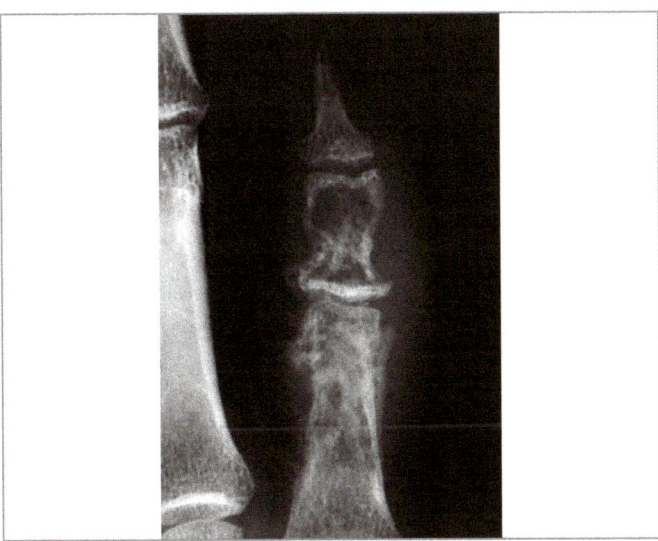

Fig. 10: Sarcoidosis. This case shows ill-defined cystic lytic lesions involving the middle phalanx. Smooth periosteal reaction along with soft tissue swelling also noted.
Source: Sellon E. Systemic disease involvement of the hand-manifestations on plain radiograph. Br J Hosp Med (Lond). 2013;74(5):275-81.

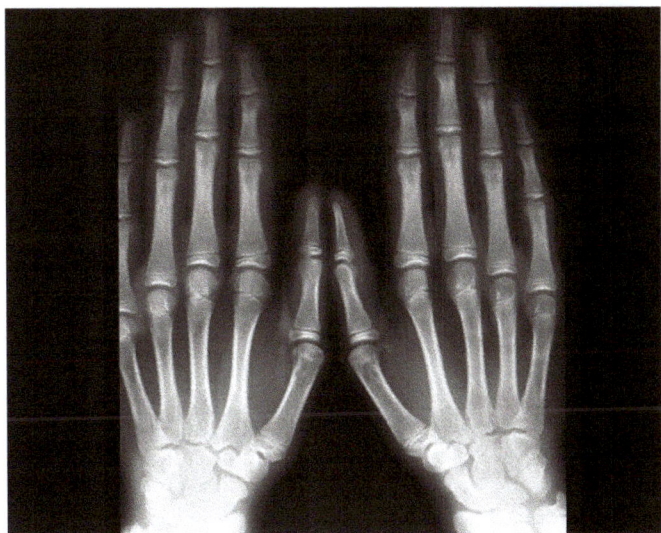

Fig. 11: Marfan syndrome. This case is showing bilateral symmetric elongation of metacarpals and phalanges.

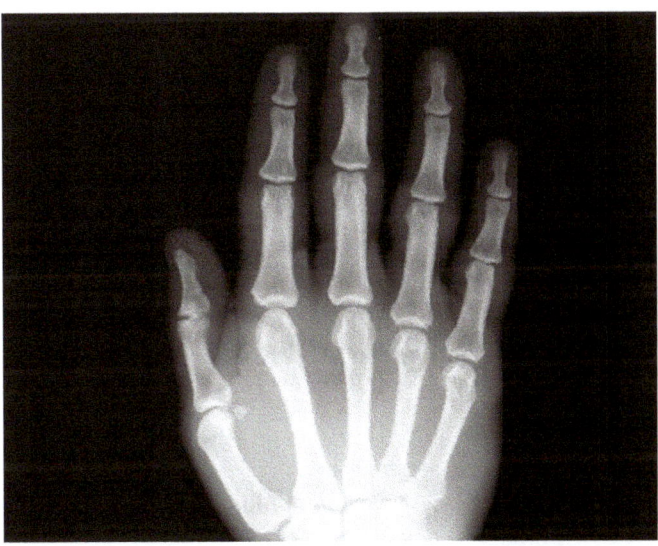

Fig. 12: Acromegaly. This case shows widening of base of distal phalanx with classic "arrow head" appearance. Mild soft tissue edema also appreciated.

- *Sarcoidosis*: Approximately 1/5th of cases have joint involvement. Ankle joint is most commonly involved. In hand it has predilection for proximal interphalangeal joint **(Fig. 10)**.
- *Tuberculous dactylitis*: It usually presents as painless swelling of hand and foot. On radiography, two distinct pattern can be seen, lytic lesion with significant sclerosis and minimal periosteal reaction, ill-defined lesion with thick periosteal reaction and minimal or no sclerosis.
- *Marfan syndrome*: It is a systemic connective tissue disorder with possible severe cardiac complications (viz., bicuspid aortic valve with aortic regurgitation, aortic dissection, and mitral insufficiency) **(Fig. 11)**.
- *Acromegaly*: It occurs due to excessive growth hormone in patients with mature skeleton. It has slow and insidious onset. Hand radiograph is characterized by enlarged hands and hypertrophied terminal phalangeal tuft which is described as spade phalanx sign **(Fig. 12)**.

FURTHER READING

1. Bassett LW, Blocka KL, Furst DE, Clements PJ, Gold RH. Skeletal findings in progressive systemic sclerosis (scleroderma). Am J Roentgenol. 1981;136 (6):1121-66.
2. Chapman S, Nakielny R. Aids Radiological Differential Diagnosis, 5th edition. New York: Elsevier Health Sciences; 2009.
3. Dixey J, Solymossy C, Young A. Is it possible to predict radiological damage in early rheumatoid arthritis (RA)? A report on the occurrence, progression, and prognostic factors of radiological erosions over the first 3 years in 866 patients from the Early RA Study (ERAS). J Rheumatol Suppl. 2004;69:48-54.
4. Jacobson JA, Girish G, Jiang Y, Resnick D. Radiographic evaluation of arthritis: inflammatory conditions. Radiology. 2008; 248(2):378-89.
5. Khan A, Bilezikian J. Primary hyperparathyroidism: pathophysiology and impact onbone. CMAJ. 2000;163(2): 184-7.
6. Magid D, Pyeritz RE, Fishman EK. Musculoskeletal manifestations of the Marfan syndrome radiologic features. Am J Roentgenol. 1990;155 (1):99-104.
7. Pineda CJ, Martinez-lavin M, Goobar JE, Sartoris DJ, Clopton P, Resnick D. Periostitis in hypertrophic osteoarthropathy: relationship to disease duration. Am J Roentgenol. 1987; 148(4):773-8.
8. Rana RS, Wu JS, Eisenberg RL. Periosteal reaction. Am J Roentgenol. 2009;193(4): 259-72.
9. Visser H, Vos K, Zanelli E, Verduyn W, Schreuder GM, Speyer I, et al, Sarcoid arthritis: clinical characteristics. Ann Rheum Dis. 2002;61(6):499-504.

Various Arthritic Joint Disorders

Madhan Jeyaraman, Rakesh Kumar, Anil Gowtham Manivannan

■ HEMOPHILIC ARTHROPATHY

Introduction
A condition characterized by repetitive hemarthroses following trivial trauma and ultimately joint deformation in patients with hereditary coagulation disorder.

Epidemiology
- *Incidence*: Rare condition, 3–4 per 100,000 population has decreased significantly due to home factor treatment
- Other comorbidities associated are HIV, hepatitis C (due to frequent blood transfusions)

Demographics
- Young males
- Affects patients between 3 and 15 years old

Etiology
Root bleeding disorders may be:
- Hemophilia A (classical hemophilia)
  - X-linked recessive
  - Decreased factor VIII
- *Hemophilia B*: Christmas disease
  - X-linked recessive
  - Decreased factor IX
- Von Willebrand's disease
  - Rare cause of joint bleeds
  - More commonly mucosal bleeding
  - Autosomal dominant
  - Abnormal factor VIII with platelet dysfunction
- Hemophilia C—deficiency of factor XI, does not cause hemophiliac arthropathy

Pathology
Accumulation of blood within the joint acts as an irritant to synovium (**Flowchart 1**).

Location
- Knee is most commonly affected
- Elbow, ankle, shoulder and spine are also involved

Mechanism of Injury
Persistent minor trauma.

Clinical Presentation
Patient gives typical history of spontaneously occurring bleeding following trivial trauma; patient gives history of uncontrollable hemorrhages following tooth extraction, minor cut or bruises.

Symptoms
- *Pain*: Severe, following acute hemarthrosis
- *Swelling*: Depending upon the joint involvement. Most commonly knee joint and it follows the lining of the synovium
- Paresthesia

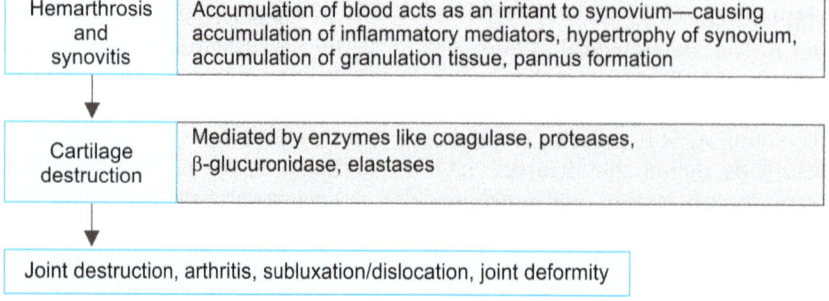

Flowchart 1: Pathogenesis of hemophilic arthropathy.

Signs

- *Attitude*: Position of ease of the joint (partial flexion of the knee and elbow, flexion/abduction/external rotation of hip joint)
- Local rise of temperature present
- Tenderness present depending upon the joint involved
- Swelling of the joints
  - *Acute phase*: It has tense swelling of hemarthrosis
  - *Chronic phase*: Boggy swelling due to synovial hypertrophy (suprapatellar area of knee joint)
- Restriction of joint movements due to capsular thickening and contracture
- Muscle wasting due to chronic immobilization of joint due to deformity (most commonly noticed in quadriceps muscles)
- Crepitus in the joint due to chronic degenerative arthritis
- Large bulbous tumor such as hematomas may be present along the shafts of long bones subperiosteally or within the muscles that envelop the long bones or between muscle and sheath producing characteristic hemophiliac pseudotumor or hemophiliac cysts >> muscle destruction chronic oozing sinus >>> secondary infection >>> fatal septicemia in children
- *Nerve compression*: Secondary to muscle hematomas, e.g., femoral nerve compression due to iliacus hematoma lateral femoral cutaneous nerve compression rarely
- *Fractures*: Due to generalized osteopenia/abnormality in healing chronology/due to compression on long shafts of bones
- *Limb length discrepancy*: Due to epiphyseal overgrowth or due to epiphyseal destruction
- *Compartment syndrome*: Especially in forearm and leg due to hemorrhage in firm fascial compartments >> ischemic necrosis >> Volkmann's contracture in forearm/ equinus deformity of ankle.

Classification

Arnold–Hilgartner Staging (Figs. 1A to D)

- *Stage 1*: Shows swelling of the soft tissues but no skeletal changes.
- *Stage 2*: Shows osteoporotic changes of epiphysis but joint integrity is preserved.
- *Stage 3*: Shows development of subchondral cysts, widening of intercondylar notch of femur and trochlear notch of ulna. Mild to moderate joint space narrowing but joint is grossly intact

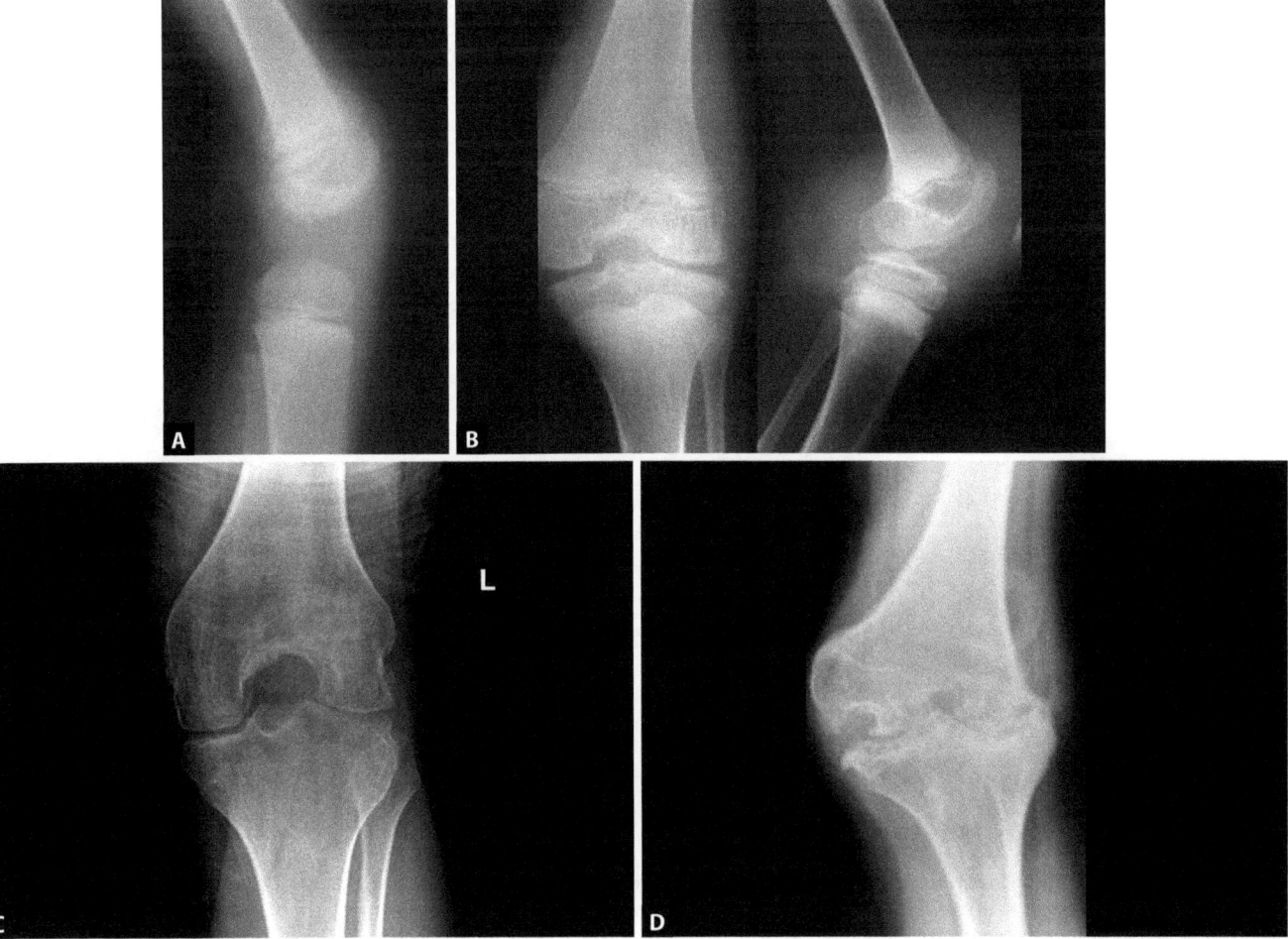

Figs. 1A to D: Arnold–Hilgartner staging. (A) Stage 1; (B) Stage 2; (C) Stage 3; and (D) Stage 4 of hemophilic arthropathy.

- *Stage 4*: Shows cartilage loss with severe narrowing of the joint along with changes of Stage 3.
- *Stage 5*: Demonstrates severe arthritis of affected joint with fibrous ankylosis. There is marked incongruity of articular structures with severe irregular hypertrophy of epiphysis.

Modified Arnold–Hilgartner staging has only 4 stages (Stage 2 is eliminated). Stages 1, 2, and 3 are reversible and can be treated conservatively but Stage 4 and 5 are irreversible.

Investigations

- *Blood investigations*: Routine investigations along with bleeding time, clotting time and factor assays, screening of factor VIII inhibitors
- Radiograph imaging
  - X-rays show decreased joint space, epiphyseal overgrowth, generalized osteopenia, fractures.
    X-ray of right knee joint:
    - Squaring of patella and femoral condyles (Jordan's sign)
    - Ballooning of distal femur
    - Widening of intercondylar notch
    - Joint space narrowing
    - Patella appear long and thin on lateral view

    X-ray of ankle joint—decreased joint space and talar widening
  - USG often helpful to follow intramuscular hematomas
  - MRI can be used to identify early degenerative joint disease **(Fig. 2)**
- Histopathology findings of synovial biopsy shows hypertrophied and hyperplastic synovium with hemosiderin laden cells in the superficial cellular layer and macrophages/leukocytes in the subsynovial stratum where disintegrating erythrocytes may be seen. Villous hypertrophy may be present. Hypervascular and reactive granulation tissue is present with perivascular cuffing with mononuclear cells and PMN cells **(Figs. 3A and B)**.

Differential Diagnosis

- *Septic arthritis*: Concomitant infection should be ruled out by physical examination and joint aspiration
- Rheumatoid arthritis

Treatment

- Nonoperative
  - Compressive dressings, ice bag application and limb elevation to prevent progress of hemarthrosis

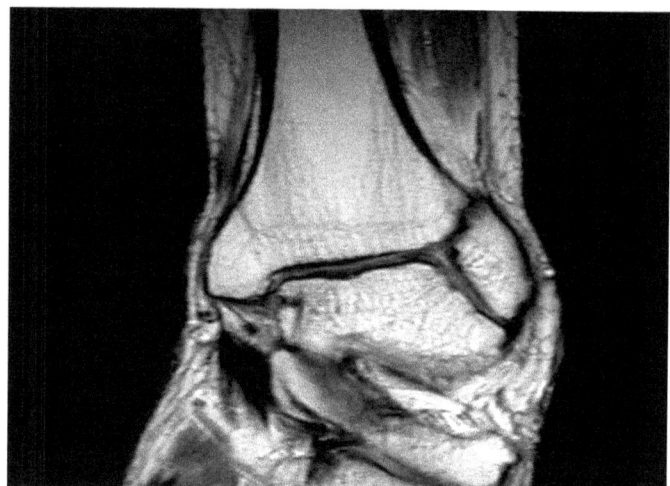

Fig. 2: Coronal MRI of a patient with hemophilic arthropathy of the ankle. Note the cartilaginous destruction of the talus.

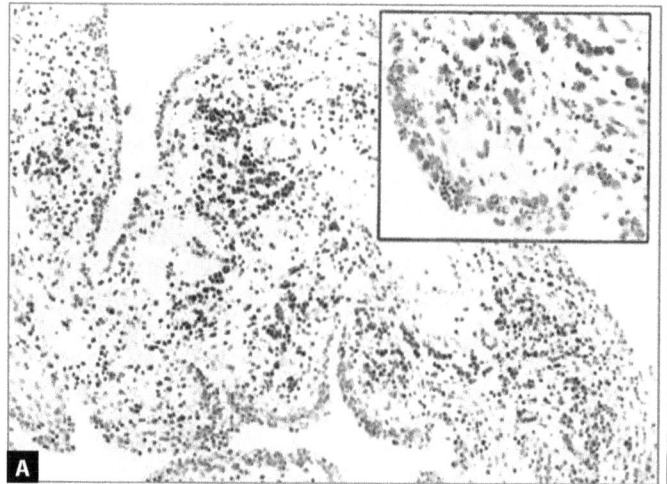
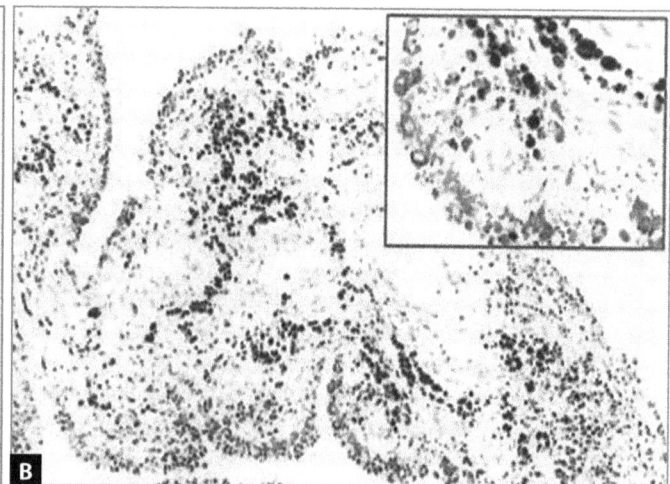

Figs. 3A and B: (A) Hemosideritic specimen showing diffuse lymphocyte infiltration and neovascularization with no follicles of lymphocytes; (B) Micrographs of synovial tissue. In haemosideritic synovium the lining cells show deposits as discrete granules, scattered throughout the cytoplasm. The deeper iron deposits are in dense intracellular and extracellular aggregates.
Source: Roosendaal G, et al. J Bone Joint Surg. 1998;80-B:540-5.

- Aspirations should be avoided for fear of reducing intra-articular counter pressure and for the fear introducing infections
- Analgesics to reduce pain
- Local Steroids to reduce inflammation
- Short term immobilization with splints and braces
- *Rehabilitation*: Physiotherapy to prevent contracture development
- Fracture management
- *Factor replacement therapy*: The dosage to correct a factor deficiency is calculated on the basis of the patients' weight and assumed plasma volume in general
    - 1 unit of factor VIII per kg body weight raises patients' plasma level of factor VIII by 2%.
    - 1 unit of factor IX per kg body weight raises patients' plasma level of factor IX by 1.5%.

It is necessary to make serial determinations of factor levels to establish rate of fall after administration.
Biological half-life of factor VIII: 6-12 hours and of factor IX is 8-18 hours. Hence for maintenance therapy, doses of factor VIII must be repeated every 8 hours and factor IX every 12 hours to maintain desired plasma level.
Indications:
- For vigorous physiotherapy flowing splinting or major surgery increase factor VIII/IX to 20%
- *Acute hematomas (including intramuscular hematomas)*: Increase factor VIII/IX to 20-30%
- *Severe bleeding in CNS/nasopharynx*: Increase factor VIII/IX to 80-100% of normal
- *Skeletal surgery*: Increase factor VIII/IX to 100% for first week following surgery then maintain at >50% for second week following surgery (a level of 100% is also needed for manipulation of fracture or joint under anesthesia or removal of pins)
- Desmopressin indicated in mild or moderate hemophillia A
- Operative—General instructions before surgery
    - Preoperatively the presence of inhibitors (antibodies) must be determined. The inhibitor titer should be checked 7-14 days after a test dose of factor has been administered. If no inhibitors are present the deficient factor must be brought to a level of 80-100%
    - As many procedures as possible has to be done at one session only (multiple operative interventions increases risk of developing inhibitors)
    - Vessels should be ligated rather than electrocoagulation
    - Tube suction necessary for minimum 24 hours
        - *Synovectomy*: Indicated in recurrent chronic hemarthroses and chronic synovitis recalcitrant to medical management.
            => Outcomes—decrease incidence of recurrent hemarthroses and limit pain and swelling
        - *Synoviorthesis*: Indicated in chronic hemophiliac synovitis that is recalcitrant to medical management
            => *Technique*: Destruction of synovial tissue with intra-articular injection of radioactive agent. Radioactive agents: Colloidal phosphorus-32 chromic phosphate, Au-198, Y-90, Dy-165.
        - *Total joint replacement*: Indicated in end stage arthropathy
        - *Arthrodesis*: Indicated in severely destroyed joints especially ankle joint involvement
        - *Supracondylar osteotomy of femur*: To correct severe flexion contracture of knee joint that does not respond to conservative treatment.
        - *Achilles tendon lengthening*: Indicated in equinus deformity of the ankle joint.
        - *Pseudotumor excision*: Under the cover of factor replacement therapy
            Radiation therapy: Indicated for small inaccessible pseudotumors. A dose of 750 rads (125 rads daily), healing is usually seen within few weeks. Higher dosage can be given those cysts present along tibia or femur.

Prognosis

Prognostic Variables

- Degree of factor deficiency—determines severity of disease
    - *Mild*: 5-25%
    - *Moderate*: 1-5%
    - *Severe*: 0-1%
- Presence of factor VIII inhibitors (including IgG antibodies)
    - IgG antibody inhibits response of therapeutic factor treatment (monoclonal recombinant factor VIII)
        - Found in 5-25% of hemophiliac patients
        - Is a relative contraindication for surgical interventions
        - Should be screened for preoperatively

NEUROPATHIC ARTHROPATHY

- First described by Jean Martin Charcot in 1868, in patients with tabes dorsalis long before the cause of syphilis was recognized
- Now Charcot joint became synonymous with neuropathic arthropathy

Definition

It is a destructive progressive arthritis associated with loss of pain sensation superadded with repeated trauma resulting in progressive cartilage and bone damage **(Figs. 4A and B)**.

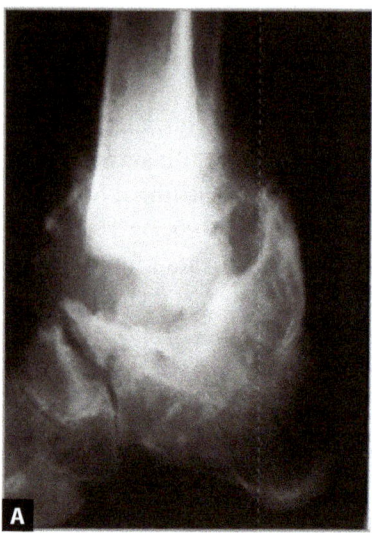 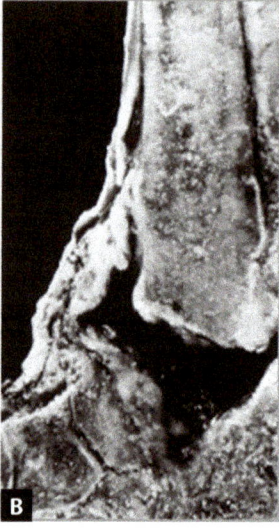

Figs. 4A and B: (A) Radiograph; and (B) MRI of left ankle joint shows severe joint destruction with the collapse of articular cartilage.

Disorders Associated with Neuropathic Arthropathy

- Diabetes mellitus—0.5%—Foot
- Tabes dorsalis—4–10%—large joints of lower limbs
- Spinal dysraphism—lower limb
- Syringomyelia—25%—upper limb
- Leprosy—lower limb
- Congenital insensitivity to pain—lower limb
- Spinal cord and peripheral nerve injury—lower limb
- Peroneal muscular atrophy
- Rheumatoid arthritis and pseudogout
- Amyloidosis and chronic liver disease
- Repeated intra-articular steroid injection
- Neuropathy associated with alcoholism and avitaminosis
- Postrenal transplant arthropathy
- Chronic intake of nonsteroidal anti-inflammatory drugs (NSAIDs)

Pathology

- Similar to severe osteoarthritic changes
- Fragmentation and eventual loss of articular cartilage
- Articular cartilage is destroyed by pannus—never seen in OA
- Eburnation of underlying bone
- Osteophytes are found at margins

Pathology in More Advanced Disease

- Subchondral fracture
- Devitalized bone, intra-articular loose bodies
- Microscopically synovial tissues show fragments of cartilage and bone
- Periosteal new bone formation around joints never seen in the OA
- Erosion over joint surface
- At times tubular bone

Mechanism

Neurovascular Theory of Allman State

- *An abnormal autonomous nervous system is the key process*: Increased blood supply to joint produce effusion that weaken capsule, ligaments and bone resorption lead to osteopenia
- Loss of sensation and proprioception lead to excessive stretching of capsule and ligament more than physiological limits
- Repeated injuries destroy cartilage, ligaments and bone
- In diabetes glycosylation make ligaments brittle, reversion of cells of capsule and bone to primitive mesenchymal state, rapid proliferation and subsequent redifferentiation as cartilage bone and osteoid tissue

Stages

- 1—Hydrarthrosis—effusion leads to capsule and ligament laxity
- 2—Atrophic—destruction of joint structures
- 3—Hypertrophic—new osseous deposit around the joint

Charcot observed two stages in 1892 in tabes dorsalis (**Figs. 5A to D**)
1. Benign—ceased to progress and disappear
2. Malignant to full-fledged disease

Clinical Course

- Starts in one joint then progress to involve other joint
- Onset is sudden, unexpected and almost painless
- Joint swollen suddenly
- Swelling increase gradually
- Diffuse edema of the limb affected
- Swelling subside gradually
- Later joint is unduly lax
- Movements of joint into abnormal direction and extend
- Later deformities arise as the result of bone end destruction and subluxation
- After few weeks or months joint become completely flail patient is now completely crippled
- Disease can be arrested at any stage or can affect other joints
- Usually there will not be any constitutional symptoms unless infected

Joints Affected

1. Foot joints—diabetic
2. Ankle ⎫
3. Knee ⎪
4. Hip   ⎬ Tabes dorsalis
5. Spine ⎪
6. Shoulder ⎭
7. Elbow ⎫ Syringomyelia
8. Wrist ⎭

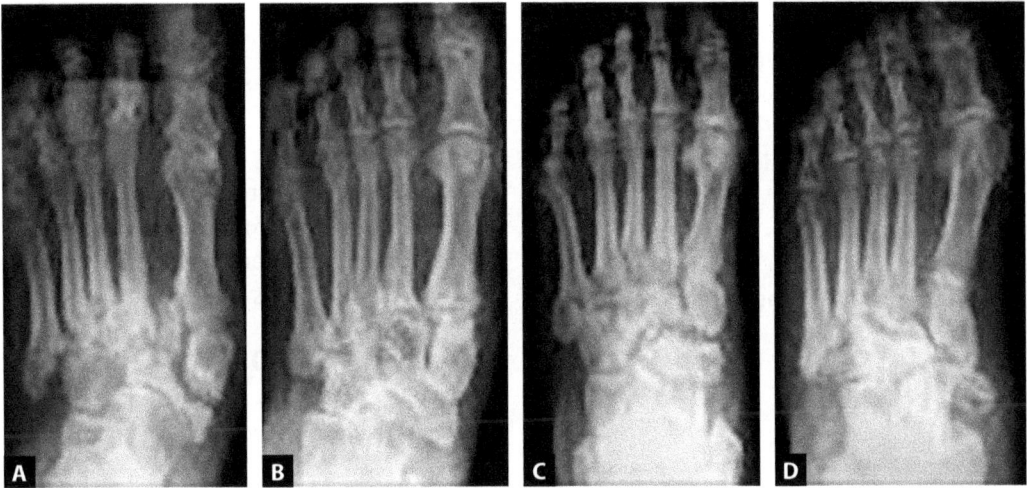

Figs. 5A to D: Modified Eichenholtz classification of neuropathic arthropathy. (A) Stage 0—normal; (B) Stage 1—fragmentation; (C) Stage 2—coalescence; and (D) Stage 3—reconstruction.

Differential Diagnosis

- Osteoarthrosis
- Osteomyelitis
- Osteonecrosis
- Hypertrophic osteoarthropathy
- Stress fractures
- Pseudogout

Differentiate from osteomyelitis:
- Difficult in diabetic foot in osteomyelitis, X-ray shows, bone ends are blurred
- In neuroarthropathy bone ends are destroyed
- MRI is helpful to distinguish
- Culture of joint fluid
- Bone scan using indium[111] labeled WBC or immunoglobulin G show increased uptake in osteomyelitis but not in neuroarthropathy

Diagnosis

Charcot's Triad
- Swelling
- Exaggerated movements
- Painlessness of joint

X-ray findings—according to stages:
- Joint space narrowing
- Subchondral bone sclerosis
- Large osteophytes
- Effusion

Later marked joint destruction
- Hypertrophic changes
- Extra-articular bone fragments
- Subluxation
- New bone formation around joint
- Lack of juxta-articular osteoporosis is the striking feature
- Margin of bony destruction is so straight and clearly defined, so as to suggest a former surgical intervention

Investigation: Blood
- ESR—normal
- Total leukocyte count and differential count—normal
- Blood sugar
- Serological test for syphilis
- Serum carboxy terminal telopeptide of type 1 collagen—increased
- Culture

Examination of joint fluid:
- Noninflammatory
- Xanthochromic
- Bloody
- Contains fragments of synovium, cartilage and bone

Treatment

General
- Treat underlying disease
- Stabilize the joint with well-padded braces and splints
- Rest and nonweight bearing till acute symptom subside
- Weight relieving calipers
- Biphosphonates reduce Charcot changes
- Therapeutic ultrasound is highly beneficial

Foot:
- Seen in diabetic and congenital sensory neuropathy, even minor injuries in diabetic patients should be carefully evaluated and observed repeatedly until symptoms and signs subside, and prevent it from proceeding to Charcot joints
- Neuropathic arthropathy of foot is complicated with ulcers so treatment of foot ulcers is very important

Prevention:
- Always use soft foot wear even inside home to avoid minor injury
- Bed rest till swelling subside following an injury
- Control blood sugar

- Goal of treatment
- To get a plantigrade foot
- Mechanically sound foot

Treatment:
- CROW (Charcot Restrained Orthotic Walker)
- Custom made shoes
- Well-padded plaster cast
- Patellar tendon bearing cast
- Very important is to protect the other foot

Ankle:
Nonoperatively by-
- Braces
- KAFO
- PTB cast
- Well-padded POP Cast
- Bed rest

Operatively by arthrodesis:
- Charnley approach
- Intramedullary ankle arthrodesis nail from calcaneum
- 6–9 months cast immobilization

Knee:
- Nonoperatively by bracing
- Operatively by
  - Total knee arthroplasty—aseptic loosening in long run
  - Arthrodesis—difficult to achieve

Points for success for arthrodesis:
- 1—complete debridement of synovium
- 2—maximum bone to bone contact
- 3—strong internal fixation
- 4—adequate external support for months

Hip:
- Nonoperatively—stable after adequate immobilization
- Operatively by
  - Arthrodesis—high failure rate
  - Total hip arthroplasty—recurrent dislocation and aseptic loosening

Spine:
- Nonoperatively by braces
- Operatively by spinal fusion
- Posterior long segmental fixation and short segment fusion
- Resection of involved segment with two stage fusion with Cotrel and Dubousset instrumentation
- Charcot involvement of spine is difficult to differentiate from degenerative spondylosis
- Multiple level malalignment of vertebral bodies with sclerosis
- Toppling brick sign, without much pain

Shoulder:
- Neuropathy arthropathy appear like soft tissue sarcoma
- Nonoperatively by splints braces and rest
- Operatively by
  - Arthrodesis
  - Arthroplasty—seldom successful

CONCLUSION

- Neuropathic arthropathy is a crippling unstable and painless problem for the patient
- But it is a highly demanding and painful problem for the stable orthopedic surgeon.

FURTHER READING

1. Botek G, Anderson MA, Taylor R. Charcot neuroarthropathy: an often overlooked complication of diabetes. Cleve Clin J Med. 2010;77(9):593-9. doi: 10.3949/ccjm.77a.09163. PMID: 20810870.
2. Frykberg RG, Belczyk R. Epidemiology of the Charcot foot. Clin Podiatr Med Surg. 2008;25(1):17-28, v. doi: 10.1016/j.cpm.2007.10.001. PMID: 18165108.
3. Gupta R. A short history of neuropathic arthropathy. Clin Orthop Relat Res. 1993; 296:43-9. PMID: 8222448.
4. James VL, Mauricio S, Carlos Rodriguez-Merchan E, Navid G, Christopher AZ, Richard SF. Hemophilic arthropathy. J Am Acad Orthop Surg. 2004;12(4):234-45.
5. Kucera T, Shaikh HH, Sponer P. Charcot neuropathic arthropathy of the foot: a literature review and single-center experience. J Diabetes Res. 2016;2016:3207043. doi: 10.1155/2016/ 3207043. Epub 2016 Aug 30. PMID: 27656656; PMCID: PMC5021483.
6. Lobet S, Hermans C, Lambert C. Optimal management of hemophilic arthropathy and hematomas. J Blood Med. 2014;5:207-18. [online] Available from https://doi.org/10.2147/JBM.S50644 [Last accessed June, 2021]
7. Luck JV Jr, Silva M, Rodriguez-Merchan EC, Ghalambor N, Zahiri CA, Finn RS. Hemophilic arthropathy. J Am Acad Orthop Surg. 2004;12(4):234-45. doi: 10.5435/00124635-200407000-00004. PMID: 15473675.
8. Melchiorre D, Manetti M, Matucci-Cerinic M. Pathophysiology of hemophilic arthropathy. J Clin Med. 2017;6(7):63. doi: 10.3390/jcm6070063. PMID: 28672826; PMCID: PMC5532571.
9. Milne TE, Rogers JR, Kinnear EM, et al. Developing an evidence-based clinical pathway for the assessment, diagnosis and management of acute Charcot neuro-arthropathy: a systematic review. J Foot Ankle Res. 2013;6(1, article 30) doi: 10.1186/ 1757-1146-6-30.
10. Munson ME, Wrobel JS, Holmes CM, Hanauer DA. Data mining for identifying novel associations and temporal relationships with Charcot foot. J Diabetes Res. 2014;2014:214353. doi: 10.1155/2014/214353. Epub 2014 Apr 27. PMID: 24868558; PMCID: PMC4020407.
11. Pulles AE, Mastbergen SC, Schutgens RE, Lafeber FP, van Vulpen LF. Pathophysiology of hemophilic arthropathy and potential targets for therapy. Pharmacol Res. 2017;115: 192-9. doi: 10.1016/j.phrs.2016.11.032. Epub 2016 Nov 24. PMID: 27890816.
12. Sohn MW, Lee TA, Stuck RM, Frykberg RG, Budiman-Mak E. Mortality risk of Charcot arthropathy compared with that of diabetic foot ulcer and diabetes alone. Diabetes Care. 2009;32(5):816-21. doi: 10.2337/dc08-1695. Epub 2009 Feb 5. PMID: 19196882; PMCID: PMC2671113.

23. Tendinopathies

Madhan Jeyaraman, Naveen Jeyaraman, Ravi VR

INTRODUCTION

In the field of sports, medicine as well other work-related disorders, tendon disorders needs a special mention, which have high incidence as well as account for a fair share in increasing morbidity. Tendinopathies includes all problems that arise from overuse or repeated use of tendons. These may affect the tendon itself as well as surrounding structures.

The treatment for tendinopathy is quite cumbersome and needs several follow-ups for months together; also the response to treatment may be poor in a number of patients. In a patient with degenerative pathology residing in a tendon, there are chances of acute rupture even during the course of treatment.

The main function of tendon is for joint movement by transmitting the force generated in muscles onto bone **(Fig. 1)**. The long course of treatment and poor response to the same even after an excellent treatment plan is one of the main reasons for substantial amount of morbidity seen in persons with tendinopathies.

FUNCTIONAL BIOMECHANICS OF TENDON

The behavior of a tendon when some deforming forces are applied on it, are best demonstrated in a *Stress-Strain curve* **(Fig. 2)**.

When no forces are acting on a tendon, the collagen fibrins present in it have a crimpy appearance when seen under a microscope, which starts to flatten up when some initial force is applied. With further forces, deformation continues in a linear way and fibers are aligned parallel to each other. This is because the triple helix formed by collagen molecules shows intermolecular sliding. The strain should be less than 4% for the tendon to retain its elastic property, otherwise the tendon may not come back to its original crimpy posture.

A tendon's tensile strength at any given time is directly proportional to the thickness of tendon and the amount of collagen in it. During sports activities and gymnastics a tendon may experience substantial amount of load. Chances for tendon rupture increase, if the force applied is in a very short amount of time or in an oblique fashion, which is seen maximum in case of eccentric type of muscle contraction.

TENDON DISORDERS (FIG. 3)

- *Tenosynovitis*: Inflammation of synovial sheath surrounding the tendon without any injury to the tendon.
- *Tendinitis*: Also called as tendonitis, refers to the acute inflammation of a tendon due to any injury or pathology.
- *Tendinosis:* It is a chronic type of tendon pathology where degeneration predominates at cellular level and inflammation, if present, is very minimal or totally absent.

TENDINOPATHIES

Tendinopathy: It refers to tendon injuries, which are chronic in nature with molecular disruption with no hint regarding etiology.

Epidemiology

About 30% of doctor visits for sports injury-related complications can be attributed to tendon injuries. Mostly

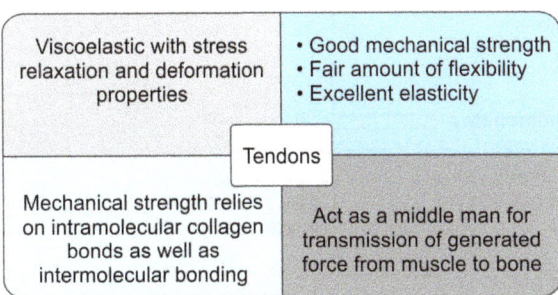

Fig. 1: Biomechanical functions of tendon.

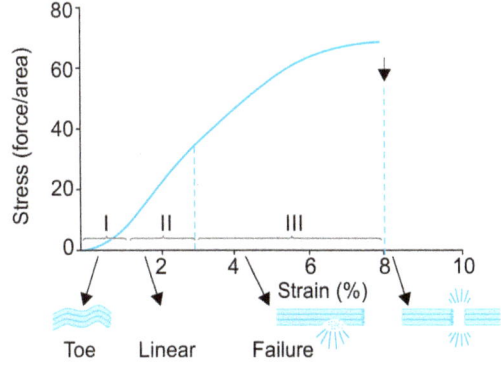

Fig. 2: Stress-strain curve.

these kinds of injuries are seen in sports persons, but there has been a surge in number of cases even in nonathletes too as well as in sedentary lifestyles.

Etiopathogenesis (Fig. 4)

- Tensile overload of the tendons
- Disruption of collagen synthesis in a tenocyte
- Neural sprouting
- Load-induced ischemia
- Thermal damage
- Adaptive compressive forces
- Intratendinous sliding motion of fascicles
- Shear forces around interface of fascicles
- *Quinolone antibiotics*: 0.08–0.2% of tendon rupture.

The most common sites at which tendon injuries occur due to overuse are:

- *Supraspinatus tendon*: Supraspinatus syndrome
- Tendinopathies involving rotator cuff
- Lateral epicondylitis aka tennis elbow
- Medial epicondylitis aka golfer's elbow
- Stenosing tenosynovitis
- *Patella tendon*: Patellar tendinopathy
- *Achilles tendon*: Achilles tendinopathy
- Peroneal tendinopathy
- Plantar fasciitis.

Molecular Mechanism in Tendinopathy

The breakdown of the extracellular matrix inside a tendon is main pathology behind tendinopathy. This degradation is the result of inflammatory molecules such as interleukin-1β, which decreases the expression of mRNA that is responsible for formation of collagen protein in tenocytes, which is a main component of the tendon.

■ TENNIS ELBOW (LATERAL EPICONDYLITIS)

Idiopathic, benign, and self-limiting disease, characterized by degeneration of musculotendinous origin at *lateral epicondyle (Origin of common extensor muscles of forearm)* **(Fig. 5)**.

Associations

- Nirschl—Mesenchymal syndrome— Genetic linkage of disease
- Higher incidence of RA factor positivity and HLA-B27 positivity
- Components
  - Rotator cuff pathology
  - Epicondylopathy
  - Carpal tunnel syndrome
  - Trigger finger
  - De Quervain's disease.

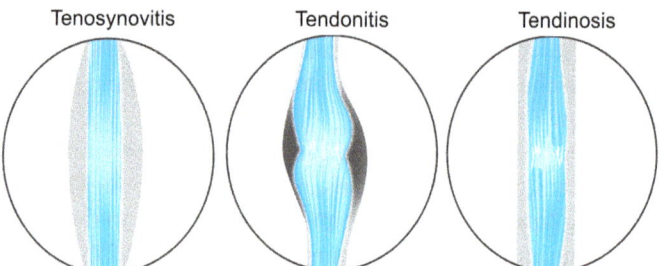

Fig. 3: Types of tendon disorders.

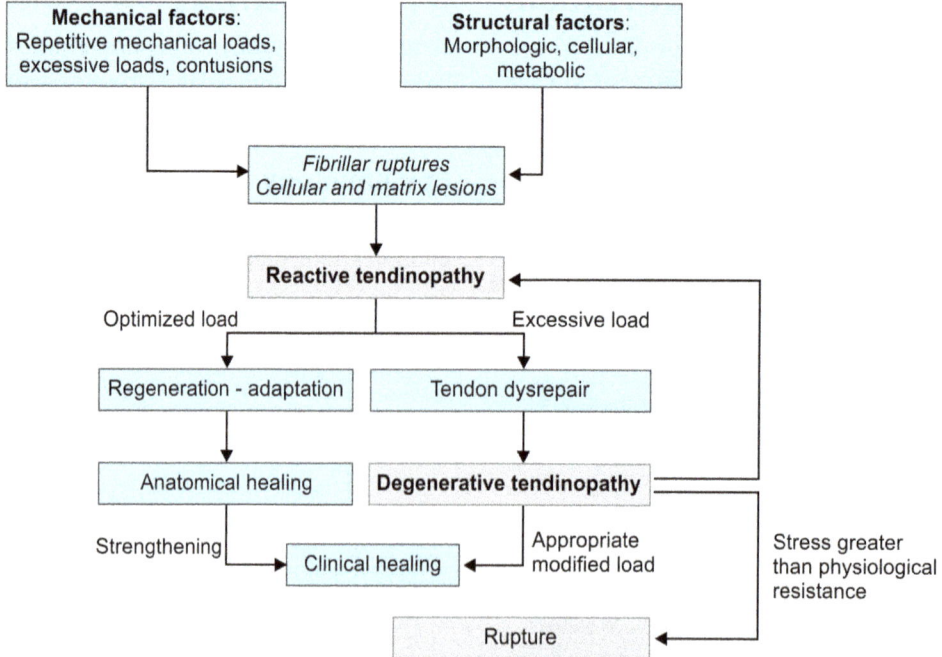

Fig. 4: Pathogenesis of tendinopathy.

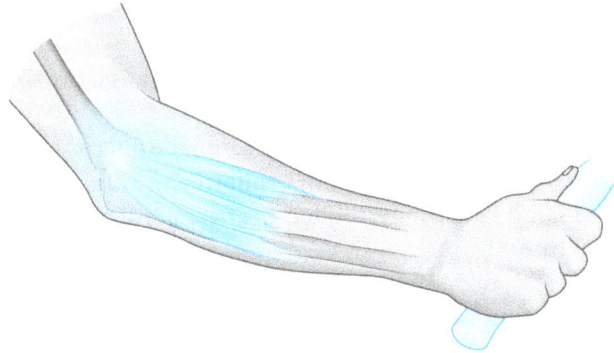

Fig. 5: Lateral epicondylitis.

Etiopathogenesis

- Altered biomechanics of elbow joint and increased activity of extensor carpi radialis brevis activity
- Underuse or stress shielding
  - Reduced intrinsic strength and structural weakening of tendon → Metaplasia of tissue due to shearing forces → Progressive fibrocartilaginous composition of extensor carpi radialis brevis enthesis → Development of tendinosis
  - HPE: Tendon defects and areas of necrosis, angio-fibroblastic hyperplasia, and signs of disorganized muscle fiber regeneration
- Compromised blood supply
  - *Tendons*: Intrinsically limited blood supply
  - Prolonged activities produce ischemia by stretching of tendons and compressing precarious blood supply rendering tendon avascular
- *Thermal injury*: Increased internal temperature by virtue of friction in collagen bundles
- *Apoptosis*: Tendon injury activates protein kinases leading to apoptosis
- *Altered tendon metabolism*: Imbalance between matrix metalloproteinases and growth factors.

Histopathologicoclinical Dissociation

- Degeneration of common extensor origin tendon with multiple tears
- *Cause of pain in lateral epicondylitis*: Increased concentration of excitatory neurotransmitter glutamate, increased levels of neurokinin-1 receptors and lactate.

Histological Stages of Tendon Injury

- *Stage 1*: Acute inflammatory response, which resolves in initial episodes and if recurrence persists, it needs medical treatment
- *Stage 2*: Sustained stage 1—angiofibroblastic hyperplasia
- *Stage 3*: Partial or complete tendon rupture
- *Stage 4*: Stage of fibrosis and calcification.

Clinical Features

- Affects approximately 1–2% of population
- Age group affected—3rd to 5th decade in dominant arm
- Pain and tenderness over the lateral condyle area
- Patient experiences pain over lateral condyle when tries to grip onto some object and also while wrist movements (e.g., using a screwdriver, sweeping floor using broom or mop) and lifting movements
- Inability to extend elbow completely after long sleep or rest
- Nonspecific symptoms
  - Radiating pain to forearm and wrist
  - Pain encountered during wrist extension
  - Weakness of forearm
  - Pain on shaking hands or opening a doorknob
- Tenderness can be elicited in anterolateral aspect of lateral epicondyle.

Provocative Tests

- *Cozen's test*: if a patient tries to do wrist extension against a resistance when wrist is in full pronation and deviated radially, it will elicit pain in anterolateral aspect of elbow
- Mill's test
  - Palpation of lateral epicondyle in one hand
  - Pronation of forearm and full flexion of wrist and the elbow extended to stretch the tendon
  - If pain present at area of insertion over lateral epicondyle, it is considered to be positive test
- *Chair lift test*: When trying to lift the back of a chair with a pinch of three finger with the elbow fully extended.

Differential Diagnosis

- Annular ligament stenosis
- Cervical spondylosis with radiculopathy
- Synovial inflammation adjacent to radial head
- Posterior interosseous nerve entrapment
- Early OA of radial head
- Radial nerve entrapment
- Osteochondritis dissecans of capitellum
- Lateral collateral ligament laxity
- Anconeus muscle inflammation.

Investigations

- *Plain elbow radiographs*: To exclude bony pathologies like loose bodies, OA, patchy calcification of soft tissues
- *Histopathology*: Presence of granulation tissue, microrupture, degenerative changes without any inflammation. When seen under a microscope, the normal tendon tissue with organized collagen is replaced with degenerated tissue with collagen arrangement totally disorganized.

- *Ultrasound of elbow*: USG elbow may reveal calcification inside and around tendon, intrasubstance tears, thickening of tendon as well as irregular margins of lateral epicondyle. If compared with a color Doppler, changes in vascularity are seen in areas of pain in extensor tendon.
- *MRI scan*: Clearly degenerative tissues replacing the normal tissues are seen with intrasubstance or even complete tears sometime.

Management Principles

- Pain control
- Preservation/restoration of movement
- Regaining grip strength and endurance
- Normalization of function
- Preventing recurrence and further clinical deterioration.

Nonoperative Management (Fig. 6)

- RICE regimen
  - *Rest*: Stopping participation in sports on heavy work activities for several weeks and activity modification
  - *Ice pack application*: Decreases inflammation, slows local metabolism, and helps to relieve pain
  - *Compression and elevation*: To assist venous return and minimize swelling
- NSAIDs: To reduce pain and swelling
- Stretching exercises for wrist with elbow extended
- *Physical therapy*: Local application of low intensity ultrasound, ice massage to improve tendinomuscular healing
- Brace application
  - Inhibit maximal contraction of wrist and finger flexor and extensor
  - Restrict full muscle expansion and reducing intrinsic muscle force to vulnerable areas
  - Reduce activity of forearm muscles decreasing overload
  - Partially fix muscle to underlying forearm bone and soft tissue, creating a new muscle origin that shortens the length of muscle pull, slightly changing the direction of force
  - Reduce stress across joint by passivating proximal muscle
- *Steroid injections*: 40 mg of triamcinolone injection given at the point of maximum tenderness. Side effects—skin and fat atrophy, tendon degeneration, and tendon rupture
- Extracorporeal shock wave therapy
  - *MOA*: Causes microtrauma that promotes body's natural healing processes
  - 2,000 shock waves of $0.04–0.12 \text{ nj/mm}^2$, three times at monthly intervals for 6 months
- *Autologous blood injection*: User dependent technique
- Platelet-rich plasma (PRP) injection
- Other nonoperative techniques
  - Cryotherapy
  - Prolotherapy with 25% dextrose
  - Radiotherapy
  - Manipulation under anesthesia
- *Open surgery*:
  - *Extensor slide*: Partial release of extensor tendon (Fig. 7)
- Making 3–4 cm incision anterior to lateral epicondyle
- Incising fascia overlying posterior edge of extensor carpi radialis longus and expose the underlying extensor carpi radialis brevis
- Identify abnormal anterior edge of extensor aponeurosis that lies just posterior to ECRL
- ECRB is elevated and released and degenerated tissue is excised
- Decortication is performed with the help of a burr.

One must be careful for the following:
- Avoid release of ECRL (Elbow weakness)
- Avoid cutting lateral collateral ligament (Chronic elbow instability)
- Defect between ECRL and extensor aponeurosis should be repaired.

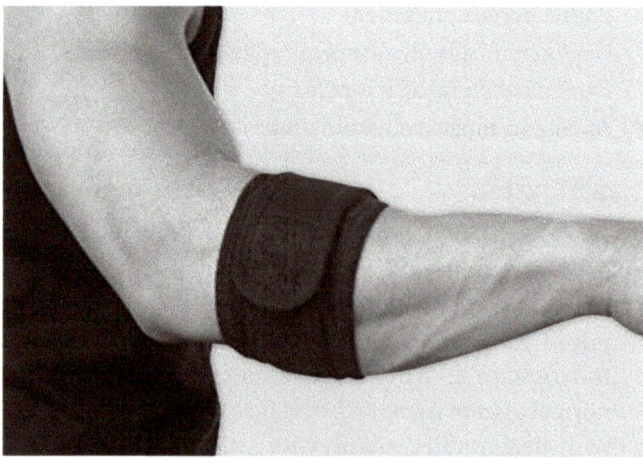

Fig. 6: Tennis elbow splint.

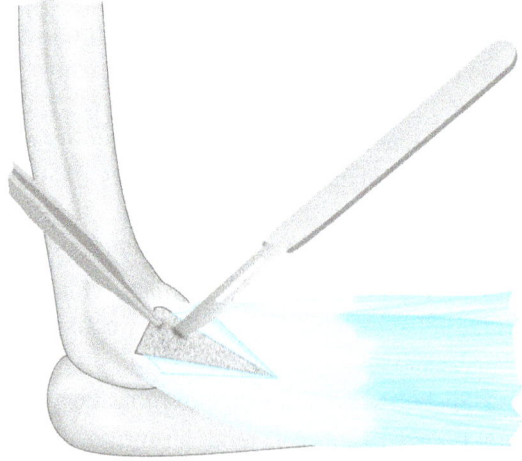

Fig. 7: Release of common extensor origin for tennis elbow.

Arthroscopic Management

- Described by Grifka, Boenke, and Kramer in 1995
- *Three portals*: Two working portals—posterolateral and anterolateral portal and one viewing portal—anteromedial portal
- Advantages
  - Any coexisting intra-articular disease can also be treated
  - Since, it is not an open procedure, damage to healthy tissue is minimal
  - The under surface of extensor carpi radialis brevis tendon can be visualized
- Disadvantages
  - Longer operative time
  - Risk of damaging the radial nerve.
- *Percutaneous release*: Extensor slide or Hohmann's epicondylar stripping
  - A local anesthesia is given surrounding the lateral epicondyle and then the common extensor tendon is incised **(Fig. 8)**.
  - The incision is taken little distal to lateral epicondyle and the incised tendon, which gets displaced can be felt or palpated through skin once the procedure is over.
  - *Postoperative regimen*: One should refrain from doing any activity, which puts strain on the operated muscle at least for a period of 3 months, following which gradual movements are started both actively and passively.
  - *Complication:* Complete tendon rupture—palpable defect in extensors results in weakness on attempted wrist extension, which needs surgical repair.

Prevention

- If any injury has previously occurred, then any activity which puts strain over outer aspect of elbow should be avoided or minimized
- A good physical health should be maintained to strengthen the core body as well as specifically for the forearm muscles and the joints around it, i.e., shoulder and upper arm.
- Any repetitive activity or sports should be avoided as it is one of the most common causes of lateral epicondylitis.

Tennis Elbow Rehabilitation

See **Figure 9**.

GOLFER'S ELBOW AKA MEDIAL EPICONDYLITIS

- It is also known as Pitcher's elbow, Climber's Elbow, and Little League Elbow
- Idiopathic, benign, and self-limiting disease, characterized by degeneration of musculotendinous origin at medial epicondyle (Origin of common flexor muscles of forearm) **(Fig. 10)**.

Historical Perspective

- *Morris' (1882)*: Radial humeral bursitis or periostitis, synovitis, or annular ligament degeneration/impingement
- *Nirschl*: Mesenchymal syndrome—genetic linkage of disease and postulated histological staging.

Biomechanics of Medial Epicondyle

The muscular and valgus forces acting on medial side of elbow sometimes are more than the sustainability of medial ligamentous and musculotendinous structures, which are borne by flexor - pronator group of muscles → Medial collateral ligament → Overloading of medial epicondyle.

Clinical Features

- Pain at medial epicondyle of the elbow.
- While trying to bend the wrist or while grasping an object will increase the pain.
- Provocative test—pronation against resistance as well as resisting wrist flexion will increase the symptoms.

Physical Examination

- Tenderness over medial epicondyle.
- There is an increase in tenderness over medial epicondyle when patient tries to extend the elbow with a supinated forearm.
- Pain increases with resisted wrist flexion and resisted forearm pronation.

Differential Diagnosis

- Cervical radiculopathy
- Elbow and forearm overuse injuries
- Ulnar collateral ligament injury.

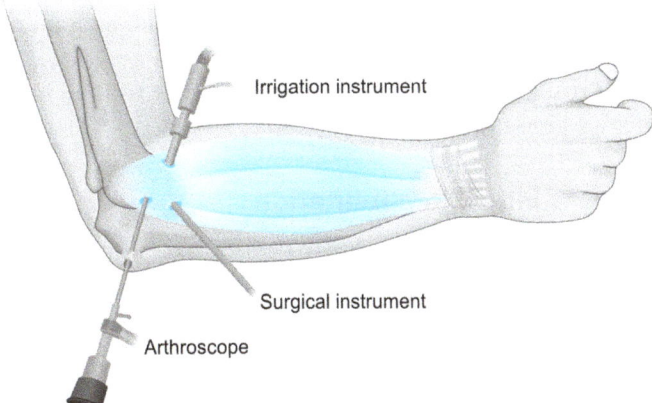

Fig. 8: Arthroscopic release of common extensor origin in tennis elbow.

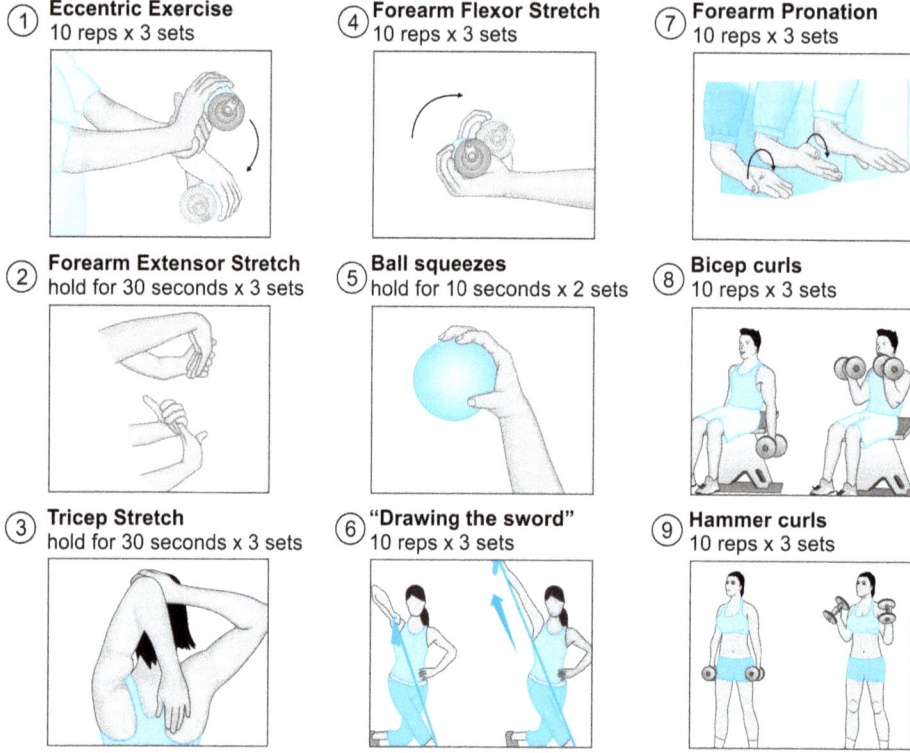

Fig. 9: Rehabilitation for tennis elbow.

Treatment

Nonoperative management: RICE regimen, NSAIDs, physical therapy, brace application, steroid injections, and PRP therapy.

Operative Management

- Surgical options
  - Release/slide of flexor origin
  - Medial epicondylectomy and excision of pathological tissue
  - Flexor pronator release
  - Enhancement of local vascularity by decortication or a couple of low intensity drill holes into epicondyle.

Procedure

- Longitudinal incision over medial epicondyle
- Careful protection of branches of medial antebrachial cutaneous nerve
- Pronator teres is separated from flexor carpi radialis by a transverse incision between them
- Resection of pathological tissue
- Medial collateral ligament lying deep must be protected as it contains ulnar nerve.

Complications

Persistent ulnar nerve symptoms, MCL injury.

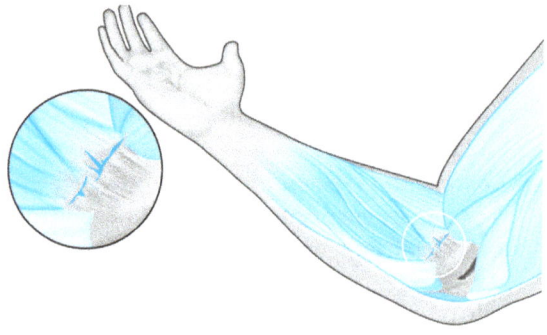

Fig. 10: Medial epicondylitis.

Postoperative Management

- With elbow flexion of 90°, an above elbow POP slab is applied with forearm kept in neutral position
- Isometric exercises started after 3–4 weeks followed by resisted exercises for wrist flexion as well as forearm pronation done at 6 weeks
- Normal full range of sporting activities usually takes 4–6 months.

Golfer's Elbow Rehabilitation

See **Figure 11**.

■ dE QUERVAIN'S TENOSYNOVITIS

- It is known by many names such as gamer's thumb, radial styloid tenosynovitis, mommy thumb, texting thumb, washerwoman's thumb, or blackberry thumb (**Fig. 12**).

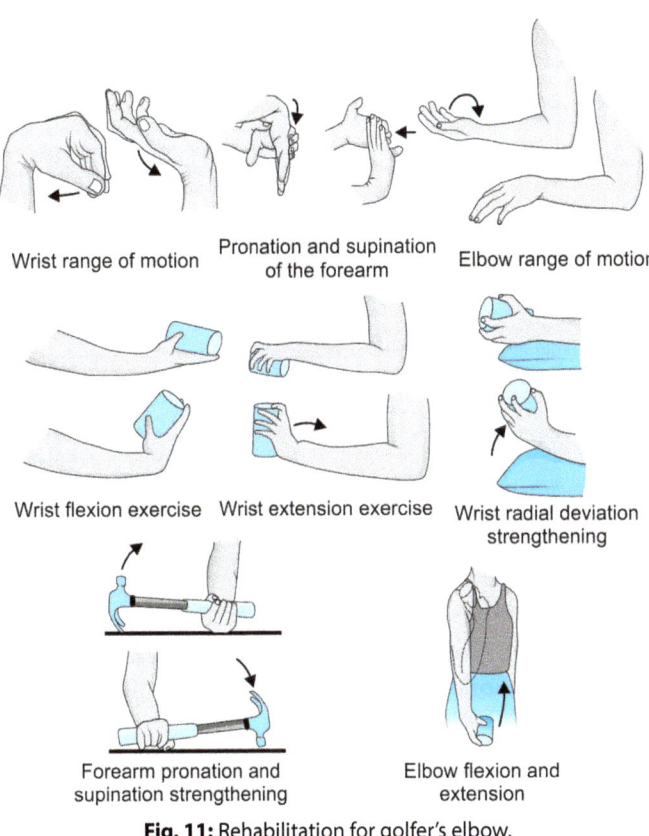

Fig. 11: Rehabilitation for golfer's elbow.

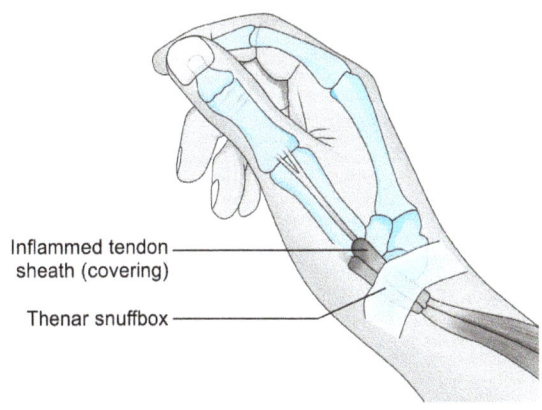

Fig. 12: de Quervain's tenosynovitis.

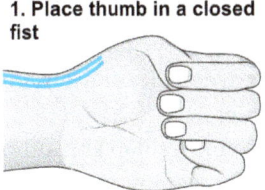

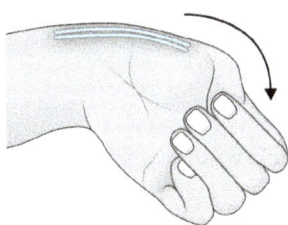

Pain felt during the Finkelstein test is a positive indicator of de Quervain's syndrome

Fig. 13: Finkelstein's test.

- In this disease, there is inflammation of the synovial sheath (tenosynovitis) covering the two tendons which are responsible for thumb movement.

Etiology
- Exact etiology is not known
- Can also be classified into an occupational disease as it involves repetitive movements.
- Repeated bending of wrist and also twisting or screwing movements are responsible as it causes a strain injury due to repetitive movement.
- Women are affected more often than men.

Pathophysiology
Due to chronic inflammatory process, there is thickening of tendon sheaths of extensor pollicis brevis and abductor pollicis longus muscles around the anatomical snuff box in the first dorsal compartment.

Clinical Features
- Pain and tenderness near the radial styloid and at base of thumb, which increases on movement of thumb
- Occasionally edema near base of thumb which may extend up to wrist
- Gripping and grasping objects is extremely painful
- Occasionally snapping sound is heard.

Diagnosis
- The disease is diagnosed clinically after a thorough history as well as physical examination. A history of previous trauma or a fracture leading to arthritis should be ruled out.
- Finkelstein's test **(Fig. 13)**.

Management
- *Nonoperative management*: RICE regimen, NSAIDs, local steroid injections, autologous blood injections, and PRP therapy.
- *Surgical management*: Longitudinal splitting of synovial sheath covering the tendons of first dorsal compartment, i.e., EPB and APL.
- *Physical therapy*: UST, SWD, infrared therapy, and cold laser treatments are effective.

TRIGGER FINGER (FIG. 14)
- Also called as stenosing tenosynovitis or locked finger
- Inflammation of tendon sheath or synovial sheath, which encases the flexor tendons of the involved digit.

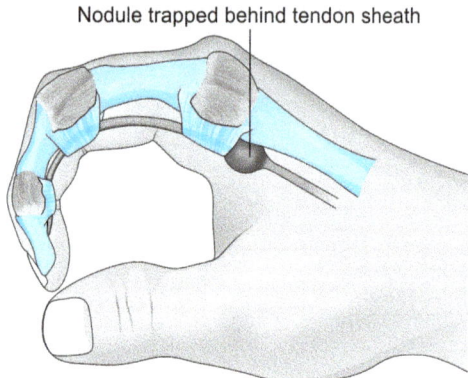

Fig. 14: Trigger finger.

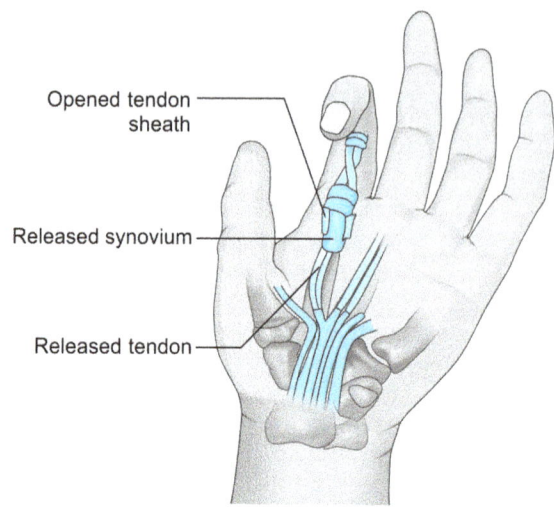

Fig. 15: Release of A1 pulley for trigger finger.

Etiopathogenesis
- Hypertrophy of A1 pulley or tendon thickening
- Discrepancy between flexor's circumference and A1 pulley at MCP level
- Pulley thickens where tendon abruptly angulates causing white ring scar thickening (Metaplastic fibrocartilage formation)
- *Triggering factors*: DM, rheumatoid arthritis, amyloidosis, and overuse.

Clinical Features
- More common in women than men in age group of 40–60 years
- *MC digit affected*: Thumb > Ring finger > Middle finger > Little finger
- Pain on finger movements and over PIP region of affected finger
- Tender nodule on volar aspect of palm near A1 pulley
- Swelling over volar aspect of palm.

Fate of Trigger Finger
- *Incarceration of tendon and adhesions in the region*: Prevents finger straightening (Finger fixed in mid flexion)
- Tendon breaks and fingers fail to flex. The patient will feel the sensation of dislocating finger and complete weakness
- *Diagnosis:* Clinical examination, USG—thickening or swollen tendon.

Staging of Trigger Finger

Stage 1 – Pretrigger	Presence of pain Positive sign of trigger finger not demonstrated On palpation, A1 pulley is tender
Stage 2 – Active	Positive trigger sign with snap when the patient able to extend finger actively
Stage 3 – Passive	A—Finger extension is possible only passively by applying external force B—Active finger flexion not possible
Stage 4 – Rigidity	Incarcerated trigger finger

Management
Nonoperative management: RICE regimen, NSAIDs, local steroid injections, autologous blood injections, and PRP therapy.

Operative Management
- *Goal of surgery*: To widen the opening of the tunnel
- Incision is taken over the A1 pulley and the flexor tendon sheath is exposed proximal and distal to it after which A1 pulley is divided completely to release triggering **(Fig. 15)**.
- Passively the tendon is inspected for any other source of triggering and if after release the tendon glides without any resistance, the wound is closed.
- If further triggering is seen, then FDS tendon is checked for etiology and tip is excised and A3 pulley is released.
- Passive range of movements are advocated and nodules are removed, if present.

Rehabilitation
- Gentle range of movement exercises are advocated after few days of surgery
- Strengthening exercises for muscles and joints in the hand
- Follow-up for 2–3 sessions each week for up to 6 weeks.

■ JUMPER'S KNEE (PATELLAR TENDINITIS)
- First described by Blazina et al., in 1973 as an insertional tendinopathy in skeletally matured athletes.
- Patellar tendinitis can be observed in young as well as in persons postclosure of the epiphysis.
- At least 20% of the athletes involved in jumping activity sustain patellar tendinitis once in their lifetime.
- Incidence is twice in males as compared to females.
- Jumping, running, and kicking put extreme tension on knee extensor muscle complex.

- The sudden repetitive forceful extensions of knee initiate inflammatory process by inciting microtrauma leading to patellar tendon degeneration.

Clinical Features
- Painful region around the inferior pole of patella
- Tenderness and swelling noted over proximal part of patellar tendon
- Worsening of pain after a strenuous activity may be seen
- Stages of pain
    - *Stage 1*: Pain only after a strenuous activity
    - *Stage 2*: Pain during as well as post activity
    - *Stage 3*: Pain during activity and prolonged after activity leads to complete rupture of tendon.

Investigations
Ultrasonogram of knee: For diagnosis and exclude and identify partial tears.

Management
Nonoperative Management
- *Rest*: Avoid sudden and explosive knee joint movements
- Ice pack application
- Topical application of ointment or gel
- NSAIDs
- Local steroid injection
- *Biological therapy*: Autologous PRP therapy.

Physical Therapy
- Phonophoresis, iontophoresis, and ultrasonic therapy
- Progressive concentric and eccentric strengthening exercises begun around 3-4 weeks
- Deep transverse friction massage at inferior patellar pole in a direction perpendicular to those of patellar tendon fibers accelerates inflammation and leads to healing by fibrosis of the patellar tendon.

Operative Management
- Surgical debridement, which need to be rested with immobilization for around 3 weeks followed by gradual movement for concentric and eccentric strengthening exercise after 3-4 weeks
- If more than half of the tendon is involved, inferior pole of patella is excised and surfaces freshened and reattachment of tendon done.

■ ACHILLES TENDINITIS
- Disorders of Achilles tendon contribute a small percentage to sports-related tendon injuries
- Most disorders result from overuse resulting in a diseased tendon symptomatically and biomechanically inferior.

Types of Achilles Tendinopathy

Insertional tendinopathy (Involves tendon–bone junction)

Noninsertional tendinopathy (Involves tendon proximal to its insertion)

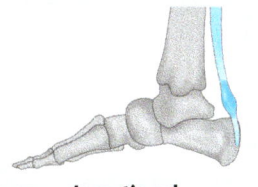
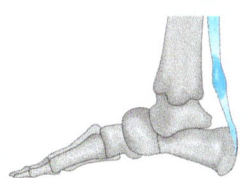

Insertional
- Insertional calcific tendinitis
- Haglund's deformity (Prominent posterior tuberosity of the calcaneum)
- Retrocalcaneal bursitis
- Precalcaneal bursitis
- Calcaneal exostosis (Skaters heel)

Noninsertional

History
- Mild to moderate pain following strenuous activities usually progresses quickly to pain
- H/o pain worse in the morning or after inactivity (start up pain is due to paratendinitis adhesions), which subsides soon after a few steps.

Physical Examination
- Inspection of the shoes worn by patient is very necessary
- Analysis of Gait
- Any valgus or varus deformity of hindfoot may lead to increased stress on Achilles tendon
- Wasting of gastrocnemius or soleus (inflicts severity of disease)
- Assessment of strength and range of motion.

Laboratory Investigations
- Serum uric acid levels for crystal arthropathy
- RA factor, CRP, and ESR for inflammatory arthropathy
- HLA-B27 for enthesopathy.

Imaging Studies
- *Plain radiograph*: Exostosis or a bony prominence such as a calcaneal spur seen on a lateral view X-ray of calcaneum
- *Ultrasound*: Demonstrates bursal inflammation and tendon degeneration
- *MRI*: Gold standard for observing any pathology of Achilles tendon as well as surrounding structures.

Management
Nonoperative Management (Fig. 16)
- RICE therapy
- Prolonged rest is not advised as it may lead to joint stiffness and further degeneration

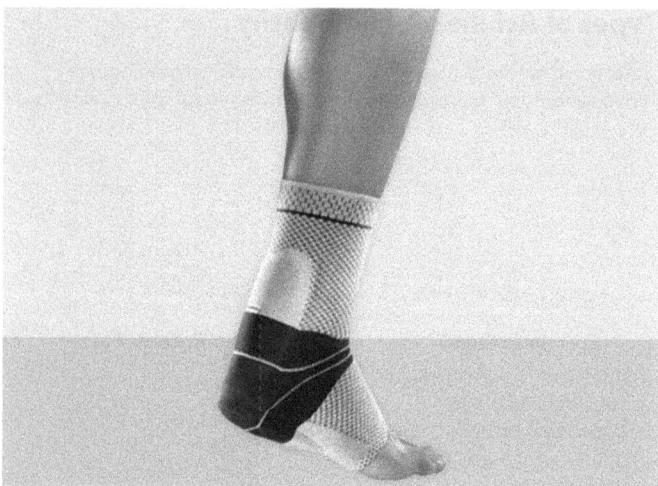

Fig. 16: Achilles guard.

- *Medications*: NSAIDs
- Avoid local infiltration of steroids (Tendon rupture)
- Custom orthotics to correct any hindfoot flexible deformities
- Shoe modifications such as Pump bump spacers can be utilized to decrease pressure areas in heel posteriorly
- Eccentric strengthening exercises.

Operative Management
- *Noninsertional Achilles tendinitis*: The grossly degenerative part of tendon can be debrided and excised.
- *Insertional Achilles tendinitis*: Excision of bony prominence, if present and resection of calcification and inflamed bursal tissues.

Achilles Tendon Exercises
See **Figure 17**.

■ TIBIALIS POSTERIOR TENDINITIS
Biomechanics
- *Primary function of tibialis posterior:* Inversion and plantar flexion of foot → Locking of midfoot transverse tarsal joints (tarsonavicular and calcaneocuboid)
- Secondary adductor of forefoot at midtarsal joint apposing action of peroneus brevis and provides support for longitudinal arch of foot.

Clinical Presentation
- Medial ankle pain and swelling
- Tenderness localized directly over navicular tuberosity or accessory navicular
- Pain over lateral aspect of sinus tarsi due to collapse of the medial arch and forefoot abduction.

Physical Examination
- Forefoot abduction
- Midfoot pes planus
- Hindfoot valgus
- On heel rising test, normal heel inversion is absent, if tibialis posterior tendon is dysfunctional.

Classification of Posterior Tibialis Tendon Dysfunction (Johnson and Strom)
- *Stage 1*: Pain localized along course of posterior tibialis tendon
- *Stage 2*: Stage 1 with functionally incompetent tendon leading to medial arch collapse
- *Stage 3*: Stage 1 + 2 with rigid deformity and passively noncorrectable
- *Stage 4*: Stage 3 + Ankle joint incongruency.

Management
Nonoperative Management
RICE regimen, activity modification, NSAIDs, physiotherapy, and medial arch support orthotics.

Operative Management
- *Stage 1*: Tendon debridement can be done which can be accompanied by a bony procedure such as a calcaneal osteotomy to shift the axis of weight-bearing more medially
- *Stage 2:* Passively correctable flatfoot is treated with combination of soft tissue reconstruction of tendon with bony procedure to reverse deformity
- *Stages 3 and 4*: Subtalar arthrodesis.

■ PERONEAL TENDINOPATHY
Clinical Features
- Swelling and tenderness in an area posteriorly to lower end of fibula because of inflammation
- On plantar flexion and inversion against resistance, there is worsening of pain
- Decrease in subtalar motion
- Difficulty in walking on uneven ground.

Management
- Activity modification, PRICE regimen, and NSAIDs
- *Orthotics and shoe wear modifications:* Decrease calcaneal fibular impingement with a medial heel wedge
- Surgical management with debridement with diseased tendon
- Stretching exercises and regular activities should be begun after 4–6 weeks.

■ PLANTAR FASCIITIS (FIG. 18)
- Also called as Plantar fasciosis or Calcaneal plantar enthesopathy.

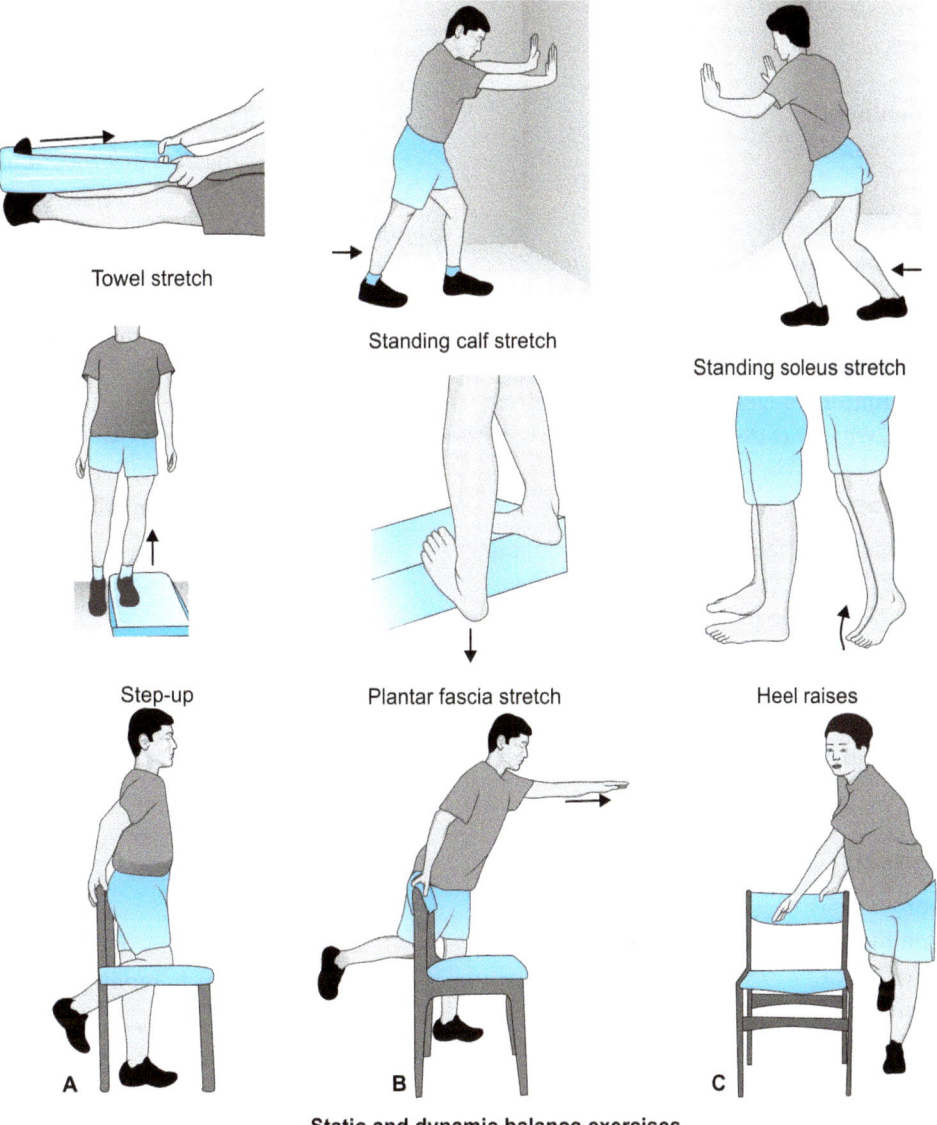

Fig. 17: Rehabilitation for Achilles tendonitis.

- Chronic self-limiting condition due to over use.
- It is mainly a disease caused by inflammation, microtears, and scarring at the attachment site of plantar fascia to the bone.
- Around 80% of the heel pain can be attributed to plantar fasciitis.
- The pain is very severe on weight-bearing after waking up from the bed or after a prolonged period of rest.
- Another feature is that the pain increases by passive or active dorsiflexion of the toes due to stretch in the already inflamed insertion site of the plantar fascia.
- Bilateral involvement is seen in around 30% of patients.

Risk Factors for Plantar Fasciitis

- Activities and occupation requiring long standing working hours.
- Decreased dorsiflexion ankle range of motion
- Pes planus
- Pes cavus
- Calcaneal spur on radiographs
- Leg length discrepancy

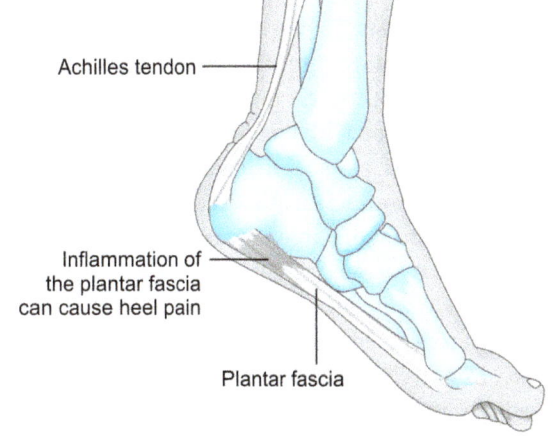

Fig. 18: Plantar fasciitis.

- Sedentary lifestyle
- An increase in exercise
- Obesity
- Achilles tendon tightness
- Inappropriate footwear.

Clinical Features

- Patient reports heel pain and tightness immediately after standing up and weight-bearing. Startup pain, which improves after taking a few steps in pain.
- When a diseased plantar fascia is examined under a microscope, myxomatous degeneration is seen along with collagen fibers, which are disorganized.

Physical Examination

- To offload the pressure on heel, patient starts walking with an equinus gait.
- On dorsiflexion of toes, a sharp pain is felt on medial side of plantar aspect of calcaneum because of attachment of plantar fascia to medial calcaneal tubercle.
- Sometimes a heel spur may be seen coincidentally on an X-ray. It is common and can be seen in around 50% of the patients.

Differential Diagnosis

- Plantar fascia tear
- Posterior tibial tendinitis
- Achilles tendinitis
- Retrocalcaneal bursitis
- SI joint radiculopathy
- Calcaneal stress fracture
- Tarsal tunnel syndrome
- Calcaneal neoplasia.

Investigations

- *Plain radiographs:* To detect calcaneal spur
- *USG:* To evaluate plantar fascia and surrounding structures. USG criteria for plantar fasciitis—thickness >4 mm associated with areas of hypoechogenicity
- *MRI:* To assess causes of recalcitrant heel pain. MRI criteria for plantar fasciitis – Thickened plantar fascia with increased signal intensity on T2-weighted and short tau inversion recovery images
- *Three-phase bone scan:* It is a very sensitive investigation which can be used to detect active disease and response to treatment, which is seen as decreased uptake following corticosteroid injections.

Management

Nonoperative Management

- Almost 95% of patients observe improvement within 6 months following conservative mode of treatment.
- RICE regimen, NSAIDs
- Local steroid infiltration at the site of maximum tenderness
- Percutaneous fenestration (dry drilling)
- Prolotherapy using 25% dextrose/lidocaine solution
- Intralesional whole blood injections
- Biological PRP therapy
- *Botulinum toxin A*: It can provide relief from pain even 14 weeks after injection.

Physical Therapy

- Extracorporeal shockwave therapy (ESWT)
  - It proves very effective in patients who do not respond to any conservative therapy for a period of 3 months.
  - Pain relief may be seen for as long as 1 year after the procedure.
  - Complications of ESWT are mild hematoma, redness, etc.
- Eccentric calf stretching
  - Eccentric calf stretching helps in slow lengthening of the muscles when put under load.
  - The plantar fascia is stretched by passive dorsiflexion of the toes until stretching load is felt in the arch of the foot.
  - Deep massage helps in increasing vascularity to the fascia and helps in repair process.
- Arch supports, silicone soft soles, and night splints
  - Further contracture of plantar fascia can be prevented by use of night splints.
  - Medial arch supports are used in combination with silicone soft soles
  - Silicone heel pads or full length soles provide an excellent pain relief **(Figs. 19 and 20)**.
  - Foot orthroses decrease the strain on plantar fascia, and also decrease the chances for collapse of medial longitudinal arch and provide symptomatic relief.

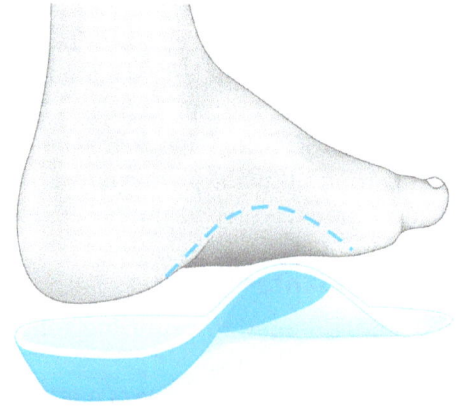

Fig. 19: Heel pad.

Operative Management

- When all sorts of conservative therapies fail for at least a period of 6 months, then operative treatment (plantar fasciotomy) may be considered **(Fig. 21)**.
- Minimally invasive surgery and endoscopic treatment are limited as they need special equipment and surgical skills.
- An alternative approach is using Coblation surgery technique, which can be used for the treatment of recalcitrant plantar fasciitis.

NEWER TREATMENT MODALITIES FOR TENDINOPATHIES

Platelet-rich Plasma Injections (Fig. 22)

- PRP is defined as a volume of plasma with an increased platelet concentration of 4–6 times above normal values (approximately 10^6/mL).
- The cell ratio in normal blood contains only 6% platelets but PRP contains 94% platelets.
- The rationale for use of PRP is to stimulate the natural healing cascade and tissue regeneration by a "Supra–physiological" release of platelet-derived factors at the site of treatment
- Autologous PRP eliminates concerns about immunogenic reactions and disease transmission.

Benefits of PRP

- Increases growth factor levels at the injury site
- Provides a provisional matrix or scaffold for healing
- Improves hemostasis
- Has anti-inflammatory and antimicrobial properties
- Processing and application patient side is simple and rapid.

Families of Platelet Concentrates

Based on presence of leukocytes and fibrin architecture:
- Pure PRP (P-PRP) or leukocyte poor PRP
- Leukocyte- and PRP (L-PRP)

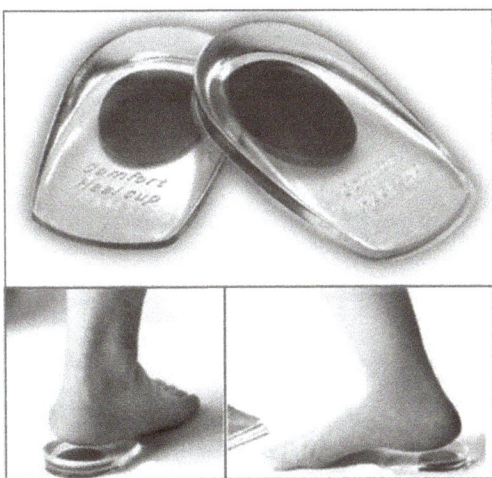

Fig. 20: Heel cup.

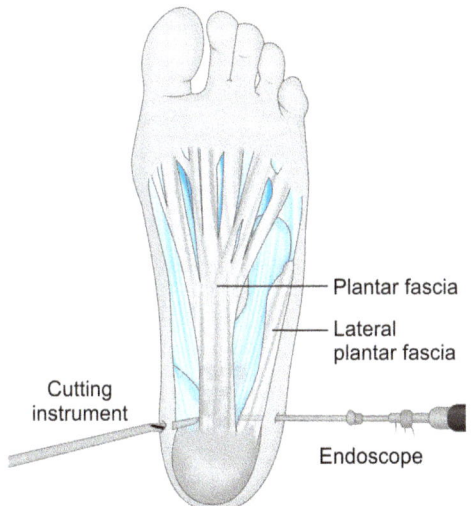

During an endoscopic plantar fasciotomy, a cut in the plantar fascia is made near the heel bone to relieve tension and pain. Fibrous tissue forms as the plantar fascia heals to bind the two parts back together resulting in longer tendon and less tension

Fig. 21: Arthroscopic release of plantar fascia.

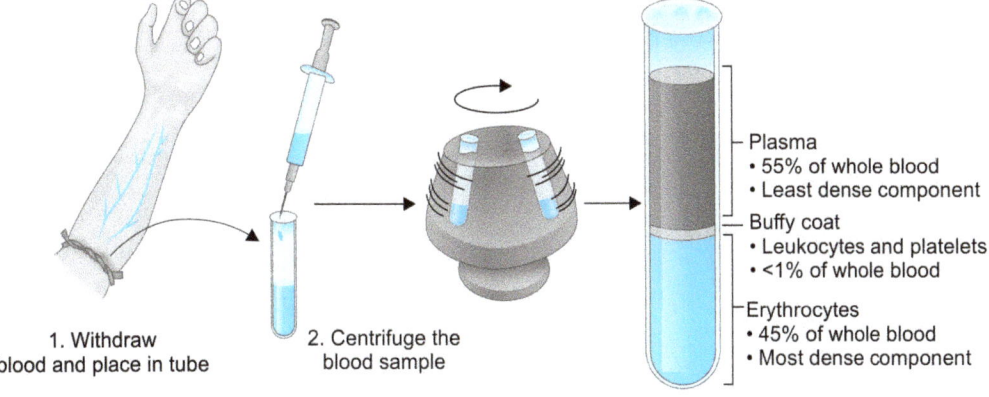

Fig. 22: Preparation of platelet-rich plasma.

- Pure platelet-rich fibrin (P-PRF) or leukocyte poor platelet-rich fibrin
- Leukocyte and PRF.

Molecular Basis of PRP

Increased HGF and TNFα activity by disrupting NF-κB-transactivating activity **(Fig. 23)**.

Uses of PRP

- *Ligament injuries*: Strains and sprains of MCL and LCL injuries.
- *Tendon injuries*: Achilles tendinitis, Rotator cuff injuries, Quadriceps tendinitis, and Patellar tendinitis
- *Overuse syndromes*: Tennis elbow, Golfer's elbow, and Plantar fasciitis
- *Muscle injuries*: Tear of quadriceps, hamstrings, biceps, triceps, and calves.
- *Cartilage injuries*: Osteoarthritis of hip, knee, and shoulder, Periarthritis of shoulder, Patellofemoral chondrosis
- *Knee injuries*: Anterior cruciate ligament (ACL) injuries and meniscal tears
- *Entrapment syndromes*: Carpal tunnel syndrome
- *Spinal injuries*: Lumbar spinal disc pain, SI joint pain
- Tendon bioengineering using mesenchymal stem cells and a silk scaffold.

Autologous Tenocyte Injection (Fig. 24)

- A needle biopsy was used on the patellar tendon, and the extracted tendon cells were expanded by in vitro culture. The autologous tenocytes were sorted and purified by real-time polymerase chain reaction, and amplified by flow cytometry.

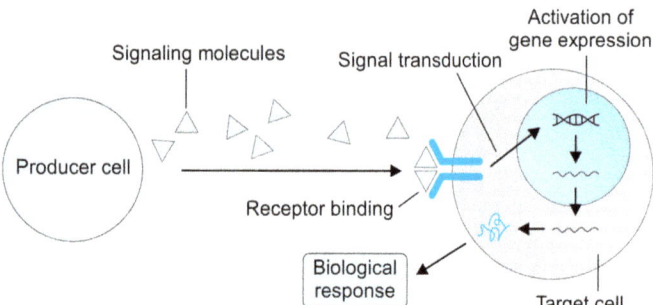

Fig. 23: Molecular basis of PRP action.

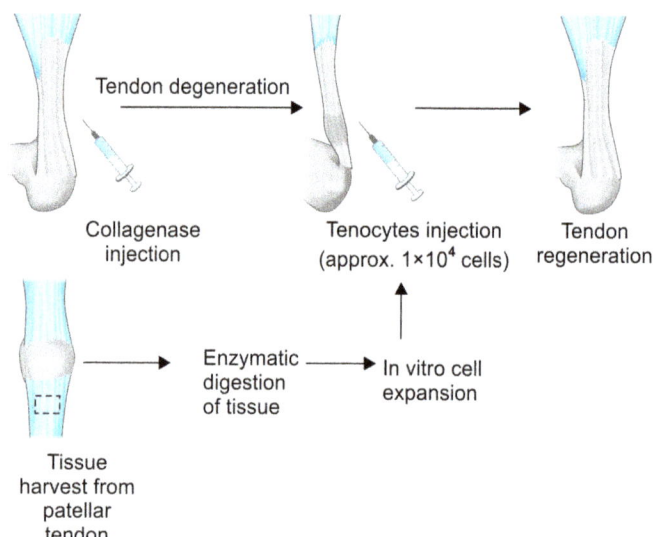

Fig. 24: Autologous tenocyte injection.

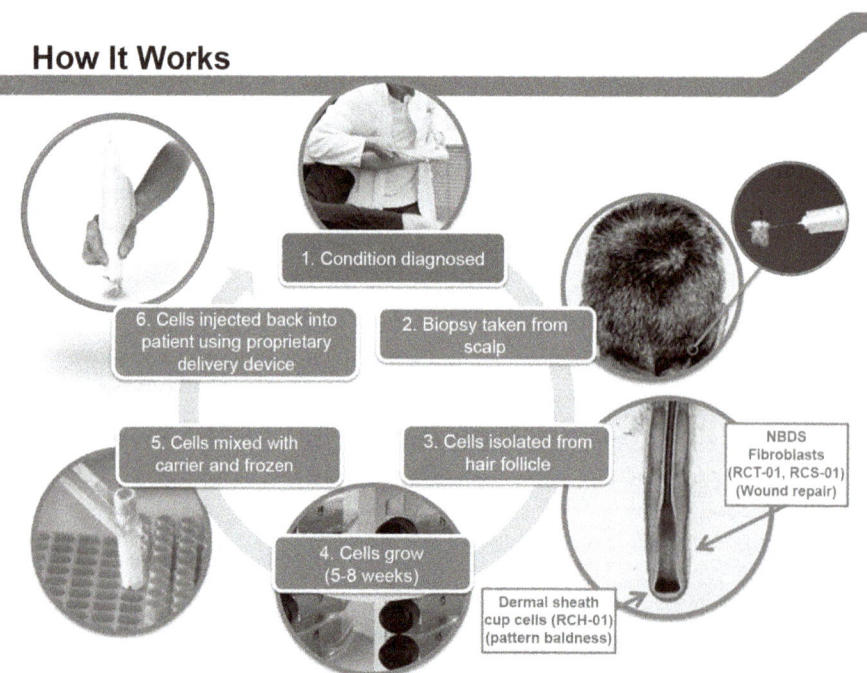

Fig. 25: Nonbulbar dermal sheath cell injection.

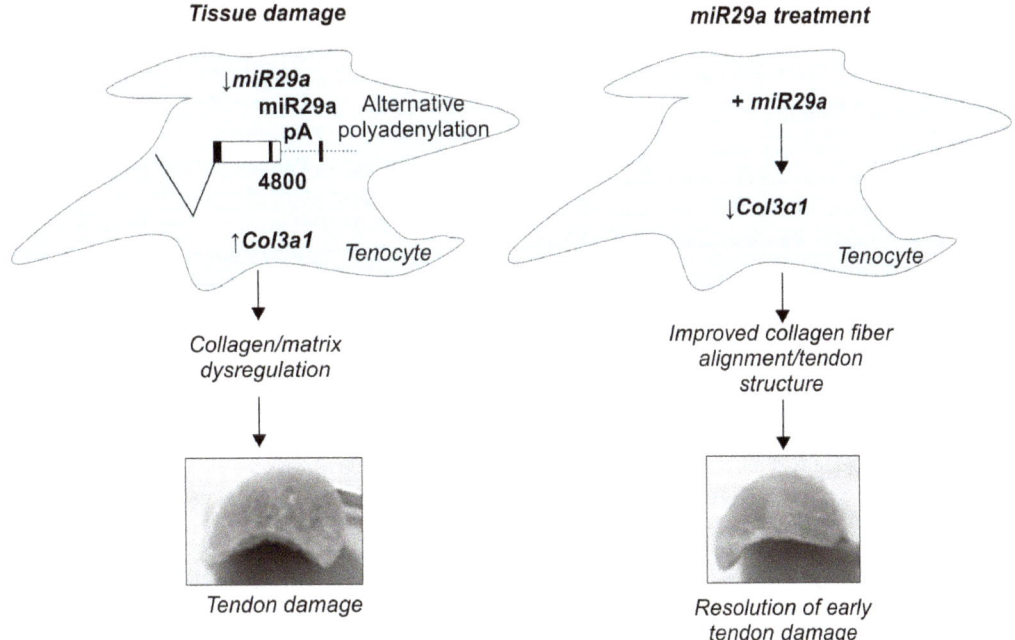

Fig. 26: Exosome therapy.

- The tenocytes were then injected into the injured tendinopathy site, which was the origin of the extensor carpi radialis brevis tendon, under the guidance of an ultrasound.
- After the autologous tenocyte injection treatment, patients with chronic lateral epicondylitis showed improved clinical function and structural repair at the origin of the common extensor tendon.

Nonbulbar Dermal Sheath Cells (Fig. 25)

- Clinical trial using fibroblasts that are isolated from the nonbulbar dermal sheath cells of a hair follicle, which produce more type I collagen than fibroblasts that are derived from adipose tissue.
- Nonbulbar dermal sheath cells will be replicated, and then reintroduced into the wounded tendons with ultrasound.
- After the injections, subjects will be assessed for pain, safety, and function, as well as changes in interstitial tears, tendon thickness, echotexture, and neovascularity.

Exosomes (Fig. 26)

- Loss of miR29a from human tendons results in an increase in collagen type 3 production, which is a key feature of tendon disease.
- The replacement of miR-29a in the damaged tendon cells in the laboratory restores collagen production to preinjury levels.
- A trial will put injections of microRNA—small molecules that help to regulate gene expression—into the tendon to decrease the production of type 3 collagen and switch to type 1.

FURTHER READING

1. Abate M, Gravare-Silbernagel K, Siljeholm C, Di Iorio A, De Amicis D, Salini V, et al. Pathogenesis of tendinopathies: inflammation or degeneration? Arthritis Res Ther. 2009;11:235.
2. Abate M, Schiavone C, Salini V, Andia I. Occurrence of tendon pathologies in metabolic disorders. Rheumatology. 2017;52:599-608.
3. Abbah SA, Spanoudes K, O'Brien T, Pandit A, Zeugolis DI. Assessment of stem cell carriers for tendon tissue engineering in pre-clinical models. Stem Cell Res Ther. 2014;5:38.
4. Ackermann PW, Renström P. Tendinopathy in sport. Sports Health. 2012;4:193-201.
5. Albers IS, Zwerver J, Diercks RL, Dekker JH, Van den Akker-Scheek I. Incidence and prevalence of lower extremity tendinopathy in a Dutch general practice population: a cross sectional study. BMC Musculoskelet Disord. 2016;17:16.
6. Andarawis-Puri N, Flatow EL, Soslowsky LJ. Tendon basic science: development, repair, regeneration, and healing. J Orthop Res. 2015;33:780.
7. Andia I, Latorre PM, Gomez MC, et al. Platelet-rich plasma in the conservative treatment of painful tendinopathy: a systematic review and meta-analysis of controlled studies. Br Med Bull 2014;110:99-115.
8. Butler DL, Juncosa-Melvin N, Boivin GP, et al. Functional tissue engineering for tendon repair: a multidisciplinary strategy using mesenchymal stem cells, bioscaffolds, and mechanical stimulation. J Orthop Res. 2008;26:5475-9.
9. Couppé C, Svensson RB, Kongsgaard M, Kovanen V, Grosset JF, Snorgaard O, et al. Human Achilles tendon glycation and function in diabetes. J Appl Physiol. 2016; 120:130-7.
10. Di Matteo B, Filardo G, Kon E, et al. Platelet-rich plasma: evidence for the treatment of patellar and Achilles tendinopathy: a systematic review. Musculoskelet Surg 2015;99:1-9.
11. Frizziero A, Oliva F, Maffulli N. Tendinopatie: Stato Dell Arte e Prospettive. Pacini Editore Medicina; Pisa, Italy; 2011.

12. Hopkins C, Fu SC, Chua E, Hu X, Rolf C, Mattila VM, et al. Critical review on the socio-economic impact of tendinopathy. Asia-Pac J Sport Med Arthrosc Rehabil Technol. 2016; 4:9-20.
13. Knobloch K. Drug-induced tendon disorders. Adv Exp Med Biol. 2016;920:229-38.
14. Krogh TP, Ellingsen T, Christensen R, et al. Ultrasound-guided injection therapy of achilles tendinopathy with platelet-rich plasma or saline: a randomized, blinded, placebo-controlled trial. Am J Sports Med. 2016;44:1990-7.
15. Lebiedziński R, Synder M, Buchcic P, et al. A randomized study of autologous conditioned plasma and steroid injections in the treatment of lateral epicondylitis. Int Orthop. 2015;39:2199-203.
16. Maffulli N, Wong J, Almekinders LC. Types and epidemiology of tendinopathy. Clin. Sports Med. 2003;22:675-92.
17. Mishra AK, Skrepnik NV, Edwards SG, et al. Efficacy of platelet-rich plasma for chronic tennis elbow: a double-blind, prospective, multicenter, randomized controlled trial of 230 patients. Am J Sports Med. 2014;42:463-71.
18. Morton S, Williams S, Valle X, Diaz-Cueli D, Malliaras P, Morrissey D. Patellar tendinopathy and potential risk factors. Clin J Sport Med. 2017;27:468-74.
19. Wesner M, Defreitas T, Bredy H, et al. A pilot study evaluating the effectiveness of platelet-rich plasma therapy for treating degenerative tendinopathies: a randomized control trial with synchronous observational cohort. PLoS One. 2016;11:e0147842.
20. Zhang J, Li B, Wang JH. The role of engineered tendon matrix in the stemness of tendon stem cells in vitro and the promotion of tendon-like tissue formation in vivo. Biomaterials. 2011;32:6972-81.

Periarthritis Shoulder

Krishna Subramanyam

Synonyms: Adhesive capsultis, Arthrofibrosis shoulder, Frozen shoulder, Periarthritis shoulder.

HISTORICAL REVIEW

Simon-Emmanuel Duplay (1896) was first person to give the initial description about periarthritis shoulder as painful restriction of range of movement of shoulder. He mentioned it as "frozen shoulder periarthritis scapula humerale". He mentioned that pathologic condition occurred in the periarticular structures. He recommended the treatment to periarthritis shoulder was manipulation under anesthesia.

Earnest Codman (1936) coined the term "frozen shoulder (FS)". He mentioned that the frozen shoulder is because of capsular pathology associated with pain and progressive loss of active and passive moments and the shoulder dysfunction is not because of calcified tendinitis.

The concept of "adhesive capsulitis" was introduced *Julius Neviaser (1945)*. He described that the basic pathology is a tight, thickened capsule adhering proximal humerus. This is due to an inflammatory reaction leading to shoulder capsular adhesion, in the axillary fold and around the neck of the humerus restricting the abduction and rotational movements of shoulder.

Simmonds (1949) further speculated that repeated wear and tear of supraspinatus tendon against acromion and coracohumeral ligament resulting increased secondary inflammation. This adds to the loss of motion at the glenohumeral joint due to continued inflammation, and therefore the disease process was not self-limiting.

Quigley (1954), observed a subgroup of patients suffering with periarthritis shoulder, had pain-free passive motion at about 45° of abduction (ABD) and near normal range of shoulder motion. This subgroup of patients is named as "Chekrein Shoulder" and have good prognosis.

Reeves (1975) observations of periarthritis shoulder after when no intervention and following the natural history disease are:
- Duration of the stiff phase and the duration of the recovery phase are directly related.
- In majority of patients the onset of the disease between 42 and 63 years.

- Management of periarthritis of shoulder is different, depending on the stage of the disease.

Periarthritis of shoulder is the result of excessive scar tissue or adhesions across the glenohumeral joint, leading to the stiffness, pain and dysfunction.

In the present clinical practice, frozen shoulder is a readily recognized by the signs and symptoms and by studying the natural course of the disease.

DEFINITION

Periarthritis is a common musculoskeletal condition involving the shoulder joint characterized by progressive painful restriction of shoulder range of movements finally resulting to shoulder stiffness. The main pathology is the formation of intra-articular and periarticular adhesions across the glenohumeral joint, leading to the stiffness, pain and shoulder dysfunction.

Frozen shoulder can be classified as either primary (idiopathic) or secondary with underlying causes. The idiopathic variety of FS has a gradual onset and slow development of symptoms, and there may not be any obvious trigger mechanisms seen. The other variety of FS is usually because of an underlying cause like shoulder trauma or prolonged shoulder immobilization which may be due to multiple shoulder pathologies.

ETIOLOGY

There is no known or obvious etiology of frozen shoulder. Commonly, FS is associated with other systemic conditions such as diabetes mellitus. Individuals with diabetes are approximately 2-4 times more likely to develop periarthritis (FS) as compared to general population. Type 1 (insulin dependent) diabetics are at higher risk for FS and it presents more severely clinically in these patients.

Other common clinical conditions associated with FS (periarthritis) are thyroid dysfunction disorders, pulmonary diseases, Parkinson's disease, surgical procedures such as radical neck dissection, neurosurgery, and cardiac surgery. In up to 60% patients with idiopathic shoulder periarthritis, history of Dupuytren's disease is seen which may suggest myeloproliferative mechanism for FS.

RISK FACTORS

Periarthritis is more common in females and among the age groups 40–60 years indicating age and gender are one of the risk factors. Patients with previous episode of shoulder periarthritis in the contralateral arm will also be more prone for the disease. Common shoulder conditions such as bicipital tenosynovitis, rotator cuff tendinitis and shoulder band syndrome results in disuse of shoulder joint and may trigger the onset of FS (periarthritis). Trauma to shoulder, be it minor or even unnoticeable is one of the known risk factors of FS pathology.

Other risk factors include immunization of the shoulder, inflammatory/autoimmune reactions, hyperthyroidism, Parkinson's disease. Universally both type 1 and 2 diabetic patients are at higher risk of developing FS (periarthritis) and prevalence of FS is approximately 10.3% and 22.4%, respectively in type 1 and 2 diabetics. The natural history of FS in diabetic patients has worse functional outcome as compared to general population without diabetes.

Although the association of FS (periarthritis shoulder) is higher in patients with the above-mentioned clinical conditions, further scientific studies need to conducted to establish the relationship between them and FS.

PATHOPHYSIOLOGY

Multiple mechanisms Immunological, inflammatory reactions have been postulated in the causation of FS (periarthritis of shoulder). The development of fibrotic changes and intra-articular adhesions appear to be mainly involved in the pathophysiology of FS (periarthritis of shoulder). The final underlying pathology in FS is capsular and intra-articular ligamentous fibrosis. The exact cause of the capsular fibrosis is not understood clearly. Basis of pathology in FS is better understood by studying the histological appearances of the synovial or subsynovial inflammatory reactions. And also increased levels of circulating immune complexes and elevation of serum C-reactive proteins levels indicating an autoimmune reaction in the development of FS. Role of cytokines in the development of FS is well studied. It was observed that both platelet-derived growth factor (PDGF) and transforming growth factor β (TGF-β) are elevated in the early stages of the disease (FS). Fibroblast proliferation is stimulated by PDGF and TGF-β promotes extracellular matrix production leading to fibrosis of capsule. The pathological process in FS is initiated by the initial hypervascular synovitis. This provokes a progressive fibroblastic response in the shoulder capsule leading to progressive capsular fibroplasias, thickening, and contracture. PDGF and TGF-β further modulate these inflammatory reactions and contribute to the pathological process in FS by both paracrine and autocrine abnormal regulation.

The series of pathological findings documented in the literature associated with periarthritis are inflammation of cytokines and adhesion of growth factors leading to rupture of tendon fibers, hypertrophy and thickening of ligamentous structures and shortening of fibrinoid changes. These lead to the immunological reactions in the synovium and finally leading to increased collagen and stiffness in the joint capsule.

In the process of pathogenesis, the cascade of immunological reactions lead to synovitis in the glenohumeral joint and finally resulting in fibrosis of shoulder joint capsule which in turn limits the glenohumeral motion and manifests as overt clinical disease.

CAUSES

Frozen shoulder (periarthritis of shoulder) can be primary (idiopathic) or secondary due to underlying shoulder or perishoulder pathology.

Shoulder joint is the articulation between head of hemerus and glenoid of scapula along with glenohumeral ligaments encased in a capsule of connective tissue. FS (periarthritis) occurs when the capsule thickens progressively and tightens around the shoulder joint. This results in restriction the shoulder joint movement associated with pain.

Any shoulder pathology resulting in chronic shoulder pain results in the development of FS. Shoulder pain can develop from any intra-articular or periarticular structures of shoulder. Common causes of chronic shoulder pain include the following:

- Rotator cuff injury to the rotator cuff tendons may develop from repetitive activity, at or above shoulder height. Usually people with rotator cuff tendinopathy may have pain in the shoulder and inhibition of shoulder movements.
- Biceps tendinopathy and an injury to the long head of tendon of the biceps muscle like in pulled shoulder may the initial triggering event for shoulder pain and thus in the development of FS.
- Damage to joint may occur from repetitive movements, active sports, aging or tedious stressful work.
- Acute injuries may cause sudden onset of shoulder pain which includes dislocations, separations, and proximal humerus fractures following which shoulder may be immobilized.
- Immobilization of upper limb following forearm and wrist fractures resulting in stiffness of shoulder (shoulder hand syndrome), if not treated may result in FS.

Along with these above causes, underlying diabetes, old age, female gender may be the different causes for the development of FS.

SIGNS

Several conditions that cause pain and the restricted shoulder joint movement. The diagnosis of FS needs the expert medical professional in shoulder maladies and differential diagnosis.

- The first and the fore most sign is pain-like burning ache in the nondermatome pattern, hyperalgesia develops, and pain does not follow a single nerve innervation pattern.
- Progressive restriction of both passive and active range of shoulder movement.
- Abduction and rotations of shoulder are more affected.
- *Trophic changes:*
  - *Early changes*: Local edema
  - *Progressive changes*: Skin thins, hair coarsens and nail thickens
  - *Late changes*: Muscle shortens and atrophies.
- Autonomic instability.
- Sensory abnormalities.
- Sleep disturbance.

SYMPTOMS

Periarthritis presents with multiple symptoms. Shoulder pain and stiffness are the primary symptoms of periarthritis. Pain may become worse during the night time or is provoked by lying in the affected side of the joint. Progressive compromise in shoulder function causes the limitation of daily activities restricting even simple activities such as combing, dressing more so with overhead activities.

Neviaser described different stages of FS as follows:
- *Stage 1*: Inflammation or pre-adhesive stage
- *Stage 2*: Freezing or painful stage
- *Stage 3*: Frozen or stiffness stage
- *Stage 4*: Thawing or chronic stage.

All these stages in FS progress typically over period of months to a year and more. Without the purposeful effort to restore the motion this may become a permanent problem. This will affect the daily activities for the living especially the external rotation. Other directional movements of shoulder are restricted depending on the area of the capsule most affected. Pain may be diffuse all over the shoulder, and occasionally extends along the biceps tendon, especially while resting in bed, however in most cases pain is not localized.

Stage 1: Stage 1 is typically mimics shoulder impingement syndrome and pain is the predominant feature. Shoulder movements are well preserved with occasional restricted movement of the joint. Sometimes underlying rotator cuff tendinitis may be the only cause of pain. This is the preadhesive phase and usually lasts for a duration of less than 3 months. This phase consists of mild-to-moderate pain, mild limitation of range of motion (ROM), and inability lying on the affected shoulder.

Stage 2: The main feature of this stage is progressively worsening shoulder pain. The characteristic features in this stage are severe night pain and significant loss of both active as well as passive shoulder movements in all directions. This phase spans over a period of 3–9 months.

Stage 3: In this stage, pain reduces. But shoulder stiffness and movement restriction continue to increase. Shoulder range of motion is typically reduced. Symptoms in this stage persist for 9–14 months. Nocturnal pain along shoulder stiffness persists.

Stage 4: This stage is featured by spontaneous "thawing". The shoulder movements improve slowly and the shoulder responds to stretching exercises and treatment. As the capsular structure remodels, there is gradual, progressive return of shoulder range of movement to normal or near normal. It occurs over a period of 15–24 months.

The natural history of FS (periarthritis shoulder) is its tendency to progress regardless of medical intervention. The crux of the treatment in FS is to maintain the shoulder movement and pain management. If this is achieved, in spite of an almost inevitable progression of this condition, the shoulder may be returned to normal or pre-disease stage avoiding the permanent loss shoulder motion that may result from a bout with a frozen shoulder **(Figs. 1A to C)**.

DIAGNOSIS

The diagnosis of FS (periarthritis) is usually done clinical. Different imaging techniques such as real-time ultrasound of shoulder, magnetic resonance imaging (MRI) and MR shoulder arthrogram (MRA) confirm the diagnosis of FS. Shoulder MRI reveals the presence of associated shoulder pathologies such as rotator cuff abnormalities and intra-articular pathologies. Assessment of severity of the disease in terms of capsular thickening and thickening of coracoacromial ligament may be done by shoulder MRI.

Imaging: Imaging is the most useful technique especially in less severe clinical symptoms and that will minimize the misdiagnosis.

Plain radiography: In patients with FS (periarthritis), plain radiographs may be normal. But sometimes plain X-rays may reveal associated features of shoulder degeneration (osteophytes and loose bodies), or calcific tendinitis and other periarticular calcifications **(Fig. 2)**.

Conventional arthrography: Shoulder arthrography consists of injecting a radiopaque dye into the shoulder joint followed by obtaining standard X-rays to study intra-articular pathology. This procedure is used for both diagnostic and therapeutic reasons.

Ultrasonography: Real time, dynamic ultrasonography of shoulder helps not only in diagnosing the various intra-articular shoulder pathologies, but also to quantify the stage of the disease. The limitation of this mode of investigation is

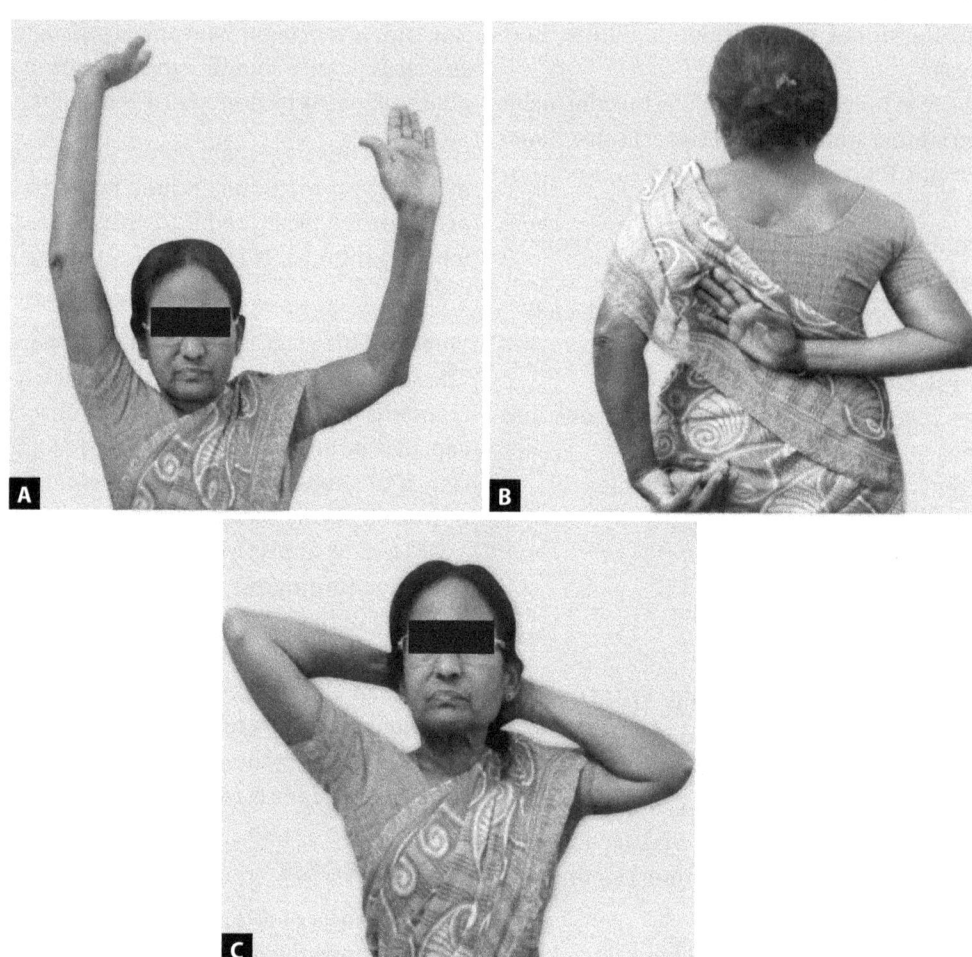

Figs. 1A to C: Clinical photographs of the patient with periarthritis shoulder showing the restriction of joint movements. (A) Restriction of abduction; (B) Restriction of internal rotation; (C) Restriction of external rotation.

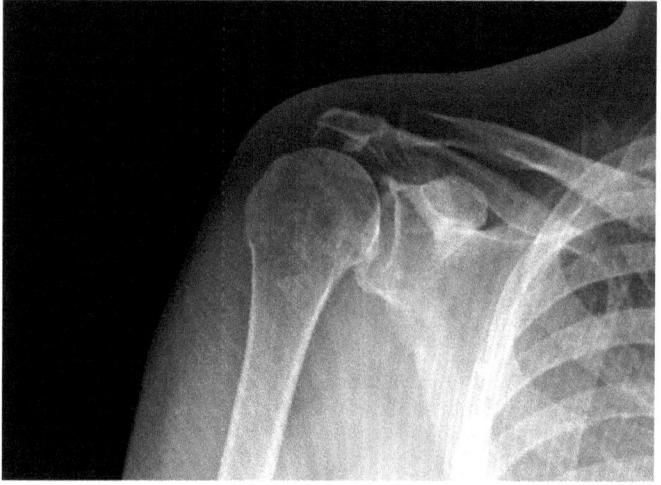

Fig. 2: X-ray anteroposterior view of right shoulder.

that it is observer dependent. Therefore role of ultrasound in the diagnosis of FS (periarthritis) is controversial and uncertain. Dynamic evaluation of shoulder helps in understanding the extent of movement of supraspinatus tendon under the acromion process and thus helps to know the extent of cuff excursion in FS. Ultrasonography also helps to measure the thickening of various intra-articular ligamentous structures **(Figs. 3A to C)**.

Magnetic Resonance Imaging and Magnetic Resonance Arthroscopy

Shoulder MRI is one of the best imaging techniques to diagnose FS (periarthritis). The specificity and the sensitivity of MRI will be very much higher. MRI with intravenous administration of contrast agents enhances the capsular and synovial structures related to the on-going inflammation. Enhancement in the postcontrast axillary pouch in MRI correlates to the reduced range of motion of the shoulder and helps in severity of the disease.

MR arthrogram of shoulder detects abnormalities of rotator cuff. Coracohumeral ligament thickening and capsular thickening at the rotator cuff interval has high specificity but low sensitivity in the diagnosis of FS (periarthritis).

The diagnosis of periarthritis is mainly based on the clinical findings. Plain radiography is usually normal and has no diagnostic value in periarthritis. Dynamic ultrasound can be used primarily to detect thickening of the coracohumeral

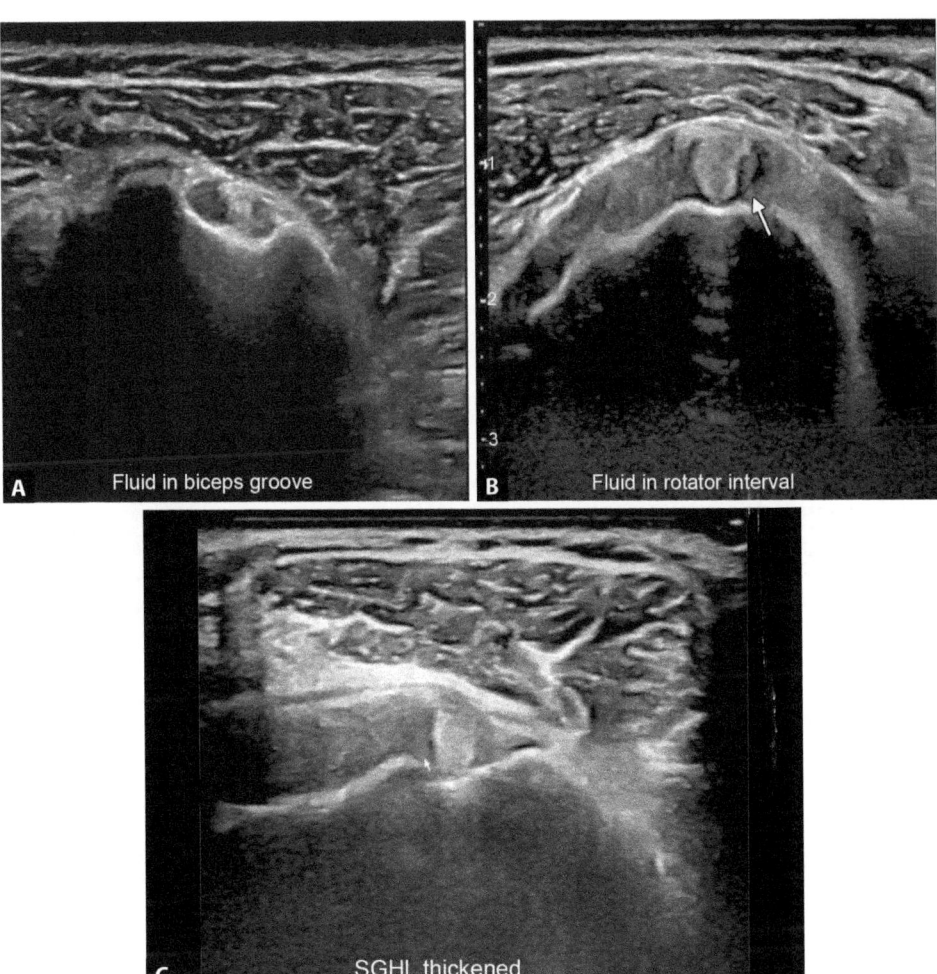

Figs. 3A to C: (A and B) Arrow showing biceps tendon with adjacent hypoechoic thickening of rotator interval suggestive of periarthritis shoulder; (C) USG image showing thickened superior glenohumeral ligament (SGHL).

ligament and synovial hypertrophy at the rotator cuff interval. MRI and MRA have demonstrated high diagnostic value in detecting the features of FS (periarthritis) **(Figs. 4A to D)**.

MANAGEMENT

Treatment in FS (periarthritis) is aimed mainly at relief of pain, improving the range of movement of shoulder, decreasing the duration of recovery and simultaneously improving the quality of the recovery. Patients with diabetes and who are undergoing shoulder, arm and cardiothoracic surgeries are the high-risk group. In these patients, early shoulder mobilization is of prime importance in the preventing the shoulder stiffness. Majority of patients of FS present in the 2nd stage of the disease with significant stiffness of shoulder. Controlling the pain is the first priority in treating these patients. Inadequate pain relief results in poor rehabilitation and poor compliance to treatment. Mode of treatment changes depending upon the stage of presentation of the disease. If the disease progresses in spite of treatment or the condition worsens, an alternate treatment protocol needs to be considered.

Mobilization of shoulder is the most important component of treating FS (periarthritis) as immobility worsens the disease. The protocols of treatment in FS include supervised physical therapy (electrotherapy and shoulder exercises), nonsteroidal anti-inflammatory medication. Intra-articular and periarticular steroid injections are given in persistent FS cases. In severe cases with stiff shoulder, manipulation under anesthesia is an alternate treatment option. From early stages to severe conditions of the disease, over all treatment options in FS (periarthritis) include shoulder movement restoring exercises, mobilization, manipulation and myofascial release, steroid injections, manipulation under anesthesia and finally arthroscopic capsular release (ACR) surgery.

Conservative Treatment

- *Oral medication:* Analgesics, i.e., nonsteroidal anti-inflammatory drugs (NSAIDs) are widely in the treatment of FS (periarthritis) as the first line of treatment particularly in the first stage of the disease. NSAIDs give only short-term pain relief during this inflammatory

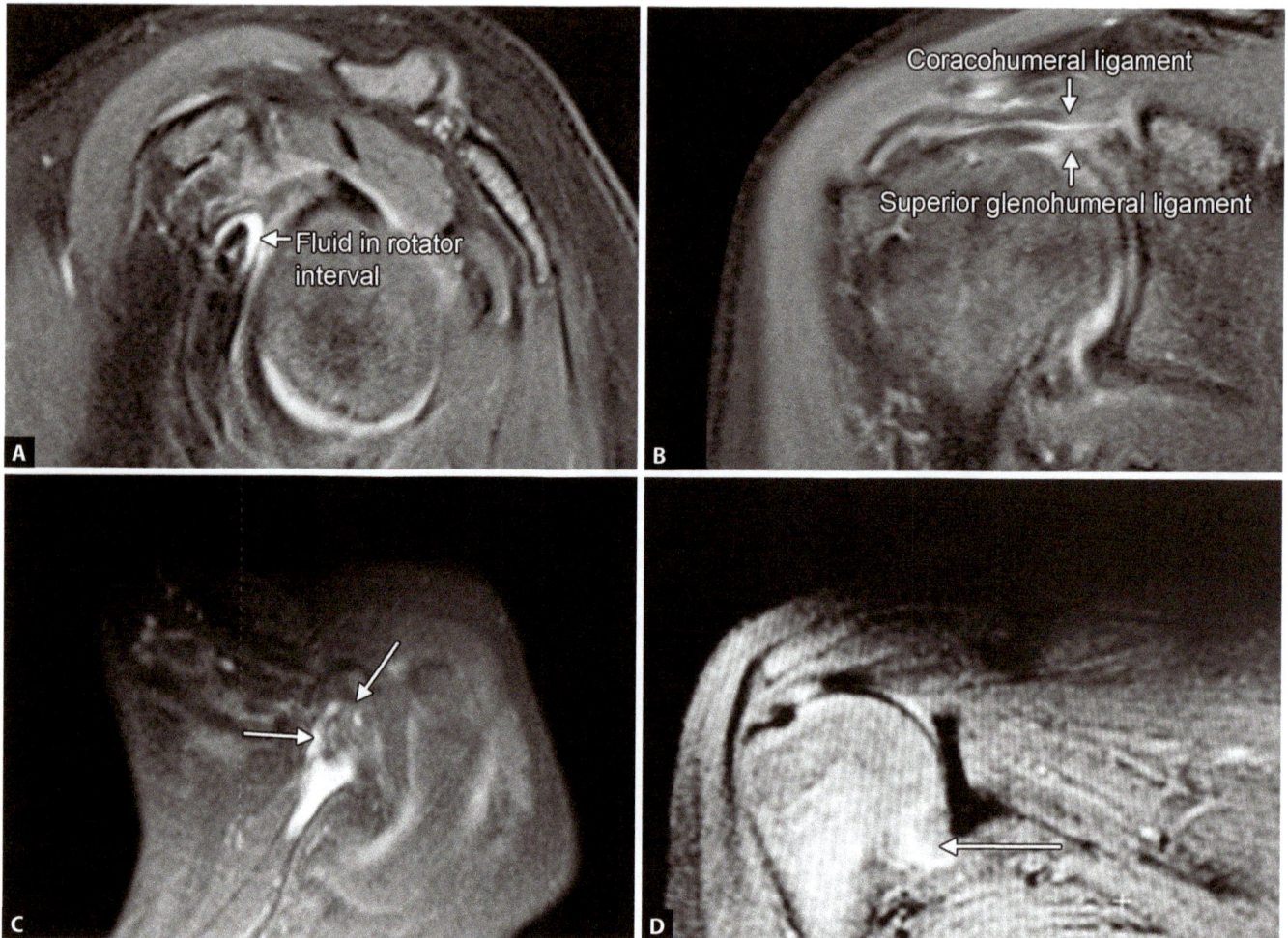

Figs. 4A to D: (A) MRI image showing fluid in rotator interval; (B) MRI image showing thickened coracohumeral ligament; (C) MRI image showing thickened superior glenohumeral ligament (SGHL); (D) MRI image showing thickened inferior glenohumeral ligament (IGHL).

stage. During this stage, oral corticosteroids are known to show to improve the pain to an extent and shoulder range of movement in short term. Associated hot fomentations and assisted manual mobilization shoulder along with NSAIDs are effective and useful. Oral medication may not be effective in stage 3 FS (periarthritis). A recent systemic review also indicated that oral steroid/medication provide significant short-term improvement but the effect may not be long lasting.

- *Intra-articular shoulder injections:* Corticosteroid injections into the shoulder joint are commonly used in the treatment of FS (periarthritis). These injections are known to decrease the inflammation process and relieve the symptoms. The immediate improvement of shoulder range of movement is attributed to the effect of the local anesthetic medication but it reduces the pain and the muscle spasm. The dose and the number of injections may vary from person to person depending on the stage of FS (periarthritis). The effect of the corticosteroid injections lasts up to 6 weeks indicating these can be used in the initial stages of the treatment. There are no uniform results in the literature. Sodium hyaluronate injection into the shoulder joint is relatively new intervention for the management of periarthritis. These are beneficial in the persistent shoulder pain especially when the main reason is osteoarthritis of the glenohumeral joint. Lin-Fen Hsiesh et al. showed that the treatment with sodium hyaluronate injections did not produce significant added benefit for the treatment of periarthritis patients.

- *Physiotherapy:* Physiotherapy is considered as a very useful part of treatment protocol in the relief of symptoms and maintaining shoulder joint movements by preventing capsular contraction or stretching the already contracted capsule. Various interventions used in physical therapy are like local hot or cold application, stretching of shoulder by both active assisted and passive shoulder exercises, gentle mobilization techniques, multidirectional stretching exercises, educating the patient about the exercises and the monitoring home exercises, laser therapy, electrotherapy like transcutaneous electrical nerve stimulation (TENS) and proprioceptive neuro-muscular facilitation techniques (PNF) **(Figs. 5A to G)**. Shoulder massaging, iontophoresis and photophoresis are not shown to be effective uniformly and therefore

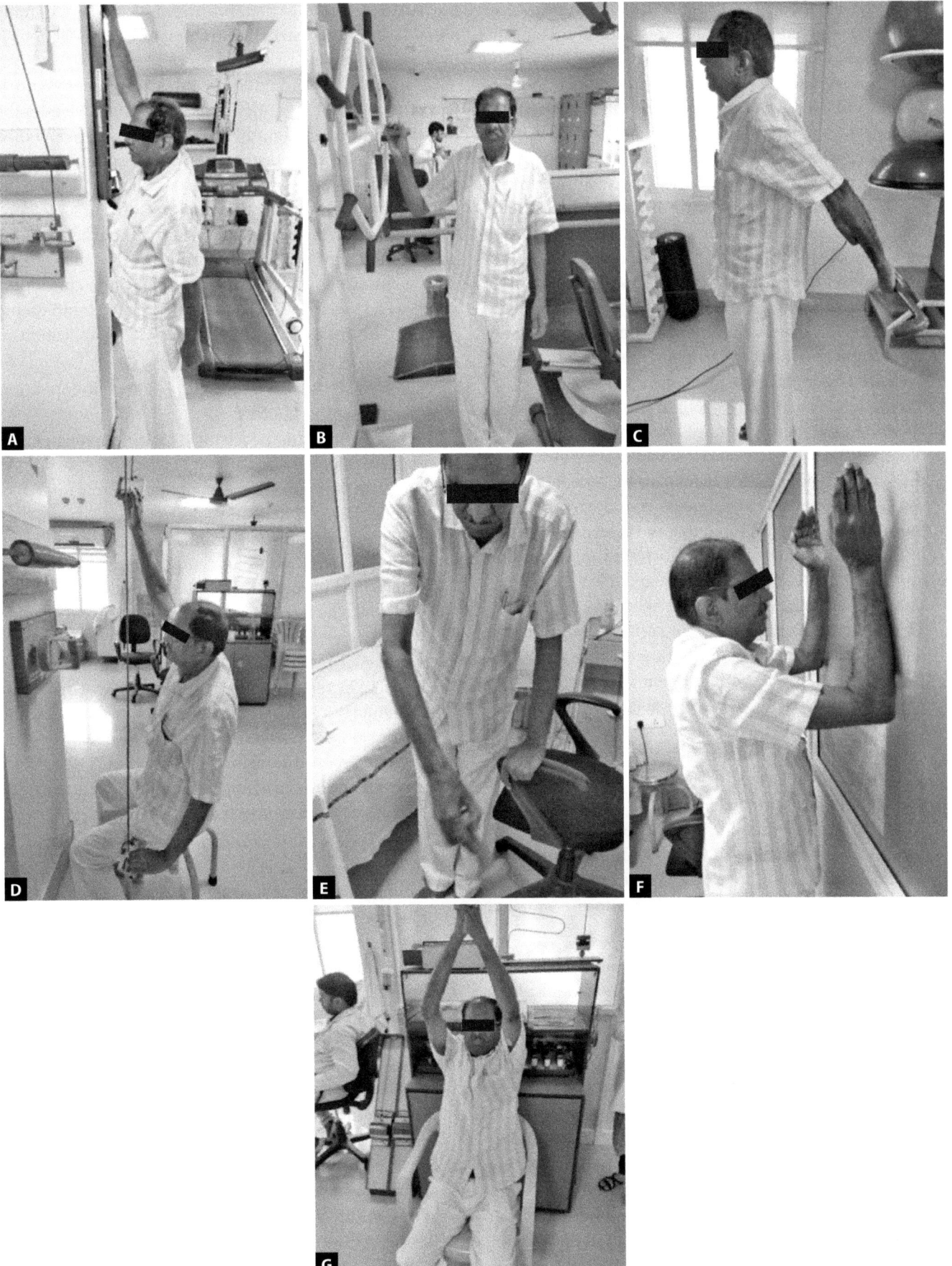

Figs. 5A to G: (A) Stepper exercises; (B) Wheel exercises; (C) Subscapular strengthening; (D) Pulley exercise; (E) Pendulum exercises; (F) Infraspinatus strengthening; (G) Active forward flexion exercises.

have no role in FS. Multidirectional stretching exercises of shoulder include pendulum stretch, towel stretch, and finger walk cross body reach, armpit reach. Therra band exercises include strengthening of periscapular muscles by outward and inward exercise band in 90° rotations.

Selection of a particular physical treatment method for FS (periarthritis) involves careful consideration patient's symptoms, stage of the disease at the time of presentation and understanding the pattern of restricted shoulder movements. Patient education is very important as a part of treatment and it is mandatory to explain and counsel the patient about the disease progression, pathology of the disease and self-limiting nature of the condition. It is equally important to convey to the patient that complete shoulder movements may not be achieved even after rigorous physical therapy.

- *Suprascapular nerve block:* Pain relief by nerve block to glenohumeral joint is achieved by suprascapular nerve block (SNB), a branch from the suprascapular nerve near the scapular notch. This block can be repeated twice weekly for a total of 2–4 treatments. A study conducted by Jonnes et al., 1999 indicated that the therapeutic effects of SNB to intra-articular corticosteroid injection and found that the technique was safe and effective and has score benefits over intra-articular injections.
- *Manipulation under anesthesia (MUA)*: Manipulation under anesthesia considered as a standard treatment for FS (periarthritis). *Duplay* in the year 1872 proposed this procedure and described the advantages of MUA such as efficient time, cost and technically easy procedure. If the conservative treatment fails, MUA can be the standard treatment for periarthritis. MUA is to be performed by a trained medical professional under anesthesia under gentle controlled manner. It may be associated with complications such as proximal humerus fractures, shoulder dislocation, rotor cuff tears or propagation of already existing cuff tear and injuries to the brachial plexus.

MUA procedure: MUA is performed in patient in supine position, under the general anesthesia and interscalene nerve block. A methodical and the fixed order of shoulder manipulation is recommended. During the entire procedure, small lever arm and scapular stabilization is highly recommended. Manipulation includes flexion, abduction, external rotation in 90° abduction, followed by internal rotation in 90° abduction and horizontal abduction with dorsal compression and external rotation in neutral. During the procedure, a typical cracking sound, definitive snap or characteristic feeling of tissue giving away is perceived. Manipulation is discontinued, if crepitant motion does not occur.

However, there are some complications involved with MUA-like fracture of the humeral shaft or the neck, scapular fracture, rotor cuff tearing, bronchial plexus nerve injury, labral lesions and osteochondral fractures. So MUA has its own advantages and risks also.

A study was conducted on MUA in patients with FS (periarthritis). The results concluded that considerable increase in ROM and improved constant score, reduction in pain and around 85% of satisfaction are possible with MUA in patient with FS (periarthritis). The overall complication rate of 0.4% was found and a reintervention rate of 14%. However, all but one study lacked a control group without intervention. Based on this review, there is hardly any evidence in favor of or against MUA. One needs to careful when considering MUA in FS (periarthritis) because the relative mild natural course of the disease and potential serious complications.

Proposed criteria before proceeding to MUA:
1. Failed conservative treatment and difficult to cope with a stiff and painful shoulder
2. Primary idiopathic periarthritis with obvious clinical progression of the disease
3. More than 50% reduction of shoulder external rotation as compared to contralateral shoulder
4. Persistent symptoms of 3 months and more and failure to respond to an intra-articular corticosteroid injection
Initiation of immediate shoulder physiotherapy after MUA is usually recommended to avoid a loss of shoulder range of movement in the initial weeks after MUA.
5. *Shoulder distension and hydrodilatation:* Andren and Lundberg in 1965 described the technique of distending the shoulder joint capsule by injecting contrast medium and/or saline solution under pressure. This procedure involves hydrodilatation of shoulder joint which result an adhesiolysis and hyluronic injection and/or corticosteroid under anesthesia.

Steps in distension and hydrodilatation procedure (**Figs. 6A to I**):
- Under anesthesia, with patient in supine position
- Shoulder arthrography is done under the guidance of image intensifier
- 80–100 mL of normal saline is infused to dilate shoulder joint
- Shoulder joint is taken through smooth arc of movement in all directions while the assistant surgeon stabilizes the scapula
- The standard steps of movements are abduction, external rotation, internal rotation, adduction and flexion and extension
- During the entire arc of movement, crepitus can be heard and a feel of giving away is felt as the intra-articular adhesions break.

Postprocedure rehabilitation involves the usage of oral antibiotics, initially assisted active and passive range of movements. Active assisted shoulder range of movements are initiated as early as possible as the pain allows. In third

Chapter 24: Periarthritis Shoulder

week, isomeric shoulder exercises are to be started followed by shoulder strengthening exercises.

Hydrodilatation of shoulder in patients with resistant FS (periarthritis shoulder) is very effective, minimally invasive, cost-effective. It is a day-care procedure with early return to physical therapy and minimization of complication of manipulation under anesthesia such as fractures, dislocations capsular tears and rotor cuff tears.

Surgical Treatment

Surgical treatment in FS is indicated in patients with resistant periarthritis of shoulder with persistent shoulder stiffness and when all the other forms of conventional treatments failed to yield improvement. The surgery involves removal of intra-articular adhesions and release of contracted capsular structures. This is achieved either by arthroscopic or open surgery.

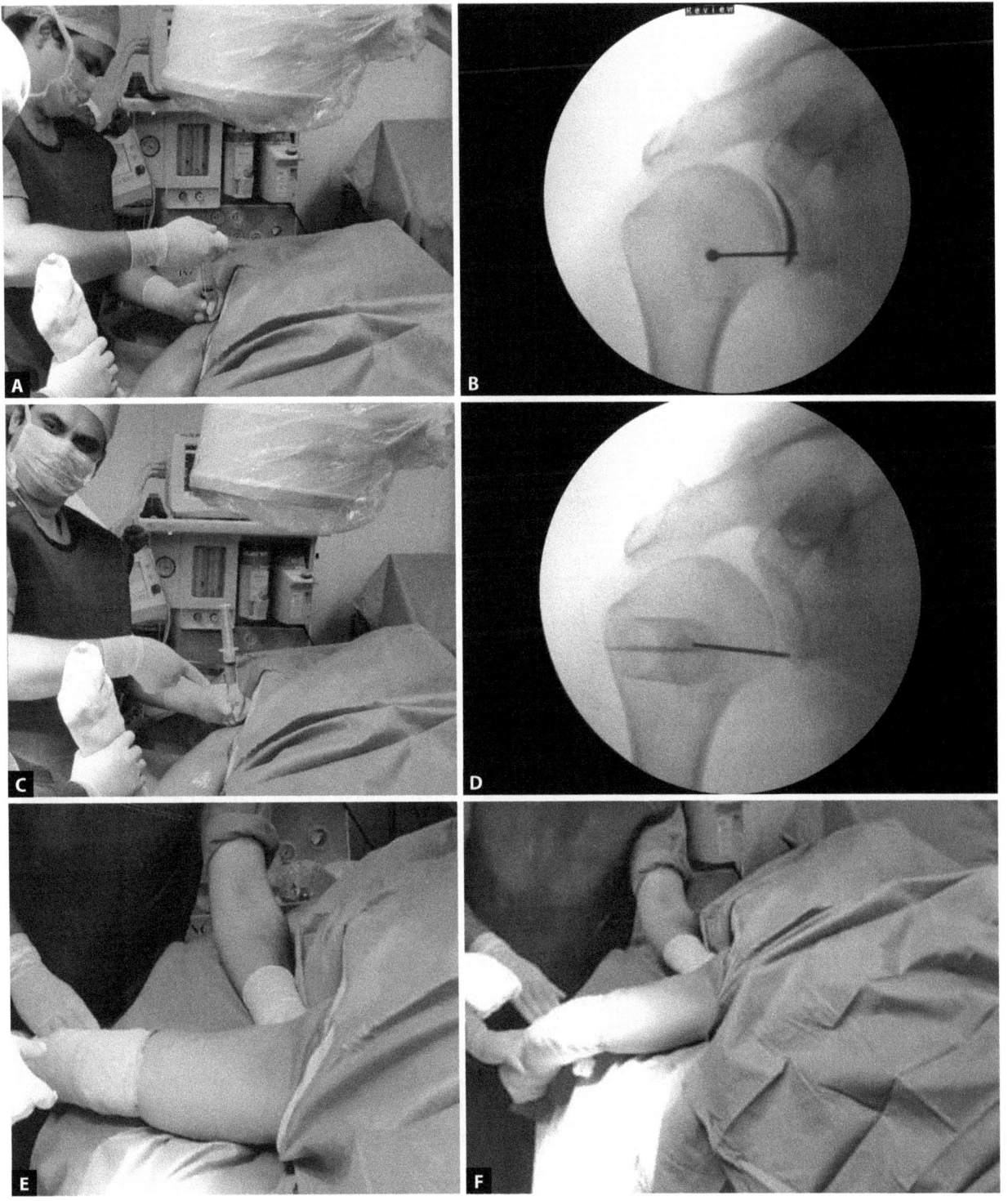

Figs. 6A to F

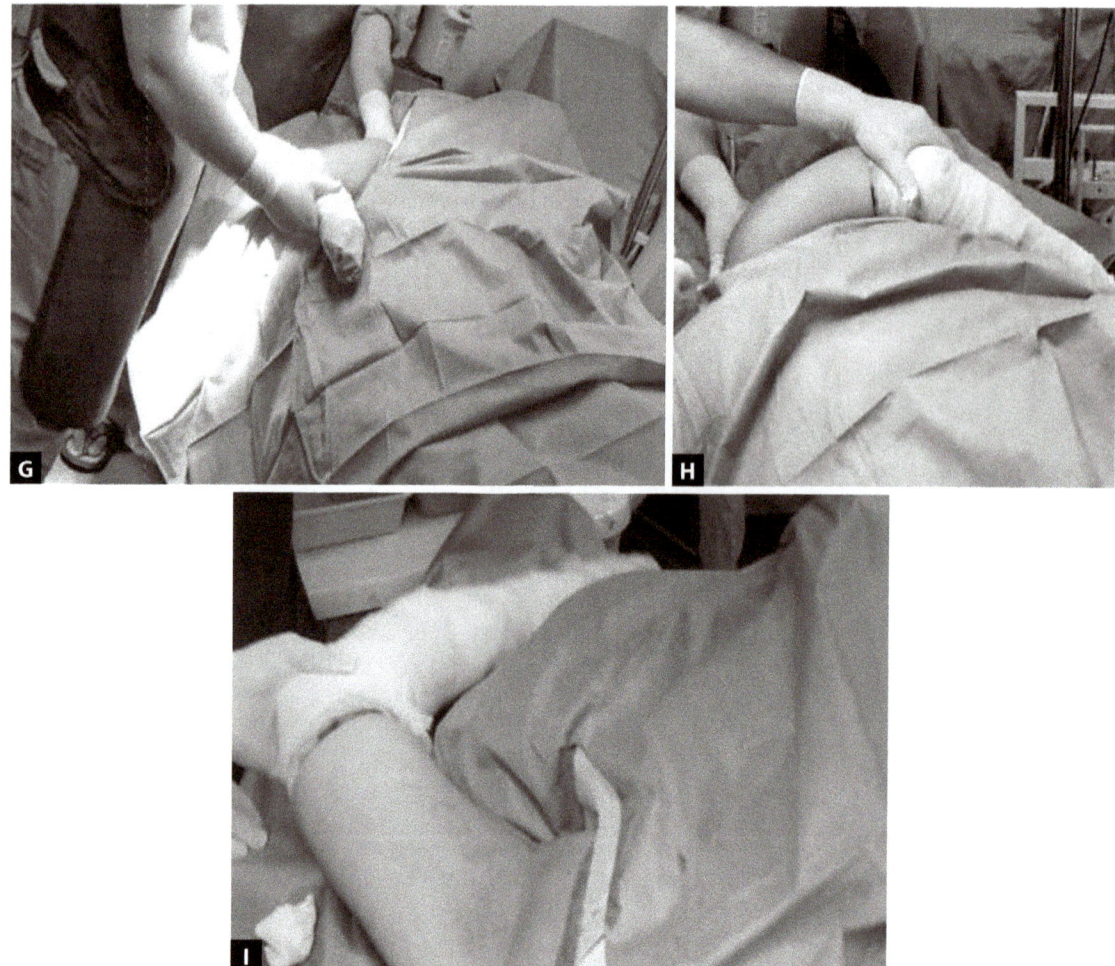

Figs. 6G to I

Figs. 6A to I: (A) Placement of needle under C-ARM guidance; (B) *C-ARM image:* Arthrography; (C) Injecting normal saline; (D) Image showing distension of shoulder joint; (E) Abduction range of movement; (F) External rotation in 90° abduction; (G) Internal rotation in 90°; (H) Complete adduction; (I) Complete abduction.

Arthroscopic Capsular Release

Conti in 1979 first described ACR. Initial techniques described only anterior and inferior shoulder capsular release arthroscopically. But recent studies favor a complete circumferential (360°) shoulder capsular release. Arthroscopic surgery is more popular nowadays which permits both evaluation of glenohumeral or subacromial disease and addresses synovitis component.

Arthroscopic capsular release procedure **(Figs. 7A to K):**
ACR involves the following steps:
- Patient is positioned either in beach-chair or the lateral decubitus position with the arm suspended in traction.
- The advantage of beach-chair position is that it is easier to assess the shoulder range of motion during surgery. But accessing the inferior capsule is difficult.
- Under arthroscopic visualization, the capsular release is performed with a radiofrequency probe and a basket punch circumferentially.
- Sequences of capsular release are the structures in the rotator interval and the anterior capsule must be released first. The anterior capsule is released along with thickened middle and inferior glenohumeral ligaments.
- The release of superior capsule is carried out parallel to the joint surface until the muscular fibers of the supraspinatus seen.
- Then release of the posterior inferior aspect of the capsule is carried out.
- The advantage of arthroscopic capsular release in the lateral decubitus position is that it provides a clear view of the inferior capsule, which facilitates a complete, 360° capsular release and mitigates the need for any manipulation under anesthesia.

Arthroscopic capsular release procedure has its own advantages and disadvantages. The ACR yields definitive results in patients with resistant FS (periarthritis) ensuring substantial and rapid improvement in shoulder range of movement and pain associated with lower risk of complications.

Open surgical capsular release: This procedure involves excision of thickened and contracted coracohumeral ligament with immediate improvement of the external rotation deficit. But with the development and advancement of arthroscopic techniques, open release is nowadays rarely performed. The literature suggests that open release could be used for recalcitrant cases of FS (periarthritis) and good results with complete pain relief and full ROM restoration is observed.

CONCLUSION

Frozen shoulder otherwise called as periarthritis of shoulder is a common shoulder problem in day-to-day clinical practice. This condition is characterized by progressive painful restriction of shoulder joint in all directions. The underlying pathology is not clearly understood, but inflammatory pathology is commonly described. The

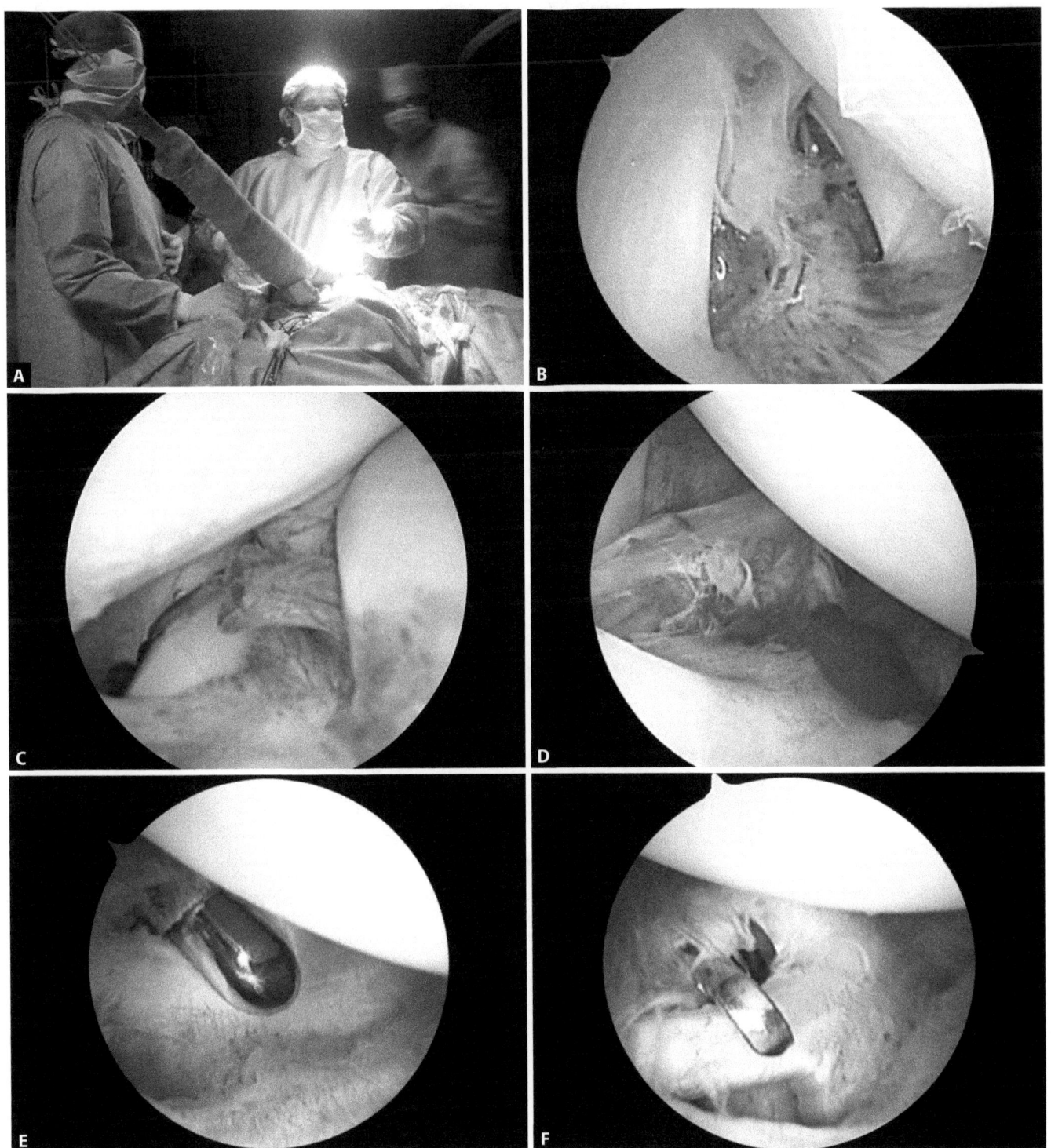

Figs. 7A to F

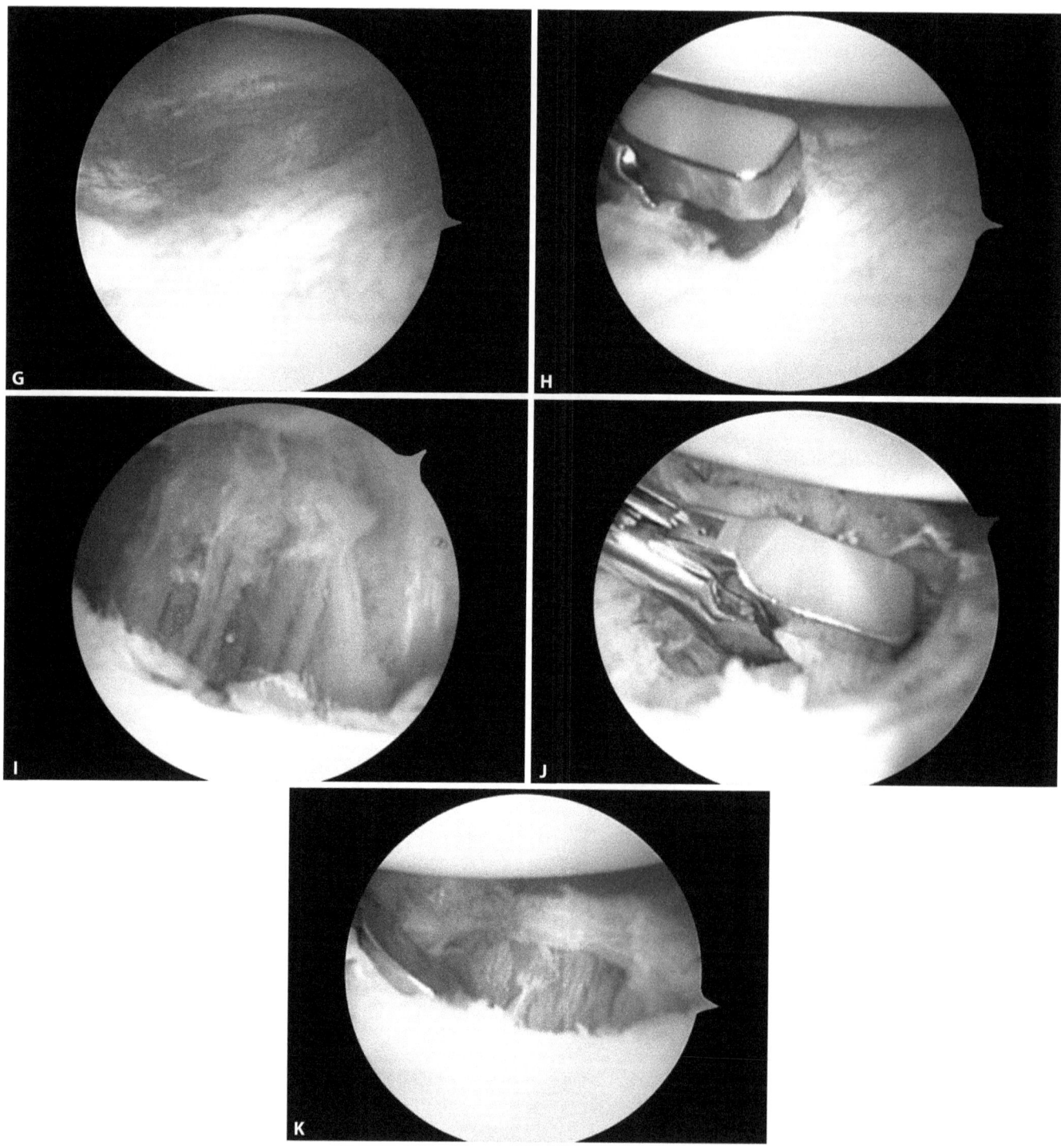

Figs. 7G to K

Figs. 7A to K: (A) Arthroscopic capsular release (ACR): Patient in lateral decubitus position; (B) Contracted rotator interval; (C) Synovitis of the rotator interval; (D) Contracted anterior capsule; (E) Middle glenohumeral ligament; (F) Dividing the middle glenohumeral ligament; (G) Contracted inferior capsule; (H) Releasing of anterior-inferior capsule; (I) Complete resection of posterior capsule; (J) Inferior capsule resection by using punch; (K) Inferior capsule resection.

main feature is thickening and contraction of shoulder capsule which along with the inflammatory reactions cause pain and restriction shoulder range of movements. FS is commonly associated with diabetes. The natural history of FS is self-limiting disease featured with four clinical stages spanning over few months. Diagnosis of FS is essentially clinical. But ultrasound of shoulder, MRI of shoulder may help in understanding the underlying intra-articular shoulder pathologies. Conservative treatment of FS includes NSAIDs, physical therapy, intra-articular steroid injections. If the conservative treatment fails careful manipulation of shoulder under anesthesia is an option followed by shoulder mobilization. More recent treatment for FS includes distention hydrodilatation of shoulder which is more effective than manipulation. In resistant cases of FS, surgical release of contracted shoulder capsular structures either by arthroscopy guided or open surgery is the choice of treatment.

FURTHER READING

1. Arkkila PE, Kantola IM, Viikari JS, Rönnemaa T. Shoulder capsulitis in type I and II diabetic patients: association with diabetic complications and related diseases. Ann Rheum Dis. 1996;55(12):907-14.
2. Arroll B, Goodyear-Smith F. Corticosteroid injections for painful shoulder: a meta-analysis. Br J Gen Pract. 2005; 55(512):224-8.
3. Codman EA. The Shoulder. Boston: Thomas Todd Co.; 1934. pp. 123-77.
4. Dehghan A, Pishgooei N, Salami MA, Nafisi-moghadam R, Rahimpour S, Soleimani H, et al. Comparison between NSAID and intra-articular corticosteroid injection in frozen shoulder of diabetic patients: a randomized clinical trial. Experiment Clin Endocrinol Diab. 2013;121(02):75-9.
5. Dennis L, Brealey S, Rangan A, Rookmoneea M, Watson J. Managing idiopathic frozen shoulder: a survey of health professionals' current practice and research priorities. Shoulder Elbow. 2010;2(4):294-300.
6. Dias R, Cutts S, Massoud S. Frozen shoulder. BMJ. 2005; 331(7530):1453-6.
7. Favejee MM, Huisstede BM, Koes BW. Frozen shoulder: the effectiveness of conservative and surgical interventions: systematic review. Br J Sport Med. 2011;45(1):49-56.
8. Green S, Buchbinder R, Glazier R, Forbes A. Systematic review of randomised controlled trials of interventions for painful shoulder: selection criteria, outcome assessment, and efficacy. BMJ. 1998;316(7128):354-60.
9. Hamdan T, Al-Essa K. Manipulation under anaesthesia for the treatment of frozen shoulder. Int Orthopaed. 2003;27(2):107-9.
10. Hanchard NC, Goodchild L, Thompson J, O'brien T, Davison D, Richardson C. Evidence-based clinical guidelines for the diagnosis, assessment, and physiotherapy management of contracted (frozen) shoulder: quick reference summary. Physiotherapy. 2012;98(2):117-20.
11. Harris G, Bou-Haidar P, Harris C. Adhesive capsulitis: review of imaging and treatment. J Med Imag Radia Oncol. 2013;57(6):633-43.
12. Holloway GB, Schenk T, Williams GR, Ramsey ML, Iannotti JP. Arthroscopic capsular release for the treatment of refractory postoperative or post-fracture shoulder stiffness. JBJS. 2001;83(11):1682-7.
13. Homsi C, Bordalo-Rodrigues M, Da Silva JJ, Stump XM. Ultrasound in adhesive capsulitis of the shoulder: is assessment of the coracohumeral ligament a valuable diagnostic tool? Skelet Radiol. 2006;35(9):673-8.
14. Hsieh LF, Hsu WC, Lin YJ, Chang HL, Chen CC, Huang V. Addition of intra-articular hyaluronate injection to physical therapy program produces no extra benefits in patients with adhesive capsulitis of the shoulder: a randomized controlled trial. Archives of Physical Medicine and Rehabilitation. 2012;93(6):957-64.
15. Kraal T, Beimers L, The B, Sievervelt I, van den Bekerom M, Eygendaal D. Manipulation under anaesthesia for frozen shoulders: outdated technique or well-established quick fix? EFORT Open Rev. 2019;4(3):98-109.
16. Lee JC, Sykes C, Saifuddin A, Connell D. Adhesive capsulitis: sonographic changes in the rotator cuff interval with arthroscopic correlation. Skelet Radiolo. 2005;34(9):522-7.
17. Lundberg BJ. The frozen shoulder: clinical and radiographical observations the effect of manipulation under general anesthesia structure and glycosaminoglycan content of the joint capsule local bone metabolism. Acta Orthopaedica Scandinavica. 1969; 40(Suppl 119):1-59.
18. Manske RC, Proshaka D. Diagnmosis and management of adhesive capsulitis. Curr Rev Musculoskelet Med. 2008; 1(3):180-9.
19. Mengiardi B, Pfirrmann CW, Gerber C, Hodler J, Zanetti M. Frozen shoulder: MR arthrographic findings. Radiology. 2004; 233(2):486-92.
20. Nesiaser AS, Neviaser RJ. Adhesive capsulitis of the shoulder. J Am Acad Orthop Surg. 2011;19:536-42.
21. Neviaser JS. Adhesive capsulitis of the shoulder: a study of the pathological findings in periarthritis of the shoulder. JBJS. 1945;27(2):211-22.
22. Omari A, Bunker TD. Open surgical release for frozen shoulder: surgical findings and results of the release. J Shoulder Elbow Surg. 2001;10(4):353-7.
23. Quigley TB. Checkrein shoulder: a type of frozen shoulder diagnosis and treatment by manipulation and ACTH or cortisone. New Engl J Med. 1954;250(5):188-92.
24. Reeves B. The natural history of the frozen shoulder syndrome. Scandinavian J Rheumatol. 1975;4(4):193-6.
25. Rizk TE, Gavant ML, Pinals RS. Treatment of adhesive capsulitis (frozen shoulder) with arthrographic capsular distension and rupture. Arch Physc Med Rehab. 1994; 75(7):803-7.
26. Rizk TE, Pinals RS. Frozen shoulder. In: Seminars in Arthritis and Rheumatism. Philadelphia: WB Saunders; 1982. pp. 440-52.
27. Sattar MA, Luqman WA. Periarthritis: another duration-related complication of diabetes mellitus. Diabetes Care. 1985;8(5):507-10.
28. Shaffer B, Tibone JE, Kerlan RK. Frozen shoulder: a long-term follow-up. J Bone Joint Surg (Am). 1992;74(5):738-46.
29. Simmonds FA. Shoulder pain with particular reference to the "frozen" shoulder. J Bone Joint Surg (British). 1949; 31(3):426-32.
30. Snow M, Boutros I, Funk L. Posterior arthroscopic capsular release in frozen shoulder. Arthroscopy. 2009;25(1):19-23.
31. Tamai K, Akutsu M, Yano Y. Primary frozen shoulder: brief review of pathology and imaging abnormalities. J Orthop Sci. 2014; 19(1):1-5.
32. Tanaka T, Morimoto Y, Masumi S, Tominaga K, Ohba T. Utility of frequency-selective fat saturation T2-weighted MR images for the detection of joint effusion in the temporomandibular joint. Dentomaxillofac Radiol. 2002;31(5):305-12.
33. Wassef MR. Suprascapular nerve block: a new approach for the management of frozen shoulder. Anaesthesia. 1992; 47(2):120-4.

25.1 Myofascial Pain Syndrome

SS Jha, Lalit Kishore

INTRODUCTION

Myofascial pain (MP) is a chronic painful condition which involves muscles and its covering fascia. Muscle pain and spasm is common presenting symptom which is usually focal and in asymmetric areas. It can originate in either single muscle or in muscle groups.

It is defined by regional pain originating from hyper-irritable spots located within taut bands of skeletal muscle, known as myofascial trigger points (MTrPs). This taut band commonly developed by repetitive strain or overuse of particular muscle or by acute injury. It usually subsides by itself within few weeks. But if it persists and require medical treatment, then it is called myofascial pain syndrome. This pain differs from fibromyalgia pain which is symmetric and widespread, however, pain arising from muscle is a potent stimulus for central sensitization, and myofascial pain foci may play a role in the initiation and maintenance of a sensitized nervous system in some fibromyalgia patients.

Myofascial Trigger Point

It is a very small localized hard spot in a discrete band of hardness in a muscle which is very tender. Characteristic features of myofascial pain syndrome are:
- Tenderness at focal point
- On palpation, similar pain can be reproduced
- Taut band palpation in adjacent muscle
- Decrease range of motion in involved muscle
- No atrophy in involved muscle but weakness may be present
- Often referred pain (RP) on continued pressure over trigger point.

Types of Trigger Points

- *Active trigger point*: A tender point which lies within the muscle causing localize or regional pain.
- *Latent trigger point*: It is not active but has potential to become turn into an active trigger point.
- *Secondary trigger point*: It is a localized point in a muscle, which is highly irritable and it may become active after stimulation or overload of a different muscle.
- *Satellite myofascial point*: It is a trigger point which becomes inactive due to involvement of muscle in another trigger pain.

HISTORY

Kellgren, in 1930, studied the pain referral patterns after injecting hypertonic saline in muscles and ligament and first used the term 'myotomal' and 'sclerotomal' pain. Glogowski and Wallraff (1951) and Glogowski and Wallraffin (1960) reported multiple club-like swelling in muscle fibers of fibrositis patients. In 1965, Mendell and Wall found that stimulus arises from muscle stimulation was more potent than stimulus arises from skin in development of central sensitization. Biopsy of trigger points in muscle was done by Simons and Trolov on dogs and found 'contraction knots'. In 1996, Windisch et al. further extended the study on fresh cadavers and found that increase in muscle fiber diameter and increased I-band and decreased A-band. Mense et al. (2003) showed the reason behind contraction knots in increased acetyl choline at muscle end plate.

EPIDEMIOLOGY

The prevalence of myofascial pain syndrome (MPS) is exactly not known but 30–85% of patients with musculoskeletal pain suffer from this condition. MPS is usually found in the population aged from 27 to 50 years. The gender difference in MPS incidence remains unclear.

ETIOLOGY

The etiology of MPS development is unclear. Common predisposing factors are:
- Trauma
- Spine-related disease
- Cumulative and repetitive strain at particular muscle
- Postural dysfunction
- Physical deconditioning
- Stress and anxiety
- Some pathological conditions such as iron-deficiency anemia, hypothyroidism, vitamins D and B_{12} deficiency, spondylosis, Lyme's disease, etc.

CLINICAL FEATURES

Pain: It can be acute or chronic but dull in nature, deep and poorly localized. Pain increases on movement of involved muscle. Muscle spasm may be present. Sometimes, it can mimic radicular or visceral pain.

Sensory disturbances: Patients can have referred pain, dysesthesias, paraesthesias and hyperesthesias. It occurs in same dermatome of nerve supplying the muscle with trigger point.

Autonomic disturbances: Common symptoms are abnormal sweating, persistent lacrimation, persistent coryza, excessive salivation, imbalance, dizziness, tinnitus, and pilomotor activities. Weight perception of lifted objects can also be distorted.

Motor disturbances: It includes spasm, weakness without any atrophy and decreased coordination. The combination of weakness in the hands and loss of forearm muscle coordination makes the grasp unreliable. Range of movements is decreased.

Sleep disturbances: Pain and muscle tenderness sometimes makes difficult for patients to sleep at night. MPS patients have poor sleep patterns with decreased recovery sleep (nonrapid eye movement sleep). This is associated with awakening feeling unrested and daytime fatigue.

DIAGNOSIS

History Taking

Detailed history should be taken about pain like history of trauma, pain site, frequency, quality of pain, involvement of other sites, any previous pain at same or different sites, progression of pain, association with movements. Any history of recent trauma, overuse of some muscles or repetitive strain is significant in diagnosis. Other causes of pain such as arthritis, bursitis, tendinitis, etc., must be ruled out. If a well-defined etiology of pain could not be established, then MPS can be a possibility.

Physical Examination

Localization and palpation of trigger point is the mainstay of diagnosis for MPS. MTrP is a focal tender point within the muscle. Features of the myofascial trigger point as described by Simons and colleagues are elicited in **Box 1**.

Sometimes involuntary flinching occurs after palpation of trigger points which is disproportionate to the amount of pressure applied, called 'jump sign'. Occasionally, trigger point palpation causes referred pain which has more diffuse distribution (myotomal) rather limiting to the area of its nerve root distribution (dermatomal). Trigger point must be firmly pressed for at least 5 seconds to produce referred pain. Procedures for identifying trigger points are elicited in **Box 2**.

Box 1: Features of the myofascial trigger point.

- Taut band within the muscle
- Exquisite tenderness at a point on the taut band
- Reproduction of the patient's pain
- Local twitch response
- Referred pain
- Restricted range of motion
- Autonomic signs [skin warmth or erythema, tearing, pilo-erection (goose-bumps)]

Box 2: Procedure for identifying trigger points.

- *History and pain diagram*: The history identifies the areas affected by pain
- Examination of muscles whose trigger points can refer pain to the affected areas
- Palpate the muscle for taut bands, using either flat palpation or pincer palpation
- Move the fingers along the taut band to find the hardest and most tender spot (the trigger point)
- Compress the trigger point manually and ask if the spot is tender or painful, and if so, does the pain resemble the patient's usual pain
- Compress the trigger point for 5–10 seconds and then ask if there is pain or some sensation away from the trigger point (referred pain)

Local twitch response (LTR) can be produced in muscle by suddenly snapping the taut band within the muscle fibers. The reason of weakness is this taut bands which limits the stretch of muscles. It can also activate autonomic activity, such as vasodilation or constriction, goose bumps, or pilo-erection.

Palpating the Taut Band

Taut band should be palpated in the direction perpendicular to muscle fiber preferably over firm or bony structure **(Figs. 1A to F)**.

Referred pain and LTR can be elicited by stimulation of center of hard area of trigger point. If we move farther from the center, then it is difficult to produce these responses, and it cannot be elicited at distance of 3 cm or more from center point. Schematic diagrams of a trigger point complex of a muscle is shown in **Figures 2A and B**.

Etiopathogenesis of Symptoms

Pain: Pain occurs at muscle and tender points due to release of various cytokines, neuropeptides, serotonin, inflammatory peptides-like substance P, interleukins, and protons that create local acidity.

Referred pain: It is caused by activation of interneurons and spreads rostrally and caudally in the spinal cord which takes some time. So, 5–10 seconds compression is necessary to produce RP.

Local twitch response: Local twitch response is produced by a brief (25–250 ms), high-amplitude, polyphasic electrical discharge causing local contraction of muscle rather entire

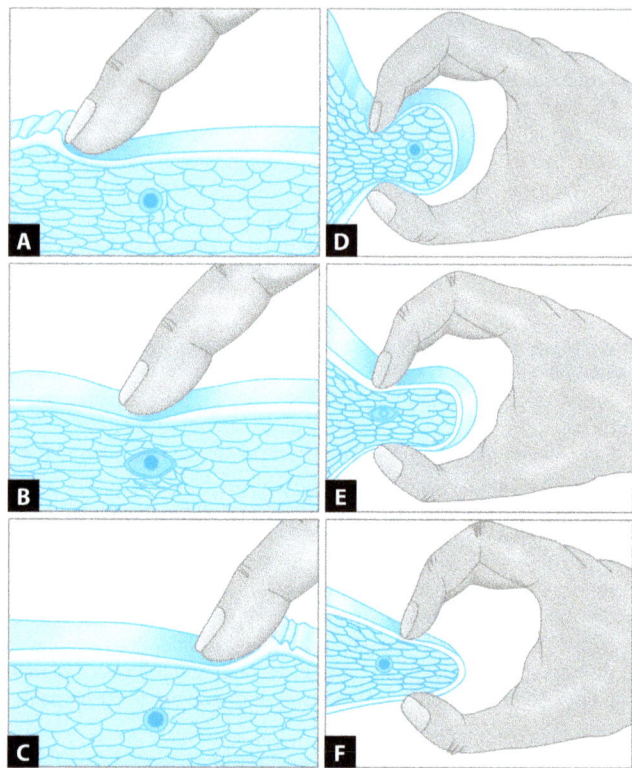

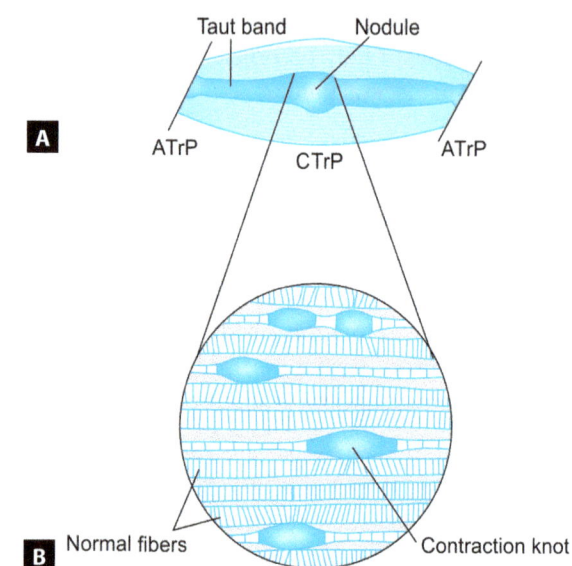

Figs. 1A to F: Cross-sectional drawing shows flat palpation of a taut band and its trigger point. (A) Skin pushed to one side to begin palpation; (B) The fingertip slides across muscle fibers to feel the cord-line texture of the taut band rolling beneath it; (C) The skin is pushed to other side at completion of movement. This same movement performed vigorously is snapping palpation; (D) Muscle fibers surrounded by the thumb and fingers in a pincer grip; (E) The hardness of the taut band is felt clearly as it is rolled between the digits; (F) The palpable edge of the taut band is sharply defined as it escapes from between the fingertips, often with a local twitch response.

Figs. 2A and B: Schematic of a trigger point complex of a muscle in longitudinal section. (A) The central trigger point (CTrP) in the endplate zone contains numerous electrically active loci and numerous contraction knots. A taut band of muscle fibers extends from the trigger point to the attachment at each end of the involved fibers. The sustained tension that the taut band exerts on the attachment tissues can induce a localized enthesopathy that is identified as an attachment trigger point (ATrP); (B) Enlarged view of part of the CTrP shows the distribution of five contraction knots. The vertical lines in each muscle fiber identify the relative spacing of its striations. The space between two striations corresponds to the length of one sarcomere. The sarcomeres within one of these enlarged segments (i.e., contraction knot) of a muscle fiber are markedly shorter and wider than the sarcomeres in the neighboring normal muscle fibers, which are free of contraction knots.

muscle as seen in Golgi tendon reflex which is also produced by stretch. LTR becomes attenuated as stimulation site moves away from trigger point. It is a type of spinal cord reflex as severing spinal cord can still produce LTR but it disappears after transacting peripheral nerves.

Limited range of motion: It occurs due to pain and shortened taut bands in muscles. Involved muscle fibers are already under substantially increased tension at rest length and further stretching of muscle causes severe pain. Range of motion returns to normal after releasing the taut band and inactivation of trigger points.

Weakness: It occurs in muscles which has MTrP. In EMG studies, it is found that muscles get early fatigue and early exhausted compared to normal muscles. It is not due to neuropathic or myopathic causes but rather by reflect reflex inhibition of the muscle by the MTrPs. Magnitude of weakness varies widely from person to person and site to site. This type of weakness get reversed after removal of taut bands and trigger points.

■ INVESTIGATIONS
Laboratory Studies
Myofascial pain syndrome cannot be diagnosed by lab studies. Lab studies only helps in diagnosing the condition associated with MPS such as deficiency of iron, vitamin B_{12}, vitamin D, hypothyroidism, parasitic and fungal infections.

Imaging Studies
It helps in diagnosing of MPS.

Ultrasound
It can localize taut bands in muscles and visualize LTR. High-resolution ultrasound imaging in combination with vibration sono-elastography localizes hypoechoic, elliptical, focal areas of trigger points in muscles. Needling of trigger points can be done under ultrasound guidance.

Magnetic Resonance Elastography
It can diagnosed varying densities of tissues. So taut bands having higher densities than normal surrounding muscle can

be localized. It uses phase contrast to identify tissue distortion when cyclic energy waves-like vibration are introduced into the muscle.

Electromyography

It is recording of the electrical activities of muscles. In electromyographic studies of muscles having trigger point, increased activity was noted after placing electrodes at trigger point, possibly arises at motor endplate, which was termed as 'endplate noise' by Simons. A characteristic persistent, low-amplitude, high-frequency discharge found at the MTrP region in active MTrP by Hubbard and Berkoff in MPS patients. It gradually diminished as electrodes moved away from trigger point. This electrical activity associated with MTrP region was called spontaneous electrical activity (SEA). This low amplitude electrical activity was thought to be produced by release of acetyl-choline at motor end plate. Endplate noise was found 5 times more frequent in trigger point zone than outside this zone. Endplate noise intensity is directly correlated with the degree of trigger point irritability as measured by pressure pain threshold.

Differential Diagnosis of Regional Pain Syndromes

A myofascial pain syndrome can have one trigger point or have multiple trigger points simultaneously producing pain in large regions. Sometimes this disease starts with one trigger point and subsequently other trigger points develop over time in same or nearby regions possibly due to prolong pain, muscle weakness and reduced range of motion. The persistence of a trigger point may lead to neuroplastic changes at the level of the dorsal horn which results in amplification of the pain sensation (i.e., central sensitization) with a tendency to spread beyond its original boundaries (i.e., expansion of receptive fields). Referred from other conditions can also be similar to RP due to MPS. To establish the diagnosis of regional pain, proper history taking and thorough physical examinations is the key. Other clinical condition may also contribute in the development of MPS and may exist as comorbidities with this condition **(Box 3)**.

Myofascial pain syndrome is commonly confused with pain of fibromyalgia. Differentiating features of both disease is given in **Table 1**.

■ TREATMENT

Treatment of MPS involves the treatment of symptoms as well as treating the cause. It is commonly seen that if a patient with a localized MPS is followed over years and if the problem is not effectively treated or resolved early enough the pain starts to spread outside the region of origin of pain. When acute pain becomes chronic, it often results in missed work, disability, and significantly high cost of care. The emphasis should be given to early, accurate diagnosis of the MPS followed by intensive, protocol-based, multidisciplinary treatment and rehabilitation.

Pharmacologic Therapy

Analgesic drugs (NSAIDs, Tramadol): Their exact role in treatment is unclear. It gives symptomatic relief to the

Box 3: Common conditions that are comorbid with myofascial pain syndrome.

- Migraine headache
- Tension-type headache
- Temporomandibular joint disorder
- Fibromyalgia
- Hypermobility syndromes
- Painful bladder syndrome
- Irritable bowel syndrome
- Pelvic pain syndrome
- Vulvovaginitis
- Prostatitis
- Endometriosis
- Dysmenorrhea
- Hypothyroidism
- Vitamin D deficiency
- Vitamin B_{12} deficiency
- Iron deficiency
- Parasitic infection
- Celiac disease of malabsorption

TABLE 1: Differentiating features of myofascial pain and fibromyalgia.

Feature	Myofascial pain (TrPs)	Fibromyalgia
Female-to-male ratio	1:1	4–9:1
Pain	Local or regional	Widespread, general
Tenderness	Focal	Widespread
Muscle	Feels tense (taut bands)	Feels soft and doughy
Motion	Restricted range of motion	Hypermobility
Examination	Examine for TrPs	Examine for tender points
LTR	Present at TrPs	Absent at tender points
Symptoms	Non-musculoskeletal symptoms occasionally occurs	Non-musculoskeletal symptoms (fatigue, sleep disturbance, IBS) usually present

(LTR: local twitch response; TrPs: trigger points; IBS: irritable bowel syndrome) patients but do not abolish the cause of the disease. It is used as initial treatment but long-term treatment with these group of drugs should be avoided as it cause many gastrointestinal and renal complication.

Tropisetron: It is a 5-HT3 receptor antagonist and alpha-7-nicotinic-receptor agonist recently used as an analgesic for fibromyalgia and myofascial pain. But its exact role in MPS treatment is not established.

Muscle relaxants: These drugs decreases muscle spasticity. Few studies suggested beneficial role of tizanidine, a centrally acting muscle relaxant, in treatment of MPS. Cyclobenzaprine is another effective muscle relaxant but it does not have statistically significant difference in pain scores after treatment. Thiocolchiside, which is a competitive GABA antagonist and glycine agonist, was found to have statistically significant improvement in pain score and range of movement after topical treatment.

Anticonvulsants: Gabapentin and pregabalin has proven role in treatment. It has anxiolytic-like, and anticonvulsant activity, which reduces the release of several neurochemicals including glutamate, noradrenaline, and substance P. It also helps in reducing pain of MPS at spinal level.

Antidepressants: Tricyclic antidepressants (TCAs) are being used for chronic pain in various conditions such as fibromyalgia, neuropathic pain. It works on central pain pathway by affecting central serotonergic and noradrenergic signals. However, its role in MSP is not clear. Duloxetine, a serotonin-norepinephrine reuptake inhibitor (SNRI), was recently found to be an evolving and possibly efficacious treatment for painful MSK conditions, may be useful in MSP.

Botulinum toxin type A (BTA): It is a very potent neurotoxin. It decreases production of substance P and glutamate. It acts on presynaptic cholinergic nerve terminals by blocking the release of acetylcholine at muscle fiber endplates. As acetylcholine is important factor in pathogenesis of MPS, so BTA has role in treatment of MPS **(Figs. 3A and B)**.

Steps of action of BTA on neuromuscular transmission:
1. It binds selectively to cholinergic nerve terminals of motor end plate through its heavy chain.
2. BTA is internalized via receptor-mediated endocytosis into the cell. When toxin-containing vesicle reaches inside cell, it releases its light chain transmission blocking domain inside cytoplasm.
3. SNAP-25 is a protein on cell membrane which is required for release of acetylcholine and causing muscle contraction. BTA acts via cleavage of this protein. It has no action on synthesis or storage of acetylcholine.

Botulinum toxin type A binds irreversibly to nerve terminal so its effect are prolonged up to 2–6 months. The nerve terminal where BTA binds become permanently nonfunctional. Later new nerve sprouts grows and gradually neuromuscular connection re-established and muscle function returns to normal. A multicenter, prospective, randomized, double-blind study demonstrated a statistically significant difference in pain intensity, duration, and reduction of trigger points of the BTA group; however, these effects were seen after 4 weeks.

Nonpharmacologic Therapy

Trigger Point Injections

Injections directly into trigger points are commonly used method for treatment. Steroids, local anesthetic or dry needling can be used as injections. Needling can mechanically disrupt taut bands and trigger zones or terminate dysfunctional activity of involved motor endplates.

Dry needling has been used for long time for treatment of pain arising from MTrPs as it is fastest and effective method. After needling by proper methods of MTrPs, pain decreases significantly. Needling should be done at trigger point in multiple direction by in-and-out technique. Proper method of needling is described in **Figures 4 and 5**.

CZ Hong described a method of needling in obese or fatty patients where there is difficulty to palpate muscle or taut bands. In his technique, he indent the skin and subcutaneous fat tissue by placing finger just beside the needle **(Fig. 6)**.

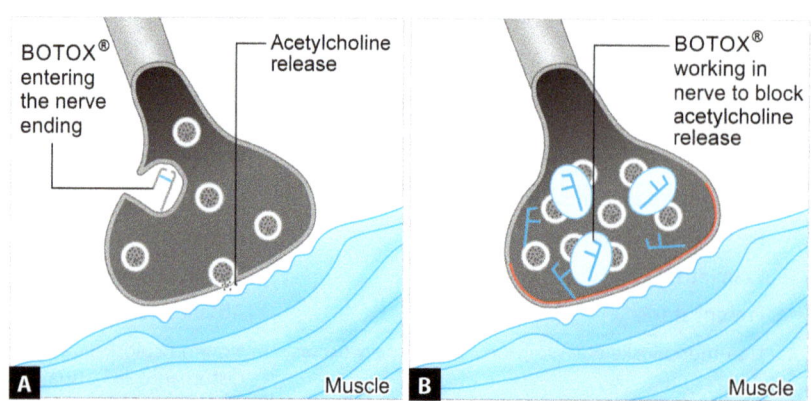

Figs. 3A and B: Mechanism of action of botulinum toxin type A.

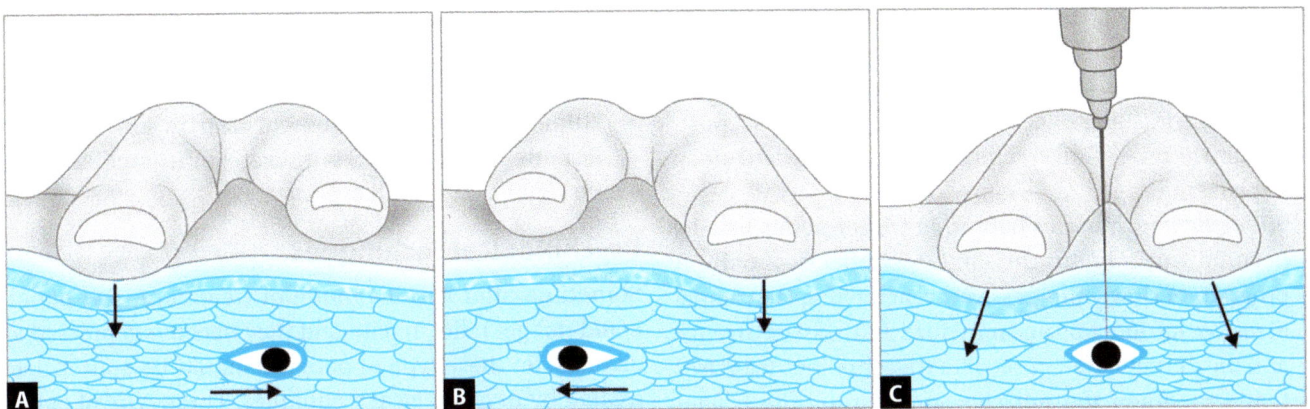

Figs. 4A to C: Trigger point injection by finger palpating method. Cross-sectional schematic drawing shows flat palpation to localize and hold the trigger point for injection. (A and B) The use of alternate pressure between two fingers to confirm the location of the palpable module of the trigger point; (C) Positioning the trigger point half way between the fingertips to keep it from sliding to one side during the injection.

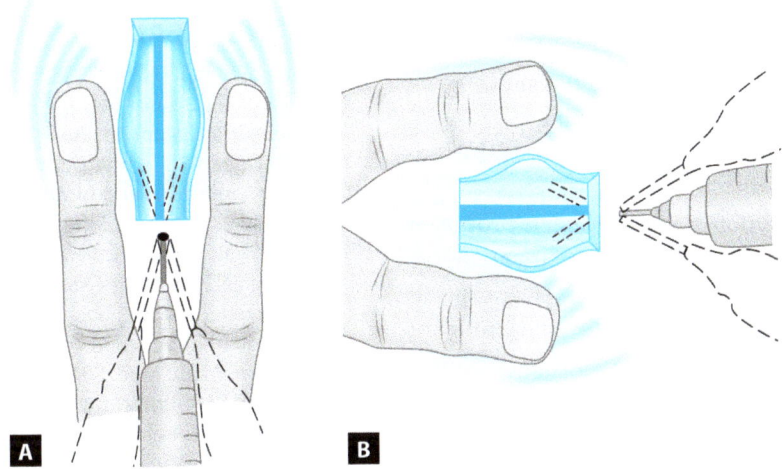

Figs. 5A and B: Trigger point injection by finger palpating method. Schematic top view in (A) of 2 approaches to the flat injection of a trigger point area in a palpable taut band. Injection away from the fingers (A) and injection toward the fingers (B).

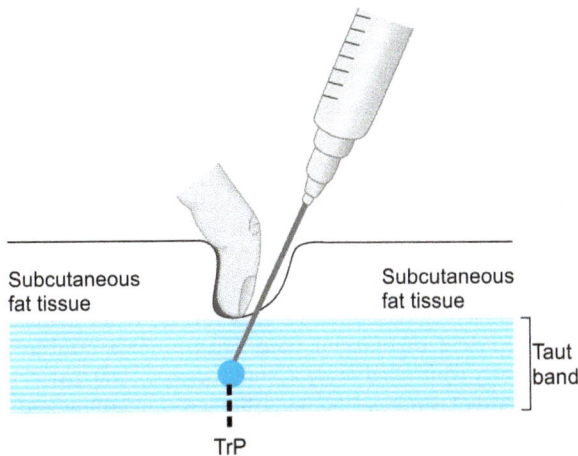

Fig. 6: CZ Hong's technique. (TrP: trigger point)

If local anesthesia-like lignocaine is used in needling, then it gives more comforts during procedure to patients, however, efficacy of the procedure remain same with or without lignocaine. It decreases pain significantly and LTR during procedure. Several studies showed that dry needling is very effective method in treatment of MPS and equal in efficacy to trigger point injections. Its only complication is soreness at injection site. Thus currently it is the mainstay of acute treatment in MPS. Benefits of steroid use as injections is not statistically proved.

Physical Therapy

Physical therapy for MPS treatment include following methods:

- *Stretching*: The muscles involved in myofascial pain syndromes are shortened due to the afore-mentioned focal contractions of sarcomeric units. It is thought that these focal contractions result in prolonged ATP consumption, and that the restoration of a muscle to its full stretch length breaks the link between the energy crisis and contraction of sarcomeric units. Effective stretching is most commonly achieved through the technique of spray and stretch. This involves the cutaneous application, along the axis of the muscle, of ethyl chloride spray while at the same time passively stretching the involved muscle. Other techniques to enhance effective stretching include trigger point to pressure release, post-isometric relaxation, reciprocal inhibition, and deep stroking massage.

- *Strengthening*: Muscles harboring trigger points usually become weak due to the inhibitory effects of pain. A program of slowly progressive strengthening is essential to restore full function and minimize the risk of recurrence and the perpetuation of satellite trigger points. Exercises that strengthen the muscles surrounding the trigger point, helps to avoid overworking of any one muscle.
- *Posture training*: It improves myofascial pain particularly of neck and back region.
- *Massage*: The physical therapist may use long hand strokes along the muscle or place pressure on specific areas of involved muscle to release tension causing relief in pain.
- *Heat*: Applying heat, via a hot pack or a hot shower, can help relieve muscle tension and reduce pain.
- *Short wave diathermy (SWD)*: It provides deep heat to muscle thus relieving pain.
- *Ultrasound*: It is a technique that has been proposed to treat myofascial pain by converting electrical energy to sound waves in order to provide heat energy to muscles. Various study showed statistically significant improvement in pain, ROM, number of trigger points, and neck pain disability index. The use of high-powered ultrasound has also been explored. A RCT study resulted in a statistically significant improvement in neck pain scores when compared to conventional ultrasound.
- *Transcutaneous electric nerve stimulation (TENS)*: It is a treatment modality that utilizes an electrical current to stimulate nerve fibers in order to provide pain relief. Various RCT showed statistically significant reduction in pain and increase in pain threshold by TENS as compared to controls. Another RCT investigated TENS versus laser therapy versus lidocaine injection versus BTA injection in patients with myofascial pain. It demonstrated no statistically significant benefit over injections. Thus TENS has been shown to have benefit among the non-invasive therapeutic modalities, however, there is currently no evidence that supports its use over trigger point injections or medication.
- *Magnetic stimulation (MS)*: It is a newer treatment that is being investigated for MSK pain and MPS. A RCT study compared MS to TENS and placebo and results showed that MS had a statistically significant improvement in pain and ROM at 1 and 3 months after treatment, longer than the beneficial effects obtained after TENS. However, only limited numbers of studies are available on MS to establish its role in treatment of MPS.
- *Laser therapy*: Laser therapy has shown some therapeutic promise, as a whole the body of evidence is mixed regarding the efficacy of this treatment strategy. Few studies showed improvement in pain and ROM after laser treatment in MPS but several other studies showed no significant benefit over placebo.

Psychological Techniques

Sometime after various mode of treatment, few patients could not get relief in pain and they become depressed and anxious. So these type of patients should be appropriately treated by psychological techniques. These type of patients need proper counseling, a rehabilitation program to improve sleep pattern and reassurance about treatment. Additional management techniques can be used such as EMG biofeedback, cognitive behavioral therapy, and hypnotic/meditation relaxation techniques.

■ FURTHER READING

1. Altan L, Bingöl U, Aykaç M, Yurtkuran M. Investigation of the effect of GaAs laser therapy on cervical myofascial pain syndrome. Rheumatol Int. 2005;25:23-7.
2. Ay S, Doğan SK, Evcik D, Baser O. Comparison the efficacy of phonophoresis and ultrasound therapy in myofascial pain syndrome. Rheumatol Int. 2011;31:1203-8.
3. Benecke R, Heinze A, Reichel G, Hefter H, Gobel H, Dysport Myofascial Pain Study Group. Botulinum type A toxin complex for the relief of upper back myofascial pain syndrome: how do fixed-location injections compare with trigger point-focused injections? Pain Med. 2011;12:1607-14.
4. Bennett RM. Emerging concepts in the neurobiology of chronic pain: evidence of abnormal sensory processing in fibromyalgia. Mayo Clinic Proc. 1999;74(4):385-98.
5. Borg-Stein J. Treatment of fibromyalgia, myofascial pain, and related disorders. Phys Med Rehabil Clin N Am. 2006;17:491-510.
6. Ceccherelli F, Altafini L, Lo Castro G, Avila A, Ambrosio F, Giron G. Diode laser in cervical myofascial pain: a double-blind study versus placebo. Clin J Pain. 1989;5:301-4.
7. Chen Q, Basford J, An KN. Ability of magnetic resonance elastography to assess taut bands. Clin Biomech. 2008;23:623-9.
8. Chen Q, Bensamoun S, Basford J, et al. Identification and quantification of myofascial taut bands with magnetic resonance elastography. Arch Phys Med Rehabil. 2007;88:1658-61.
9. Dundar U, Evcik D, Samli F, Pusak H, Kavunca V. The effect of gallium arsenide aluminum laser therapy in the management of cervical myofascial pain syndrome: a double blind, placebo-controlled study. Clin Rheumatol. 2007;26:930-4.
10. Edwards J, Knowles N. Superficial dry needling and active stretching in the treatment of myofascial pain: a randomised control trial. Acupunct Med. 2003;21:80-6.
11. Fallah H, Currimbhoy S. Use of botulinum toxin A for treatment of myofascial pain and dysfunction. J Oral Maxillofac Surg. 2012;70:1243-5.
12. Gam A, Warming S, Larsen L, et al. Treatment of myofascial trigger-points with ultrasound combined with massage and exercise: a randomised controlled trial. Pain. 1998;77:73-9.

13. Gerwin RD, Duranleau D. Ultrasound identification of the myofascial trigger point. Muscle Nerve. 1997;20:767-76.
14. Glogowski G, Wallraff J. Clinical and histologic aspects of myogelosis (German). Zeitschrift fur Ortho-padie und Ihre Grenzgebiete. 1951;80(2):237-268.49.
15. Graff-Radford S, Reeves J, Baker R. Effects of transcutaneous electrical nerve stimulation on myofascial pain and trigger point sensitivity. Pain. 1989;37:1-5.
16. Graven-Nielsen T, Arendt-Nielsen L. Peripheral and central sensitization in musculoskeletal paindisorders: an experimental approach. Current Rheumatology Reports. 2002;4(4):313-21.
17. Gur A, Sarac A, Cevik R, Altindag O, Sarac S. Efficacy of 904 nm gallium arsenide low level laser therapy in the management of chronic myofascial pain in the neck: a double-blind and randomize-controlled trial. Lasers Surg Med. 2004;35:229-35.
18. Gül K, Onal SA. Comparison of non-invasive and invasive techniques in the treatment of patients with myofascial pain syndrome. Agri. 2009;21:104-21.
19. Hakgüder A, Birtane M, Gürcan S, Kokino S, Turan F. Efficacy of low level laser therapy in myofascial pain syndrome: an algometric and thermographic evaluation. Lasers Surg Med. 2003;33:339-43.
20. Hong C. Lidocaine injection versus dry needling to myofascial trigger point. The importance of the local twitch response. Am J Phys Med Rehabil. 1994;73:256-63.
21. Hong CZ, Simons DG. Pathophysiologic and electrophysiologic mechanisms of myofascial trigger points. Arch Phys Med Rehabil. 1998;79:863-72.
22. Hong CZ, Torigoe Y, Yu J. The localized twitch responses in responsive taut bands of rabbit skeletal muscle fibers are related to the reflexes at spinal cord level. J Muscoskel Pain. 1995;3(1):15-33.
23. Hong CZ, Torigoe Y. Electro-physiologic characteristics of localized twitch responses in responsive taut bands of rabbit skeletal muscle. J Muscoskel Pain. 1994;2:17-43.
24. Hou C, Tsai L, Cheng K, Chung K, Hong C. Immediate effects of various physical therapeutic modalities on cervical myofascial pain and trigger point sensitivity. Arch Phys Med Rehabil. 2002;83:1406-14.
25. Hsueh C, Cheng P, Kuan T, Hong C. The immediate effectiveness of electrical nerve stimulation and electrical muscle stimulation on myofascial trigger points. Am J Phys Med Rehabil. 1997;76:471-6.
26. Hubbard DR, Berkoff M. Myofascial trigger points show spontaneous needle EMG activity. Spine. 1993;18:1803-7.
27. Kellgren JH. Observations on referred pain arising from muscle. Clin Sci. 1938;3:175-90.
28. Ketenci A, Basat H, Esmaeilzadeh S. The efficacy of topical thiocolchicoside (Muscoril) in the treatment of acute cervical myofascial pain syndrome: a single-blind, randomized, prospective, phase IV clinical study. Agri. 2009;21:95-103.
29. Kuan TS, Hsieh YL, Chen SM, et al. The myofascial trigger point region: correlation between the degree of irritability and the prevalence of endplate noise. Am J Phys Med Rehabil. 2007;86:183-9.
30. Leite F, Atallah A, El Dib R, Grossmann E, Januzzi E, Andriolo RB, et al. Cyclobenzaprine for the treatment of myofascial pain in adults. Cochrane Database Syst Rev. 2009;3:CD006830.

Fibromyalgia

SS Jha, Lalit Kishore

INTRODUCTION

Fibromyalgia (FM) is a persistent and debilitating chronic, generalized, painful disorder, widespread in the body; fatigue, muscle and joint stiffness and rigidity, disturbed sleep cycle are usually various presenting symptoms of the disease. The clinical sign of tenderness is located at classically designed multiple spots. Psychological, cognitive affections have negative influence on their ability to work usually leading to disturbed daily routine. Aberrant interpersonal relationship can have devastating repercussion in workplace and family life. This disease is a lifetime phenomenon with symptomatic pain spread out in whole body.

THE PREDISPOSING FACTORS

- Association of neck and back pain with history of headache, irritable bowel, disorders of temporomandibular (TM) joint are usual. Females predominate with the dysmenorrhea, endometriosis, cystitis either interstitial or due to painful bladder syndrome.
- Other associated pathologies are:
  - Osteoarthritis
  - Lupus
  - Rheumatoid arthritis
- Contribution of psychosocial features such as depression, anxiety and other psychiatric illnesses
- Family members and first degree relatives
- History of chronic pain and similar diseases

Fibromyalgia is the second most common disease after osteoarthritis. Seventy-five percent remains undiagnosed.

PATHOGENESIS

The underlying mechanisms are involved:

- *Neurogenic origin*: "Central amplification" of pain perception due to neurochemical imbalances in central nervous system. Allodynia and hyperalgesia are two essential elements of the chronic pain. While allodynia brings forth the heightened sensitivity to suboptimal painful stimuli whereas hyperalgesia involves increased response to painful stimuli. A much lower stimulus elicit pain response.
- Psychosocial and behavioral issues are contributory-response to simple measures such as improving the sleep pattern, reduction of stress, continued physical exercises and activities are usually encouraging in management of such patients.

HISTORICAL LANDMARKS

- *Mid nineteenth century*: German-Cluster of symptoms were grouped as "generalized body tenderness with rheumatism" and were labeled as "Muskelschwiele"—meaning "muscle callus".
- *1904*: Gowers coined the term "fibrositis".
- *1950*: Graham called "fibrositis syndrome" and sought attention to the fact of "in the absence of a specific organic disease".
- *Mid 1970s*: Smythe and Moldofsky first coined this term "fibromyalgia" and identified the classical "tender points".
- *1978*: Published evidence of fibromyalgia, sleep pathology and central pain sensitization.
- *1990*: American College of Rheumatology (ACR) defined the new nomenclature "Fibromyalgia syndrome" and put forward the diagnostic criteria.
- *1994*: Russell demonstrated three-fold increase in substance P in the cerebrospinal fluid in such patients.
- *2007*: Landmark approval of pregabalin use.
- *2008*: Duloxetine approval.
- *2009*: Milnacipran was approved.
- *2010*: ACR criteria was modified.
- *2011*: ACR criteria further modified.
- *2014*: Bennet proposed an alternative criteria.
- *2016*: ACR criteria revision.

EPIDEMIOLOGY

Female versus male: Women are seven times more prone.

Incidence: Depending on the diagnostic criteria used, the prevalence is from 2 to 8% of the population.

- One study showed global prevalence of 2.7%, female: male = 4.2:1.4.
- Other study showed 2% prevalence.
- In USA, female: male = 3.4:0.5.

- While using ACR diagnostic criteria 2010, Vincent et al. found 6.4% prevalence in USA.
- Brazil had a prevalence of up to 2.5% with females predominating in the age group of 35 to 44 years.
- A study in France found prevalence of 1.4%.

Geographical Prevalence

The geographical prevalence of fibromyalgia is shown in **Figure 1**.

Age

No age is immune including childhood but the peak prevalence is at 60 and 79 years. Persons younger than 39 or older than 40–59 have worse symptoms with poor quality of life as compared to the older population of 60 years or more.

Urban versus Rural Population

In a review study of literatures on epidemiology of FM, the prevalence found by the authors ranged between 0.69 and 11.4% in the urban area, and between 0.06 and 5.2% in the rural area. It is difficult to diagnose fibromyalgia in primary care centers because of its gradual evolution and extensive basket of symptoms resulting into this condition remain undiagnosed.

Delay in Diagnosis

It usually takes more than 2 years for diagnosis of fibromyalgia to be established. During this period, an average of 3.7 physicians were consulted.

Preceding Stressor

Viral diseases such as Lyme disease or hepatitis C or injury can be responsible in 50% of cases.

Etiopathogenesis

Affective spectrum disorder (ASD) is a family of related disorders which are either existing simultaneously or get aggregated together. They commonly share among themselves the physiologic abnormalities along with genetic risk factors. These two constitute the central core of etiological factors. Besides FM, ASD includes:
- Bulimia nervosa
- Generalized anxiety disorder
- Obsessive-compulsive disorder
- Post-traumatic stress disorder
- Social phobia and medical disorders such as irritable bowel syndrome (IBS), migraine, etc.
- Attention-deficit/hyperactivity disorder
- Dysthymic disorder
- Major depressive disorder
- Panic disorder
- Premenstrual dysphoric disorder

PATHOPHYSIOLOGY

Numerous abnormal factors are inherently responsible for the pathophysiology of fibromyalgia:
- Central nervous system
- Autonomic nervous systems (ANS)
- Neuroendocrine system
- Genetic factors
- Psychosocial variables
- Environmental stressors

Central Nervous System

Enhanced sensitivity is displayed against a wide range of stimuli, such as cold and heat, mechanical and ischemic pressure. Pain is produced as a result of these stimuli which

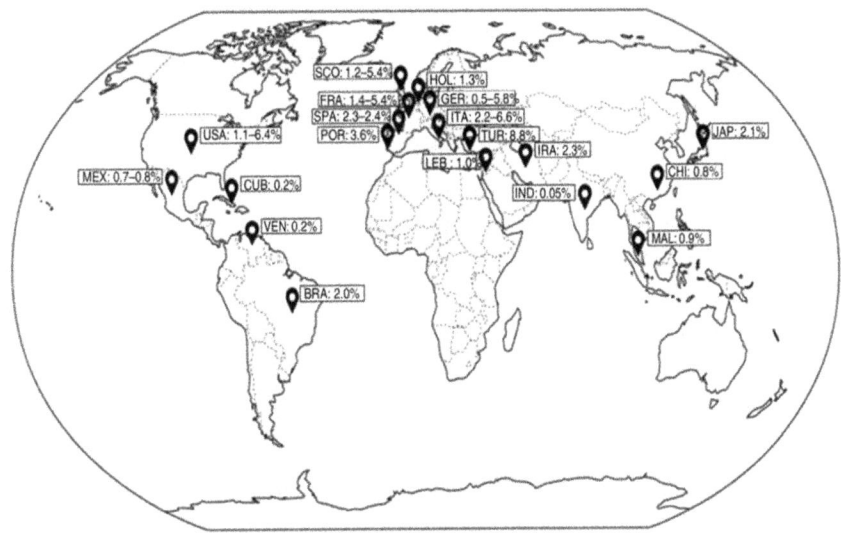

Fig. 1: Geographical prevalence of fibromyalgia.
Source: Marques AP, Santo AS, Berssaneti AA, Matsutani LA, Yuan SL. Prevalence of fibromyalgia: literature review update. Rev Bras Reumatol. 2017;57(4):356-63.

ordinarily will not produce pain responses in normal healthy persons. Main mechanism involved is central sensitization and is an exaggerated response as a result of CNS signaling. This results in "set point" or "volume control" for the pain being produced. Central sensitization is transmitted by primary afferent fibers and consequently has
- Spontaneous nerve activity
- Enlarged receptive fields
- Augmented stimulus responses

Earlier central sensitization described specific spinal mechanism for pain where an initial nociceptive focus brings about regional pain amplification. Amplification is the correct terminology.

Mechanism of Pain Perception

The sensory input transmitted in the form of stimulus to either the skin or the muscle stimulate the nerve receptors in these tissues along primary afferents A-δ and C nerve fibers to its intermediate destination in the dorsal horns presynaptic terminals of the spinal cord. The second order spinal neurons after alterations in the dorsal horns carry the sensory input to the brain after depolarization of the dorsal horn neurons extracellular Ca^{2+} diffuse into neurons resulting in release of pain associated glutamate and substance P neurotransmitters. They in turn activate postsynaptic receptors in the second order pain transmission neurons (PTN). Various regions in the brain receive the sensory inputs through this pathway. Thalamus, somatosensory cortices and the limbic system finally result into perception of pain (**Figs. 2A to C**).

Both facilitatory and inhibitory signals then descend from the brain to the spinal cord and finally to the periphery via pain modulatory pathways. It can regulate the "volume control" either way resulting into increasing or decreasing the response. Number of neurotransmitters and neurochemicals such as norepinephrine, serotonin, endorphins mediate the signals along the pathways.

Pain Processing in Fibromyalgia

Fibromyalgia has the unique credential of operating the pain pathways abnormally leading to central amplification. Though, the mechanism is not fully explained but is likely to be multifactorial. "Volume control setting" is no doubt disproportionately high. Not only the excitability of central neurons is increased but simultaneous reduced pain inhibitory mechanisms are also brought into play. Genetics and modified environmental influences determine the central amplification. Intense or prolonged exposure to the painful stimuli results in abnormal pain processing thereby sensitization of PTNs become operative.

Central sensitization is exacerbated because the descending inhibitory pain pathways get impaired in patients with fibromyalgia (**Fig. 3**).

One of the mechanisms underlying this sensitization is the over activation of postsynaptic nitric oxide production, which in turn increases the presynaptic release of excitatory amino acids and causes the PTNs to become hyperexcitable. The role of spinal glia cells in central sensitization and enhanced pain sensitivity has been demonstrated in preclinical studies. Dorsal horn glia are activated by the

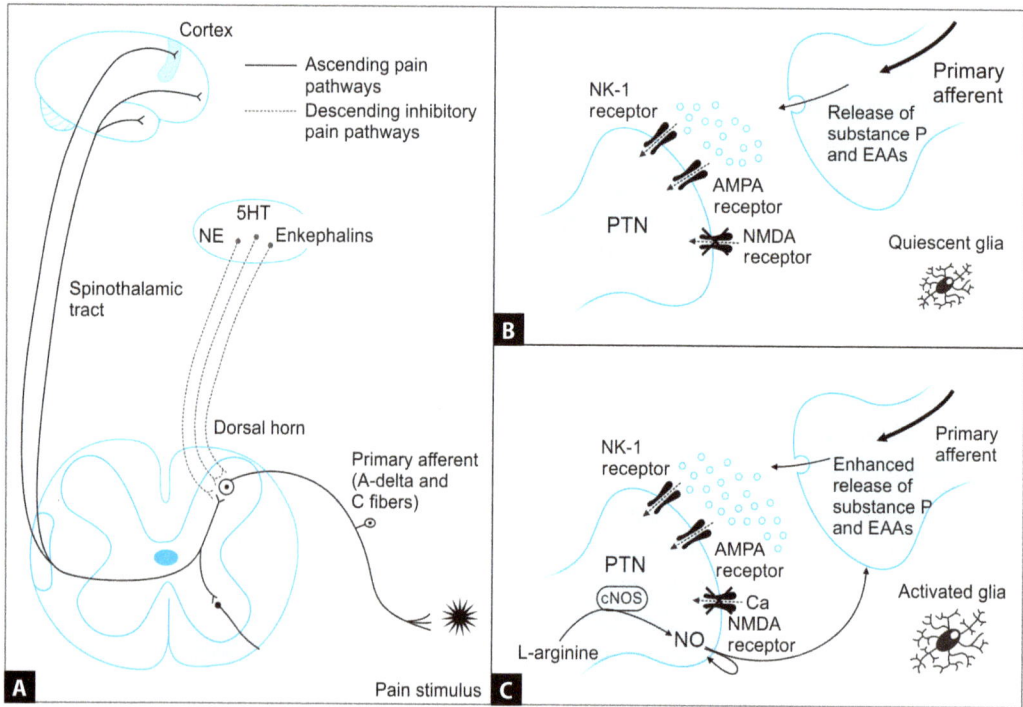

Figs. 2A to C: (A) Pain pathways; (B) Normal pain processing; (C) Abnormal pain processing. (PTN: pain transmission neuron; EAAs: excitatory amino acids; 5-HT: serotonin; NE: norepinephrine; NMDA: N-methyl-D-aspartic acid; AMPA: alpha-amino-3-hydroxy-5-methyl-4-isoxazolepropionic acid; NK-1: neurokinin; cNOS: constitutive nitric oxide synthase; NO: nitric oxide)

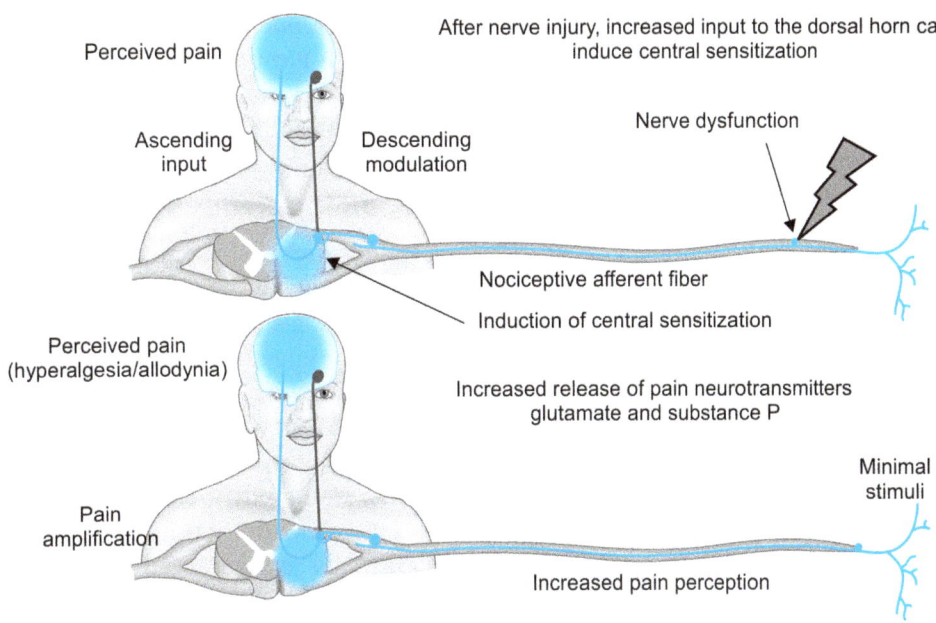

Fig. 3: Central sensitization produces abnormal pain signaling.

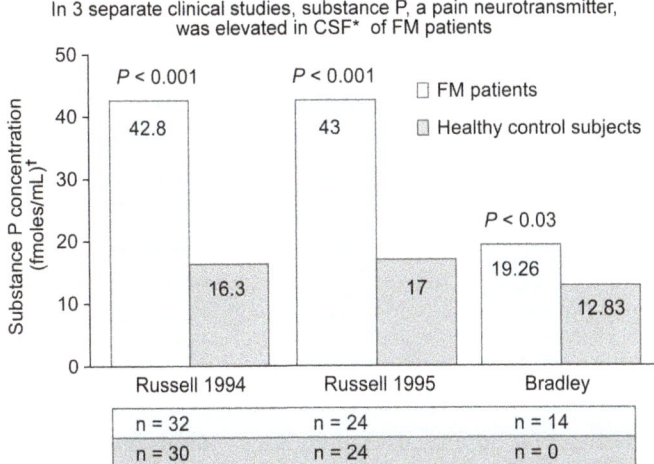

Fig. 4: Patients with fibromyalgia have elevated pain transmitter substance P in their cerebrospinal fluid. (CSF: cerebrospinal fluid)
*CSF sample collected via lumbar puncture in fibromyalgia (FM) and healthy controls and SP levels assessed by radioimmunoassay
†fmoles/mL = femtomole/mL = 10–15 mole/mL

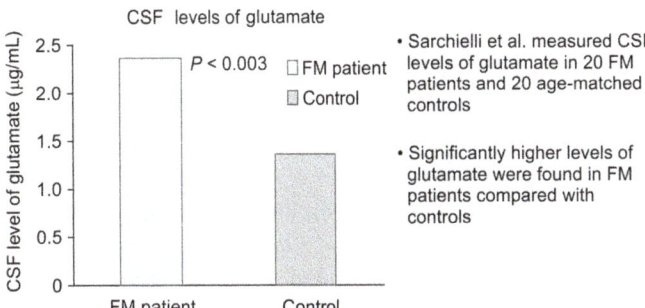

Fig. 5: Patients with fibromyalgia (FM) have elevated pain transmitter glutamate in their cerebrospinal fluid (CSF).
Source: Sarchielli P, Mancini ML, Floridi A, Coppola F, Rossi C, Nardi K, et al. Increased levels of neurotrophins are not specific for chronic migraine: evidence from primary fibromyalgia syndrome. J Pain. 2007;8:737-45.

release of nitric oxide, prostaglandins, fractalkine, substance P, adenosine triphosphate (ATP), and excitatory amino acids from PTNs and primary afferents. The glia, in turn, releases proinflammatory cytokines, nitric oxide, prostaglandins, reactive oxygen species, ATP, and excitatory amino acids. In addition to further increasing the release of substance P and glutamate from the A-δ and C afferents, these substances enhance or prolong the hyperexcitability of the PTNs. In different clinical studies, pain neurotransmitter substance P and glutamate were found elevated in cerebrospinal fluid (CSF) of FM patients **(Figs. 4 and 5)**.

Another possible mechanism in central sensitization is "wind up" phenomenon in which spinal cord neurons have increased excitability. After a painful stimulus, subsequent stimuli of the same intensity are perceived as stronger. This occurs normally in everyone but it is excessive in FM patients. These phenomena are the expression of neuroplasticity and are mainly mediated by N-methyl-D-aspartate (NMDA) receptors located in the postsynaptic membrane in the dorsal horn of the spinal cord.

In patients with FM, the activity of descending, antinociceptive pathways is also decreased, as evidenced by lower CSF levels of metabolites of serotonin, norepinephrine, and dopamine. Serotonin (5-HT) has a significant role in the modulation of pain. Serotonin is involved also in the regulation of mood and sleep and this could explain the association between fibromyalgia and sleep and mental disorders.

In contrast to low levels of these antinociceptive neurotransmitters, opioid levels are increased and opioid receptor binding is decreased, with the net effect that baseline endogenous opioidergic activity is increased in fibromyalgia. The findings of decreased opioid receptor availability (likely due to the high endogenous release of opioids) may explain why opioids, are overall less effective in treating FM.

Functional neuroimaging studies support the involvement of the brain in the pathogenesis of this condition. Neuroimaging data demonstrate greater regional cerebral blood flow in areas of the brain associated with pain processing at lower pain-producing pressures than healthy controls. Mountz et al. demonstrated decreased regional cerebral blood flow (rCBF) in bilateral thalamus and caudate nucleus in the fibromyalgic group of patients in a neuroimaging study by single-photon-emission computed tomography (SPECT). In a study by Wik et al. using positron emission tomography (PET), fibromyalgic patients showed higher rCBF than controls in the retrosplenial cortex bilaterally, while lower rCBF in the left frontal, temporal, parietal, and occipital cortices. This could reflect increased attention towards subnoxious somatosensory signaling and a dysfunction of the normal cognitive processing of pain in patients affected by fibromyalgia. Jensen et al. showed attenuated response to pain in the rostral anterior cingulate cortex, an important region of the descending pain regulating system in a functional magnetic resonance imaging study. This also explains the impairment in descending inhibitory pathway in pain perception.

Neuroendocrine System

Hypothalamic-pituitary-adrenal (HPA) axis is abnormal functioning in FM patients as it is a stress related disorder. Fibromyalgia has been associated with the inability to suppress cortisol. As compared to patients with RA, patients with fibromyalgia have significantly higher overall plasma cortisol and exhibits higher peak and trough levels of plasma cortisol. Different studies showed elevated cortisol levels, particularly in the evening, associated with a disrupted circadian rhythm. These patients showed high values of adrenocorticotropic hormone (ACTH) both basally and in response to stress, most likely as a consequence of a chronic hyposecretion of corticotropin-releasing hormone (CRH). These alterations are probably related to low levels of 5-HT observed in cases of fibromyalgia, because serotoninergic fibers regulate the HPA axis function.

Hypothalamic-pituitary-growth hormone (HPGH) axis disturbance may play a role in a deficiency of insulin-like growth factor-1 (IGF-1). Growth hormone (GH) levels are increased in sleep time in normal persons while it tends to be normal during the day, reduced during sleep in FM patients. It can be explained by two ways, first—GH is mainly secreted during stage 4 of sleep and this phase is disrupted in patients affected by fibromyalgia; second—these patients have high levels of somatostatin, a GH inhibitor, induced by ACTH whose levels are high as previously mentioned.

Hypothalamic-pituitary-thyroid (HPT) axis is also disturbed in FM patients as explained by hypothyroid status in FM patients. There is some evidence suggesting an association with abnormal thyrotropin-releasing hormone (TRH) stimulation tests.

Hypothalamic-pituitary-gonadal (HPG) axis may be disturbed in FM patients as explained by dysmenorrhea in some FM patients but several studies found normal gonadotropin and gonadal steroid secretion.

Autonomic Nervous System

Autonomic nervous system abnormalities may contribute to enhanced pain and other clinical problems associated with fibromyalgia via the alteration of physiologic responses required for effective stress management (e.g., increases in blood pressure) and pain inhibition via diminished production of growth hormone (GH) and IGF-1. In FM the sympathetic nervous system is hyperactive but hypoactive to stress. In a study, patients with fibromyalgia showed blunted vasoconstriction responses to cold presser tasks as well as decreased microcirculatory responses to auditory stimulation. During tilt-table testing, 60% of patients with fibromyalgia exhibited an abnormal drop in blood pressure compared with 0% of controls, and all of the patients who tolerated the tilt-table test for more than 10 minutes reported a worsening of pain symptoms, whereas control subjects remained asymptomatic. Difficulty in maintaining blood pressure levels may directly contribute to some of the unpleasant symptoms frequently associated with fibromyalgia, such as fatigue and dizziness, as well as affect physiologic responses to stressors. High serum levels of neuropeptide Y, which is normally secreted along with norepinephrine, are supposed to be a sign of this dysautonomic state.

Sleep Disturbances

Patients with fibromyalgia often have problems with sleep, including nonrestorative sleep, insomnia, early morning awakening, and poor quality of sleep. In polysomnography studies, alpha-delta sleep patterns associated with interrupted and nonrestorative sleep were frequently observed in patients with fibromyalgia. Sleep disturbances may be related to the reduced energy, fatigue and enhanced pain often found among patients with fibromyalgia. Frequent alpha-wave intrusions during delta-wave sleep have been associated with the reduced production of GH and IGF-1. GH and IGF-1 are necessary for the repair of muscle microtrauma, sleep disturbances may impair the healing of muscle tissue damage, thereby prolonging the transmission of sensory stimuli from damaged muscle tissue to the CNS and enhancing the perception of muscle pain. This enhanced pain may contribute to increases in sleep disturbance, thereby maintaining the patient's fatigue and continuing the inadequate muscle tissue repair. These findings suggest that pharmacologic and nonpharmacologic therapies that improve sleep quality may also help to reduce pain.

Genetic Factors

Genetic predisposition is likely to be an important factor as suggested by several familial studies and transmission is thought to be polygenic. The findings from these family studies also suggested that genetic factors contribute to the enhanced sensitivity to pain in patients with fibromyalgia. Among the various genes investigated, the most important are associated with neurotransmitters (serotonin transporter gene) and *catechol-O-methyltransferase (COMT) gene* variants.

Single nucleotide polymorphism (SNP) in the serotonin transporter (5-HTT) gene may contribute to enhanced pain sensitivity among patients with fibromyalgia. Short (S) allele of this SNP (i.e., S/S genotype) in the regulatory region of the *5-HTT* gene occurs significantly more frequently in patients with fibromyalgia than in healthy controls.

The *COMT gene* encodes an enzyme that metabolizes catecholamines (norepinephrine and dopamine) and thereby influences several cognitive-affective phenotypes, including pain phenotypes. Initial studies focused on the *val158met* polymorphism, an SNP in codon 158 of the *COMT gene* that substitutes valine for methionine and results in reduced activity of the enzyme. Individuals who are homozygous for the *met158* allele of this polymorphism have shown diminished regional μ-opioid system responses to tonic pain compared to heterozygotes; these responses have been accompanied by increased pain intensity ratings and more negative internal affective states. Findings from the COMT studies suggest a potential clinical role for pharmacologic agents that affect catecholaminergic activity.

Another gene studied in relation to FM is dopamine D4 receptor (DRD4) gene. An association between fibromyalgia and the DRD4 exon III 7 repeat genotype has been demonstrated and it was found that the frequency of the 7 repeat genotype was significantly lower in persons with fibromyalgia relative to healthy controls.

Other various genes whose link to FM was found were angiotensin converting enzyme and *methylenetetrahydrofolate reductase (MTHFR) gene* C677T polymorphism, tachykinin receptor 1 (TACR1) mutation gene, leukocyte mRNA gene, mitochondrial DNA mutation (m.15804T>C) in the mtCYB gene in peripheral blood cells, epigenetic modification of DNA- three 5'-C-phosphate-G-3' islands (CpGs) (including the genes for malate dehydrogenase 2, tetranectin, and heat shock protein beta-6), and the HLA-region gene. However further studies are needed to prove their exact association.

Psychosocial Stressors

Dissatisfaction with social support from colleagues and monotonous work were the strongest psychosocial predictors of new-onset widespread pain as found by Harkness et al. Psychosocial stress may also affect the severity or aversiveness of pain associated with fibromyalgia, as demonstrated in a study by Davis and colleagues. The prevalence of psychiatric conditions among patients affected by fibromyalgia is higher than among subjects complaining of other rheumatic diseases. The most common disorders associated are anxiety, somatization, dysthymia, panic disorders, posttraumatic stress, and overall depression. Depression is more frequently associated with fibromyalgia and it worsens fibromyalgic symptoms. Of patients with fibromyalgia, 50% have had or will have depression at some time in their lives. 25% of FM patients will meet criteria for depression at the time of diagnosis.

Physical Stressors and Trigger Factors

Physical trauma, injury, manual work, exercises like heavy weight lifting exercise, repetitive motions, squatting for extended periods can be associated factors for occurrence of widespread pain in FM. Infections can be potential trigger factors for FM. In particular, viruses such as HCV, HIV, coxsackie B, and parvovirus and bacteria like *Borrelia* could be involved. Vaccinations and chemical substances may also be trigger factors.

Other Factors

- Fibromyalgia is common in patients affected by autoimmune diseases such as SLE, Sjögren's syndrome. Association between FM and antipolymer antibodies (APAs) had also been studied but results were controversial.
- Vascular dysregulation in muscles, inadequate response to oxidative stress, exacerbated by the nocturnal fall in saturation, increased IL-1 in cutaneous tissues, increased substance P in muscles, and DNA fragmentations of muscle fibers are all suspected to possibly play a role in this condition.
- Vitamin D supplementation improves pain in fibromyalgia pateints. However, because of the lack of well-designed trials, the real importance of vitamin D supplementation in FM is still unclear, and it is only recommended in the case of deficiency.
- Neuroinflammation may be a factor in pathology of FM as there are increased levels of neuropeptides CRH, SP, HK-1, and inflammatory cytokines IL-6 and TNF in serum of patients with fibromyalgia syndrome (FMS). Activated monocytes from FM patients release more eotaxin, C-C Motif Chemokine Ligand 22 (CCL22) and C-X-C Motif Chemokine Ligand 1 (CXCL1) than those of healthy subjects.
- Mitochondrial superoxide production was significantly increased in FM fibroblasts in comparison with controls, and this may be related to impairment of the AMPK pathway, which plays a protective role against oxidative damage.

- Diet is one of the environmental factors that may influence the onset and course of FM. A Puerto Rican study of 144 FM patients found that obese patients were more likely to develop self-reported memory impairments and urinary disturbances than nonoverweight patients, and visceral adiposity also correlated with a higher tender point count. Another study found that being overweight was associated with increased serum levels of C-reactive protein (CRP), apolipoprotein B and triglycerides in FM patients.

CLINICAL FEATURES

1. *Pain*: Either alone or in combination has variously described: Sharp and shooting, stabbing and throbbing, burning and tingling, deep aching and aching in bones, exhausting and feeling bruised all over.
   a. *Other highlights of pain*: Allodynia, hyperalgesia, persistent pain with pronounced summation effect and after-reaction two painful stimuli.
   b. *Tenderness*: Classical tender points on palpation, more localized than radiating to a distant region are generally located at sites of attachment of ligaments and muscles and tendons to the bone.

   Other features of pain:
   - Bilateral pain above and below the waist defines the pain to be widespread.
   - Pain often migratory gets located in nonanatomical or global regions.
   - Pain even over joints are unassociated with swelling and redness.
   - Angina like a typical chest pain with or without breathlessness.
   - Sciatica like radiating pain can be associated with low back pain.
   - 40% patients do have calf cramps
   - Recurring stiffness during daytime following in activity but the morning stiffness persisting from 15 minutes or more is prevalent in 79–83%
   - Severe headache persists in more than half of the patients.
   - TM joint pain should also be considered a forewarning symptom.

2. *Neurological manifestations*: There are three levels of neurological dysfunctions.
   a. Neurotransmitters
   b. Receptors
   c. Abnormal Gating

   These dysfunctions result into dysregulation of sensory information. The neurological manifestations are reflected as follows: Process whereby the prefrontal cortex assigns relative importance to sensory input) resulting in dysregulation of the signal to noise ratio.
   - *Romberg test*: Positive
   - *Dysesthesia and tingling*: 65% involve feet and hands
   - Myofascial pain syndrome may be associated—abnormal twitch response
   - Gait-Tandem Gait
   - Fasciculation along with generalized or muscle weakness
   - Temporal instability—performance of sequencing action becomes difficult
   - Spatial instability—difficult to walk on uneven surfaces due to accommodation inabilities
   - Aberrant perception-gradual loss of
     - Visual focus and accommodation
     - Visual depth perception
   - Hyper-reactive to light, noise, odors and even speed—overload phenomenon.

3. *Neurocognitive dysfunction*:
   "*Fibro frog*": Confusion, forgetfulness or short-term memory consolidation and even lack of concentration. All these are result of either misinterpretation or failing integration of information.

4. *Fatigue*:
   Glucose and muscles
   a. Lowered glucose utilization
   b. Accelerated glucose backflow from tissues to the vascular channel
   c. Deceleration of phosphorylation—results into loss of steady supply of oxygen to muscles.

   Movements initiate paresis or spastic dysfunction and prolonged rest helps recover the muscle fatigue.

5. *Sleep dysfunction*:
   a. Inadequate time spent in nonrapid eye movement (NREM) sleep is represented by deep restorative delta wave stages 3 and 4 in EEG and the alpha waves gets rapidly intruded.
   b. Genesis of tender points has an important contribution from disturbed sleep. This is brought out by observations that normal persons not getting stage 4 sleep due to auditory stimuli do have painful tender joints.
   c. Nocturnal myoclonus—50%
   d. Restlessness syndrome—3%

6. *Autonomic dysfunctions*: Patients of FM shows various symptoms of autonomic dysfunction.
   a. *Neurally-mediated hypotension (NMH), dizziness, and vertigo*: Symptoms of NMH occur upon rising from a prone or sitting position, or standing, and include lightheadedness, cognitive difficulties, blurred vision, severe fatigue, pallor, tremulousness, and syncope. Vertigo, dizziness, tinnitus, nausea and vomiting may also occur. Low resting blood volume, decreased venous return of blood, and/or disturbances of cerebral blood flow may be

involved. Abnormal autonomic response to postural orthostatic stress is common.
   b. *Loss of thermostatic and vasomotor stability*: Body temperature may be subnormal and vasomotor instability often has an unusual distribution. Neuropathic pain may be associated with vasoconstriction and result in part of the body becoming colder. Painful movements may be followed by excessive sweating, and chilling may precipitate pain.
   c. *Neurogenic or trophic edema*: It is common in hands and feet. Changes in shape and loss of flexibility of red blood cells may reduce the rate of blood flow, and oxygen and nutrient delivery into the tissues and inhibit the ability to dispose of metabolic waste.
   d. *Sicca syndrome*: Approximately 30% of FM have symptoms of dry eyes and mouth.
   e. *Respiratory and cardiac irregularities*: Breathing dysregulation may occur, chest wall pain and contractures of chest muscles may contribute to alveolar hypoventilation. Patients may experience regulation abnormalities of heart rate and/or cardiac arrhythmias. Heart abnormalities are suggested by increased sympathetic and decreased parasympathetic basal tones identified by electrocardiograms.
   f. *Intestinal irregularities and bladder dysfunction*: IBS, occurring in approximately 40% of FMS patients. Bladder dysfunction may be associated with allodynia and pain sensitivity.
7. *Neuroendocrine dysfunctions*:
   a. Dysregulation of the HPA axis may be involved in diurnal rhythm abnormalities with hypocortisolemia and blunted response to physiological stress.
   b. Elevated production of prolactin and deficiencies in the production of thyroid stimulating hormone, tetra-iodothyronine (T4), and triiodothyronine (T3) in response to the administration of thyrotropin-releasing hormone suggest a disturbance in the HPT axis. Hypothyroidism is 3–12 times more common in FM patients.
   c. A deficiency of IGF-1 is mediated by hypothalamic-pituitary-growth hormone (HPGH) axis.
   d. Dysmenorrhea is the likely fall out of hypothalamic-pituitary-gonadal (HPG) axis. Premenopausal women are less symptomatic than postmenopausal.
8. *Stiffness*: Limited movements with morning stiffness lasting more than 15 minutes has been attributed to correlate with dramatic increase in hyaluronic acid (HA) but in rheumatoid arthritis hyaluronic acid is not elevated to such higher extent.
9. *Musculoskeletal changes*: These patients usually have muscle shortening and postural imbalance which develops over prolonged period of time from months to years to blow out. Continuous increased muscle tension and spasm due to non-voluntary motor activity in early phase is perceptible on EMG, whereas in later stage spontaneous muscle shortening or contractures are visible in EMG as nonaction potentials in localized bands. Fibrotic cord like bands can be palpated in the muscle belly or groups. The muscles with tout bands are weak with resultant stiffness. Enthesopathy can be usual accompaniment along with various deformities of the spine like kyphosis, scoliosis, exacerbated lumbar lordosis, etc.

DIAGNOSIS

Clinical evaluation alone is the guide to proper diagnosis. Neither any lab test nor any biomarker has evolved to establish the diagnosis. No imaging modality is facilitatory, either.

Rheumatic diseases, hypothyroidism and degenerative osteoarthritis are closely mimicking the symptoms and should be evaluated and ruled out.

Evolution of Diagnostic Criteria by American College of Rheumatology

The diagnostic criteria of ACR evolved in 1990 as research classification criteria and were not meant for use in clinical practice as strict tool for diagnosis.

As per these criteria, the following requirements are necessary prerequisites for diagnosis of fibromyalgia:
   i. Widespread pain in axial skeleton above and below the waist with bilateral involvement of the body.
   ii. Duration of symptoms ≥3 months.
   iii. Tenderness at 11 or more of 18 possible sites of "tender points"
   iv. Palpating digital pressure of 4 kg/cm² for 4 seconds just enough for the examiner's thumbnail.

Every patient of fibromyalgia may not have widespread pain all over the body as well as may not also have at least 11 tender points (**Fig. 6**). This diagnostic criterion has sensitivity of 88% and specificity of 81%. This also has 25% false negatives. Primary care physicians did rely more on tender points and did not consider other symptoms.

In 2010, ACR introduced newer diagnostic criteria. They were put forward as an alternative to clinical diagnosis. 19 painful spots were identified along with 41 somatic symptoms. They were not intended to replace the 1990 criteria. In this modification, tender points examination were not required. It was based on widespread pain index (WPI) and symptom severity (SS) score. The widespread pain index had a scale of 0–19 with a cutoff >8. The diagnosis has sensitivity of 83.2%, specificity of 87.6%, and accuracy of 85.4%.

Table 1 shows the differences between the ACR 1990 and the revised ACR 2010 criteria for FM.

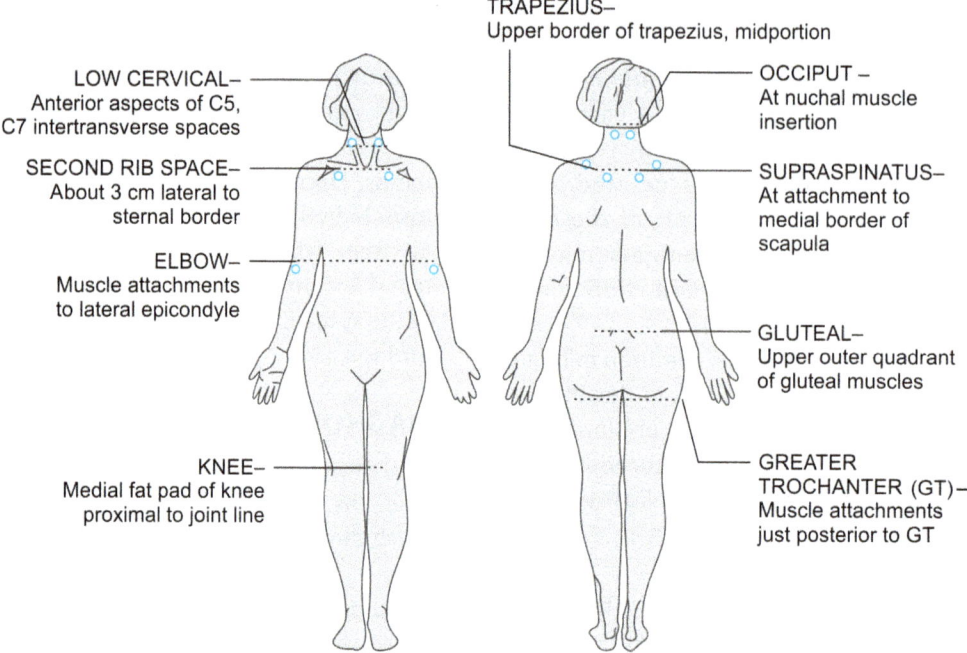

Fig. 6: Tender points based on 1990 American College of Rheumatology (ACR) criteria.
Source: Chakrabarty S, Zoorob R. Fibromyalgia. Am Fam Physician. 2007;76(2):247-54.

TABLE 1: Differences between the American College of Rheumatology (ACR) 1990 and the revised ACR 2010 criteria for fibromyalgia (FM).

1990	2010
History of widespread pain	WPI ≥ 7 and SS ≥ 5 or WPI 3–6 and SS ≥ 9
Pain of ≥3 months' duration	Symptoms have been present at a similar level for ≥3 months
Pain in 11 of 18 tender points on digital palpation	Patient does not have a disorder that would otherwise explain the pain
Definitions	
• Widespread pain • Pain on left side of body, right side of body, above waist, below waist and axial skeletal pain	• WPI score • The number of areas in which patient has had pain over the last week (six lower extremities, six upper extremities, seven axial skeleton) • *Final score*: Between 0 and 19
• Tender points (all bilateral) • Occiput, low cervical, trapezius, supraspinatus, second rib, lateral epicondyle, gluteal, greater trochanter, knee	• SS score • The sum of severity of fatigue, waking un-refreshed and cognitive symptoms, plus the severity of general somatic symptoms • Each symptom is rated on a scale of 0–3, where 0 = no symptoms/problem and 3 = severe symptoms/problems • *Final score*: Between 0 and 12

(SS: symptom severity; WPI: widespread pain index)
Source: Arnold LM, Gebke KB, Choy EH. Fibromyalgia: management strategies for primary care providers. Int J Clin Pract. 2016;70(2):99-112.

The WPI assessment points and symptoms severity scale are described in **Boxes 1 and 2**.

In 2011, ACR criteria was modified further to do away with the ambiguity of 2010 criteria for coming to a clinical diagnosis. This was put forward to simplify and make it clinician friendly for use. These criteria retained the 19 sites WPI and have a scope for self-reporting by the patient of their specific symptoms. It eliminated the physician's estimation of SS score. It was replaced by three "Yes/No" of dichotomous nature concerning depression, abdominal pain and headaches in previous 6 months. Hence, 2011 criteria took into consideration the presence of severity and location of self-survey of various symptoms faced by the patients **(Fig. 7)**.

The symptoms included:
- Fatigue
- Sleep disturbances
- Headache
- Mood problems
- IBS
- Memory problems

Box 1: Widespread pain index.

Note the number of areas in which the patient has had pain over the last week.
- Shoulder girdle, left
- Shoulder girdle, right
- Upper arm, left
- Upper arm, right
- Lower arm, left
- Lower arm, right
- Hip (buttock, trochanter), left
- Hip (buttock, trochanter), right
- Upper leg, left
- Upper leg, right
- Lower leg, left
- Lower leg, right
- Jaw, left
- Jaw, right
- Chest
- Abdomen
- Upper back
- Lower back
- Neck

Total score (will be 0 to 19)

Box 2: Symptoms severity scale.

Score is the sum of the severity of the three symptoms plus the extent (severity) of somatic symptoms in general. Score will be between 0 and 12.
1. Fatigue
2. Waking unrefreshed
3. Cognitive symptoms

For each of the 3 symptoms above, indicate the level of severity over the past week using the following scale:

0 = no problem
1 = slight or mild problems, generally mild or intermittent
2 = moderate, considerable problems, often present and/or at a moderate level
3 = severe: pervasive, continuous, life-disturbing problems

Considering somatic symptoms in general, indicate whether the patient has:

0 = no symptoms
1 = few symptoms
2 = a moderate number of symptoms
3 = a great number of symptoms

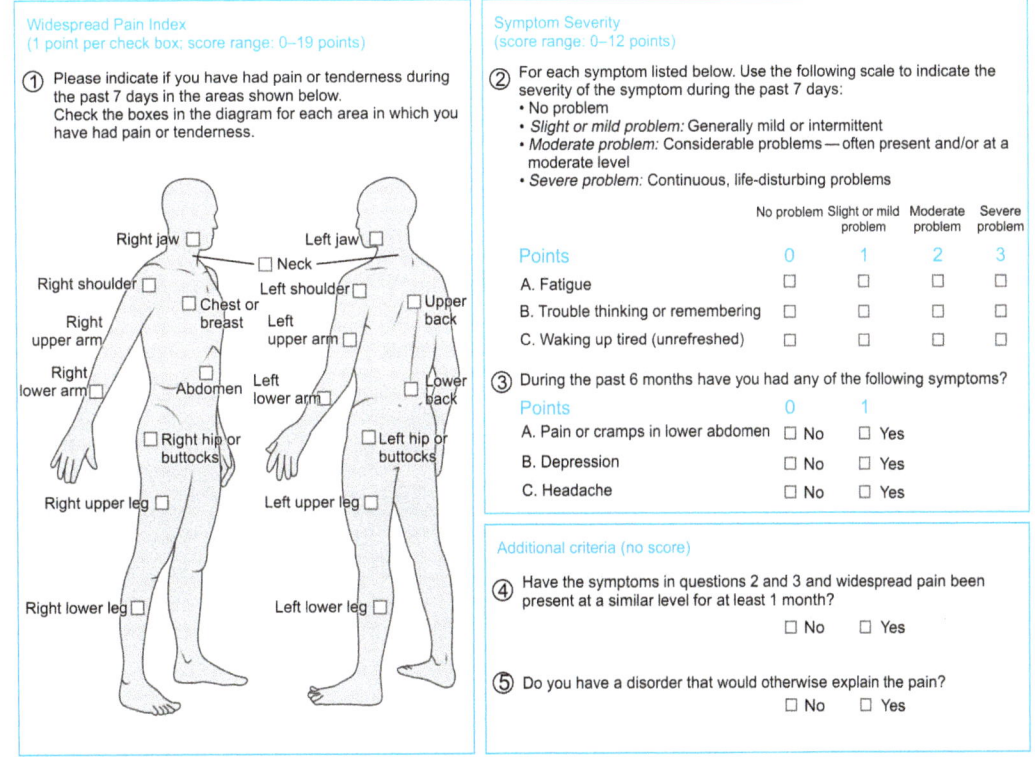

Fig. 7: Example of a patient self-report survey for the assessment of fibromyalgia based on criteria in the 2011 modification of the American College of Rheumatology (ACR) preliminary diagnostic criteria for fibromyalgia. Scoring information is shown in blue. The possible score ranges from 0 to 31 point; a score ≥13 points is consistent with a diagnosis of fibromyalgia.

These criteria were thought to be a practical approach involving the patients themselves. A score of ≥13 points out of 0–31 points is in favor of diagnosis of fibromyalgia. Inadequate number of tender points, helped in identifying some male patients who did not meet the 1990 criteria.

Fibromyalgianess was a word coined for the core symptoms of pain centralization-this new criteria had evolved this concept. It had 83% sensitivity and specificity of 67%. Bennett in 2014 graded this as 74% of correct classification. Bennett further proposed on alternative criteria same to 19 points. The 16 modified locations were added in pain location inventory (PLI):

i. Jaw
ii. Neck
iii. Mid-upper back
iv. Front of the chest

v. Mid-lower back
vi. Upper back
vii. Lower back
viii. Shoulders
ix. Arms
x. Hands
xi. Wrists
xii. Hips
xiii. Thighs
xiv. Knees
xv. Ankles
xvi. Feet.

It had 10-item questionnaire regarding symptom impact (SIQR) **(Fig. 8)**.

Final evolution reported 81% sensitivity, 80% specificity. For diagnosis of fibromyalgia, 80% correct classification score was achieved. Among patients meeting 1990 or 2010/2011 criteria, those with fibromyalgia cannot be clearly distinguished from others with illnesses like chronic fatigue and IBS if such patients also satisfy fibromyalgia criteria. Another problem with the 2010/2011 criteria was, misclassifying a small fraction of patients who did not have generalized pain. So, a further modification in ACR 2010/2011 criteria was done in 2016.

The fibromyalgia syndrome (FS) scale is synonymous polysymptomatic distress (PSD) scale. It has been excluded in generalized pain definition. The changes in these criteria from previous criteria are listed in **Box 4**.

Pain location inventory (PLI)
Directions: For each of the following 28 sites, select those locations where you have experienced persistent pain during the past 7 days. The score will be between 0 and 28.

10-item SIQR symptoms:
Directions: For each of the following 10 questions, check the one box that best indicates the intensity of the following common symptoms over the last 7 days:

Criteria:

		0 1 2 3 4 5 6 7 8 9 10	
1. Pain	No pain	☐☐☐☐☐☐☐☐☐☐☐	Unbearable pain
2. Energy	Lots of energy	☐☐☐☐☐☐☐☐☐☐☐	No energy
3. Stiffness	No stiffness	☐☐☐☐☐☐☐☐☐☐☐	Severe stiffness
4. Sleep	Awoke rested	☐☐☐☐☐☐☐☐☐☐☐	Awoke very tired
5. Depression	No depression	☐☐☐☐☐☐☐☐☐☐☐	Very depressed
6. Memory problems	Good memory	☐☐☐☐☐☐☐☐☐☐☐	Very poor memory
7. Anxiety	Not anxious	☐☐☐☐☐☐☐☐☐☐☐	Very anxious
8. Tenderness to touch	No tenderness	☐☐☐☐☐☐☐☐☐☐☐	Very tender
9. Balance problems	No imbalance	☐☐☐☐☐☐☐☐☐☐☐	Severe imbalance
10. Sensitivity to loud noises, bright lights, odors and cold	No sensitivity	☐☐☐☐☐☐☐☐☐☐☐	Extreme sensitivity

Note: Summate the 10 individual scores; the range will be between 0 and 100. Divide this summated score by 2 to obtain the SIQR symptom score.

A patient fulfilling the following guidelines has a high likelihood of having fibromyalgia:*

1. The symptoms and pain locations have been persistent for at least the last 3 months
2. Pain location score is ≥17
3. SIQR symptom score is ≥21

*1. Fibromyalgia patients have a continuum of symptoms; a diagnosis based on a strict numerical cutoff is subject to error.
*2. The presence of another pain disorders or related symptoms does not rule out a diagnosis of fibromyalgia.
*3. A careful clinical evaluation is always required in order to identify any condition that could fully account for the patient's symptoms and/or contribute to the severity of the symptoms.

Fig. 8: The 2013 alternative criteria for diagnosing fibromyalgia.

Box 3: Fibromyalgia criteria—2016 revision.

Criteria:
A patient satisfies modified 2016 fibromyalgia criteria if the following FIRST 3 conditions are met:
1. Widespread pain index (WPI) ≥ 7 and symptom severity scale (SSS) score ≥ 5 OR WPI of 4–6 and SSS score ≥9
2. Generalized pain, defined as pain in at least 4 of 5 regions, must be present. Jaw, chest, and abdominal pain are not included in generalized pain definition
3. Symptoms have been generally present for at least 3 months
4. A diagnosis of fibromyalgia is valid irrespective of other diagnoses. A diagnosis of fibromyalgia does not exclude the presence of other clinically important illnesses

Ascertainment:
1. **WPI**: Note the number of areas in which the patient has had pain over the last week. In how many areas has the patient had pain? Score will be between 0 and 19
   Left upper region (Region 1)
   Left jaw[a], left shoulder girdle, left upper arm, left lower arm
   Right upper region (Region 2)
   Right jaw[a], right shoulder girdle, right upper arm, right lower arm
   Left lower region (Region 3)
   Left hip (buttock, trochanter), left upper leg, left lower leg
   Right lower region (Region 4)
   Right hip (buttock, trochanter), right upper leg, right lower leg
   Axial region (Region 5)
   Neck, upper back, lower back, chest[a], abdomen[a]
2. **Symptom severity scale (SSS) score:**
   Fatigue
   Waking unrefreshed
   Cognitive symptoms
   For the each of the 3 symptoms above, indicate the level of severity over the past week using the following scale:
   0 = No problem
   1 = Slight or mild problems, generally mild or intermittent
   2 = Moderate, considerable problems, often present and/or at a moderate level
   3 = Severe, pervasive, continuous, life-disturbing problems

The symptom severity scale (SSS) score: It is the sum of the severity scores of the 3 symptoms (fatigue, waking unrefreshed, and cognitive symptoms) (0–9) plus the sum (0–3) of the number of the following symptoms the patient has been bothered by that occurred during the previous 6 months:
1. Headaches (0–1)
2. Pain or cramps in lower abdomen (0–1)
3. And depression (0–1)
The final symptom severity score is between 0 and 12
The fibromyalgia severity (FS) scale is the sum of the WPI and SSS

[a]Not included in generalized pain definition

Box 4: 2016 Changes to modified ACR fibromyalgia diagnostic criteria.

This revision makes the following changes to the fibromyalgia criteria shown in **Box 3**
1. Changes criterion 1 to "widespread pain index (WPI) ≥ 7 and symptom severity scale (SSS) score ≥ 5 OR WPI 4–6 and SSS score ≥ 9" (WPI minimum must be ≥4 instead of previous ≥3)
2. Adds a generalized pain criterion (criterion 2), and one that is different from the 1990 widespread pain definition. The definition is: "Generalized pain is defined as pain in at least 4 of 5 regions. In this definition, jaw, chest, and abdominal pain are not evaluated as part of the generalized pain definition"
3. Standardizes and makes 2010 and 2011 criterion (criterion 3) wording the same: "Symptoms have been generally present for at least 3 months"
4. Removes the exclusion that regarding disorders that could (sufficiently) explain the pain (criterion 4) and adds the following text: "A diagnosis of fibromyalgia is valid irrespective of other diagnoses. A diagnosis of fibromyalgia does not exclude the presence of other clinically important illnesses"
5. Adds the fibromyalgia symptom scale as a full component of the fibromyalgia criteria
6. Creates one set of criteria instead of having separate physician and patient criteria by replacing the physician estimate of somatic symptom burden with ascertainment of the presence of headaches, pain or cramps in lower abdomen, and depression during the previous 6 months

A multifocal pain without any background of injury or inflammation, suspect fibromyalgia in clinical practice setup. Most prominently, musculoskeletal pain is the iconic symptom. Pain can be perceived anywhere in the body for the mere fact that there is existence of amplification of pain pathways. The usual accompaniments are:
- Chronic headache
- Sensory hyper-responsiveness
- Visceral pain
- Sore throat

Unearthing depression, symptomatic myofascial trigger points, and arthritis will rule out the mimicking pathologies on thorough clinical evolution. This finally will modify the approach the further treatment. Apart from the awareness of presence of fibromyalgia, in presence of diffuse chronic myofascial pain, it requires that any comorbid association with rheumatic diseases is to be unearthed. Thyroid dysfunction SLE, RA and ankylosing spondylitis must especially be hunted for any such association.

Any patient repeatedly presenting himself before the physician for examination because of progression of symptoms, it is apt to suspect fibromyalgia. The progressive symptoms includes:
- Chronic pain spread out in body
- Fatigue
- Sleep disturbances

Comorbid disorders such as IBS, pelvic or genitourinary pain, TM joint disorders, mood disorders, migraine could provide a key lead in diagnosis.

For diagnosis of FM, a detailed physical examination must be carried out by physician. Finally it is worthwhile to repeatedly mention that detailed physical examination must include:
- Evaluation of joints to rule out inflammation
- Looking for tenderness or pain threshold by prescribed digital pressure
- Neurological examination
- Rule out possible potential contributory factors responsible for symptoms

Laboratory Investigations

Laboratory tests are generally not necessary for confirming the diagnosis of FM, but rather it should be done to rule out other diseases. Routine tests such as CBC, ESR, CRP, routine serum chemistry, thyroid function tests should be done for causes of fatigue and hypothyroidism. CPK can be done for myalgia and various serological tests can be done for other autoimmune and chronic inflammatory conditions, if suspected.

Differential Diagnosis
- Polyarticular arthritis
  - Rheumatoid arthritis
  - Systemic lupus erythematosus (SLE)
  - Polymyalgia rheumatica
- Endocrine disorders
  - Hypothyroidism
  - Hyperparathyroidism (hypercalcemia)
- Myopathies
  - Polymyositis
  - Rhabdomyolysis
- Neuropathies
- Depression
- Chronic fatigue syndrome
- Myofascial pain syndrome
- Anemia

Overlapping Syndromes and Symptoms

Common comorbidities:
- Rheumatoid arthritis (12%)
- SLE
- Hepatitis C
- Myofascial pain syndrome
- Temporomandibular joint syndrome
- IBS
- Osteoarthritis (7%)
- Depression
- Migraine headaches
- Obstructive sleep apnea (OSA)
- Restless legs

Common Symptoms
- Fatigue
- Subjective joint/muscle swelling
- Difficulty sleeping
- Night sweats
- Dyspnea
- Palpitations
- Pelvic pain
- Dysmenorrhea
- Noncardiac chest pain
- Diarrhea/constipation (IBS)

■ TREATMENT

Over long time, a large variety of modalities have been tested for treating FMS but no single modality has been found to be universally effective for all FMS patients or all FMS symptoms in an individual patient. Because pain, depression, and other symptoms of fibromyalgia are linked to inherited and environmental causes, a multifaceted treatment approach is often required including both nonpharmacological pain management strategies and medication **(Table 2)**.

TABLE 2: Pharmacological and nonpharmacological therapy for fibromyalgia syndrome.

Pharmacological therapy	Nonpharmacologic therapy

• FDA approved drugs
  – Pregabalin
  – Duloxetine
  – Milnacipran
• Amitriptyline
• Cyclobenzaprine
• Gabapentin
• Venlafaxine
• Selective serotonin reuptake inhibitors
  – Fluoxetine
  – Paroxetine
  – Citalopram
• Dopamine agonist
  – Pramipexole
  – Ropinirole
• Opioids
• Pain medications
• Tramadol
• Tropisetron
• Sodium oxybate
• Monoamine oxidase inhibitors
  – Pirlindole
  – Moclobemide
• Growth hormone
	• Patient education
	• Exercise
	• Biofeedback
	• Cognitive behavioral therapy
	• Nutrition
	• Hypnotherapy
	• Tai chi, Yoga
	• Massage
	• Balneotherapy
	• Chiropractic
	• Capsaicin
	• S-adenosyl methionine
	• Hydrotherapy/spa therapy
	• Multicomponent therapy

The goals of fibromyalgia treatment are to alleviate pain, increase restorative sleep, and improve physical function through a reduction in associated symptoms. The identification and treatment of all pain sources that may be present in addition to fibromyalgia such as peripheral inflammatory or neuropathic pain generators (e.g., comorbid osteoarthritis or neuropathic pathologies) or visceral pain (e.g., comorbid IBS) are central to the proper clinical management of fibromyalgia.

Pharmacological Therapy

FDA Approved Drugs

Currently, only three drugs are FDA approved: Pregabalin, duloxetine and milnacipran which were approved in 2007, 2008 and 2009, respectively **(Table 3)**. These medications work either to increase the activity of inhibitory neurotransmitters (to "turn down the pain volume") or to reduce the activity of facilitatory neurotransmitters (which "turn up the pain volume").

Pregabalin is a γ-aminobutyric acid (GABA) analog and antiepileptic agent. A systematic review evaluating the efficacy of pregabalin found a benefit of pregabalin relative to placebo in pain reduction, improvement in sleep and quality of life measures (except for mood variables). A meta-analysis of 4 randomized controlled trials (RCTs) with more than 3,000 patients has shown that a 30% pain reduction was reported by 40% of patients receiving pregabalin versus 28% of those receiving placebo.

Duloxetine and *Milnacipran* both are serotonin norepinephrine reuptake inhibitors (SNRIs). Double-blind RCTs evaluating duloxetine doses ranging between 60 and 120 mg per day have typically shown greater improvement in pain reports and self-report functioning than those in the placebo arm. Analysis of pooled data from the 4 RCTs indicates that 48% of treated patients and 32% of patients receiving placebo reported >30% pain reduction. However, low doses duloxetine less than 30 mg per day failed to show improvement in pain severity relative to placebo, mostly due to marked placebo effects.

A double-blind RCTs evaluating *milnacipran* (100–200 mg daily) showed significant improvement in pain reports and a range of symptoms as compared to placebo. Pooled data from two RCTs showed approximately 52–61% of treated patients reporting >30% pain reduction, versus 36% of the placebo group.

Figure 9 shows the results (percentage of patients reporting >30% pain reduction) from the three trials by dose.

Amitriptyline: It is a tricyclic antidepressant (TCA). It has long been the mainstay therapy for FM. Their low cost and benefit in chronic neuropathic pain has supported its use. By inhibiting the reuptake of both serotonin and norepinephrine, tricyclic compounds enhance norepinephrine and serotonin neurotransmission in the descending inhibitory pain pathways, resulting in a reduction in pain. A systematic review of 10 RCTs evaluated amitriptyline, at dosages of 25 or 50 mg daily, in 615 patients. Six of the 10 trials used 25 mg

TABLE 3: A comparison of FDA approved pharmacological medications for fibromyalgia (pivotal studies).

Drug	FDA approval	Mechanism of action	Efficacy studies	Primary end points	dosing	Adverse events[a]
Pregabalin	June 21st 2007	γ-aminobutyric acid (GABA) analog and antiepileptic agent	• 14 weeks, randomized, double blind, placebo controlled • 6 months, randomized, withdrawal	Pain reduction, improvements in PGIC and FIQ	300–450 mg/day; start at 75 mg bid (might increase to 150 mg bid within 1 week); maximum dose 225 mg bid	300–450 mg/day; start at 75 mg bid (might increase to 150 mg bid within 1 week); maximum dose 225 mg bid
Duloxetine	16 June 2008	SNRI	• 3 months, randomized, double blind, placebo controlled • 6 months, randomized, double blind, placebo controlled	Pain reduction, improvements in PGIC and FIQ	60 mg/day; start 30 mg/day for 1 week then increase to 60 mg/day	Nausea, dry mouth, somnolence constipation, decreased appetite, hyperhidrosis
Milnacipran	14 January 2009	SNRI	• 3 months, randomized, double blind, placebo controlled • 6 months, randomized, double blind, placebo controlled	Composite end point that concurrently evaluated improvement in pain (VAS), physical function (SF 36 PCS) and PGIC	100 mg/day; start 12.5 mg/day, increasing incrementally to 50 mg bid in 1 week; maximum dose 100 mg bid	Nausea, constipation, hot flush, hyperhidrosis, vomiting, palpitations, increased heart rate, dry mouth, hypertension

(bid: twice daily; FDA: US Food and Drug Administration; FIQ: Fibromyalgia Impact Questionnaire; FM: fibromyalgia; PGIC: patient global impression of change; SF36 PCS: Short Form 36 Physical Component Summary; SNRI: serotonin norepinephrine reuptake inhibitor; VAS: visual analog scale)

[a]The most commonly reported adverse events are shown.

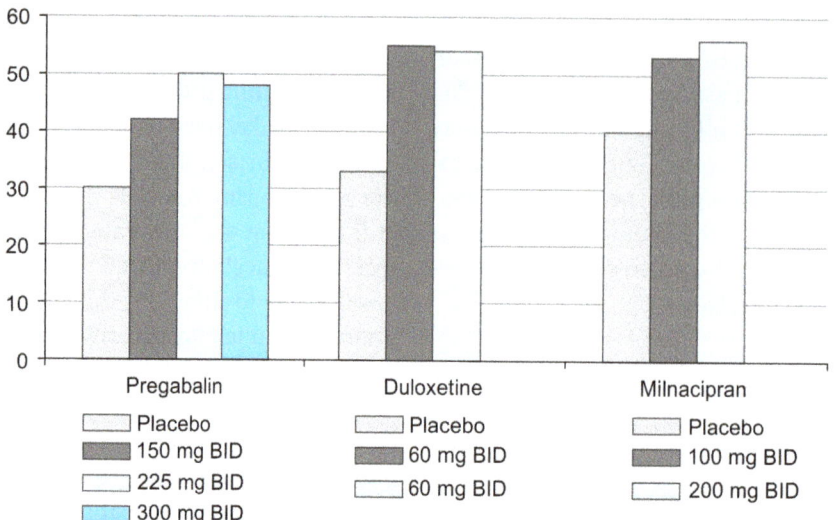

Fig. 9: Percentage of patients reporting >30% pain reduction by dose for pregabalin, duloxetine, and milnacipran versus placebo. (BID: twice daily; QD: every day)

daily, which significantly improved pain, sleep disturbances, and fatigue. Amitriptyline 50 mg daily did not show a benefit over placebo, possibly because of a large adverse event-related drop-out rate. Häuser et al. reported that patients receiving amitriptyline were more likely to achieve 30% pain reduction, equivalent to a "number needed to treat (NNT)" of 3.54. In a meta-analysis by Arnold et al., the largest improvement was associated with measures of sleep quality; the most modest improvements were found in measures of stiffness and tenderness.

Tricyclic antidepressants possess significant affinity for histaminergic, cholinergic, and adrenergic receptor systems, which contribute to their strong side effects such as sedation, dry mouth, gastrointestinal disturbance, weight gain and constipation at higher doses. No dosage adjustments are required for impaired kidney function.

Cyclobenzaprine: It is structurally similar to TCAs. Five trials were included in a meta-analysis comparing cyclobenzaprine, at dosages of 10–30 mg daily, with placebo. Sleep and pain symptoms improved for three times the number of patients taking cyclobenzaprine versus placebo. Fatigue or tender points did not improve with cyclobenzaprine, and 85% of the patients taking cyclobenzaprine reported adverse effects. Its NNT is 4.8.

Gabapentin: It is not extensively studied but its similarity to pregabalin suggests a potential benefit. Compared with placebo, gabapentin titrated to a dosage of 1,200–2,400 mg/day significantly improved the pain severity score. Other scales for symptom severity, including an assessment of sleep, showed benefits with gabapentin compared with placebo. Dizziness, weight gain, and sedation were noted with gabapentin.

Venlafaxine: Venlafaxine is a selective serotonin and norepinephrine reuptake inhibitor (SSNRIs) antidepressant. It is used as an off-label treatment for fibromyalgia. Its mechanism of action is still not fully understood, but it is thought that it affects positively the communication between nerve cells in the central nervous system and/or restores chemical balance in the brain. Two small open-label studies with venlafaxine have been conducted, one using immediate release venlafaxine 37.5–375 mg daily in 15 patients and one using venlafaxine 75 mg daily in 20 patients. In both trials, pain improved from baseline using a visual scale and pain questionnaire. In another study venlafaxine treatment improved fibromyalgia symptoms and pain severity particularly in women. Venlafaxine is taken orally, two or three times a day. It is usually started on a lower dose then gradually increased. It may take 1–4 weeks or longer before its effects are effective. This drug may also give withdrawal symptoms, so it should not be suddenly stopped. Common venlafaxine side effects may include vision changes, nausea, vomiting and diarrhea, changes in appetite or weight, dry mouth, yawning, dizziness, headache, anxiety, nervousness, fast heartbeats, tremors or shaking, etc.

Selective Serotonin Reuptake Inhibitors

Fluoxetine, paroxetine, and citalopram are common drugs in this group of SSRIs. They are antidepressants that increase the concentration of serotonin in the brain. In a study by Arnold et al., a flexible placebo controlled dose study of fluoxetine (dose <80 mg/day) demonstrated significant efficacy in women with FM. Improvement was noted in FIQ total score as well as sub-scores for pain, fatigue and depression. Pain in tender points and total myalgic scores were not significantly improved. Cochrane meta-analysis reviewed eight double-blind randomized controlled trials that included 383 patients. Six of the eight studies showed superior efficacy than in placebo in global improvement measures and pain in patients who had >30% pain reduction while two studies did not show a statistically significant difference. SSRIs were found to be superior to placebo for depression symptoms in patients with fibromyalgia. SSRIs were also superior to placebo for improvements in pain intensity as well as disease-specific quality of life. Although a small, statistically significant benefit was detected for 30% pain reduction, global improvement, and depression with SSRIs versus placebo in this meta-analysis, the quality of evidence was very low because of the limited numbers of patients and the potential for attrition and reporting bias. Its doses are 20–40 mg/day citalopram, 20–80 mg/day fluoxetine and 20–60 mg/day paroxetine. Its major side effects are increased suicidal tendency in young adults aged 18–24, with major depressive disorders. Other side effects are drowsiness, nausea, dry mouth, insomnia, diarrhea, nervousness, agitation or restlessness, dizziness, etc.

Dopamine Agonists

Pramipexole and ropinirole are common drugs in this group. Dopamine agonists may decrease adrenergic arousal that may contribute to disordered sleep in patients with fibromyalgia. In a small 14-week trial of 60 patients initiated on treatment with pramipexole, 42% of patients had a 50% or more reduction in their pain score using a visual analog scale, compared with 14% of patients taking placebo. A trial of ropinirole found no benefit; however, the discontinuation rate was high (63%) for both intolerance and lack of efficacy. Dose of pramipexole is 4.5 mg/day. Common adverse effects are transient anxiety and weight loss.

Opioids

Opioids are not recommended for fibromyalgia because these drugs may actually worsen symptoms such as fatigue and cognitive impairment. A 1-year observational study evaluated the use of opioids in 1,700 adults with fibromyalgia and found that patients taking nonopioid pain relievers demonstrated greater improvements in assessments such as the BPI and FIQ.

Pain Medications

Although pain is a characteristic feature of fibromyalgia, analgesics are often of limited clinical value. Nonsteroidal anti-inflammatory drugs and acetaminophen act peripherally and are therefore less likely to be of benefit for the centrally mediated pain mechanisms that are associated with fibromyalgia. A single review identified two small trials with no evidence of improved outcome compared with placebo.

Tramadol

Tramadol is a weak opioid with mild serotonin-noradrenalin reuptake inhibitor (SNRI) activity. In a study it showed statistically significant improvements in pain intensity, pain relief and myalgic scores. The recommended dose of tramadol is 50–100 mg (immediate release tablets) every 4–6 hours as needed for pain with maximum dose is 400 mg/day. Its common side effects are nausea, constipation, dizziness, headache, etc. A careful consideration of adverse effects and the abuse potential should be considered before tramadol is used for fibromyalgia pain relief.

Tropisetron

It is a serotonin 5-HT3 receptor antagonist. 28 days treatment of fibromyalgia patients with 5 mg tropisetron resulted in significant pain reduction, which was most pronounced after 10 days with a further reduction up to day 28. Psychometric tests showed significant improvements in depression and anxiety state scores, while functional symptoms improved with extended tropisetron treatment. At higher doses (15 mg/day) the decrease in pain was less than in the placebo group but side effects increased. Its common side effects are headache, constipation, and dizziness.

Sodium Oxybate

It is a commercially produced form of the sodium salt of γ-hydroxybutyric acid (GHB). Its ability to restore slow wave sleep (SWS) has led to a series of trials to evaluate the efficacy of sodium oxybate for treating FMS and an application to the FDA. An early small, crossover RCT showed that sodium oxybate 6 g a day at bedtime for 4 weeks significantly improved pain, fatigue, and sleep (restored SWS) as compared to placebo. Multicenter studies have shown that sodium oxybate 4.5–6 g per night significantly improved clinical pain and FMS-related symptoms relative to placebo. This drug has potential for abuse and misuse.

Monoamine Oxidase Inhibitors

Pirlindole and moclobemide are common among this group. Its doses are pirlindole 150 mg/day and moclobemide 150–300 mg/day. Häuser et al. reported a moderate effect on pain across the studies but the single studies that evaluated fatigue and sleep showed no effect. Monoamine oxidase inhibitors (MAOIs) are known to cause potentially fatal hypertensive crises, serotonin syndrome and psychosis when they interact with foods containing tyramine and medications (many of which are commonly used in the treatment of FM), including SSRIs, TCAs and tramadol.

Growth Hormone

There is evidence of functional growth hormone (GH) deficiency, expressed by means of low IGF-1 serum levels, in a subset of fibromyalgia patients. Regarding fibromyalgia patients with low IGF-1 levels, GH administration demonstrated efficacy and a good tolerability profile in a placebo-controlled study. In another study GH group showed a 60% reduction in the mean number of tender points (pairs) compared to the control group and improvements in FIQ score and EQ-VAS scale. A single systematic review of two studies involving 74 patients reported an effect size on pain of 1.36 (0.01 to 1.34). The improvement in functional deficit was not statistically significant. Its recommended dose is 0.0125 mg/kg/day. Common adverse effects are sleep apnea, carpal tunnel syndrome.

Nonpharmacologic Therapy

Patient Education

As with any chronic condition that requires ongoing management, patient education is critical in aiding patient understanding, acceptance and self-management of their condition. The use of familiar terminology might help the patient better understand the clinical picture and provide reassurance. However, because time for patient education is likely to be limited during a consultation, the use of clinical support staff to provide supplementary information is the key, along with details of useful educational sources (books, websites, advocacy groups, etc.). It is also recommended that physicians partner with patients to decide on treatments, set goals and manage their expectations of symptom improvement and impact on daily life. Poor communication between patient and physician is likely to lead to frustration and over-reliance on pharmacological interventions with limited benefit; whereas shared decision making and positive interactions might help patients engage with their treatment and actively manage their pain.

Exercise

Exercise as a therapy for fibromyalgia may appear paradoxical given the syndrome's classic symptoms of pain and fatigue. However, strong evidence supports exercise as an effective treatment. Aerobic exercise is most often recommended, but resistance and flexibility exercise may also be of benefit. Physical exercises (PE) have a direct positive impact on joint rigidity, muscle stiffness, widespread pain and tenderness, and fatigue and secondary positive effects on cognitive dysfunction. Evidence-based aerobic exercise programs focus on increasing strength and flexibility, but they cannot have high-intensity or be performed too frequently. Low-impact exercise programs and the constant ability to individualize the protocol are crucial in ensuring optimal adherence to such regimens to promote a shift to a more physical lifestyle with a good attitude. Isometric contractions are not recommended, because they increase muscle pain, discouraging further exercise in someone who already engages in little physical activity.

Generally, exercise activates the endogenous opioid and adrenergic systems but does not consistently mitigate pain in FM patients, possibly due to sensitization of the primary afferent pathways or the dysfunction of endogenous systems that modulate afferent activity in FM and the overall increase in sensitivity. Pain has seemingly infinite interindividual variability, wherein a complex relationship exists between proprioceptive capacity, tactile acuity, pain intensity, and cortical organization. Thus, as reported, a specific tactile and proprioceptive rehabilitation program, comprising somatosensory stimuli to the painful area, patient-specific perceptive exercises, and motor imagery, can reduce pain and sensory dysfunction.

A review of 16 trials, by Busch et al. involving a total of 724 patients, that focused on exercise as a treatment for fibromyalgia divided exercise interventions into categories of single exercise (aerobic training, strength training, flexibility training) or more than one type of exercise (mixed training). Benefits were noted in all exercise groups compared with control groups with regard to aerobic performance, tender-point pain pressure threshold, and pain. A review that focused specifically on resistance training showed improvements in overall well-being, physical function, pain reporting, tenderness, and muscle strength, thereby supporting a role for resistance training in fibromyalgia treatment.

The general recommendations for providing exercise therapy include:
- Starting at a low level where patients can engage without significant distress.
- Gradual increase of the intensity level.
- Incorporating different types of exercise.
- Reduction of exercise intensity/duration, while maintaining the frequency of exercise, if not tolerated.

Biofeedback

Biofeedback is a mind-body technique used to teach people how to control involuntary body functions such as heart rate, blood pressure and muscle clenching. It is a very popular intervention alone or within cognitive-behavioral or multidisciplinary pain treatments. Biofeedback is a procedure in which patients' bodily responses such as muscle tension, heart rate, or skin temperature are monitored and reported to the patient through an auditory or visual modality. The information it provides can help patients be more aware of how his/her body reacts to physical or psychological stress. Once they are aware of their reactions, they can work on changing them. Various biofeedback modalities are used, electromyographic feedback (EMG-FB) being the most common for treatment of fibromyalgia and another is electroencephalographic feedback (EEG-FB).

Biofeedback is often called a "psychophysiological intervention," although its change mechanisms are more psychological than physiological: it has been repeatedly demonstrated that the effectiveness of EMG biofeedback is mediated by cognitive changes, such as increases in self-efficacy and coping strategies induced through biofeedback training, rather than primarily by learned physiological control. Glombiewski et al. reviewed seven studies, comprising 321 participants. Treatment sessions varied from 6 to 22; with control therapy comprising sham biofeedback, attention control, medication and treatment as usual. Biofeedback was effective in reducing pain intensity (Hedges' g = 0.79; 0.22 to 1.36). Only EMG-FB and not EEG-FB significantly reduced pain intensity in comparison to control groups. Biofeedback did not reduce sleep problems, depression, fatigue, or health-related quality of life in comparison to a control group.

Cognitive Behavioral Therapy

Cognitive behavioral therapy (CBT) is a type of short-term psychotherapy that is typically used to change the way of thinking and behavior toward something, such as sleep. For example, years of insomnia can create negative mental images of what it means to go to bed (i.e., frustration, anxiety, rising pain levels), and that may cause patients to stay up late and become stressed about even attempting to sleep. In CBT, a therapist would try to help them by changing their thoughts and attitudes about going to bed and also change their behavior by helping them to establish and follow a better night time routine. Several RCTs of 6-30 months in duration found that CBT improved function and decreased the severity of pain in fibromyalgia. Two other systematic reviews showed improved pain, mood, fatigue, and function when CBT was used for fibromyalgia treatment. In another high-quality review which included 23 trials, comprising >2,000 patients showed CBTs were effective in reducing pain and disability at the end of treatment compared with a variety of controls groups, and results were sustained long term. However, CBTs alone is insufficient and it needs other forms of combined therapy.

Nutrition

Nutritional deficiencies have been described in FM patients and the benefits of specific diet and nutritional supplementation are shown. Obesity and overweight, often present in FM patients, are related to the severity of FM worsening the quality of life in terms of higher pain, fatigue, worsened sleep quality and higher incidence of mood disorders. Weight control is thus an effective tool to improve the symptoms. According to the National Fibromyalgia Research Association, symptoms of fibromyalgia tend to be alleviated when refined sugar, caffeine, alcohol, fried foods, red meat, and highly processed foods are eliminated or kept to a minimum, due to the potential of these foods to irritate muscles and stress the immune system.

Eliminating certain food items like these not only contributes to a healthier overall diet and lifestyle, but also allows patients to see if the foods are contributing to their fibromyalgia symptoms. To evaluate systematically which foods are problematic for fibromyalgia patients, the "elimination diet" can be used. Elimination diets focus on the foods most commonly implicated in allergy and other adverse reactions (wheat and other glutinous grains, dairy products, eggs, corn, soy and tofu, peanuts, citrus fruits, yeast and refined sugars, as well as highly processed foods, chemical additives, preservatives, artificial colorings, flavorings, caffeine, and alcohol), removing them singly or in groups. If symptoms improve with elimination of a food, its role in the condition is suggested.

Supplementation with some food items in diet is also important in FM. The dietary deficiencies present in fibromyalgia are supported by a large body of peer-reviewed data which supports the basis for increased requirements of specific amino acids in conditions which are impacted by neurotransmitter imbalances. Patients with fibromyalgia show decreased blood levels of certain amino acids despite maintaining a normal protein intake such as L-carnitine, malic acid, tryptophan. This deficiency has been documented in fibromyalgia patients by clinical studies which reported statistically significant improvements in musculoskeletal pain, fatigue and memory in patients after consuming 1,000-2,000 g/day of acetyl-L-carnitine over an 8-24-week period. Individuals with fibromyalgia might have difficulty creating or utilizing malic acid. Such a deficiency could interfere with normal muscle function. So malic acid (in the form of green apples) is sometimes prescribed to fibromyalgia patients to enhance energy production. Glutamine plus probiotics are also among the supplements often used for fibromyalgia.

Because fibromyalgia may be triggered by inflammation, ginger, turmeric, and fish oil are often prescribed due to their anti-inflammatory properties. Vegan diets may also help relieve pain, improve quality of sleep, and enhance overall health in fibromyalgia patients. Vitamin D supplementation improves pain in fibromyalgia pateints but it is not routinely recommended for treatment in all FM patients. It is recommended only in documented vitamin D deficiency patients.

Vitamins and minerals may be used as nutritional therapy for fibromyalgia to combat stress, replace deficiencies, and support the immune system. Intravenous micronutrient therapy (IVMT) and specifically use of the "Myers' Cocktail" is a popular approach among complementary and alternative medicine physicians. It was developed by Dr John Myers, and later modified by Dr Alan Gaby. RCT is currently going on to establish its role in treatment of FM.

The modified Myers' Cocktail consists of:
- Magnesium chloride hexahydrate (200 mg/mL) 5 mL (1,000 mg magnesium)
- Calcium gluconate (100 mg/mL) 3 mL (300 mg calcium)
- Hydroxocobalamin (B12) (1,000 µg/mL) 1 mL (1,000 µg)
- Pyridoxine hydrochloride (B6) (100 mg/mL) 1 mL (100 mg)

- Dexpanthenol (B5) (250 mg/mL) 1 mL (250 mg)
- B-complex 100* 1 mL (see below)
- Vitamin C (500 mg/mL) 5 mL (2500 mg)
- Sterile Water 20 mL

Hypnotherapy

It comes from the Greek word meaning "sleep". Hypnosis is an intense state of concentration used to control pain, stress, sleep problems or alter negative behaviors. A hypnotherapist puts patients in an extremely relaxed state and then uses the power of suggestion to trigger changes in their brain that are believed to improve both physical and mental health. The therapist may also use role-play, imagination, motivation, and the power of suggestion in this therapy to enhance the session. With hypnosis, they concentrate deeply on a single thought. Success might be greater in those patients who are more convinced that they can change behavior. While even experts are unsure as to how hypnosis works to resolve pain, it is thought that hypnosis changes their expectations about how intense the pain will be, which alters the pain they actually feel. It may also be that when they focus their attention on a competing image that helps to block their perception of pain.

Bernardy et al. reviewed four trials of hypnotherapy and/or guided imagery. Median treatment duration (where reported) was 360 minutes and hypnotherapy was compared with a variety of control therapies: cognitive intervention, active control (physical therapy/massage/relaxation/autogenic training) and treatment as usual. In meta-analysis, two of the four hypnotherapy trials report some significant benefit in terms of pain, the other two demonstrate null, nonsignificant results. In another study, eight sessions of hypnotherapy, delivered over 12 weeks, improved visual analog scale pain ratings, fatigue, sleep, and global assessment. In another study using hypnotically induced analgesia found that patients experienced less pain during hypnosis than at rest.

Tai Chi and Yoga

Tai chi is originally a Chinese martial art. It is a mind-body practice that combines meditation, slow movements, and deep breathing. It is thought to move energy throughout the body. It is a useful modality in treatment of FM. Tai chi compared to wellness education and stretching improves symptoms, physical function, quality of sleep, self-efficacy, and functional mobility for people with fibromyalgia. Benefits seen at 12 weeks were sustained at 24 weeks. Significant improvements in static balance, dynamic balance, and timed get-up-and-go had been seen. It may help decrease risk for falls and minimize difficulties in performing essential daily physical activity tasks. Yoga is also a meditative movement. In a review which included seven trials, with 362 participants randomized to tai chi, yoga, qigong or body awareness therapy, showed improvements in sleep and fatigue.

Acupuncture

Acupuncture, defined as the stimulation of specific points of skin on the body using heat, pressure, laser, or small needles, has been suggested as a complementary treatment for fibromyalgia. A review of nine trials concluded acupuncture had no better effect for pain relief, suggesting a placebo effect. In another review of 16 trials of accupoint stimulation including acupuncture, cupping therapy, moxibustion, point injection, point embedding, or a combination showed similar findings. One high quality RCT of electroacupuncture found that along with positive changes in pain perception and sleep quality, pain threshold improved by 70% in the treated group compared with only 4% in the sham acupuncture control group.

Massage

Massage therapy, as one of complementary and alternative treatments, has been widely used for FM. It may improve pain, anxiety, depression, and sleep disturbance by complex interplay of both physical and mental modes of action. When massage therapy is delivered to soft and connective tissues, local biochemical changes would be stimulated. This helps to improve muscle flexibility, and modulate local blood and lymph circulation. As a result, local nociceptive and inflammatory mediators may be reabsorbed. Some studies found that massage therapy improved pain by modulating serotonin levels in patients with FM. The local effects may change neural activity at the spinal cord segmental level, which is responsible for both mood and pain perception. One meta-analysis including 9 RCTs involving 404 patients showed massage therapy sessions lasting 25–90 minutes, and treatment duration ranging from 1 to 24 weeks (median 5 weeks) had beneficial immediate effects on improving pain, anxiety, and depression in patients with FM. Overall, massage was not associated with a significant improvement in pain.

Hydrotherapy/Balneotherapy/Spa Therapy

Hydrotherapy or aquatic exercises (water-based exercises, aquatic therapy) are exercises that are performed in the water. The Chartered Society of Physiotherapists defined aquatic exercises as a therapy program using the properties of water, designed by a suitably qualified physiotherapist, to improve function, ideally in a purpose-built and suitably heated pool. It remains unclear whether aquatic exercises are more effective than other active interventions such as land-based exercises. Furthermore there is a lack of evidence for specific doses and timing of exercise programs because most RCTs and SRs did not provide enough information to address these issues. The term balneotherapy (seated immersion or spa therapy) is used for bathing in water without exercise. In spa therapy generally hot water is used.

Hot stimuli produce analgesia on nerve endings by increasing the pain threshold. It causes relief of muscle spasms through the γ fibers of muscle spindles and activates the descending pain inhibitory system. According to the "gate theory," pain relief may be due to the temperature and hydrostatic pressure of water on the skin. Spa therapy provokes a series of endocrine reactions, particularly in the release of adrenocorticotropic hormone (ACTH), cortisol, prolactin, and growth hormone (GH), although it does not alter the circadian rhythm of these hormones. A dysregulation of the HPA axis, marked by mild hypocortisolemia and glucocorticoid feedback resistance, has been demonstrated in fibromyalgia patients. These findings can explain the beneficial clinical effects of spa therapy in fibromyalgia. One high-quality review included 10 trials, 446 participants and compared a median of 4-hour hydrotherapy (range 200–300 minutes) against various comparators showed significant improvement in pain at the end of therapy. Other studies also supports the beneficial effects of hydrotherapy/spa therapy in treatment of FM.

Chiropractic

The term "chiropractic" combines the Greek words cheir (hand) and praxis (practice) to describe a treatment done by hand. Chiropractic is based on the notion that the relationship between the body's structure (primarily that of the spine) and its function (as coordinated by the nervous system) affects health. During initial visit, doctors of chiropractic perform a thorough physical and neurological evaluation of the patient and later they may perform one or more of the many different types of adjustments and other manual therapies used in chiropractic care for treatment. A chiropractic adjustment involves using the hands or a device to apply a controlled, rapid force to a joint. The goal is to increase the range and quality of motion in the area being treated and to aid in restoring health. Other different types of therapies are therapeutic exercise and stretching, spinal traction, manual soft tissue therapy, transcutaneous electric nerve stimulation (TENS), ultrasound, diet and nutritional counseling, and lifestyle modification. A review study summarized three studies. One study was an open pilot study, one quasi-randomized and in the third no between-group differences were observed in terms of pain. The studies were poor quality and lacked robust interpretable data.

Capsaicin

It is a naturally occurring compound that is commonly found in chili peppers. It is used as topical ointment as 0.025% capsaicin cream. It diminishes pain by acting on substance P. Capsaicin forces the cells in the tissue it touches to release all of their substance P, and that is causing burning pain on skin after application. Once the substance P is gone, those cells can no longer send pain messages. Another possibility is that it actually desensitizes the peripheral nerves, which tend to be hypersensitive in fibromyalgia patients. Two reviews included two trials and 153 participants showed some evidence of positive effect in terms of pain relief, although results were not consistent for other outcomes.

S-adenosyl Methionine

It is a naturally occurring methyl donor compound that plays a role in many chemical reactions in the body. There are many reactions in the body that involve the transfer of a methyl group from S-adenosyl methionine (SAMe) to substrates such as proteins, nucleic acids, and other metabolites. Its starting dose is 400 mg/day and can be increased up to 800 mg/day. In terms of safety, SAMe is typically well-tolerated. Most of the reported adverse effects are short-lived and are of mild to moderate severity. Common adverse effects of oral SAMe include gastrointestinal distress, dizziness, and hypomania. De Silva et al. reported that, after the end of treatment, significant improvements were observed in pain and fatigue compared with placebo. Another study which compared the efficacy of oral SAMe with that of a placebo showed decrease in clinical disease activity, a decrease in morning stiffness, reductions in fatigue, and improvements in mood among the SAMe-treated patients compared with the placebo group. However, there was no significant difference in tender point score, depression (BDI score) or muscle strength.

Multicomponent Therapy

Fibromyalgia is complex, multifactorial disease and associated with varying nature of symptoms. No single treatment modality will be able to target each one of them, hence a multimodal therapy is expected to target the multiple factors and should work effectively. Wide variability in the parameters of management does not make it possible to critically analyze the systematic evaluation of various multimodal therapies. In spite of these limitations, five RCTs of multidisciplinary management based on combined education and/or CBT with exercises found improved results on overall FMS impact and patient self-efficacy. On measurement by FIQ, there were significant decrease in pain and 6-minute walk showed encouraging trend. Häuser et al. in his review meta-analysis of nine trials over 1,119 patients concluded that multicomponent therapy effectively immediately reduced pain and fatigue. Another RCT study on the effects of a 6-week biofeedback therapy suggested that in combination with education, CBT, and exercise, and concluded that this combination is better than the education attention control group on self-efficacy and tender points.

RECOMMENDATIONS AND GUIDELINES FOR FIBROMYALGIA TREATMENT

Three evidence-based guidelines for the management of FMS was published:
1. The American Pain Society (APS) (2005)
2. The European League Against Rheumatism (EULAR) (2007)
3. The Association of the Scientific Medical Societies in Germany (AWMF) (2008)

Details of the methodologies used for establishing the three guidelines included in this synthesis are presented in **Table 4**.

The primary recommendations of the three guidelines are outlined in **Table 5**.

Revised EULAR 2016 Recommendations

In 2016 EULAR finally revised its recommendations. They recommended "overarching principles" and specific recommendations comprising nonpharmacological and pharmacological management.

EULAR Overarching Principles

A prompt diagnosis is the first prerequisite to optimal management. Comprehensive assessment of pain, function and psychosocial status leads to full understanding of fibromyalgia. Abnormal pain processing and other secondary features should emphasize on recognizing fibromyalgia as *complex and heterogeneous* condition. *Graduated approach* is the ideal modality in general management of fibromyalgia.

Specific Recommendations (Table 6)

Primary aim is directed towards balancing the benefit and risk involved of treatment by health-related quality of life (HRQoL). A multidisciplinary approach combining dual treatment modality of nonpharmacological and pharmacological, the therapy is tailored as per the symptoms

TABLE 4: Comparison of the categorization of evidence and recommendations of the three guidelines.

	American Pain Society	European League Against Rheumatism	Association of the Scientific Medical Societies in Germany
Evidence level I	Meta-analysis of multiple well-designed controlled studies	Randomized controlled double-blind trials	Ia–SR (with homogeneity) of RCTs Ib-Individual RCT (with narrow Confidence Interval) Ic-All or none
Evidence level II	Well-designed experimental studies	Randomized, blinded crossover trials	IIa-SR (with homogeneity*) of cohort studies IIb-Individual cohort study (including low quality RCT; e.g., <80% follow-up) IIc-"Outcomes" Research; Ecological studies
Evidence level III	Well-designed quasi-experimental studies, such as nonrandomized controlled studies, single-group pre-/post, cohort, time series, or matched controlled studies	Randomized single blind trials	IIIa-SR (with homogeneity) of case-control studies IIIB-Individual case-control study
Evidence level IV	Well-designed non-experimental studies, such as comparative and correlational descriptive and case studies	Randomized open trials/nonrandomized single blind	Case-series (and poor quality cohort and case-control studies)
Evidence level V	Case reports and clinical examples	Nonrandomized open trials	Expert opinion without explicit critical appraisal, or based on physiology, bench research or "first principles"
Recommendation Strength A	Evidence level I or consistent findings from multiple studies of level II, II or IV	Directly based on evidence level I*	Based on evidence level I**
Recommendation Strength B	Evidence of level II, II or IV with generally consistent findings	Directly based on evidence level II or extrapolated recommendation evidence level I	Based on evidence level II**
Recommendation Strength C	Evidence of level II, II or IV with inconsistent findings	Directly based on evidence level III or extrapolated recommendation from evidence levels I, II or III	Based on evidence levels III, IV and V**
Recommendation Strength D	Evidence level V or little/no evidence	Directly based on evidence level IV or extrapolated recommendation from evidence level I, II or III	
Panel consensus	Expert opinion		

(RCT: randomized controlled trial; SR: systematic review or meta-analysis)
*The levels of evidence underlying these recommendations differ between the literature and the levels of evidence defined by EULAR
**An up- or down-grading is possible by taking into consideration the following factors: consistency of study results, clinical relevance of outcome measures and effect sizes, benefit-risk-ratio, ethical obligations, patients' preferences, and practicability.

TABLE 5: Primary recommendations of American Pain Society (APS), European League Against Rheumatism (EULAR) and Association of the Scientific Medical Societies in Germany (AWMF).

	APS		EULAR		AWMF	
	Level of evidence	Strength of recommendation	Level of evidence	Strength of recommendation	Level of evidence	Strength of recommendation
Aerobic exercise	I	A	IIb	C	Ia	A
Cognitive-behavioral therapy	I	A	IV	D	Ia	A
Amitriptyline	I	A	Ib	A	Ia	A
Cyclobenzaprine	I	A	-	-	Ia	C
Multicomponent therapy	I	A	-	-	Ia	A
Tramadol	II	B	Ib	A	IIb	C
Balneotherapy	II	B	IIa	B	IIb	B
Patient education alone	II	B	-	-	Ia	Not B
Hypnotherapy	II	B	-	-	IIb	B
Biofeedback	II	B	-	-	IIb	Not B
Massage therapy	II	B	-	-	IIb	B
Anticonvulsants	II	B	Ib	A	IIb	B
SSRI (Fluoxetine)	II	B	Ib	A	IIb	B
SNRI (Duloxetine)	II	B	Ib	A	IIb	B
Opioids	III	C	IV	Not D	IV	Not C
Acupuncture	II	C	-	-	Ia	Not A
Trigger point injection	III	C	-	-	IV	Not C

(Not = Not recommended; - = No statement)

TABLE 6: Specific recommendations.

Specific recommendations	Level of evidence	Grade	Strength of recommendation	Agreement (%)*
Nonpharmacological management				
Aerobic and strengthening exercise	Ia	A	Strong for	100
Cognitive behavioral therapies	Ia	A	Weak for	100
Multicomponent therapies	Ia	A	Weak for	93
Defined physical therapies: acupuncture or hydrotherapy	Ia	A	Weak for	93
Meditative movement therapies (Qigong, yoga, tai chi) and mindfulness-based stress reduction	Ia	A	Weak for	71–73
Pharmacological management				
Amitriptyline (at low dose)	Ia	A	Weak for	100
Duloxetine or milnacipran	Ia	A	Weak for	100
Tramadol	Ib	A	Weak for	100
Pregabalin	Ia	A	Weak for	94
Cyclobenzaprine	Ia	A	Weak for	75

*Scoring of working group on 0–10 numerical rating scale: desirable score = minimum 7

and comorbidities. Shared decision making involving the patients into confidence about their preferences should focus on nonpharmacological therapies. The overall management will take into account the intensity of pain and functional limitations of the patients. Other important clinical features such as fatigue, depression and sleep disturbances will also determine the priorities in close consultation with the patient.

EULAR recommended specific management in their various categories.

A. Strong recommendations for aerobic and strengthening exercise
B. Weak recommendations for
   i. Amitriptyline
   ii. Pregabalin
   iii. Cyclobenzaprine
   iv. SNRI (duloxetine and milnacipran)
   v. Tramadol
   vi. Acupuncture
   vii. CBT
   viii. Hydrotherapy/spa therapy/balneotherapy
   ix. Meditative movements (tai chi, Yoga)
   x. Mind body therapy
   xi. Multicomponent therapy.
C. Weak recommendations against:
   i. MAOIs
   ii. NSAIDs
   iii. SSRI
   iv. Capsaicin
   v. Massage
   vi. Biofeedback
   vii. Hypnotherapy
   viii. SAMe
D. Strong recommendations against:
   i. Growth hormone
   ii. Sodium oxybate
   iii. Chiropractic
   iv. Homeopathy
   v. Guided imagery
   vi. Strong opioids
   vii. Corticosteroids.

EULAR versus Other Recommendations

Three recommendations from Canada, Israel and Germany are in agreement with EULAR 2016 recommendations on the followings three issues:
1. Requirement for tailored therapy
2. Basics of approach to the therapy
3. Utility of nonpharmacological therapies as first line

In relation to use pharmacological therapies, use of recently available evidence has brought about the differences in the strength of recommendations as follows:
1. Canadian and Israeli guidelines strongly favors use of SNRIs anticonvulsants but EULAR and German guidelines have a weaker recommendations for them

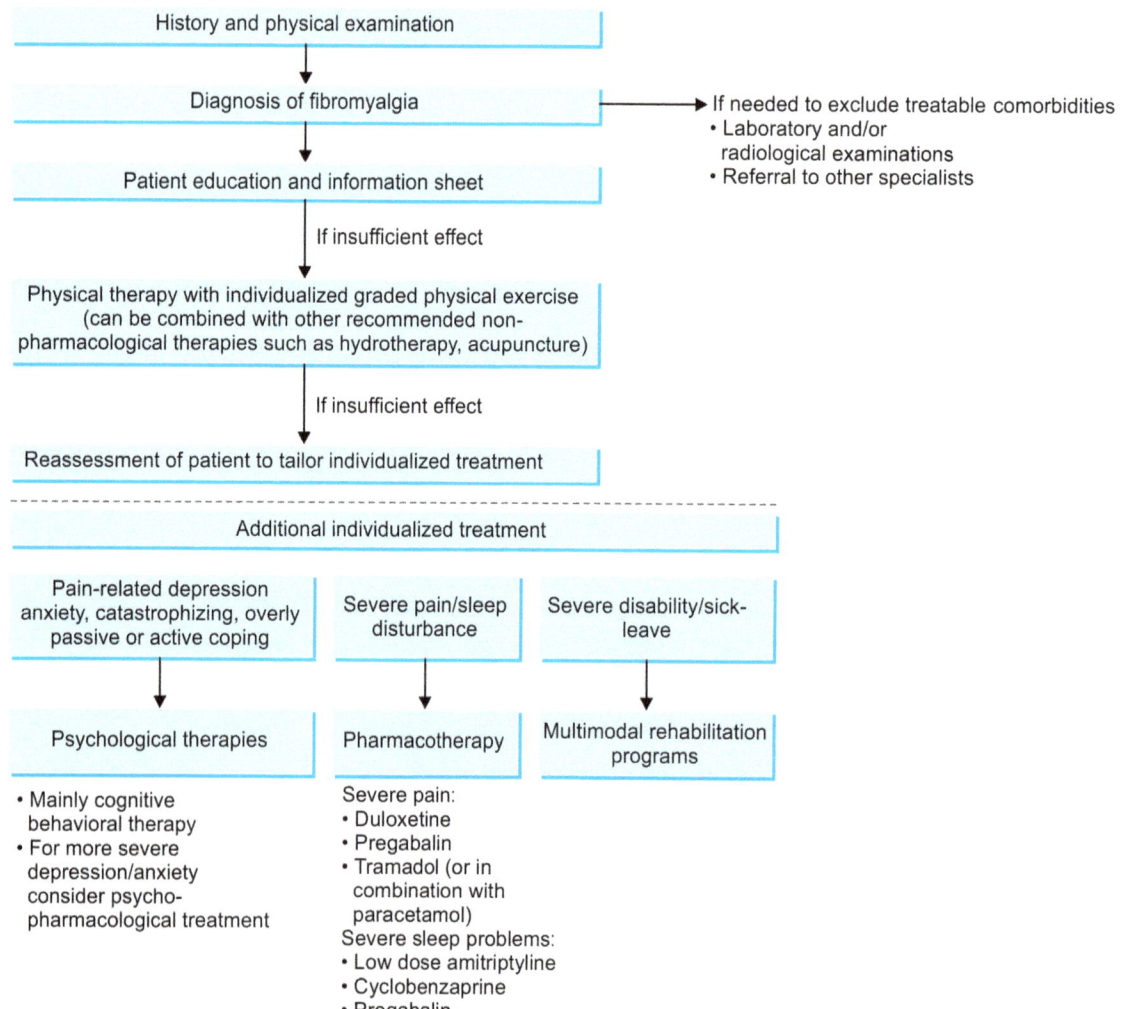

Flowchart 1: Management recommendations.

2. "Meditative movement" vary in their approval rating and it is strongly favored by German but "weak for" approval by EULAR and is reserved for a "minority" by Israel guidelines

The future of management guidelines in coming decade is likely to evolve around five identified relevant questions as under:

Q1. *Exercises:* Strengthening and/or aerobic training more effective?

Q2. *Single modality or multimodal therapy:* Which one is more effective?

Q3. *Predictive characteristics of fibromyalgia:* Which ones respond favorably to therapies?

Q4. *Inflammatory arthritis associated fibromyalgia:* How to manage?

Q5. *Optimal outcome for patients:* Which healthcare system provides best management?

Management recommendations are finally summarized to be followed as per the **Flowchart 1**.

FURTHER READING

1. Ablin JN, Shoenfeld Y, Buskila D. Fibromyalgia, infection and vaccination: two more parts in the etiological puzzle. J Autoimm. 2006;27(3):145-52.
2. Arnold LM, Clauw DJ, Dunegan LJ, Turk DC. A framework for fibromyalgia management for primary care providers. Mayo Clin Proc. 2012;87:488-96.
3. Arnold LM, Clauw DJ, McCarberg BH. Improving the recognition and diagnosis of fibromyalgia. Mayo Clin Proc 2011;86:457-64.
4. Arnold LM, Clauw DJ, Wohlreich MM, Wang F, Ahl J, Gaynor PJ, et al. Efficacy of duloxetine in patients with fibromyalgia: pooled analysis of 4 placebo-controlled clinical trials. Prim Care Companion J Clin Psychiatry. 2009;11(5):237-44.
5. Arnold LM, Crofford LJ, Mease PJ, Burgess SM, Palmer SC, Abetz L, et al. Patient perspectives on the impact of fibromyalgia. Patient Educ Couns. 2008;73(1):114-20.
6. Arnold LM, Gebke KB, Choy EH. Fibromyalgia: management strategies for primary care providers. Int J Clin Pract. 2016;70(2): 99-112.
7. Arnold LM, Goldberg DL, Stanford SB. Gabapentin in the treatment of fibromyalgia: a randomized, double-blind, placebo-controlled, multicenter trial. Arthritis Rheum 2007;56:1336-44.
8. Arnold LM, Hess EV, Hudson JI, Welge JA, Berno SE, Keck PE, Jr A randomized, placebo-controlled, double-blind, flexible-dose study of fluoxetine in the treatment of women with fibromyalgia. Am J Med. 2002;112(3):191-7.
9. Arnold LM, Hudson JI, Hess EV, Clauw DJ. Family study of fibromyalgia. Arthritis Rheum. 2004;50(3):944-52.
10. Arnold LM, Keck PE, Welge JA. Antidepressant treatment of fibromyalgia. A meta-analysis and review. Psychosomatics. 2000;41(2):104-13.
11. Arnold LM, Lu Y, Crofford LJ, Wohlreich M, Detke MJ, Iyengar S, et al. A double-blind, multicenter trial comparing duloxetine with placebo in the treatment of fibromyalgia patients with or without major depressive disorder. Arthr Rheum. 2004;50(9):2974-84.
12. Arnold LM, Rosen A, Pritchett YL, D'Souza DN, Goldstein DJ, Iyengar S, et al. A randomized, double-blind, placebo-controlled trial of duloxetine in the treatment of women with fibromyalgia with or without major depressive disorder. Pain. 2005; 119(1-3):5-15.
13. Arnold LM, Russell IJ, Diri EW, Duan WR, Young JP Jr, Sharma U, et al. A 14-week, randomized, double-blinded, placebo-controlled monotherapy trial of pregabalin in patients with fibromyalgia. J Pain. 2008; 9(9):792-805.
14. Arnold LM, Zhang S, Pangallo BA. Efficacy and safety of duloxetine 30 mg/d in patients with fibromyalgia: a randomized, double-blind, placebo-controlled study. Clin J Pain. 2012;28(9):775-81.
15. Arnold LM. Strategies for managing fibromyalgia. Am J Med. 2009;122(12): S31-S43.
16. Bannwarth B, Blotman F, Roué-Le Lay K, Caubère JP, André E, Taïeb C. Fibromyalgia syndrome in the general population of France: a prevalence study. Joint Bone Spine. 2009;76(2):184-7.
17. Baraniuk JN, Whalen G, Cunningham J, Clauw DJ. Cerebrospinal fluid levels of opioid peptides in fibromyalgia and chronic low back pain. BMC Musculoskelet Disord. 2004;5:48.
18. Bennett R, Friend R, Marcus D, Bernstein C, Han BK, Yachoui R, et al. Criteria for the diagnosis of fibromyalgia: validation of the modified 2010 preliminary ACR criteria and the development of alternative criteria. Arthritis Care Res. 2014;66(9):1364-73.
19. Bennett RM, Bushmakin AG, Cappelleri JC, Zlateva G, Sadosky AB. Minimal clinically important difference in the fibromyalgia impact questionnaire. J Rheumatol. 2009; 36(6):1304-11.
20. Bullón P, Alcocer-Gómez E, Carrión AM. AMPK phosphorylation modulates pain by activation of NLRP3 inflammasome. Antioxid Redox Signal. 2016;24:157-70.
21. Burri A, Marinova Z, Robinson MD, Kühnel B, Waldenberger M, Wahl S, et al. Are epigenetic factors implicated in chronic widespread pain? PLoS One. 2016;11:e0165548.
22. Busch AJ, Schachter CL, Peloso PM, Bombardier C. Exercise for treating fibromyalgia syndrome. Cochrane Database Syst Rev. 2003;3,CD003786.
23. Busch AJ, Webber SC, Brachaniec M, Bidonde J, Bello-Haas VD, Danyliw AD, et al. Exercise therapy for fibromyalgia. Curr Pain Headache Rep. 2011;15(5):358-67.
24. Busch AJ, Webber SC, Richards RS, Bidonde J, Schachter CL, Schafer LA, et al. Resistance exercise training for fibromyalgia. Cochrane Database Syst Rev. 2013;12,CD010884.
25. Buskila D, Cohen H, Neumann L, Ebstein RP. An association between fibromyalgia and the dopamine D4 receptor exon III repeat polymorphism and relationship to novelty seeking personality traits. Mol Psychiatry. 2004;9:730-1.
26. Buskila D, Sarzi-Puttini P, Ablin JN. The genetics of fibromyalgia syndrome. Pharmacogenomics. 2007;8(1):67-74.
27. Cao H, Li X, Han M, Liu J. Acupoint stimulation for fibromyalgia: a systematic review of randomized controlled trials. Evid Based Complement Alternat Med. 2013;2013:362831.
28. Chakrabarty S, Zoorob R. Fibromyalgia. Am Fam Physician. 2007;76(2):247-54.
29. Choy E, Marshall D, Gabriel ZL, Mitchell SA, Gylee E, Dakin HA. A systematic review and mixed treatment comparison of the efficacy of pharmacological treatments for fibromyalgia. Semin Arthritis Rheum. 2011;41:335-45.

SECTION 7

Hand and Wrist Involvement in Orthopedic Rheumatology

- **Anatomy of Wrist and Hand**
  Vipul Sud

- **Approach to Inflammatory Arthritis of Hand**
  Alok Chandra Agrawal, Mukund Madhav Ojha, Harshal Sakale

- **Arthrodesis and Arthroplasty of the Rheumatoid Wrist and Small Joints of Hand: Where do We Stand?**
  Abhay Elhence, Mahaveer Mali

- **Pain in Hand: Carpal Tunnel Syndrome, Ulnar Nerve Entrapment at Wrist, Kienböck's Disease, and Osteoarthrosis of Carpometacarpal Joint of the Thumb**
  RB Kalia

- **Common Hand Disorders**
  Alok Chandra Agrawal, Bikram Kar, Anupam Inamdar

26. Anatomy of Wrist and Hand

Vipul Sud

INTRODUCTION

The anatomy of hand and wrist is a complex interplay of bones, ligaments, extrinsic and intrinsic muscles, and tendons. Despite physically being smaller in comparison to the rest of the body, it has a relatively large representation in the cerebral cortex. This is because the hand needs to perform a wide range of complex functions that require minute control over the smaller parts to enable it to carry out all of its functions smoothly.

When we look at it from the point of view of rheumatoid arthritis, the functioning of the hand depends on the interplay between the neuromuscular apparatus, the bony and the ligamentous structures of the hand and the wrist and disturbance of any one of these upsets the balance.

Twenty-eight muscle groups, controlled by predominantly three nerves with their motor and sensory pathways act upon the bone and joint system consisting of 29 bones and the similar number of joints and innumerable short and long ligaments. This gives rise to tremendous mechanical possibilities giving the hand a capability of performing unlimited actions.

BONES AND JOINTS

The wrist consists of 8 carpal bones arranged in 2 rows of 4 each in a cup fashion facing palmary to accommodate the tendons, nerves and vessels. They articulate proximally with the distal end of ulna and radius and distally with metacarpals (**Fig. 1**). The radius and ulna also articulate with each other forming the distal radioulnar joint (DRUJ). These bones are held together by ligamentous attachments which not only permit the major wrist movements of dorsi and palmar-flexion and radio and ulnar deviation but also restrict excessive movement so as to stabilize and translate the force from the hand to the forearm and arm. The triangular fibrocartilaginous complex (TFCC) between the triquetral and distal ulna and partly between sigmoid notch of the radius and distal ulna also acts as a major shock absorber and stabilizer for the wrist as the ulna faces the major brunt of the force of transmission.

The configuration of the various carpals and their articulation with each other and the metacarpals allow increased mobility of the wrist despite the compact fitting (**Fig. 2**).

The design of all metacarpals is essentially the same with volar arching and hemispherical distal ends. The arching augments the cupping of palm which is further accentuated by the thumb metacarpal being positioned at almost right angles to the other 4 digits.

The metacarpophalangeal (MCP) joint of the thumb is a hinge joint and allows unidirectional movement of flexion

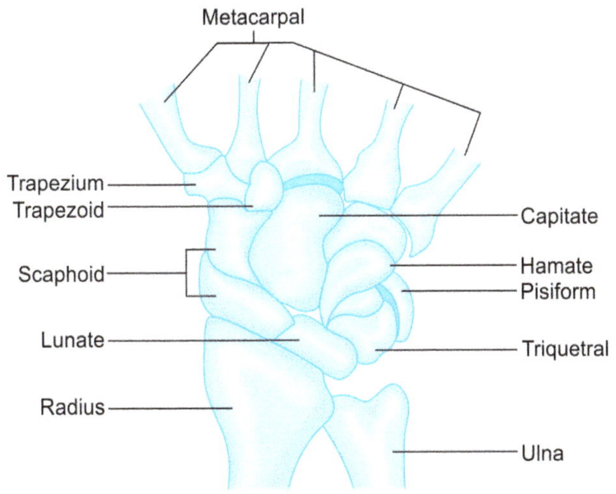

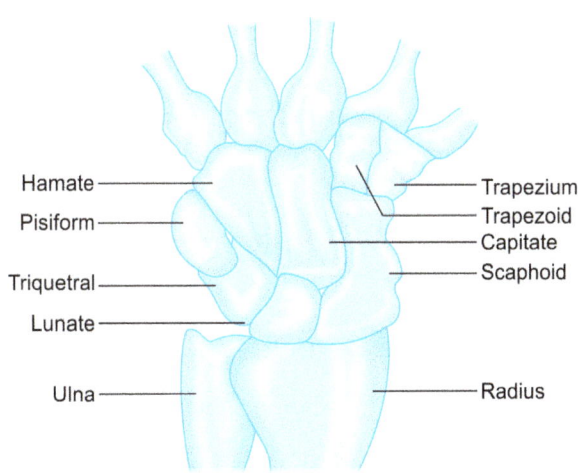

Fig. 1: Skeletal articulations of wrist—dorsal view.

Fig. 2: Skeletal articulations of wrist—palmar view.

and extension and rarely, hyperextension while the MCP joints of 2nd to 5th fingers are ball and socket joints with a hemispherical distal end of metacarpal and concave cup-shaped end of proximal phalanx supported by a lax capsule. This should ideally allow multidirectional movements but strong palmar and collateral ligaments restrict them to mainly flexion and extension with limited abduction and adduction. The rotatory movement is only possible in index finger to a certain extent partly due to the attachment and functioning of intrinsic muscles.

The interphalangeal joints are hinge joints that allow unidirectional movement of flexion and extension. However, the range of motion varies from 90 to 135° increasing from index to little finger, both in proximal as well as distal interphalangeal joints. This configuration allows us to form a strong grasp while making a fist.

The configuration of carpometacarpal (CMC) and MCP joint of the thumb permits greater mobility. This is important because the thumb by virtue of its position contributes 50% to the strength and power of the hand as compared to the rest of the fingers.

■ MUSCLES AND TENDONS

The extrinsic muscles controlling the hand originate at the elbow or the forearm as a fleshy muscle belly which becomes tendinous in nature in the distal part of the forearm. Their excursion is kept under control at various junctures in the wrist, palm and fingers in the form of fibro-osseous tunnels before its distal attachment to the fingers **(Fig. 3)**. This creates a pulley system and permits individual balancing of different tendons, allowing the different units of hand to work individually as well as cohesively together to produce myriad and often complex actions.

The intrinsic muscles of the hand originate either from the carpus or distal to it, some from the extrinsic tendons and help in balancing the fine movements of the hand.

■ DORSAL EXTRINSIC MUSCLES

The extrinsic tendons of extensor muscles pass through the wrist under extensor retinaculum which by its intermittent attachment to bony protuberances of radius and ulna creates six fibro-osseous tunnels **(Fig. 4)**:

- *Tunnel 1*: It contains the abductor pollicis longus (APL) and extensor pollicis brevis (EPB). Both are attached on the thumb helping in its abduction and extension along with radial deviation and palmar flexion of the hand. They also form the radial border of "snuffbox". Travelling together in a tight tunnel may at times give rise to synovitis due to overuse.
- *Tunnel 2*: It contains the extensor carpi-radialis brevis and longus which attach on the base of metacarpals. They primarily perform the wrist function, assisting in its radial deviation and dorsiflexion.
- *Tunnel 3*: It contains the extensor pollicis longus (EPL) which curves around the dorsal tubercle of radius to attach on the base of distal phalanx of the thumb forming the ulnar border of "snuffbox". The curvilinear excursion allows hyperextension of thumb but may lead to attrition and rupture of EPL in certain attenuating circumstances such as rheumatism.
- *Tunnel 4*: It contains extensor digitorum and extensor indicis.
- *Tunnel 5*: It contains extensor digiti minimi (EDM) and they all merge with the dorsal aponeurosis at the base of proximal phalanx. Both the accessory extensors are on the ulnar side of the digitorum slip and so can be identified easily in case of need for a donor for tendon transfer.
- *Tunnel 6*: It contains the extensor carpi ulnaris, lying in the ulnar groove in the distal ulnar head. It is an ulnar deviator and accessory dorsiflexor of the wrist.

Another point to note is that some of these tendons may be in multiple number (APL, EPB, EDM) which must be kept in mind during exploration. Also, they have intertendinous connections which are called junctura tendinae which may mislead during examination **(Fig. 5)**.

■ PALMAR/FLEXOR MUSCLES

The long flexors originate from the forearm and pass underneath the flexor retinaculum over the cup-shaped

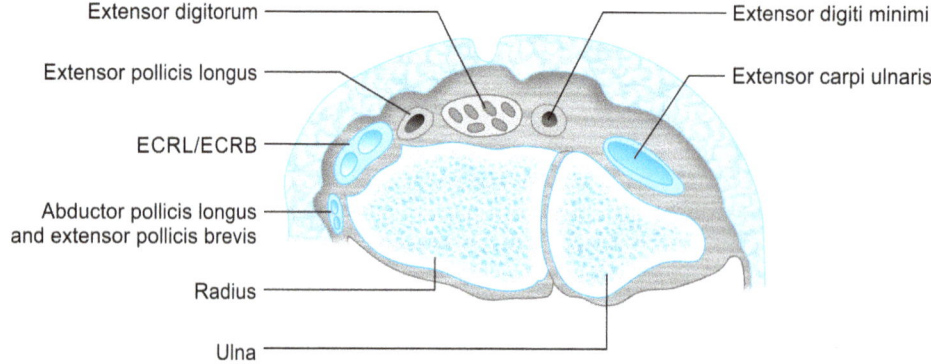

Fig. 3: Distribution of extensor tendons in the wrist. (ECRB: extensor carpi radialis brevis; ECRL: extensor carpi radialis longus)

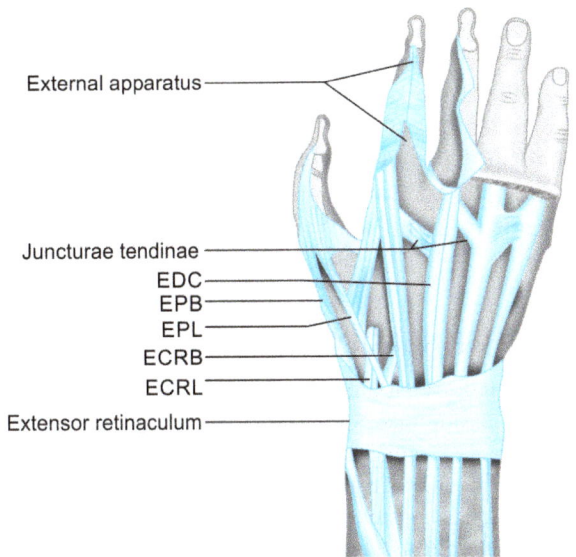

Fig. 4: Extensor tendons in their tunnels in forearm and wrist. (EDC: extensor digitorum communis; EPB: extensor pollicis brevis; EPL: extensor pollicis longus; ECRB: extensor carpi radialis brevis; ECRL: extensor carpi radialis longus)

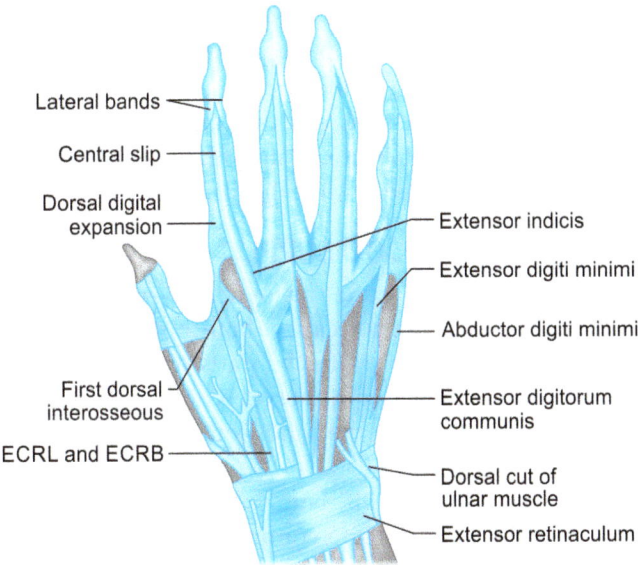

Fig. 5: Incision for carpal tunnel release and its relation to flexor tendons.

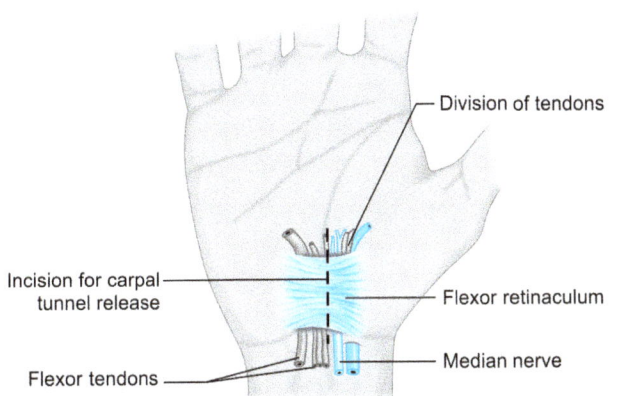

Fig. 6: Distribution of flexor tendons in hand along with pulleys.

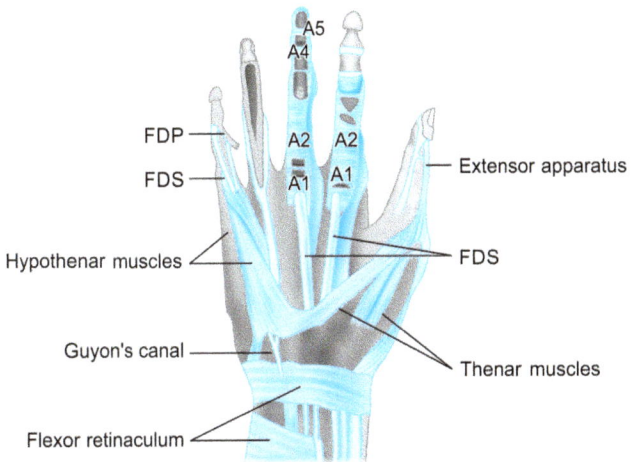

Fig. 7: Extensor apparatus in dorsum of hand along with expansion. (FDP: flexor digitorum profundus; FDS: flexor digitorum superficialis)

concavity formed by the carpus along with the median nerve. As they are all confined in a narrow space in the wrist, they are covered with synovium to allow smooth gliding of the tendons. Narrowing of the canal or inflammation of the synovium may lead to compression of the nerve leading to carpal tunnel syndrome **(Fig. 6)**.

The flexors of the wrist are the flexor carpi radialis and ulnaris along with palmaris longus while that of the fingers are flexor digitorum superficialis and profundus. The latter are further confined to their fibro-osseous tunnel with the help of annular and cruciate pulleys **(Fig. 7)**. This helps in guided excursion of the fingers and allows distinctive fine movements.

The Guyon's canal is on the ulnar side of the hand. It allows the passage of ulnar neurovascular bundle which can get compressed due to inflammation of the synovium.

The intrinsic muscles are the thenar and hypothenar muscles along with palmar and dorsal interossei and the lumbricals. They assist the extrinsic muscles and at times are either antagonistic or synergistic to allow the hand to perform fine movements while restraining the other joints for stability.

INTEGUMENT

The palmar surface of the hand has a thick padding of subcutaneous fat covered with a thickened skin which has innumerable folds. The glabrous skin allows a better grip while the subcutaneous fat underneath cushions the pressure when holding these objects firmly. The palmar skin is firmly attached to subcutaneous fat which is further attached to the tendinous sheaths and skeletal elements with the help of fibrillary structures. The skin is further emphasized with furrows which re-ensures that the subcutaneous fat is limited in between the two sulci or furrows. All these factors ensure that the hand has a secure and firm grasp.

However, the dorsal skin is thin and pliable with an equally mobile subcutaneous tissue. This allows the skin the elasticity to drape properly when the hand makes a firm grip.

■ NERVE AND BLOOD SUPPLY

The hand is supplied by three major nerves—median, ulnar and radial nerve. These nerves have both motor and sensory components and supply different parts of the hand. This ensures that even if one of the nerves is not functioning, the other nerves ensure that the hand would be at least partly functional.

The hand is supplied by both radial and ulnar arteries which have numerous interconnections to form dorsal carpal arch, superficial and deep palmar arch. These then give individual branches to digits and rest of the hand. This ensures that the hand continues to get good blood supply despite minor obstructions.

The venous drainage is done by basilic vein from the medial side and cephalic vein from the radial side and is placed superficially on the volar aspect of the forearm.

Thus, we can see that the various components of the hand are intricately attached to each other to able to perform complex actions. Disturbance or failure of any component can result in inability of the hand to perform optimum function.

■ FURTHER READING

1. Apergis E. Wrist anatomy. In: Fracture-Dislocation of the Wrist. Basingstoke: Springer; 2013. pp. 7-41.
2. Ombregt L. Applied anatomy of the wrist thumb and hand. In: A System of Orthopaedic Medicine, 3rd edition. Philadelphia: Churchill Livingstone; 2013. pp. 102-11.
3. Pechlaner S, Hussl H, Kerschbaumer F, Poisel S. Atlas of Hand Surgery. Stuttgart: Thieme Medical Publishers; 2000.
4. Taylor CL, Schwartz RJ. The anatomy and mechanics of human hand. In: Artificial Limb, 2nd edition. Philadelphia: Lippincott Williams and Wilkins; 1955. pp. 22-35.

27. Approach to Inflammatory Arthritis of Hand

Alok Chandra Agrawal, Mukund Madhav Ojha, Harshal Sakale

OVERVIEW

The word "arthritis" has its genesis from Greek in which *arthro-* means joint and *itis-* means inflammation. Inflammatory arthritis comprises rheumatoid arthritis (RA), systemic lupus erythematous (SLE), psoriatic arthropathy, and arthritis in ulcerative colitis and Crohn's disease, Still's disease, scleroderma and juvenile idiopathic arthritis. One can say that in usual practice, joint pains are pretty quotidian which can be healed if clinical acumen applied aptly. Needless to say, human hands are unique as no other creature in the world has hands with the ability to grasp, hold, move, and manipulate objects like we do. Hand arthritis can be really painful thus incapacitating daily routine activities. Manifestations of different arthritis appearing over the small joints of hands if visualized with a good clinical eye can lead to early diagnosis and prompt treatment. In this chapter, we will focus on the clinical approach of different types of inflammatory arthritis affecting the hands.

EPIDEMIOLOGY AND PATHOPHYSIOLOGY

The course of any inflammatory response is influenced by the immune condition of the host and the fine tuning of the local tissue reaction, which may be influenced by individual genetic factors and environmental factors. Inflammatory arthritis is characterized by inflammation affecting joint structures, such as synovium, synovial cavity, articular cartilage or enthuses. The classical signs and symptoms of inflammation are pain, warmth, swelling, and erythema which may not be present in all patients.

Rheumatoid arthritis is more prevalent among inflammatory arthritis, affecting 1% of the population worldwide; resulting from T cell-mediated autoimmune process. The exact etiology of RA is unknown but there are theories suggesting genetic predisposition and environmental influence behind it. Studies reveal two genes in particular, associated with RA. One is *PTPN22 gene* on which non-synonymous single nucleotide polymorphism leads to RA pathogenesis and second one is HLA-DRB1, giving a contribution of 37% in development of RA, whose multiple alleles coding for a shared epitope at 70–74 positions of amino acid accounting for propensity and severity of RA. Interestingly with advent of industrial age, various toxins such as silica dust, carcinogens have increased proneness for RA development. Smoking is also a risk factor.

Psoriatic arthritis is second most common after RA, affecting one in five patients. There is complex communication between genetic and environmental factors resulting in persistent immune response. Arthropathy in psoriasis is a late feature to develop.

Lupus arthritis is chronic inflammatory disease with potential involvement of type 2 and 3 hypersensitivity reactions, triggered by unknown environmental factors.

Pathophysiologic mechanisms for gouty arthritis are crystal deposition, acute crystal induced inflammation and chronic destructive lesions of joints.

CLINICAL APPROACH

The diagnosis of the etiology of the inflammatory arthritis depends primarily on good history taking and physical examination. An imperative job is to differentiate arthralgia from arthritis. In simple layman language, arthralgia is nonspecific pain without swelling and often seen in various pathological conditions such as systemic diseases, hypothyroidism, etc., while arthritis presents typically with joint swelling and tenderness.

HISTORY

Pain and Stiffness

The most characteristic symptom of arthritis is joint pain. In inflammatory type, pain is worse at the beginning thereby subsiding at the end of usage. Usually pain is present both at rest and with movement. While in noninflammatory, pain ameliorates with rest and occurs mostly during motion. Patients with arthritis tend to hold the joint in partial flexion; hence contractures may develop which is a sign of inflamed joint. Morning stiffness lasting for at least thirty minutes is quintessential in inflammatory arthritis which improves with movement. It is a sensation of tightness during an attempt to move joints after a period of inactivity. Joint swelling is related to synovial hypertrophy, effusion, and/

or inflammation of periarticular structures in inflammatory while in noninflammatory cases, mild degrees of soft tissue swelling occur.

Joint Involvement, Symmetry and Distribution

Single joint arthritis is monoarthritis. Involvement of 2–3 joints is oligoarthritis, while polyarthritis is defined as pain involving 4 or more joints. Symmetry is manifested as involvement of the same joints on each side of the body which is typically seen in RA and SLE while asymmetry is pathognomonic of psoriatic arthritis, reactive arthritis and Lyme arthritis. The distal interphalangeal (DIP) joints of the fingers are usually involved in psoriatic arthritis, gout, or osteoarthritis but are usually spared in RA. Joints of the lumbar spine are typically involved in ankylosing spondylitis but are spared in RA.

Duration

Conventionally if the duration of arthritis is less than 6 weeks, it is acute arthritis, and more than 6 weeks it is chronic arthritis.

Inflammatory arthritis is usually manifested as spontaneous flares. In clinical scenario, many patients with inflammatory arthritis are often symptom free but then they present with arthritis flare. So, a spontaneous up and down course is indicative of inflammatory process.

Deformities

- *Rheumatoid arthritis*: Small joints of hands and feet are affected first as an early manifestation of RA leading to multiple deformities. Common deformities of hand are as follows:
  - *Boutonniere's deformity*: Flexion of proximal interphalangeal (PIP) joint and hyperextension of DIP joint.
  - *Swan neck deformity*: Hyperextension of PIP joint and flexion of DIP joint. Nalebuff classification (1989) is used for describing this deformity:
    - Type I—flexibility of PIP joints in all positions, normal integrity and function
    - Type II—limited flexibility of PIP joints at certain positions, intrinsic muscle tightness
    - Type III—limited flexibility of PIP joints in all positions, near normal X-ray.
    - Type IV—stiff PIP joints with poor X-ray appearance.
  - *Hitchhiker's thumb*: Also known as Z-deformity, characterized by flexion at metacarpophalangeal joint of thumb and hyperextension at the interphalangeal joint below thumb nail.
  - *Ulnar drift*: Also known as ulnar deviation in which the swelling of the metacarpophalangeal (MCP) joints causes displacement of fingers bending them toward the little finger.
- *Psoriatic arthropathy*:
  - Moll and Wright described psoriatic arthritis into five clinical courses
  - Involvement of DIP joints is the classic one in psoriatic arthropathy
  - *Arthritis mutilans*: Multiple radiographic changes evident in metacarpophalangeal and interphalangeal joints resembling "pencil-in-cup' appearance.
  - Symmetric polyarthritis with negative rheumatoid factor.
  - *Asymmetric polyarthritis*: It is most common form resembling ankylosing spondylitis.
- *Lupus arthritis*: Lupus arthritis deformities strike similarities with RA. The only difference is nonerosive bone damage, hence easily correctable. This condition is also known as "Jaccoud's arthropathy". Various deformities are non-erosive carpal collapse and ulnar deviation, subluxation of MCP joints, Z deformity, parametacarpophalangeal joint hook formation.

Extra-articular Manifestations

Inflammatory arthritis is often associated with constitutional symptoms such as fatigue, low grade fever indicating an underlying systemic illness. This feature is unlikely in degenerative pathologies. Other manifestations may be in the form of skin lesions like in scleroderma, SLE and Psoriasis and ocular signs like anterior uveitis in AS, iridocyclitis in juvenile RA, etc.

Pathology

Progression of RA passes through four stages:
- Stage I (Synovitis)—initial stage RA, mild inflammation of synovial tissue
- Stage II (Early arthritis)—moderate stage RA, severe inflammation of synovial tissue
- Stage III (Late arthritis)—severe RA, advanced inflammation of synovial tissue with bone destruction leading to specific deformities
- Stage IV (Destruction)—end stage, severely crippled and damaged hand

■ PHYSICAL EXAMINATION

The musculoskeletal examination helps to distinguish joint inflammation from degenerative joints and gives an access to information about site and distribution of joint involvement. General conditions and vitals should be assessed. Joint examination mainly comprises inspection, palpation, range of motion and special tests. Articular and extra-articular sites should be observed like butterfly rash on face indicative of SLE, tophi a common finding in gout, etc. Passive and active movements should be checked. Any instability or deformity should be looked for. Crepitus during active or passive range of motion indicates a derangement of bone, cartilage, or menisci. Range of motion (ROM) should be assessed well. Increased ROM indicates an unstable joint while decreased ROM represents effusion, capsule fibrosis or any bony abnormality.

Warning Signs

- Demand immediate workup
- Swelling, warmth, redness of the joint may point out to infection, rheumatic process and crystal induced arthropathy.
- Other joints and spine should be checked out.
- Associated features, e.g., nails pitting, tenosynovitis, ear nodules, conjunctivitis, mouth ulcers etc., should be kept in mind while reaching a diagnosis.

■ MANAGEMENT

Investigations cannot replace the diagnostic clue one can get from detailed history and clinical examination. On investigations, a patient of inflammatory arthritis may have one or more of the following: high erythrocyte sedimentation rate (ESR), high C-reactive protein (CRP) levels. Blood picture may be indicative of normocytic normochromic anemia with thrombocytosis—a sign of inflammation. The total leukocyte count may be high. Reversal of the albumin:globulin ratio with moderate elevations of serum alkaline phosphatase are common in inflammatory arthritis.

In clinical suspicion of RA, rheumatoid factor (RF) with anti-citrullinated peptide antibodies (ACPA) plus plain radiographs of both hands should be recommended to look for bony erosions. Presence of both RF and ACPA are poor prognostic markers with ACPA being more disease specific and sensitive than RF. The sensitivity and specificity of ACPA for RA are 66% and 90.4% as compared with sensitivity and specificity of RF for RA is 71.6% and 80.3%.

Elevated serum uric acid levels are usually observed in gout but do not confirm the diagnosis.

In suspected cases of connective tissue diseases such as SLE, ANA is a very good screening test by indirect immunofluorescence technique but not routinely recommended in all cases of arthritis as it is also found in systemic scleroderma, dermatomyositis, even in normal individuals and elderly population. Other routine and relevant tests including complete hemogram to check for cytopenias (sign of active SLE), with baseline liver function tests, renal function tests, urine examination for proteinuria and sediments, plain chest radiograph, ECG and echocardiogram should be advocated.

Synovial Fluid Analysis (Table 1)

It is an urgent indication in case of warm, red joint with effusion in absence of history of trauma.

The aspirated synovial fluid should be collected in three tubes:

1. Heparinized tubes—chemistry and immunology
2. Sterile tubes—microbiology
3. EDTA tubes—cytology and hematology

Few specific inclusions are observed:

- *Rice bodies*: Free floating tissue aggregates seen in RA, fibrin enriched degenerated synovium
- *Ochronotic shards*: Ground pepper like debris from joint prosthesis

Procedure done at Wrist and MCP Joints

- *Wrist*: 21-gauge, 1-inch needle is introduced perpendicularly via dorsal approach. Wrist is kept in neutral position and in line with forearm and dimple over radiocarpal joint is palpated.
- *MCP joint*: 25-gauge, 1-inch needle is inserted to about 0.3–0.5 cm in a site which is created by giving distal traction on finger producing depression on either side of extensor tendons.

"Ropes" Or "Mucin Clot Test"

Basis of this test lies in checking integrity of hyaluronic acid-protein complex. It is done by adding 2–5% acetic acid to

TABLE 1: Synovial fluid analysis.

Parameters	Normal	Noninflammatory	Inflammatory	Septic
Clarity	Transparent	Transparent	Cloudy	Cloudy
Color	Clear	Yellow	Yellow	Yellow
WBC	<200	<200–2,000	200–50,000	>1,100
PMN	<25%	<25%	>50%	>64%
Lactate	<5.6 mmol/L	<5.6 mmol/L	<5.6 mmol/L	>5.6 mmol/L
LDH	<250	<250	<250	>250
Culture	Negative	Negative	Negative	>50% positive
Crystals	None	None	Multiple or none	None

(LDH: lactate dehydrogenase; PMN: polymorphonuclear cells)

normal synovial fluid which causes clot formation. Poor clot formation occurs in variety of inflammatory conditions such as RA, gout, etc.

Imaging

Plain radiography is the least expensive imaging modality though during acute cases of inflammatory arthritis, they are often normal but in chronic inflammatory cases, plain radiographs of hands are indicated to look out for soft tissue swelling, osteopenia, bone erosion, widened joint epiphysis, loss of joint space, any malalignment or fracture.

Radiographic features of some arthritis are as follows:
- RA
  - *Early changes*: Soft tissue swelling, periarticular demineralization
  - *Later changes*: Juxta-articular osteoporosis, marginal erosions caused by pannus of the bony "bare areas", symmetrical joint space narrowing, subchondral cyst formation, carpal instability
  - *Advanced changes*: Joint subluxation, foreshortening of digits
- Gout
  - Punched out erosions with sclerotic border and overhanging edges
- Lupus arthritis
  - Subchondral sclerosis, ulnar deviation of phalanges without erosions, joint space loss
- Psoriatic arthritis
  - Predilection for interphalangeal joint, marginal erosions, classic pencil-in-cup deformity
  - Osteoporosis not found.

Musculoskeletal ultrasonography uses ultrasonic waves for imaging of soft tissues manifestations of RA, including tendons, bursae, ligaments, and components of the joint. Joint aspirations and injections are greatly facilitated when performed under ultrasound guidance as it ensures correct positioning of the needle.

Computed tomography is most useful for assessment of degenerative disk disease, herniations and trauma of spine and pelvis, evaluation of arthritis in axial joints, pain evaluation in complex joints like in hands where overlying structures peripheral RA.

Magnetic resonance imaging (MRI) is the best modality for assessing subtle features of RA. Synovial hyperemia, synovial hyperplasia (rice bodies), pannus formation, decreased cartilage thickness, subchondral cysts, and erosions are best seen in MRI than radiography. MRI dynamic enhancement pattern may differentiate psoriatic arthritis from RA.

Arthrography is most useful for defining abnormal communication between the synovial space and adjacent bursae and soft tissue.

TREATMENT

Treating the arthritic hand is somewhat similar to Herculean job with constant discrepancy between physicians and hand surgeons over the ideal line of treatment.

Many physicians particularly rheumatologists often considered surgery ineffective for hand deformities due to inflammatory arthritis, thereby advocating for medication for the same. The main objective of medical management is to prevent progression of chronic inflammation and structural protection of affected joints.

Nonsteroidal anti-inflammatory drugs (NSAIDs), corticosteroids, and disease modifying antirheumatic drugs are the three classes of drugs used for the treatment of this pathology. NSAIDs work by reducing inflammation resulting in pain amelioration and functional improvement but they do not change the disease course or further progression to joint destruction.

Corticosteroids come into role when NSAIDs are unable to relieve symptoms. Corticosteroids such as prednisone and methylprednisolone are usually very effective by reducing inflammation and regulating immune system activity but there is always a risk-benefit ratio which should be balanced while prescribing it owing to its adverse effects ranging from mild irritability to life threatening cardiac and adrenal complications.

Only disease-modifying antirheumatic drugs (DMARDs) are effective in improving radiographic outcomes which both NSAIDs and corticosteroids failed to do. As soon as the diagnosis of inflammatory arthritis is made, DMARDs should be started without any delay as it possess anti-inflammatory effects with structural modifying properties with long lasting control of disease activity. The two subgroups of DMARDs are nonbiologic and biologic. The former one is more common. Methotrexate is nonbiologic DMARD qualifying as gold standard for treatment of inflammatory arthritis with little toxicity but with recent advancements, methotrexate works best when used as an adjunct with biologic agents.

Two classes of biologic agents are used for treatment. Tumor necrosis factor (TNF) inhibitors act by neutralizing cytokines that specifically mediate the inflammatory process. They significantly slow down radiographic progression with side by side improving functional status of hands. TNF inhibitors include etanercept, infliximab and adalimumab. Anakinra is an IL-1 receptor antagonist used where there is inadequate response to DMARD therapy.

The only problem lies in using biologic agents is their high cost. New advances in medical research are still going on. Medications are considered a failure when administered in late stages of disease hence hand surgery may still be indicated in certain cases. Hence, rheumatologists and surgeons should work in sync in order to provide best available care to the patients.

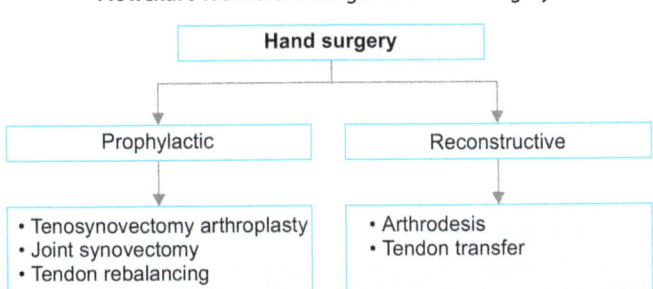

Flowchart 1: Different categories of hand surgery.

Through Surgeon's Lens

The traditional approach in managing hand deformities due to arthritis is based on the individual surgeon's experiences. For years, surgeons have been working constantly in devising new surgical techniques to improve functional outcomes for various hand deformities. From a hand surgeon's perspective, referral to hand surgeon does not mean failure of medical management or immediate surgical intervention but a welcome of planning of present and future care. An expert in arthritic hand surgery will understand the priority of treatment and avail various surgical options which may improve functional status of patients. Certain considerations in hand surgery are important while planning a surgical action in order to solicit the patient's input regarding his or her needs.

First-line treatment for the inflammatory arthritic hand is to control systemic disease without which any surgical attempt will be considered a complete fiasco. Different categories of hand surgery are described in **Flowchart 1**.

Prophylactic procedures usually slow down the destruction process of disease thereby extending the life span of tendon and joints. They are often simpler as compared to reconstructive techniques which are complex though normal functional restoration of arthritic hand is next to impossible.

■ PREOPERATIVE EVALUATION

This is a mandatory step which should be kept in mind before planning any surgical procedures. The surgeon should keenly assess patient's hand and religiously enquire any hindrance in their daily routine activities because deformity alone is not an indication for proposing surgical treatment and with time, many patients can attune to their hand deformities by certain lifestyle modifications.

Patient should be treated as a whole and an experienced surgeon will consider the priority of reconstruction. Lower extremity corrective procedures performed first to avoid stress on the reconstructed upper limbs while in upper extremity; proximal joints should be addressed before the distal joints. The elbow should be treated first, followed by the wrist and the hand.

Orthogonal radiograph of wrist and hand are of utmost importance to understand the stage of disease and planning the extent of repair. Preoperative evaluation of neck and cervical spine is necessary because a substantial proportion of patients have atlantoaxial subluxation.

Wrist

The most commonly affected joint in RA is wrist due to progressive synovitis there is continuous damage to the triangular fibrocartilage ligament (TFCC) and dorsal and palmar ulnocarpal ligaments resulting in collapse of the ulnar column and erosion of distal radioulnar joint as a consequences distal ulna is dislocated dorsally and there is volar subluxation of extensor carpi ulnaris and proximal carpal row is supinated collectively called caput ulnae syndrome.

Wrist deformity progression is well described by Taleisnik who postulated the sequential, predictable events in the RA wrist. The scapholunate ligament is susceptible to weakening from the synovitis, which leads to scaphoid flexion and radial column collapse. Stretching of the wrist ulnar collateral ligament attenuates the ulnar column support. These events ultimately lead to characteristic carpal supination pattern, the consequence of which leads to the collapse of the radial wrist, which contributes to the radial deviation of the metacarpals and attenuates the ulnar deforming forces on the fingers at the MCP joints.

As previously mentioned in this chapter, treatment for wrist deformities can be prophylactic or reconstructive. Chamay described radiolunate fusion procedure which helps in retaining the stability of wrist along with permitting the movement through midcarpal joint. The Darrach and the Suave-Kapandji procedures are performed for the distal radioulnar joint (DRUJ) pathologies, in former there is resection of distal ulna while in latter, distal radioulnar joint is fused and proximal ulnar osteotomy is done. The Masada's shelf arthroplasty procedure is a modified technique in which there is 90° turning of excised distal ulna with fusion into the radius. Radiocarpal fusion is reserved for patients in whom midcarpal joint is maintained by fusing scaphoid and lunate to the radius with retention of mobility in the midcarpal joint. For achieving wrist stability and pain alleviation, total wrist fusion is executed with pins or plates. Procedure related complications can be reduced by using Kirschner wires or buried Steinman pins. In cases of bilateral wrist disease, wrist arthroplasty for dominant hand and fusion in neutral or 10–15° of extension for non-dominant hand is suggested. Studies revealed that total wrist fusion (TWF) is preferable than total wrist arthroplasty (TWA) for the rheumatoid wrist owing to high cost of the latter and better outcomes in the former.

Metacarpophalangeal Joints

Chronic synovitis at the MCP joints distorts the ligamentous support and radial stress on digits cause ulnar deviation of the fingers. MCP joint synovectomy paired with ulnar lateral bands shift to either proximal phalanges or extensor tendons is successful in preventing ulnar subluxation recurrence. For chronic MCP subluxation and complete joint destruction, arthroplasty is recommended as it shortens the bone length resulting in releasing tension to the adjoining ligaments and soft tissues thereby correcting ulnar deformity more effectively. In silicone metacarpophalangeal joint arthroplasty (SMPA), silicone implants creates space between the metacarpal and the proximal phalanx. By overlapping edges of stretched radial sagittal bands and liberating tense ulnar sagittal bands, the extensor tendon is centralized. For satisfactory reduction results, alignments of index and middle fingers are somewhat easy but a tough call for ring and little fingers, requiring division of deformed abductor digiti minimi tendon. Sometimes medullary cavity is opened by using bur for implant accommodation. Earlier volar plate arthroplasty method (described by Tupper) was employed in these cases, where there is detachment of proximal volar plate and its fixation to the dorsum of the metacarpal by providing buffer. This procedure can be done to attain a pseudarthrosis between bone ends in cases where implant arthroplasty cannot be performed. The shortcomings of this technique are recurrent deviation and dubious joint stability. In SMPA, 6 weeks splinting or dynamic extension exercise is indicated as a part of the procedure.

Tendon Rupture

The reasons for tendon rupture are abrasion over bony prominences and tendon attenuation by synovial invasion. The little finger extensor tendon is often the first to rupture subsequently leading to movement of ring finger tendon toward ulna causing rupture. By removing the ulnar head and resection of hypertrophic synovial tissue over the extensors is the ultimate cure for tendon rupture. Tendon transfer is the key step while doing corrective surgeries for tendon rupture. In case of little finger extensor tendon rupture, transfer of distal end of intact tendon is done end to side to the intact ring finger. Transfer of extensor indicis proprius (EIP) to strengthen ring and little fingers is done in cases where the tendons of both the ring and little fingers are damaged. EIP transfer to power ring and little fingers with simultaneous transfer of extensor tendon of middle finger to the index communis extensor tendon is employed in cases where tendons of middle, ring and little fingers are ruptured. Other way out is FDS transfer from middle or ring finger to strengthen ring and little fingers and for middle finger, EIP tendon is used.

Finger Deformities

Proximal point deformity affects distal joints as hand and wrist joints are interlinked. Boutonniere's deformity due to trauma is difficult to treat but next to impossible in case of rheumatoid arthritis—quoted by Dr Adrian Flatt due to the functional limitation of flexed PIP joint. While assessing finger deformities, surgeons need to categorize the deformity into flexible and fixed type in order to plan surgical strategy. Soft tissue reconstruction is the answer to cure flexible type while for fixed deformities, joint fusion or implant arthroplasty is the satisfactory remedy. Joint synovectomy, central tendon tightening with dorsal shifting of collateral bands are performed with doubtful outcomes for flexible chronic Boutonniere's deformities therefore chronic PIP joint synovitis should be prevented by medication initially, failure of which leads to surgical interventions such as synovectomy, fusion, and implant arthroplasty. While doing implant arthroplasty for Boutonniere's deformity, excessive excision of PIP joint results in joint instability by removal of collateral ligaments.

Swan neck deformities can occur at the DIP joint, the PIP joint, or the MCP joint so exact deformity site should be identified. Release of tight intrinsic tendon of ulna, restriction of PIP joint via volar plate advancement or FDS tenodesis method can be employed for flexible swan neck deformities while fusion or implant arthroplasty is the only option for fixed deformities.

Thumb Deformities

It is very rewarding to correct a thumb deformity as 50% function of the hand is executed by thumb. For correcting boutonniere thumb deformity, fusion of MCP joint is done which will shorten the thumb which leads to create balance in extensors giving somewhat normal stance to thumb. Fusion of carpometacarpal (CMC) joint or arthroplasty by tendon or implant is done for correcting swan-neck deformity.

■ CONCLUSION

Evaluation of inflammatory arthritis is quite challenging, reason attributed to multiple differential diagnosis. The keystone to arrive at diagnosis is good history, assessment of all systems, identification of pattern of arthritis and pertinent investigations. Treatment plan should be carved out systematically keeping in mind the priorities of the concerned patients. Both physicians and surgeons should work in harmonious way and carry out the treatment process by applying knowledge and skills from respective domains to cater to the needs of the patients which should be individual based rather than conforming to the standard norms.

■ FURTHER READING

1. Abu-Shakra M, Buskila D, Shoenfeld Y. Osteonecrosis in patients with SLE. Clin Rev Allergy Immunol. 2003;25:13-7.
2. Alderman AK, Chung KC, Kim HM, Fox DA, Ubel PA. Effectiveness of rheumatoid hand surgery: contrasting perceptions of hand surgeons and rheumatologists. J Hand Surg. 2003;28A:3-11.

3. Anderson J, Caplan L, Yazdany J, American College of Rheumatology. Rheumatoid arthritis disease activity measures: American College of Rheumatology Recommendations for use in clinical practice. Arthritis Care Res (Hoboken). 2012;64:640-7.
4. Balint P, Sturrock RD. Musculoskeletal ultrasound imaging: a new diagnostic tool for the rheumatologist? Br J Rheumatol. 1997;361141-2.
5. Begovich AB, Carlton VE, Honigberg LA, Schrodi SJ, Chokkalingam AP, Alexander HC, et al. A missense single-nucleotide polymorphism in a gene encoding a protein tyrosine phosphatase (PTPN22) is associated with rheumatoid arthritis. Am J Hum Genet. 2004;75:330-7.
6. Buckley TJ. Radiographic features of gout. Am Fam Physician. 1996;54:1232-38.
7. Cavaliere CM, Chung KC. A systematic review of total wrist arthroplasty compared with total wrist arthrodesis for rheumatoid arthritis. Plast Reconstr Surg. 2008;122:813-25.
8. Cerezal L, Abascal F, Garcia-Valtuille R, Del Pinal F, Wrist MR. Arthrography: how, why, when. Radiol Clin North Am. 2005;434: 709-731.
9. Chamay A, Della Santa D. Radiolunate arthrodesis in rheumatoid wrist (21 cases). Ann Chir Main Memb Super. 1991;10:197-206.
10. Chen YF, Jobanputra P, Barton P, Jowett S, Bryan S, Clark W, et al. A systematic review of the effectiveness of adalimumab, etanercept and infliximab for the treatment of rheumatoid arthritis in adults and an economic evaluation of their cost-effectiveness. Health Technol Assess. 2006;10:1-229.
11. Chung K. Tendon transfers for the rheumatoid arthritis patient. In: Operative Techniques: Hand and Wrist Surgery. Philadelphia: Saunders/Elsevier; 2007. pp. 757-70.
12. Chung KC, Kotsis SV, Kim HM. A prospective outcomes study of Swanson metacarpophalangeal joint arthroplasty for the rheumatoid hand. J Hand Surg. 2004;29A:646-53.
13. Chung KC, Kowalski CP, Kim HM, Kazmers IS. Patient outcomes following Swanson silastic metacarpophalangeal joint arthroplasty in the rheumatoid hand: a systematic overview. J Rheumatol. 2000; 27:1395-402.
14. Cornelis F, Faure S, Martinez M, Prud'homme JF, Fritz P, Dib C, et al. New susceptibility locus for rheumatoid arthritis suggested by a genome-wide linkage study. Proc Natl Acad Sci U S A. 1998;95:10746-50.
15. Currey HL, Vernon- Roberts B. Examination of synovial fluid. Clin Rheum Dis. 1976;2: 149-77.
16. Cush JJ, Dao KH. Polyarticular arthritis. In: Firestein GS, Budd RC, Gabriel SE, McInnes IB, O'Dell JR (Eds). Kelly's Textbook of Rheumatology, 9th edition. Philadelphia: Elsevier Saunders; 2013. pp. 587-98.
17. Cush JJ. Approach to Articular and musculoskeletal disorders. In: Kasper DL, Fauci AS, Longo DL, Hauser SL, Jameson JL, Loscalzo J (Eds). Harrison's Principles of Internal Medicine, 19th edition. New York: McGraw-Hill; 2015. pp. 2216-25.
18. Deighton CM, Walker DJ, Griffiths ID, et al. The contribution of HLA to rheumatoid arthritis. Clin Genet. 1989;36:178-82.
19. Fardet L, Kassar A, Cabane J, Flahault A. Corticosteroid-induced adverse events in adults: frequency, screening and prevention. Drug Saf. 2007;30:861-81.
20. Fujita S, Masada K, Takeuchi E, Yasuda M, Komatsubara Y, Hashimoto H. Modified Sauve-Kapandji procedure for disorders of the distal radioulnar joint in patients with rheumatoid arthritis. Surgical technique. J Bone Joint Surg Am. 2006;88(Suppl 1 Pt 1):24-8.
21. Furst DE, Schiff MH, Fleischmann RM, Strand V, Birbara CA, Compagnone D, et al. Adalimumab, a fully human anti-tumor necrosis factor-alpha monoclonal antibody, and concomitant standard antirheumatic therapy for the treatment of rheumatoid arthritis: results of STAR (Safety Trial of Adalimumab in Rheumatoid Arthritis). J Rheumatol. 2003;30:2563-71.
22. Gibofsky A. Combination therapy for rheumatoid arthritis in the era of biologicals. HSS J. 2006;2:30-41.
23. Gladman DD, Chaudhry-Ahluwalia V, Ibanez D, Bogoch E, Urowitz MB. Outcomes of symptomatic osteonecrosis in 95 patients with systemic lupus erythematosus. J Rheumatol. 2001;28:2226-9.
24. Grainger AJ, McGonagle D. Imaging in rheumatology. Imaging. 2003;15:286-97.
25. Greenstein B, Greenstein A. Concise clinical pharmacology. London: Pharmaceutical Press; 2007. p. 102.
26. Gregersen PK, Silver J, Winchester RJ. The shared epitope hypothesis. An approach to understanding the molecular genetics of susceptibility to rheumatoid arthritis. Arthritis Rheum. 1987;30:1205-13.
27. Harris H, Joseph J. Variation in extension of the metacarpophalangeal and interphalangeal joints of the thumb. J Bone Joint Surg. 1949;31:547-59.
28. Iizuka H, Sorimachi Y, Ara T, Nishinome M, Nakajima T, Iizuka Y, et al. Relationship between the morphology of the atlanto- occipital joint and the radiographic results in patients with atlanto-axial subluxation due to rheumatoid arthritis. Eur Spine J. 2008;17(6):826-30.
29. Klareskog L, Stolt P, Lundberg K, Källberg H, Bengtsson C, Grunewald J, et al. A new model for an etiology of rheumatoid arthritis: smoking may trigger HLA-DR (shared epitope)-restricted immune reactions to autoantigens modified by citrullination. Arthritis Rheum. 2006;54:38-46.
30. Kotsis SV, Chung KC. A qualitative assessment of rheumatoid hand surgery in various regions of the world. J Hand Surg. 2005;30A:649-57.
31. Lard LR, Visser H, Speyer I, vander Horst-Bruinsma IE, Zwinderman AH, Breedveld FC, et al. Early versus delayed treatment in patients with recent-onset rheumatoid arthritis: comparison of two cohorts who received different treatment strategies. Am J Med. 2001;111:446-51.
32. Lau FH, Chung KC. William Darrach, MD: his life and his contribution to hand surgery. J Hand Surg. 2006;31A:1056-60.
33. Lee AT, Li W, Liew A, Bombardier C, Weisman M, Massarotti EM, et al. The PTPN22 R620W polymorphism associates with RF positive rheumatoid arthritis in a dose-dependent manner but not with HLA-SE status. Genes Immun. 2005;6:129-33.
34. Lee DM, Schur PH. Clinical utility of the anti-CCP assay in patients with rheumatic diseases. Ann Rheum Dis. 2003;62:870-4.
35. Maini RN, Breedveld FC, Kalden JR, Smolen JS, Furst D, Weisman MH, et al. Sustained improvement over two years in physical function, structural damage, and signs and symptoms among patients with rheumatoid arthritis treated with infliximab and methotrexate. Arthritis Rheum. 2004;50:1051-65.
36. Malaviya AN. Approach to the Patient with Polyarthritis. In: Medicine Update. Mumbai: Association Physicians of India; 2008.

37. Malaviya AN. Clinical approach to patients with joint disease: importance of distinguishing inflammatory from non-inflammatory conditions. APLAR J Rheumatol. 2006;9:11-7.
38. Peh WC. Tophaceous gout. Imaging consultation. Am J Orthop. 2001;30:665.
39. Pipili C, Sfritzeri A, Cholongitas E. Deformity arthropathy in systemic lupus erythematosus. Eur J Int Med. 2008;19(7):482-7.
40. Reichman EF, Larkin J. Euerle B. Arthrocentesis. In: Reichman EF (Ed). Emergency Medicine Procedures, 2nd edition. New York: McGraw-Hill; 2013.
41. Ring D, Simmons BP, Hayes M. Continuous passive motion following metacarpophalangeal joint arthroplasty. J Hand Surg Am. 1998;23:505-11.
42. Santiago, Mittermayer B. Miscellaneous non-inflammatory musculoskeletal conditions. Jaccoud's arthropathy. Best Pract Res Clin Rheumatol. 2011;25(5):715-25.
43. St Clair EW, van der Heijde DM, Smolen JS, Maini RN, Bathon JM, Emery P, et al. Combination of infliximab and methotrexate therapy for early rheumatoid arthritis: a randomized, controlled trial. Arthritis Rheum. 2004;50:3432-3443.
44. Stack HG, Vaughan-Jackson OJ. The zig-zag deformity in the rheumatoid hand. Hand. 1971;3:62-7.
45. Stastny P, Fink CW. HLA-Dw4 in adult and juvenile rheumatoid arthritis. Transplant Proc. 1977;9:1863-6.
46. Steenland K, Goldsmith DF. Silica exposure and autoimmune diseases. Am J Ind Med. 1995;28:603-8.

Arthrodesis and Arthroplasty of the Rheumatoid Wrist and Small Joints of Hand: Where do We Stand?

Abhay Elhence, Mahaveer Mali

INTRODUCTION

Wrist and small joint affection occurs as a component of the systemic, autoimmune inflammatory process observed in rheumatoid arthritis (RA). Advanced progressive RA severely handicaps the affected population in many ways. Wrist involvement is observed in more than 90% cases. Wrist involvement leads to severe pain, deformation and grossly affects hand function. The disease causes bilateral involvement in 95% cases with more wrist destruction and deformity than osteoarthritis. Wrist pain is observed in more than 50% patients in less than 2 years of diagnosis of RA and an excess of 90% of these patients develop wrist disease within 10 years of diagnosis.

Total joint replacement and wrist fusion has been quoted as the only significant solution to disabling wrist arthritis by a significant section of world literature.

As part of a research on functional outcomes of hand surgery, Cavaliere and Chung pointed out that working with a painful and dysfunctional wrist for 12 years equates to working with a normal wrist for 30 years. In current day scenario, it is very difficult to advise on the best surgical treatment for a severely destroyed wrist joint in RA. Wrist fusion has good results in patients desirous of performing hard manual labor, but leads to loss of wrist motion and difficulty in performing personal hygiene. On the other hand, in endoprosthetic total wrist arthroplasty, range of motion is fairly preserved but risk of loosening and infection always persists. Classical end stage disease of metacarpophalangeal (MCP) joint in RA entails subluxation and/or dislocation of the wrist following destruction and loss of articular surface and loss of structural support around the joint due to proliferative synovitis; as such in advanced disease, excision of the hypertrophic synovium and soft tissue reconstruction alone are not sufficient. Patient centric outcome evaluation methods demonstrate that total joint arthroplasty of MCP joint restores reasonable function but may require additional proximal realignment procedures considering the deformities observed in a rheumatoid hand.

WRIST ARTHRODESIS IN RHEUMATOID ARTHRITIS

A stable pain-free wrist is the primary end point of treatment in a rheumatoid wrist with severe damage and loss of articular geometry. Wrist arthrodesis has demonstrated optimal deformity correction, remarkable pain relief, and significant improvement of function.

A normal wrist moves through a functional flexion-extension arc of motion of 10–30°, though most activities related to personal care and hygiene can be reliably executed with flexion alone at the wrist joint. Therefore in cases of bilateral affection, one side wrist arthrodesis and contralateral wrist arthroplasty has been documented to provide satisfactory results, as the arthrodesed wrist provides strength and the wrist which has undergone arthroplasty provides dexterity of function. The correct choice of surgical procedure in the above subset of patients requires a detailed evaluation of ipsilateral shoulder and elbow function, especially range of motion. Patients requiring walking aids for ambulation are better suited for wrist arthrodesis than wrist arthroplasty. Wrist arthrodesis is the optimal procedure for patients with advanced disease, viz., wrist instability due to articular destruction, osteoporosis, patients with history or stigmata of infection and in high demand patients requiring to perform heavy manual labor. Multiple techniques for surgical arthrodesis have been described in the literature, mostly all with favorable rates of fusion. Surgical wrist arthrodesis was first described by Clayton in 1965. Clayton performed stabilization of the wrist with an intramedullary device. This technique was popularized by Mannerfelt (1971), who utilized a rush nail for fixation and added a staple for additional stability of the construct. The original technique was further modified and dynamic compression plates were used, which give good primary stability to the damaged and deformed rheumatoid wrists.

Partial Wrist Arthrodesis

Rheumatoid arthritis predominantly involves the radiocarpal and midcarpal joints which can be successfully treated with partial or complete fusion of the wrist joint complex.

Partial fusion is indicated in cases where disease is restricted to radiocarpal joint with sparing of the midcarpal joint; the procedure of choice, therefore involves arthrodesis of the scapholunate and radiolunate joints. The keystone to the success of this operation is to avoid undue flexion or extension of the lunate and avoid overcorrection of the carpal height. The arthrodesed radiocarpal joint is stabilized by either K-wires, plate and screws, interfragmentary screws in compression mode, staples or tension band fixation. The fusion mass is augmented by grafted bone sourced from the iliac crest or lower end of radius. Results of partial wrist arthrodesis are reliable in terms of achieving fusion and preservation of some motion at the wrist. Complications of the procedure include nonunion, malunion, extensor tendon irritation or rupture by malplaced hardware, progressive midcarpal arthritis, and pain due to the implant. Midcarpal degeneration following partial wrist fusion is usually well tolerated. Partial wrist fusion is to be avoided in patients with preexisting midcarpal arthritis and in patients with a severe and progressive inflammatory pathology.

Total Wrist Arthrodesis

Complete wrist fusion is indicated in patients with pan carpal disease with severe deformity and cases of failed wrist arthroplasty.

Total wrist arthrodesis involves fusion of radiolunate, radioscaphoid, scaphocapitate, capitolunate, and capitometacarpal joints. The optimal position of wrist arthrodesis depends on the patient's need and should be discussed with the patient and family preoperatively. Fusion is usually performed with wrist in dorsiflexion and ulnar deviation. Clayton and Smyth, discuss that some surgeons make a case for wrist fusion in neutral position quoting easier pronosupination at the wrist and a better balance of the flexors and extensors of the wrist. The position of the wrist at fusion is tailored to the individual patient depending on hand dominance and the level of involvement of the nondominant wrist. In patients with bilateral involvement of wrists, the dominant side should be fused in 5–30° of wrist dorsiflexion and the nondominant side in neutral or mild palmar flexion in order to balance and optimize function on both sides. The fusion mass may be augmented by bone graft sourced from the iliac crest or lower end of radius. In order to achieve the desired position, dorsal plates have been designed which can provide moderate extension and ulnar deviation of wrist **(Fig. 1)**. The volar lip of distal radius is left which helps in maintaining length and tension and therein preventing compromise of the dimensions of the carpal tunnel. This procedure is safe and provides reliable functional outcomes as published in most scientific literature. Meads and colleagues document excellent wrist fusion achieved with precontoured commercially available dorsal fusion plates. However, using intramedullary

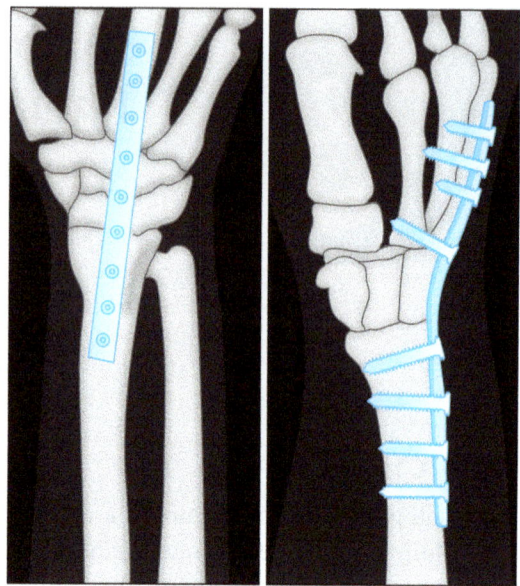

Fig. 1: Diagrammatic representation of wrist arthrodesis by dynamic compression plate.

Steinmann pins also shows excellent results. Comparative study between intramedullary pins and dorsal fusion plates has demonstrated that both methods lead to excellent fusion rates; however, higher complication rates were observed with intramedullary Steinmann pins. Dorsal plates have shown to provide superior stability and are able to position the wrist better. Complications of wrist fusion include pseudarthrosis of the carpometacarpal joint, implant failure, pain due to implant irritation, tendon irritation, and limitation of finger movements.

ARTHROPLASTY OF THE RHEUMATOID WRIST

- Total wrist arthroplasty
- Ulnar head arthroplasty
- Midcarpal resection interposition arthroplasty

Total Wrist Arthroplasty

Arthroplasty is a good alternative for patients with advanced disease and severe deformation of the wrist. The first reported, total wrist arthroplasty had an ivory socket and ball articulation, performed by Themistocles Gluck (1890).

The first wrist arthroplasty was a semi-constrained prosthesis by design. Early results of this design were favorable but loosening of metacarpal and radial components was observed. For achieving better outcomes one needs to have an improved understanding of patient selection along with better instrumentation, implants, and a more refined surgical technique **(Fig. 2)**.

Arthrodesis is an effective salvage operation for failed arthroplasty situations but has higher complications rates. Patients with failed wrist arthroplasty usually need revision surgery in the form of wrist arthrodesis. However, in failed

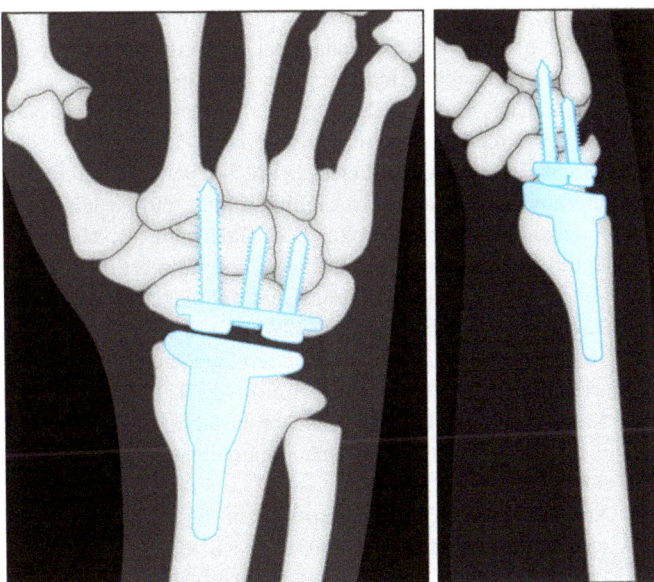

Fig. 2: Diagrammatic representation of total wrist arthroplasty.

arthroplasty situations bone stock is inadequate for fusion, there is inadequate lever arm for functioning of hand tendons as length is lost due to bone loss; these problems are overcome by using autologous iliac crest bone graft or fresh frozen femoral head allograft for correcting the length and deformity. Presently, wrist arthroplasty is considered a valid alternative for treating advanced rheumatoid arthritis of wrist but it needs a highly skilled surgeon and improved quality implants.

Ulnar Head Arthroplasty

Ulnar head replacement is usually indicated in select cases of rheumatoid arthritis in which other salvage procedures, viz. hemi or complete resection of ulna, Suave-Kapandji procedure have failed. The replacement armamentarium comprises of fully constrained and minimally constrained ulnar head designs; partial head and total ulnar head replacement designs are also part of the available inventory. Compared to distal ulnar resection surgery, ulnar head replacement offers the benefit of better stability and improved function of the forearm. The procedure is contraindicated in cases of severe destruction of the ulnar head, gross distal radioulnar joint instability and known allergies or metal hypersensitivities to implants.

Midcarpal Resection Interposition Arthroplasty

In progressively increasing arthritis Larsen, Dale and Eek defined a classification for midcarpal joint involvement wherein, midcarpal resection arthroplasty is indicated. Good outcome can be achieved by combining radiocarpal fusion along with resection and interposition arthroplasty at the Luno-capitate articulation (proximal resection interposition arthroplasty).

However, in a subset of arthritic patients, arthrodesis of the proximal carpal row may additionally be required. In these patients, 5 mm of the damaged articular surface of capitate and hamate is resected to create a pseudoarticulation and either the dorsal capsule or extensor retinaculum are interpositioned at the level of the proximal carpal row so as to retain some motion at the midcarpal joint (distal resection interposition arthroplasty).

It has been observed that where the integrity of the articular cartilage of the midcarpal joint is preserved, radiocarpal fusion is chosen over midcarpal fusion to preserve whatever function can be retained at the midcarpal joint. The stability obtained with radiocarpal fusion combined with a functional arc of motion from distal resection interposition arthroplasty (RIAP) fulfills most demands of activities of daily living for a rheumatoid wrist.

SILICONE METACARPOPHALANGEAL JOINT ARTHROPLASTY

Typical end stage deformity of MCP joint involves flexion and ulnar deviation of MCP with or without subluxation or dislocation of the articulation. Arthroplasty is indicated when a severely destroyed joint limits function. An MCP joint arthroplasty will be preceded by proximal realignment procedures, predominantly wrist surgeries. In case of an associated wrist deformity, partial or complete wrist fusion is performed to stabilize and axially realign the wrist joint before an MCP endoprosthetic replacement can correct MCP deformity, relieve pain, and restore function. These designs can be grouped into three basic types:

1. Hinged prosthetic joint
2. Flexible prosthetic joint
3. Third generation prosthetic joint

The hinged prosthetic joint is no longer in use due to its high failure rate. Flexible silicone implants have a usership of over four decades and remain the gold standard for MCP arthroplasty. Shortening of the metacarpal and proximal phalanx and periarticular osteolysis are the noted problems at long-term follow-up.

PROXIMAL INTERPHALANGEAL JOINT ARTHROPLASTY

Advanced rheumatoid changes in joint, severe disabilities, destroyed, subluxed, stiff joints in which only soft tissue release procedure will not be beneficial are candidates for proximal interphalangeal joint (PIP) arthroplasty. Involvement of the index and middle fingers in an occupationally employed patient requires arthrodesis of the proximal interphalangeal joint of the index finger in functional position (20–40° of flexion) and arthroplasty of the proximal interpalangeal joint of middle finger to provide a functional hand. There is little published literature for the ideal indications of PIP joint flexible silicone rubber implant resection arthroplasty in end stage rheumatoid PIP joint disease, as such, we discuss here the surgical technique and the relevant outcomes in severely affected PIP joint disease.

A C-shaped dorsal incision is usually preferred for arthroplasty to avoid the site of tendon repair. The central slip of the tendon is incised along with lateral attachment release from the middle phalanx; collateral ligaments are initially exposed but not released from their insertion. After exposure of the joint, cartilage is removed with adequate soft tissue release for better visualization; additional bony resection may be required from the proximal and middle phalanges if severe soft tissue contracture is encountered at surgery. Collateral ligament take down may be performed if necessary for optimizing exposure but the collaterals should be reattached to bone at the time of surgical closure. The intramedullary canals of proximal and middle phalanx are prepared by using blunt leader tip burr. After preparation of canal, the implant is seated on the smoothened bone ends.

Postoperatively, active flexion and extension movements are started after 3–5 days. Complications can occur in the form of infection, implant dislocation and revision surgery. In isolated end stage involvement of the PIP joint, arthroplasty results in near normal restoration of arc of motion. Flexible implant arthroplasty of the PIP joint, if performed well and for the right indications, can give stable painless motion in the medium and long term.

FURTHER READING

1. Barbier O, Saels P, Rombouts JJ, Thonnard JL. Long-term functional results of wrist arthrodesis in rheumatoid arthritis. J Hand Surg Br. 1999;24:27-31.
2. Beer TA, turner RH. Wrist arthrodesis for failed wrist implant arthroplasty. J Hand Surg. 1997;22A:685-93.
3. Bhamra J, Bhamra K, Hindocha S, Khan W. The role of wrist fusion and wrist arthroplasty in rheumatoid arthritis. Curr Rheumatol Rev. 2017;13(1):23-8.
4. Borisch N, Haussmann P. Radiolunate arthrodesis in the rheumatoid wrist: a retrospective clinical and radiological long term follow-up. J Hand Surg Br. 2002;27:61-72.
5. Carroll RE, Dick HM. Arthrodesis of the wrist for rheumatoid arthritis. J Bone Joint Surg. 1971;53A:1365-9.
6. Cavaliere CM, Chung KC. Outcomes of hand surgery in the patient with rheumatoid arthritis. J Hand Surg Am. 2010;28(4):570-6.
7. Chamay A, Della Santa D. Radiolunate arthrodesis in rheumatoid wrist [21 cases]. Ann Chir Main Memb Super. 1991;10:197-206.
8. Chung KC, Kotsis SV, Kim HM. A prospective outcomes study of Swanson metacarpophalangeal joint arthroplasty for the rheumatoid hand. J Hand Surg Am. 2004;29(4):646-53.
9. Clayton ML, Smyth CJ. Surgery for rheumatoid arthritis. New York: Churchill Livingstone; 1992. pp. 182-5.
10. Dinges H, Furst M, Ruther H, Schill S. Operative differential therapy of rheumatic wrists. Z Rheumatol. 2007;66:388-94.
11. Esenwein S, Fritz J, Klinger HM, Gaissmaier C, Martini F, Sell S. Radiolunate and radioscapholunate arthrodeses in rheumatoid arthritis—a clinical and radiological follow-up in 32 cases [in German]. Chirurg. 2003;75:176-84.
12. Herzberg G. Management of bilateral advanced rheumatoid wrist destruction. J Hand Surg Am. 2008;33(7):1192-5.
13. Kane PM, Stull JD, Culp RW. Concomitant total wrist and total elbow arthroplasty in a rheumatoid patient. J Wrist Surg. 2016;5(2): 137-42.
14. Kumar K, Cox QG. Pin arthrodesis of the wrist: a modified technique. J Hand Surg Br. 2005;30(5):461-3.
15. Lee DH, Carroll RE. Wrist arthrodesis: a combined intramedullary pin and autogenous iliac crest bone graft technique. J Hand Surg Am. 1994;19:733-40.
16. Meads BM, Scougall PJ, Hargreaves IC. Wrist arthrodesis using a Synthes wrist fusion plate. J Hand Surg Br. 2003;28(6):571-4.
17. Murphy DM, Khoury JG, Imbriglia JE, Adams BD. Comparison of arthroplasty and arthrodesis for the rheumatoid wrist. J Hand Surg. 2003;28A:570-6.
18. Papp SR, Thaw GS, Pichora DR. The rheumatoid wrist. JAAOS. 2006;14(2):65-77.
19. Rauhaniemi J, Tiusanen H, Sipola E. Total wrist fusion: a study of 115 patients. J Hand Surg Am. 2005;30(2):217-9.
20. Swanson AB, de Groot Swanson G, Maupin BK. Flexible implant arthroplasty of the radiocarpal joint. Surgical technique and long-term study. Clin Orthop Relat Res. 1984; (187):94-106.
21. Taleisnik J. Combined radiocarpal arthrodesis and midcarpal (lunocapitate) arthroplasty for treatment of rheumatoid arthritis of the wrist. J Hand Surg. 1987;12:1-8.
22. Trieb K. Treatment of the wrist in rheumatoid arthritis. J Hand Surg Am. 2008;33:113-23.
23. V Schoonhoven J, Herbert TJ, Fernandez DL, Prommersberger KJ, Krimmer H. Ulnar head prosthesis. Orthopade. 2003; 32:809-15.
24. Wei DH, Feldon P. Total wrist arthrodesis: indications and clinical outcomes. J Am Acad Orthop Surg. 2017;25(1): 3-11.
25. Willis AA, Berger RA, Cooney WP 3rd. Arthroplasty of the distal radioulnar joint using a new ulnar head endoprosthesis: preliminary report. J Hand Surg Am. 2007;32: 177-89.
26. Wright CS, McMurtry RY. AO arthrodesis in the hand. J Hand Surg. 1983;8:932-5.

Pain in Hand: Carpal Tunnel Syndrome, Ulnar Nerve Entrapment at Wrist, Kienböck's Disease, and Osteoarthrosis of Carpometacarpal Joint of the Thumb

RB Kalia

CARPAL TUNNEL SYNDROME

DEFINITION

Carpal tunnel syndrome (CTS) is a group of symptoms related to compression of median nerve at the wrist in the carpal tunnel caused by increased pressure. Median nerve is compressed where it passes, along with the flexor tendons, beneath the volar ligament of the carpus.

ETIOLOGY

The cause of CTS is largely idiopathic. It can be caused by repetitive strain or overuse of the hand or wrist, and prolonged, improper positioning (typically work-related). Occupational hazards seems to be the most frequent identifiable cause of CTS. An association with repetitive tasks causing flexion of the wrist and transmission of excessive forces are implicated. Common risk factors include obesity, pregnancy, hypothyroidism, diabetes, and fractures.

PATHOLOGY

The median nerve lies within the confines of the carpal tunnel, which has very little room to accommodate swelling of any of the structures passing through it. Initially in the course of the syndrome, the median nerve injury is reversible. However, prolonged compression results in demyelination followed by axonal degeneration. Sensory fibers often are affected first, followed by motor fibers. Autonomic nerve fibers in the median nerve also may be affected.

AGE AND GENDER

Carpal tunnel syndrome is seen most commonly between 45 and 60 years. Only 10% of CTS patients are younger than third decade. CTS has a predilection for female sex and the female-to-male ratio is about 7:1.

CLINICAL FINDINGS

History and physical examination form the basis of the diagnostic evaluation; include provocative testing (e.g., Phalen test, Tinel sign) in the diagnostic evaluation. However, none of the provocative tests have been established as a gold standard. It is important to understand that duration of symptoms and examination findings does not always correlate with degree of nerve injury or treatment outcomes.

SYMPTOMS

Typically, patients awaken in the middle of the night or morning with numb fingers. Numbness is the pathognomonic symptom of CTS. Typical symptoms include pain, paresis, and/or paresthesia of palmer aspect of the radial three and half finger, which is typically worsens after sleeping probably due to unconscious flexion of the wrist during sleep. Pain sometimes radiate into forearm and, less commonly, into upper arm and shoulder.

Motor involvement of the thenar muscles causes decreased grip strength, resulting in loss of dexterity; patients may complain of dropping things and having difficulty with opening jars. Some patients complain of sensation of swelling, tightness in the absence of edema, or sensation of extreme temperature in the affected hand.

Symptoms sometimes appear intermittently and during performance of specific manual activities and can vary day-to-day. Dominant hand can be affected initially and/or with greater severity, but bilateral CTS occurs frequently. Patients sometimes report flicking or shaking their wrist in an attempt to relieve symptoms (flick sign). However, the flick sign should not be used as an independent factor for diagnosis, because this sign alone has only weak association with diagnosing CTS.

SIGNS

Various clinical signs such as Phalen's sign, Tinel's sign, Hoffmann-Tinel sign, median nerve compression test, the square wrist sign, and the Durkan's test are described and may be useful in confirming CTS. Phalen test is deemed to be positive, if induction of symptoms in median nerve distribution occur with 90 degree flexion of wrists for 1 minute. Tinel sign is positive, if induction of symptoms occur in median nerve distribution with tapping over carpal tunnel. Carpal compression test is elicited by direct compression of carpal tunnel and is deemed to be positive if induction of symptoms occurs in the anatomical distribution of the median nerve. Reverse Phalen test is positive, if induction of symptoms occur with full extension of wrists.

Decreased sensation on palmer side of thumb, second finger, third finger, and radial side of fourth finger; other areas of the hand should demonstrate normal sensation. Sensory abnormalities however, have a week association with diagnosis as the positive predictive value or negative predictive value is low. In more severe cases, a 2-point discrimination test with calipers will demonstrate inability to discriminate points less than 6 mm apart as two distinct points in volar pads of affected fingers. The Semmes-Weinstein monofilament test measures the response to a touching sensation of the monofilaments. The milligrams of force required to bend the heaviest filament is converted by a logarithmic scale to a numerical value. Semmes-Weinstein testing is useful in detecting moderate-to-severe CTS when the criterion of 3.22-CM is applied. In patients where other diagnostic methods are not preferred or are inconclusive Semmes-Weinstein testing could be an option for diagnosing CTS.

Thenar atrophy may be observable, usually in more severe cases. There is strong evidence to support the presence of thenar atrophy in ruling in CTS but only weakly associated with ruling it out. In severe CTS thenar wasting, weakness of thumb abduction and trophic ulcers may be seen in later stages. Weakness of abductor pollicis brevis is demonstrated when the patient raises the affected thumb perpendicular to the palm when downward pressure is applied on the distal phalanx by the examiner (demonstrates weakness of abduction and opposition). Measure pinch and grip strength on both hands either manually or by using a dynamometer; weakness is commonly demonstrated. Ecchymosis or abrasions on hands and wrists may be present in cases caused by acute injury.

■ SPECIAL TESTS

Electromyography and nerve conduction velocity testing (EMG/NCV) are excellent test for CTS with an accuracy ranging from 85 to 90%. EMG/NCV are extremely useful to detect the presence or absence of nerve dysfunction and quantify it. When physical examination and/or provocative test results are positive and, in patients with thenar atrophy and/or persistent numbness (to document more severe nerve injury), to exclude differential diagnosis and if surgical management is being contemplated obtaining needle EMG and nerve conduction studies is highly desirable. Measurements are obtained from a needle electrode placed in muscle tissue; a reference electrode is placed some distance away on skin.

Electrical activity data are collected from the following points:
- Across muscle membrane
- Muscle at rest
- Active muscle contraction

Nerve conduction velocity is measured by stimulating a peripheral nerve and measuring the latency and amplitude of the muscle response recorded at a known distance from the stimulation site. Relative contraindications to EMG, which require extra caution during needle insertion and removal, are coagulopathy or blood dyscrasias, patients on anticoagulation.

■ INTERPRETATION OF RESULTS

Slowed median NCV supports the diagnosis of CTS. Abnormal electrophysiological findings suggesting CTS are categorized into three grades according to Stevens' classification: prolonged median sensory distal latency >3.5 ms—mild; abnormal median sensory latency >3.5 and prolonged median motor distal latency >4.2 ms—moderate, the absence of median sensory nerve action potential, or low amplitude of thenar compound muscle action potential <5 mV—severe. Decreased or absent sensory or motor responses on EMG/NCV distal to carpal tunnel on needle EMG are indicative of severe CTS **(Box 1)**.

■ IMAGING

Ultrasonography or magnetic resonance imaging (MRI) may be used to diagnose space-occupying lesions in and around the carpal tunnel. Routine use of MRI or CT scans has no role in the diagnosis of CTS.

■ DIFFERENTIAL DIAGNOSIS

Pronator teres syndrome causes median nerve compression in the forearm. It causes aching pain in the forearm, hand weakness, and sensory alteration in the median nerve distribution of the hand and mimic CTS. Since, the palmar cutaneous nerve arises before the median nerve enters behind the transverse carpal ligament sensory dysfunction of the thenar eminence is an important distinguishing feature.

Box 1: Risk factors and associations.

- Repetitive movements—computer use and occupations involving vibrating machinery, assembly on a production line, and construction
- Flexor tenosynovitis
- Obesity
- Pregnancy
- Arthritis
- Hypothyroidism
- Diabetes mellitus
- Fracture or acute injury of the wrist
- Mass lesions (e.g., ganglion cyst, lipoma)
- Amyloidosis
- Congenitally small carpal tunnel
- Sarcoidosis
- Multiple myeloma
- Leukemia
- Acromegaly
- Gout

Sensory symptoms in pronator teres syndrome occur with resisted pronation of the forearm and wrist flexion or with direct pressure on the leading edge of the pronator while the forearm is in maximum supination and the wrist is in a neutral position. Pronator compression test is elicited by manual compression of the median nerve over pronator muscle. It usually causes development of paresthesia in the hand within 30 seconds of manual compression.

Cervical radiculopathy causes neck pain with associated radiation to upper extremity in a specific dermatomal distribution. Cervical radiculopathy can cause numbness, weakness, and decreased reflexes in upper extremities. Cervical radiculopathy can be differentiated by positive result on Spurling's test (foraminal compression test). Cervical radiographs typically shows disk space narrowing, sclerosis, and osteophyte formation. Cervical MRI scan is the imaging method of choice and shows disk herniation, compression of neurological tissues, and signal changes.

Ulnar neuropathy is caused by nerve compression in the cubital tunnel medially in the elbow or the ulnar side of the wrist. Symptoms can occasionally affect the third finger, and weakness is a common finding; sensory symptoms affect the fourth and fifth fingers. It can be differentiated by EMG, which reveals abnormalities of the ulnar nerve physiology.

Raynaud phenomenon causes recurrent vasospasm of fingers and toes; usually occurs in response to stress or cold exposure. Typical symptoms include numbness and pain occurs in affected area, which also demonstrates at least two color changes: white (pallor), blue (cyanosis), and red (hyperemia).

Primary osteoarthritis (OA) wrist occurs because of articular cartilage degeneration in wrist while secondary OA can result from fractures and dislocations. OA of the wrist results in severe pain and restricted movement of wrist. OA can be differentiated by plain radiographs of wrist which demonstrate degenerative changes.

Diabetic peripheral neuropathy is a distal polyneuropathy caused by chronic prolonged hyperglycemia and is frequently bilateral; causes tingling and numbness in a stocking-and-glove distribution. It can be differentiated from CTS by elevated levels of hemoglobin A1C and fasting plasma glucose.

■ TREATMENT

The goal of treatment in CTS is to relieve symptoms and prevent further nerve compression and injury. Initially, conservative therapy like splinting (neutral or cock-up wrist splints), local steroid injections are appropriate in patients with mild to moderate CTS (75–81% achieve short-term relief). Splints are worn nightly or full-time; optimal splinting duration has not been established, but 6–8 weeks of usage is suggested.

Local steroid injection are indicated, if unresponsive to splinting and symptoms have been persisting for at least 3 weeks. 40–80 mg of methylprednisolone acetate is instilled as a single injection adjacent to the carpal tunnel in adults. If first injection provides relief, second injection can be considered after a few months. Use of more repeat injections is not advisable as local damage may occur to the tendons traversing the carpal tunnel.

Oral corticosteroids are optional conservative therapy. Usual oral dosage of steroids is prednisolone 20 mg PO once daily for 2 weeks, then 10 mg PO once daily for 2 weeks. It is pertinent to remember that the definitive treatment for established median-nerve entrapment is surgery. Corticosteroids are at best temporary measures and can be tried on patients who have intermittent pain and paresthesias without fixed motor-sensory deficits not responding to splintage and activity modification.

If first line conservative treatment methods fail to resolve symptoms in 2–6 weeks, implement alternative non-operative or surgical treatment options. Surgical release is recommended when symptoms do not respond to conservative treatment.

Generally, CTS is a gradually progressive condition that can progress to permanent median nerve damage; it may be reversible in the early stages, so early treatment is recommended. If symptoms resolve with conservative treatment recurrence can be prevented through avoidance of repetitive movements and overuse activities, particularly in certain occupations; ergonomic interventions can mitigate physiologic stresses. It is important that the patient stop repetitive movements and overuse activities to avoid exacerbating symptoms. Ergonomic interventions, such as using wrist supports with computer keyboards, can help relieve symptoms. Symptoms that develop during pregnancy often resolve spontaneously within several months after delivery.

Patients who fail to respond to conservative treatment and patients who initially are in the severe CTS category (as defined by EMG) are candidates for surgery. Surgical release of the transverse carpal ligament provides high initial success rates (greater than 90%) with low rates of complications. Success rates after surgical release also considerably lower for individuals with normal EMG studies. Surgical release of flexor retinaculum in recalcitrant or severe CTS is effective treatment **(Figs. 1 to 7)**.

Strong evidence supports that surgical release of CTS relieves symptoms and improve function. Surgical treatment is recommended when symptoms do not respond to conservative treatment. Early surgery is an option with clinical evidence of median nerve denervation on NCV/EMG or if patient elects to proceed directly to surgery. Acute, severe CTS occurs very rarely (e.g., after a wrist injury); in such cases, immediate surgery may be the best option for symptomatic relief.

Section 7: Hand and Wrist Involvement in Orthopedic Rheumatology

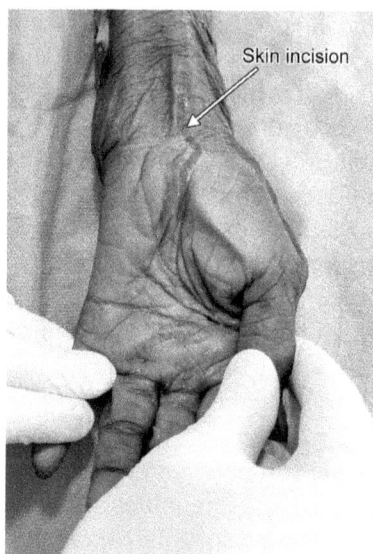

Fig. 1: Cadaveric dissection: Skin incision.

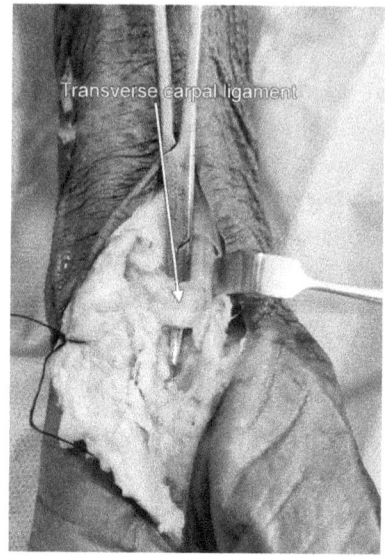

Fig. 2: Superficial dissection.

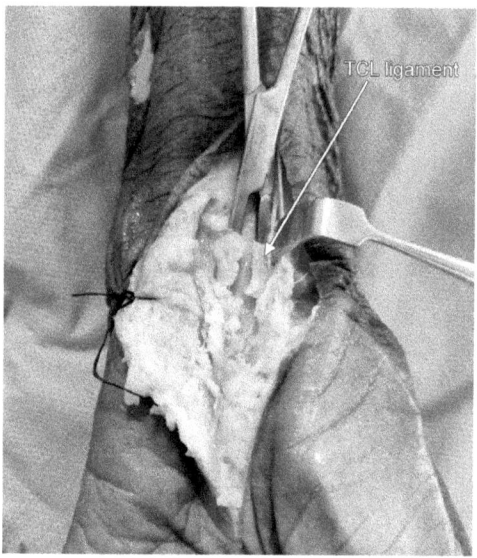

Fig. 3: Release of transverse carpal ligament.
(TCL: transverse carpal ligament)

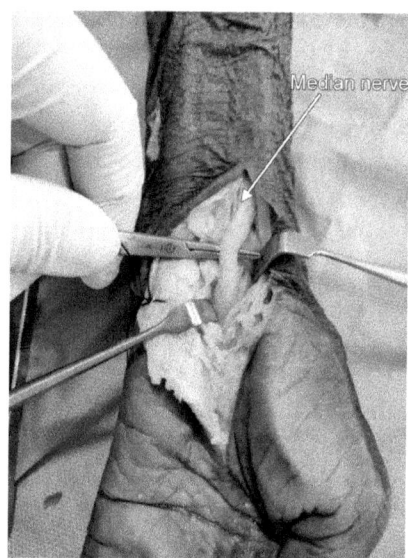

Fig. 4: Dissection of median nerve (Hooked up by the artery forceps).

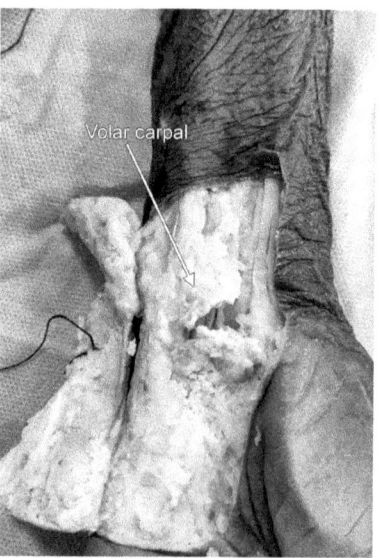

Fig. 5: Dissection of the Guyon's canal.

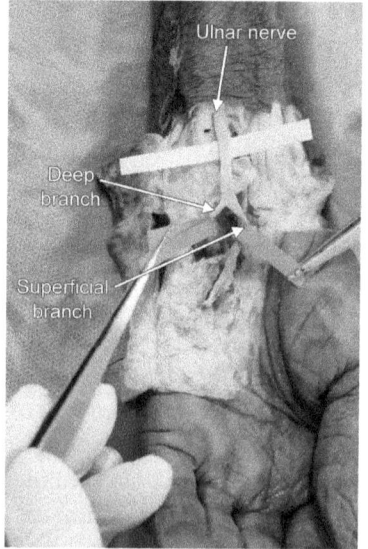

Fig. 6: Deep dissection of the Guyon's canal showing the superficial and deep branch of the ulnar nerve.

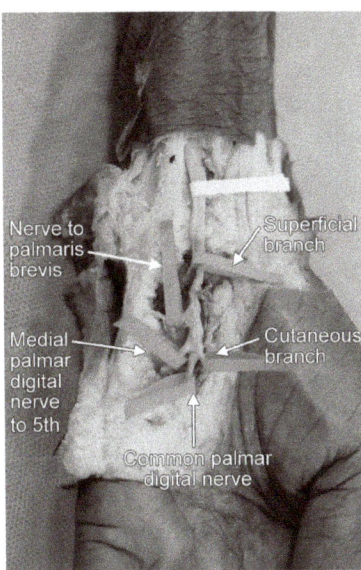

Fig. 7: Deep dissection of the branches of the ulnar nerve.

■ COMPLICATIONS

The compressive neuropathy may continue to increase median nerve damage leading to permanent impairment and disability. The permanent nerve damage does not respond favorably to surgical release.

■ PITFALLS

Patients with more severe or prolonged CTS may not benefit from ill advise prolonged, nonoperative treatment. It is important to consider the location of the median nerve when performing injections and surgery to avoid iatrogenic injury; the median nerve is the most superficial structure in the carpal tunnel.

■ SURGICAL CARPAL TUNNEL RELEASE

Surgical CTS release is an outpatient procedure, which reduces pressure on the median nerve by completely releasing the transverse carpal ligament (flexor retinaculum of hand) typically under regional anesthesia. Two methods of surgical release can be used: (1) Open release of the carpal tunnel (interthenar incision and release of the transverse carpal ligament) and (2) endoscopic release (minimally invasive techniques with the use of an endoscope to release the ligament without incision of interthenar skin). Both methods of surgical release have comparable similar efficacy. Strong evidence exists that surgical release of this ligament relieve symptoms and improves function in patients with documented CTS.

Contraindications to endoscopic release method include rheumatoid arthritis, mass lesions, and repeated surgery. In such situations open-surgical release is preferable and safer.

Complications

The complications of surgical release include median nerve damage resulting in pain, permanent loss of sensation, denervation of thenar muscles with loss of thumb opposition and abduction, and difficulty moving thumb, hypertrophic scarring of the surgical scar, iatrogenic laceration of superficial palmar arch, tendon adhesion, and stiffness and reflex sympathetic dystrophy. A systematic review found that endoscopic release has a higher incidence of transient nerve injury.

Untreated CTS can result in permanent atrophy of the thenar muscles and related grip weakness with difficulty performing some activities of daily living, such as opening jars.

■ PROGNOSIS

Generally, CTS is a progressive condition, which can lead to permanent median nerve damage. Spontaneous resolution occurs in some patients when predisposing factors are avoided. Disease course can be reversible in the early stages, so early treatment is recommended. In later stages, permanent nerve damage may occur owing to chronic nerve compression, if compression is unrelieved.

In mild to moderate cases, surgical release results in success in most cases, with complete recovery in patients who fail initial conservative treatment methods. In severe cases, complete recovery is unlikely, but most patients have experienced partial recovery. Patients with an underlying condition (e.g., diabetes, trauma) often have poorer prognosis.

ULNAR NERVE ENTRAPMENT AT THE WRIST

Distal nerve entrapment of the ulnar nerve at the wrist in the Guyon's canal is a relatively uncommon condition. The space in the hypothenar region of the wrist where the ulnar nerve divides was described first by Guyon in 1861 who suggested compression to the ulnar nerve could occur in this region. Ulnar nerve entrapment in the Guyon's canal occurs much less frequently than in the cubital tunnel at the elbow.

Compression to the ulnar nerve in the Guyon's canal besides direct trauma and laceration is most commonly caused by a ganglion cyst. Other causes of ulnar nerve neuropathy are chronic or repeated external pressure by hand tools used in occupations, bicycle handlebars, the handles of canes, or excessive push-ups in exercise enthusiasts. Compression also may be caused by degenerative wrist joint changes, rheumatoid arthritis, or distal space-occupying vascular lesions including thrombosis, and pseudo-aneurysms of traversing vessels or anomalous muscles.

The unique anatomy of the Guyon's canal influences the symptoms. If the nerve is compressed proximal to the bifurcation of the ulnar nerve (zone I) a mixture of both motor and sensory deficits occurs. If the compression is on the deep motor branch of the ulnar nerve in the piso-hamate hiatus (zone II) characteristically pure motor loss occurs. This is in contrast to compression on superficial sensory

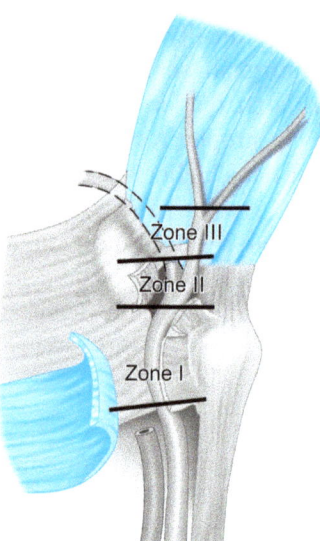

Fig. 8: Anatomy of the Guyon's canal showing the three zones.
Source: Wolfe SW, Hotchkiss RN, Pederson WC, Kozin SH Green's Operative Hand Surgery, 6th edition. Philadelphia: Elsevier; 2011. pp. 939.

branch distally (zone III), which is associated with pure sensory dysfunction. If the compression results in intrinsic weakness, the functional motor loss in the hand can be profound and manifested by a strongly positive Froment's sign, clawing of the ring and small digits, and severe atrophy of the innervated interossei muscles **(Fig. 8)**.

In most cases of ulnar nerve entrapment motor fibers at zone II in the Guyon's canal are involved and this involvement presents with painless unilateral hypothenar and interossei weakness or muscle atrophy. Sensory dysfunction in the proximal hypothenar region and the dorsum of little and ring fingers is not evident as the palmar cutaneous and dorsal cutaneous branches leave the ulnar nerve in the distal forearm before the ulnar nerve enters the Guyon's canal. The sensory dysfunction is confined to the palmar surface of the ulnar-innervated fingers (the little finger and usually the ulnar half of the ring finger) and the distal part of the hypothenar region.

Electrodiagnostic studies are confirmatory and usually reveal low amplitude (with or without prolonged distal motor latencies) to the first dorsal interosseous or abductor digiti minimi muscles or both. Motor denervation of the ulnar-innervated hand muscles is also revealed by electro-diagnostic studies consistent with the clinical manifestations. Ulnar sensory nerve action potentials (SNAP) may or may not be abnormal depending on the involvement of the sensory component. Electrodiagnostic studies are also important in excluding more proximal ulnar neuropathy at the elbow. Several features consistent with an ulnar neuropathy at a proximal level are low amplitude or absent dorsal ulnar SNAP, focal slowing, or conduction block across the elbow, or denervation of the flexor carpi ulnaris or the flexor digitorum profundus.

IMAGING

A carpal tunnel view with standard AP and lateral views of the wrist are required and may reveal a fracture of the pisiform or hook of the hamate bone as the cause of compression in patients with wrist trauma. MRI or ultrasound of the Guyon's canal may demonstrate a structural lesion such as a ganglion cyst. MRI scores over ultrasound as the latter is more operator dependent.

NONOPERATIVE MANAGEMENT

If chronic or repeated external pressure by hand tools, bicycle handlebars, cane handles, or excessive push-ups are the inciting reason for the neuropathy-activity modification is effective. A removable wrist splint may be helpful in the neutral position and can be worn for a few weeks with avoidance of the inciting known cause. Electrodiagnostic studies may be used to monitor improvement in the nerve.

OPERATIVE TREATMENT

In patients with fracture causing crowding in the Guyon's canal, ganglia, or mass lesions causing compressive neuropathy surgical intervention is usually necessary. Guyon's canal is opened by an incision slightly ulnar to the incision used in accessing the transverse carpal ligament in Carpal tunnel release. The hook of the hamate is confirmed by palpation and the neurovascular bundle is dissected from proximal to distal along its length through the Guyon's canal. The leading tendinous edge of the hypothenar muscles is identified under which the deep motor branch of the ulnar nerve is passing. The deep motor branch of the ulnar nerve located just below the leading tendinous edge of the hypothenar muscle origin is released. The prognosis is usually good after surgical decompression with effective reinnervation.

KIENBÖCK DISEASE

In 1843, Peste noticed a collapsed lunate in cadaver dissections and his was the first description of AVN lunate. The radiographic changes associated with avascular necrosis (AVN) lunate was first described by Robert Kienböck, a radiologist and the disease has been associated with his name.

ETIOLOGICAL FINDINGS

The relationship between acute lunate fractures and Kienböck disease is controversial. Doubts persist whether some lunate fractures are actually pathologic fractures in patients with pre-existing Kienböck disease. Lunate fractures in a follow-up study failed to show AVN changes even though 50% of the patients studied had ulnar-negative variance. AVN after a fracture of the lunate cause signal loss of a portion on MRI. In Kienböck disease, the signal loss on MRI is homogeneous for the entire lunate rather than localized and is progressive, which is very different from the findings of AVN after fracture. The cause of Kienböck disease is multifactorial as the exact origin and natural progression of Kienböck disease remain unclear. Despite extensive study no consistent correlation with any specific disease process has been clearly demonstrated. Primary circulatory abnormality, trauma, and ligamentous injury with collapse have all been attributed to the loss of blood supply and leading to the avascular changes in the lunate. Kienböck disease has been associated with various medical conditions such as scleroderma, sickle cell anemia, SLE, and prolonged corticosteroid use.

The causal relationship of negative ulnar variance and Kienböck disease is also controversial. A significant relationship between the presence of ulnar-negative variance and Kienböck disease was found that was refuted by another study, which found no statistically significant relationship between ulnar variance and Kienböck disease. No statistically significant difference in ulnar variance between a sex and age-matched control group and a group of patients affected with Kienböck's disease was found suggesting that negative ulnar variance is not an important etiological factor. The variation in the distal radial slope has been postulated as a potential etiological cause of Kienböck disease and a study found a correlation between lower radial inclination and Kienböck disease.

■ CLINICAL FEATURES

Patient presents with insidious onset of dull aching pain and stiffness in the wrist. Typically, Kienböck's disease involves the dominant wrist of young males. On palpation bony tenderness is usually elicitable in the dorsum of the wrist over lunate and patients have a decreased strength on grip testing. Activity aggravates the pain and rest and immobilization relieves the pain. Progression of the disease may cause radiocarpal effusion with boggy synovitis of the radiocarpal joint and restricted range of motion of the wrist.

■ RADIOLOGICAL FEATURES

With the wrist in neutral rotation plain PA and lateral radiographs of the wrist are provide a lot of information. Although radiographs may be normal in early disease, increased radio-opacity of the lunate is the earliest sign of avascularity on plain radiographs. The most sensitive imaging study for detection of Kienböck's disease is MRI and is especially useful in patients with no abnormality on plain radiographs.

■ CLASSIFICATION

Staging of Kienböck's disease is most commonly done by the Lichtman classification. Stage 1 disease has no abnormality on plain radiographs and signal changes on MRI. Stage 2 typically reveals sclerosis on plain radiographs, maintenance of joint articular space, and sometimes a fracture line **(Fig. 9)**. Stage 3 is marked by articular involvement, which manifests as decreased joint space and this stage is subdivided into 3A with no carpal collapse and 3B with carpal collapse, loss of carpal height, proximal migration of the capitate, and fixed deformity of the scaphoid **(Figs. 10A to C)**. Stage 4 disease has pan carpal arthritis **(Figs. 11A and B)**.

Stage 4 presents with lunate collapse along with radiolunate or midcarpal arthritis **(Figs. 11A and B)**.

Several studies have assessed the inter observer reliability and intra observer reproducibility of the Lichtman classification scheme. Staging according to Stahl (1947), Lichtman et al. (1977), and Voche et al. (1992) was performed independently by three observers on 39 radiographs. Interobserver reliability by kappa values after classification of the 76 sets of radiographs, according to Stahl and Lichtman varied between 0.45 and 0.52. Authors concluded that current staging systems of Kienböck's disease are inadequate as the kappa values of the interobserver reliability and the intraobserver reproducibility demonstrated by these staging systems is poor. In contrast a study of 64 radiographs of patients with Kienböck's and 10 control subjects were reviewed independently by four observers on two separate occasions disease indicated substantial reliability and reproducibility of the Lichtman classification for Kienböck's disease. Paired comparisons for reliability among the four observers showed an average absolute percentage agreement of 74% and an average paired weighted kappa coefficient of 0.71. Furthermore, all the controls were correctly classified as stage I, which is in accordance with the Lichtman system.

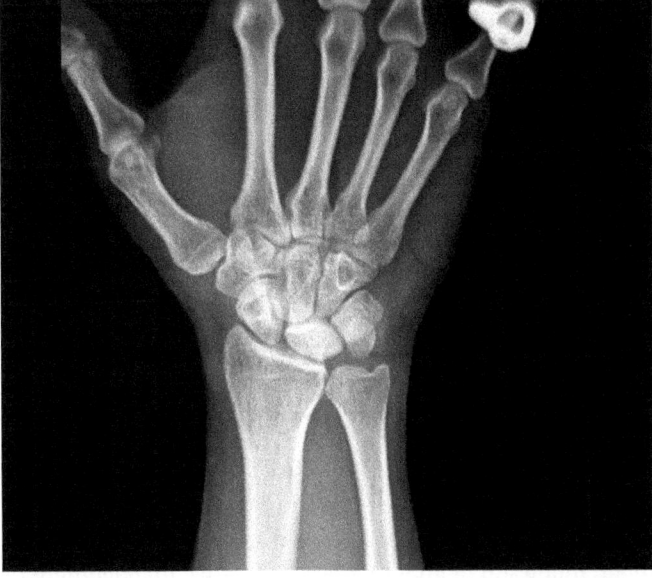

Fig. 9: A posterior–anterior radiograph of a 45-year-old male with stage 2 Kienböck's disease showing sclerosis of the lunate with preserved radio-lunate joint space.
Courtesy: Dr V Singh.

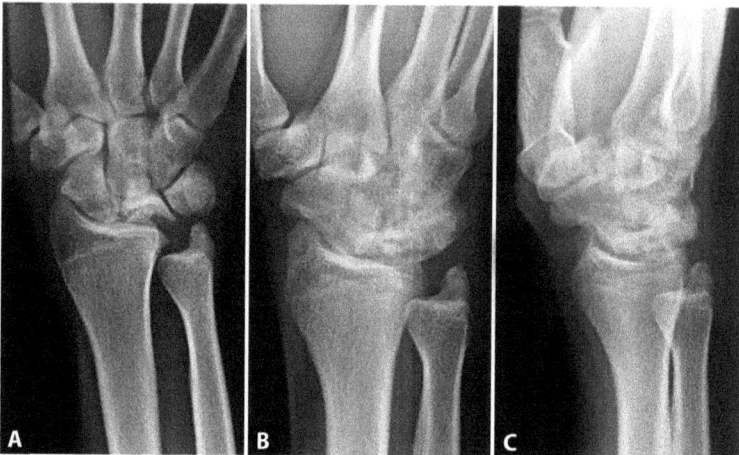

Figs. 10A to C: A posterior–anterior, oblique and lateral radiograph of stage 3B with lunate collapse, loss of carpal height, proximal migration of the capitate, and fixed deformity of the scaphoid.
Courtesy: Dr V Singh.

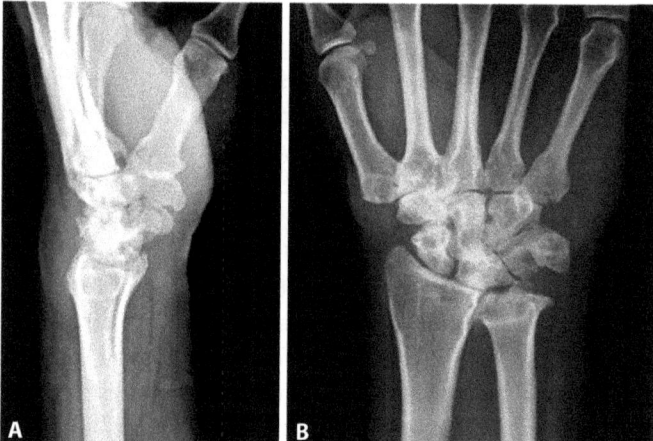

Figs. 11A and B: A posterior–anterior and lateral radiograph of stage 4 showing radiolunate and midcarpal arthritis.

With regard to reproducibility, observers duplicated their initial readings 79% of the time with an average weighted kappa coefficient of 0.77.

In another study on 43 radiographs: The interobserver reliability of the Lichtman classification was substantial (kappa coefficient 0.63), but stage 3A was less reliably identified (kappa coefficient 0.38). Differentiating between stages 3A and 3B was improved after the additional criterion that the radio-scaphoid angle be greater than 60° to qualify as stage 3B to a kappa of 0.75.

SURGICAL OR NONSURGICAL TREATMENT

In a retrospective study on Kienböck's disease, a comparison was made between 21 cases operated on by various techniques and 22 cases treated conservatively, with a mean follow-up of about 5 years. Operative management of the disease did not show any superiority over conservative treatment. Moreover, surgery was responsible for a loss of mobility of 24%, and for a change in social activities in about a quarter of the patients, while grip strength was only slightly improved. Authors concluded that surgical indications for Kienböck's disease need careful consideration keeping in mind their side effects, and the relative benignity in some cases of the natural course of the disease. More advanced cases in the surgical treatment group, most likely owing to selection bias and could be responsible for poorer results than the nonsurgically treated patients.

In a comparative study on 33 patients followed for a mean duration of 3.6 years: 18 were treated nonsurgically and 15 treated with radial shortening osteotomy, the authors concluded that although there was progression of the disease in both groups, the rate of progression was slower in the surgical group who also had less pain and better grip strength, especially in stage 3. The larger negative ulnar variance in the surgical groups (-2.5 mm vs. -1.7 mm) probably suggests a selection bias.

TREATMENT

Treatment of Kienböck's disease is broadly based on the Lichtman stage. For stage 1 nonsurgical treatment like splinting and below elbow casting with close follow-up is appropriate. The goal of treatment in stages 2 and 3A is to limit carpal collapse and arthritis while the bone vascularizes. Recommended interventions include casting, external fixation, free or pedicled vascularized grafting, and shortening of the radius especially in patients with negative ulnar variance and drilling of the radius and ulna in an attempt to increase vascularity and revascularization. In stages 3B and 4 collapse of the lunate and variable amounts of radiocarpal arthritis are present and are usually treated with palliative salvage procedures such as proximal row carpectomy and wrist arthrodesis. Some surgeons use disease modifying procedures even for patients in stage 3B in an attempt to preserve the biomechanical function of the radiocarpal joint.

As Kienböck's disease is uncommon, it is difficult to determine whether the disease is progressing or has run its course at the time of initial diagnosis. It may evolve slowly over many years, and the natural history is still incompletely understood. The evidence that surgical treatment alters progression of Kienböck's disease is limited and of low-quality. Many prospective case series have documented slight improvements in motion and grip after surgical treatment, but it is not clear that this is better than conservative treatment. It is difficult to emphatically suggest with conviction that the minimal clinically important differences in motion and grip after surgery can justify the risk, discomfort, inconvenience, rehabilitation, and cost of surgical interventions. Even more difficult is to recommend among the plethora of surgical techniques.

Asymptomatic stage 1 Kienböck's diseases, which are identified incidentally, do not need treatment and close observation suffices. Symptomatic patients who present with stages 2 or 3A disease are optimally treated with an initial 6-week period of immobilization in a splint or below elbow cast. If symptoms persist despite conservative treatment, radial shortening is appropriate for patients who are ulnar negative or neutral. Patients with positive ulnar variance can be treated with 4, 5 extensor compartmental vascularized bone graft with temporary external fixation. Percutaneous pinning as a temporary offloading or permanent procedure like capitate shortening, scapho trapezium-trapezoid (STT) fusion, or capitate-hamate fusion are also feasible procedures.

The disease-modifying procedures are based on largely unproved hypothesis. The assumption that the ulnar negative variance creates an unfavorable mechanical environment is based on limited, low-quality scientific evidence. Collapse in osteonecrosis is probably due to so weakening of lunate microstructure with revascularization and the presence of varying amounts of dead bone. As revascularization is a part of the normal evolution of the disease process, it is difficult to clearly that vascular bone transfer hastens the revascularization without adequately powered high-quality studies.

The main vascularized bone grafts currently used for the treatment of Kienböck's disease include 4, 5 extensor compartment artery (ECA) bone graft, second or third metacarpal base bone grafts, 2, 3 ICSRA and 1, 2 ICSRA bone grafts, pisiform bone graft, volar bone grafts from the distal radius, and free pedicle bone grafts from the medial femoral condyle. A recent systematic review on vascularized bone grafting included 917 patients, 825 with scaphoid nonunion, and 92 with Kienböck disease concluded that vascularized grafts lead to revascularization of the lunate in most of the cases with concomitant improvement of the clinical parameters.

In a study on 26 patients, 10 Lichtman stage 2, 12 stage 3A, and 4 stage 3B underwent vascularized bone grafting and external fixation or pinning of the scaphoid to the capitate 20 patients had no radiographic signs of progression after an average of 31 months after surgery. There was statistically significant improvement in grip strength. A total of 17 patients had MRI scans; of these there were 12 documented revascularization.

A study on free vascularized transfers based on the iliac crest with concomitant temporary external fixation reported osteointegration in 16 of 18 patients. The range of motion and grip strength improved and did not deteriorate over the next 10 years.

A 12-year follow-up study of vascularized pisiform transfer found that pain was improved in 20 of 23 patients. Grip strength and motion were 84% and 80% of the contralateral side, respectively. A total of 6 patients had progression of Lichtman staging and 7 had mild arthritis on radiographs. In a study on 68 patients had improved pain, grip strength, and motion; an average of 52 months after radial recession osteotomy.

Another long-term study evaluated 12 patients an average of 21 years after radial shortening osteotomy, noting 81% flexion and 88% grip compared with the opposite side and progression of 1 Lichtman stage in 6 patients. Another study found comparable Nakamura ratings an average of 85 months after radial shortening osteotomy in 13 patients with stage 3A and 10 patients with stage 3B disease.

Drilling the metaphysis of the distal radius and ulna was proposed as an effective disease-modifying treatment for Kienböck's disease in a retrospective review of 48 patients (2 stage 0, 4 stage 1, 17 stage 2, and 25 stage 3A) with an average follow-up of 9 years, 3 patients progressed 1 Lichtman stage.

The need at present is a well-designed prospective multicenter, open-label, prospective, long-term cohort studies to help define the natural history of Kienböck's disease and determine the best treatment options for the various stages.

OSTEOARTHROSIS OF THE CARPOMETACARPAL JOINT OF THE THUMB

Carpometacarpal (CMC) joint OA of the thumb is a common radiographic finding, particularly in postmenopausal women, but is symptomless in most cases. Only a minority of symptomatic patients consult a physician, and most can be managed nonoperatively.

PATHOGENESIS OF THE DISEASE

The human CMC joint of the thumb is a biconcave saddle joint that allows flexion, extension, abduction, adduction, pronation, and supination. These movements allow opposition, a uniquely human movement. The greater mobility however produces stresses on the articular cartilage due to the less stability of the articulation and predisposes the CMC joint to degenerative OA.

Multiple ligaments stabilize the CMC joint of the thumb. The beak ligament and the dorsoradial ligament are important stabilizers of the joint. Weakening of these ligaments alter the biomechanics of the articulation, with migration of the point of maximal contact from volarulnar to dorsoradial resulting in distinct patterns of cartilage wear.

Osteoarthritis can either be primary or secondary with both types being common in the hand and wrist. OA of the CMC joint of the thumb is usually oligoarticular. Primary CMC arthritis commonly develops at the base of the thumb while secondary disease occurs at the base of the little finger. CMC OA is far more common in women (female:male ratio 15:1). In primary disease, it classically affects multiple DIPJs. Clinically, a combination of thumb CMCJ, PIPJ, and DIDJ joint involvement is commonly seen. The left CMC joint tends to become arthritic before the right, which could be caused by the protective effect of greater thenar muscle strength in the usually dominant right hand. Fractures of fingers and thumb may all lead to secondary degenerative joint disease, if there is significant damage to the joint surface. Malunion of intraarticular fractures is a theoretical cause of secondary CMC joint arthritis but is rarely seen. Hypermobility is a known risk factor. There is no racial predilection or association with socioeconomic status or occupation. A positive family history is common; however, no hereditary pattern has been recognized.

■ CLINICAL HISTORY

The patient of CMC joint OA presents with pain and swelling at the base of the thumb. The symptoms wax and wane over time, but with gradual deterioration. The typical presentation is a postmenopausal woman with a history of gradually worsening pain at one or both thumb bases. Activities that require strong grip, twisting, or tripod pinch cause exacerbations of sharp pain on a background of a dull ache at rest. Eventually, the movement of the joint decreases and it becomes stiff. The pain may occasionally improve at this point as the joint progresses to autofusion.

■ ASSESSMENT OF THE HAND AND WRIST

History

General: Which is the dominant hand?

What are their occupational usages or hobbies?

Pain

- Site
- Nature
- Duration
- Intensity
- Aggravating/Relieving factors

Function: How does the arthritis affect their occupations/hobbies/activities of daily living (ADL)?

Sensation: Do they have any numbness or tingling in the hand?

Past history of trauma or infection?

Do they have any relevant systemic diseases or affliction of other joints?

Drug history (disease modifiers, anti-tumour necrosis factor agents).

Examination

- *Inspection*: Skin, swelling, deformity, previous operations.
- *Palpation*: Tenderness, crepitus, lumps, sensation (Tinel's test, two point discrimination).

Movements

Specific: Active/passive.

Investigations

- *Blood tests*: ESR, CRP, rheumatoid factor/anti-CCP antibodies.
- *Imaging*: Plain X-rays, computed tomography, MRI.

■ EXAMINATION

The joint line is usually tender on palpation at the base of the thumb and this can be differentiated from scapho-trapezial tenderness, which is 1 cm proximal. The patient with advanced arthritis has a broad thumb base which gives the hand a "squared" appearance caused by dorsal subluxation and adduction deformity, with compensatory hyperextension of the metacarpophalangeal joint—the Z deformity. The grind test is positive, if pain is present, often with crepitus, on axial compression and rotation of the thumb metacarpal (specificity 97% and sensitivity 30%). More sensitive is the "traction-shift test", in which the metacarpal is passively subluxated and then relocated, causing pain (67% sensitivity and 100% specificity).

■ RADIOLOGICAL ASSESSMENT

Twenty one percent of adults after the fifth decade have radiographic evidence of basal thumb OA, however, most are asymptomatic. Standard posteroanterior, lateral, and oblique radiographs of the hand reliably demonstrate advanced but not early osteoarthritic change. The Eaton and Littler staging system (**Box 2**) is the accepted radiological classification system and a fifth stage has been added to incorporate scapho-trapezial trapezoid joint arthritis and subdivision based on the amount of CMC joint subluxation.

■ NONOPERATIVE TREATMENT

For patients with mild symptoms, reassurance, and explanation of the disease and its natural history is all that is necessary. For patients with moderate symptoms,

> **Box 2:** The Eaton and Littler radiographic staging system.
>
> - Normal articular contours; slight widening of joint space (joint capsule distension)*
> - Slight narrowing of joint space; calcific/bony debris <2 mm in diameter; minimal sclerotic changes*
> - Marked joint space narrowing; sclerotic bone and cystic changes; varying degrees of subluxation; debris >2 mm in diameter; STT joint spared*
> - Obliteration of TMCJ as in stage III with STT joint narrowing associated with sclerosis and cystic changes*
> - Pantrapezial arthritis†

(STT: scaphotrapezial trapezoid; TMCJ: trapeziometacarpal joint)
Source: Shin E, Meals R. Green's Operative Hand Surgery, 5th edition. In: Green DP, Hotchkiss RN, Pederson WC, Wolfe SW (Eds). New York: Churchill Livingstone; 2005. pp. 461-85.
*From Wajon A, Vinycomb T, Carr E, Edmunds I, Ada L. Surgery for thumb (trapeziometacarpal joint) osteoarthritis. Cochrane Database Syst Rev. 2015;2:CD004631.
†From Tomaino MM. Thumb basilar joint arthritis. In: Green DP, Hotchkiss RN, Pederson WC, Wolfe SW (Eds). Green's Operative Hand Surgery. Philadelphia, PA: Elsevier; 2005.

activity modification, analgesics, splints, and reassurance may suffice. Conservative initial treatment begins with occupation or activity modification, splints and analgesics or nonsteroidal anti-inflammatory drugs (NSAIDs). Oral analgesics can be supplemented by topical diclofenac gel, which has been shown in a randomized controlled trial to reduce pain.

Patients may be benefit by a removable brace which can be custom-made thermoplastic splints or a neoprene splints which are more comfortable and as effective. Physical therapy can be used as it temporarily reduces pain. Intra-articular steroid injections into the CMC can be tried and gives long lasting relief in patients. Injections can be repeated, if required every 3 months. Patients who fail conservative treatment are candidates for surgery.

OPERATIVE TREATMENT

The indication for surgery is unresponsiveness to conservative treatment. Patients should be reassured that delaying surgery does not risk the procedure becoming technically impossible. Although the outcomes of numerous procedures have been published, high quality evidence is lacking, and a recent Cochrane review update failed to show that any operation produced better outcomes than another. Surgical options for base of thumb OA include excision of the trapezium with or without a ligament suspension, arthrodesis or replacement. Trapeziectomy is often supplemented with a ligament suspension using a portion of flexor carpi radialis, with the objective to prevent collapse of the thumb metacarpal, however, studies suggest that simple excision has similar results as the more complicated procedures.

Interposition with a tendon graft (such as Palmaris longus) after excision of the Trapezium is also an option. In the younger more active population CMC arthrodesis can be considered. Arthrodesis of the CMC joint is fraught with complications such as non-union, stiffness, and STT arthritis. Arthroplasty of the CMC is becoming increasingly popular, and options include hemiarthroplasty, total joint replacement or an interposition arthroplasty using a pyrocarbon disc.

FURTHER READING

1. Allan CH, Joshi A, Lichtman DM. Kienböck's disease: Diagnosis and treatment. J Am Acad Orthop Surg. 2001;9:128-36.
2. Altay T, Kaya A, Karapinar L, Ozturk H, Kayali C. Is radial shortening useful for Litchman stage 3b Kienböck's disease? Int Orthop. 2008;32:747-52.
3. Altman RD, Dreiser RL, Fisher CL, Chase WF, Dreher DS, Zacher J. Diclofenac sodium gel in patients with primaryhand osteoarthritis: A randomized, double-blind, placebo controlled trial. J Rheumatol. 2009;36:1991-9.
4. American Academy of Orthopaedic Surgeons (2018). Management of carpal tunnel syndrome: Evidence-based clinical practice guideline [online] Available from https://aaos.org/globalassets/quality-and-practice-resources/carpal-tunnel/management-of-carpal-tunnel-syndrome-7-31-19.pdf. [Last accessed on June, 2021].
5. Armstrong AL, Hunter JB, Davis TR. The prevalence of degenerative arthritis of the base of the thumb in postmenopausal women. J Hand Surg Br. 1994;19:340-1.
6. Armstrong T, Dale AM, Franzblau A, Evanoff BA. Risk factors for carpal tunnel syndrome and median neuropathy in a working population. J Occup Environ Med. 2008;50(12):1355-64.
7. Arora R, Lutz M, Deml C, Krappinger D, Zimmermann R, Gabl M. Long-term subjective and radiological outcome after reconstruction of Kienböck's disease stage 3 treated by a free vascularized iliac bone graft. J Hand Surg. 2008;33A:175-81.
8. Becker SJ, Bot AG, Curley SE, Jupiter JB, Ring D. A prospective randomized comparison of neoprene vs thermoplast hand-based thumb spica splinting for trapezio- metacarpal arthrosis. Osteoarthritis Cartilage. 2013;21:668-75.
9. Calandruccio JH, Thompson NB. Carpal tunnel syndrome: making evidence-based treatment decisions. Orthop Clin North Am. 2018;49(2):223-9.
10. Choa RM, Parvizi N, Giele HP. A prospective case-control study to compare the sensitivity and specificity of the grind and traction-shift (subluxation-relocation) clinical tests in osteoarthritis of the thumb carpometacarpal joint. J Hand Surg Eur Vol. 2014;39:282-5.
11. Cranford CS, Ho JY, Kalainov DM, Hartigan BJ. Carpal tunnel syndrome. J Am Acad Orthop Surg. 2007;15(9):537-48.
12. D'Arcy CA, McGee S. The rational clinical examination. Does this patient have carpal tunnel syndrome? JAMA. 2000;283(23):3110-7.
13. D'Hoore K, De Smet L, Verellen K, Vral J, Fabry G. Negative ulnar variance is not a risk factor for Kienbock's disease. J Hand Surg. 1994;19(2):229-31.
14. Daecke W, Lorenz S, Wieloch P, Jung M, Martini A-K. Vascularize dos pisiform for reinforcement of the lunate in Kienböck's disease: an average of 12 years of follow-up study. J Hand Surg. 2005;30A:915-22.
15. Davis TR, Brady O, Barton NJ, Lunn PG, Burke FD. Trapeziectomy alone, with tendon interposition or with

ligament reconstruction? A randomized prospective study. J Hand Surg. 1997;22B:689e94.
16. Davis TR, Brady O, Dias JJ. Excision of the trapezium for osteoarthritis of the trapeziometacarpal joint: A study of the benefit of ligament reconstruction or tendon interposition. J Hand Surg Am. 2004;29:1069-77.
17. Davis TR, Pace A. Trapeziectomy for trapeziometacarpal joint osteoarthritis: Is ligament reconstruction and temporary stabilisation of the pseudarthrosis with a Kirschner wire important? J Hand Surg Eur Vol. 2009;34:312-21.
18. Delaere O, Dury M, Molderez A, Foucher G. Conservative versus operative treatment for Kienböck's disease: A retrospective study. J Hand Surg. 1998;23A:33-6.
19. Deniz FE, Oksüz E, Sarikaya B, Kurt S, Erkorkmaz U, Ulusoy H, et al. Comparison of the diagnostic utility of electromyography, ultrasonography, computed tomography, and magnetic resonance imaging in idiopathic carpal tunnel syndrome determined by clinical findings. Neurosurgery. 2012; 70(3):610-6.
20. Downing ND, Davis TR. Trapezial space height after trapeziectomy: Mechanism of formation and benefits. J Hand Surg Am. 2001;26:862-8.
21. Faucher GK, Daruwalla JH, Seiler JG 3rd. Complications of surgical release of carpal tunnel syndrome: a systematic review. J Surg Orthop Adv. 2017;26(1):18-24.
22. Gangopadhyay S, McKenna H, Burke FD, Davis TR. Five- to 18-year follow-up for treatment of trapeziometacarpal osteoarthritis: A prospective comparison of excision, tendon interposition, and ligament reconstruction and tendon interposition. J Hand Surg Am. 2012;37:411-7.
23. Goldfarb CA, Hsu J, Gelberman RH, Boyer MI. The Lichtman classification for Kienböck's disease: an assessment of reliability. J Hand Surg. 2003;28A:74-80.
24. González del Pino J, Delgado-Martínez AD, González González I, Lovic A. Value of the carpal compression test in the diagnosis of carpal tunnel syndrome. J Hand Surg Br. 1997; 22(1):38-41.
25. Goodyear-Smith F, Arroll B. What can family physicians offer patients with carpal tunnel syndrome other than surgery? A systematic review of nonsurgical management. Ann Fam Med. 2004;2(3):267-73.
26. Graham B, Peljovich AE, Afra R, Cho MS, Gray R, Stephenson J, et al. The American Academy of Orthopaedic Surgeons evidence-based clinical practice guideline on: management of carpal tunnel syndrome [guideline summary]. J Bone Joint Surg Am. 2016;98(20):1750-4.
27. Haugen IK, Englund M, Aliabadi P, Niu J, Clancy M, Kvien TK, et al. Prevalence, incidence and progression of hand osteoarthritis in the general population: The Framingham Osteoarthritis Study. Ann Rheum Dis. 2011;70:1581-6.
28. Hegmann KT. Upper extremity disorders. In: Occupational Medicine Practice Guidelines, 3rd edition. Elk Grove Village, IL: American College of Occupational and Environmental Medicine; 2011. pp. 655-6.
29. Illarramendi AA, De Carli P. Radius decompression for treatment of Kienböck's disease. Tech Hand Up Extrem Surg. 2003; 7:110-3.
30. Incebiyik S, Boyaci A, Tutoglu A. Short-term effectiveness of short-wave diathermy treatment on pain, clinical symptoms, and hand function in patients with mild or moderate idiopathic carpal tunnel syndrome. J Back Musculoskelet Rehabil. 2015;28(2):221-8.
31. Jafarnia K, Collins ED, Kohl HW III, Bennett JB, Ilahi OA. Reliability of the Lichtman classification of Kienböck's disease. J Hand Surg. 2000;25A:529-34.
32. Jensen CH, Thomsen K, Holst-Nielsen F. Radiographic staging of Kienböck's disease: poor reproducibility of Stahl's and Lichtman's staging systems. Acta Orthop Scand. 1996;67:274-6.
33. Jónsson H, Valtýsdóttir ST, Kjartansson O, Brekkan A. Hypermobility associated with osteoarthritis of the thumb base: A clinical and radiological subset of hand osteoarthritis. Ann Rheum Dis. 1996;55:540-3.
34. LeBlanc KE, Cestia W. Carpal tunnel syndrome. Am Fam Physician. 2011;83(8):952-8.
35. Lee HJ, Kim IS, Sung JH, Lee SW, Hong JT. Intraoperative dynamic pressure measurements in carpal tunnel syndrome: correlations with clinical signs. Clin Neurol Neurosurg. 2016;140:33-7.
36. Lin JD, Karl JW, Strauch RJ. Trapeziometacarpal joint stability: The evolving importance of the dorsal ligaments. Clin Orthop Relat Res. 2014;472:1138-45.
37. Moran SL, Cooney WP, Berger RA, Bishop AT, Shin AY. The use of the 4-5 extensor compartmental vascularized bone graft for the treatment of Kienböck's disease. J Hand Surg. 2005;30A:50-8.
38. Page MJ, O'Connor D, Pitt V, Massy-Westropp N. Therapeutic ultrasound for carpal tunnel syndrome. Cochrane Database Syst Rev. 2013;3:CD009601.
39. Peste JL. Discussion. Bull Soc Anat. 1843; 18:169.
40. Quenzer DE, Dobyns JH, Linscheid RL, Trail IA, Vidal MA. Radial recession osteotomy for Kienböck's disease. J Hand Surg. 1997;22A:386-95.
41. Salem H, Davis TR. Six year outcome excision of the trapezium for trapeziometacarpal joint osteoarthritis: Is it improved by ligament reconstruction and temporary Kirschner wire insertion? J Hand Surg Eur Vol. 2012;37:211-9.
42. Salmon J, Stanley JK, Trail IA. Kienböck's disease: Conservative management versus radial shortening. J Bone Joint Surg. 2000; 82B:820-3.
43. Shiri R. Arthritis as a risk factor for carpal tunnel syndrome: a meta-analysis. Scand J Rheumatol. 2016;45(5):339-46.
44. Stevens JC. AAEM mini monograph #26: the electrodiagnosis of carpal tunnel syndrome. American Association of Electro-diagnostic Medicine. Muscle Nerve. 1997;20(12):1477-86.
45. Swindells MG, Logan AJ, Armstrong DJ, Chan P, Burke FD, Lindau TR. The benefit of radiologically-guided steroid injections for trapeziometacarpal osteoarthritis. Ann R Coll Surg Engl. 2010;92:680-4.
46. Teisen H, Hjarbaek J. Classification of fresh fractures of the lunate. J Hand Surg. 1988;13(4):458-62.
47. Tsantes AG, Papadopoulos DV, Gelalis ID, Vekris MD, Pakos EE, Korompilias AV. The efficacy of vascularized bone grafts in the treatment of scaphoid nonunions and Kienbock disease: A systematic review in 917 patients. J Hand Microsurg. 2019;11(1):6-13.
48. Tsuge S, Nakamura R. Anatomical risk factors for Kienböck's disease. J Hand Surg. 1993;18(1):70-5.

49. Van Nortwick S, Berger A, Cheng R, Lee J, Ladd AL. Trapezial topography in thumb carpometacarpal arthritis. J Wrist Surg. 2013;2:263-70.
50. Vasiliadis HS, Georgoulas P, Shrier I, Salanti G, Scholten RJ. Endoscopic release for carpal tunnel syndrome. Cochrane Database Syst Rev. 2014;1:CD008265.
51. Verdugo RJ, Salinas RA, Castillo JL, Cea JG. Surgical versus non-surgical treatment for carpal tunnel syndrome. Cochrane Database Syst Rev. 2008;(4):CD001552.
52. Vermeulen GM, Spekreijse KR, Slijper H, Feitz R, Hovius SE, Selles RW. Comparison of arthroplasties with or without bone tunnel creation for thumb basal joint arthritis: A randomized controlled trial. J Hand Surg Am. 2014;39:1692-8.
53. Viera AJ. Management of carpal tunnel syndrome. Am Fam Physician. 2003;68(2): 265-72.
54. Villafañe JH, Cleland JA, Fernández-de-Las-Peñas C. The effectiveness of a manual therapy and exercise protocolin patients with thumb carpometacarpal osteoarthritis: A randomized controlled trial. J Orthop Sports Phys Ther. 2013;43:204-13.
55. Wajon A, Vinycomb T, Carr E, Edmunds I, Ada L. Surgery for thumb (trapeziometacarpal joint) osteoarthritis. Cochrane Database Syst Rev. 2015;2:CD004631.
56. Watanabe T, Takahara M, Tsuchida H, Yamahara S, Kikuchi N, Ogino T. Long-term follow-up of radial shortening osteotomy for Kienböck's disease. J Bone Joint Surg. 2008;90A:1705-11.
57. Wilder FV, Barrett JP, Farina EJ. Joint-specific prevalence of osteoarthritis of the hand. Osteoarthritis Cartilage. 2006;14:953-7.
58. Wolfe SW, Hotchkiss RN, Pederson WC, Kozin SH. Green's Operative Hand Surgery. 6th edition. Philadelphia: Elsevier; 2011.
59. Woodward JF, Heller JB, Jones NF. PyroCarbon implant hemiarthroplasty for trapeziometacarpal arthritis. Tech HandUp Extrem Surg. 2013;17:7-12.
60. Yildirim P, Gunduz OH. What is the role of Semmes-Weinstein monofilament testing in the diagnosis of electrophysiologically graded carpal tunnel syndrome? J Phys Ther Sci. 2015;27(12):3749-53.

30 Common Hand Disorders

Alok Chandra Agrawal, Bikram Kar, Anupam Inamdar

■ INTRODUCTION

The hand plays a very vital role in almost all the activities. Many disorders affect directly or indirectly the hand and thus affect the function of the hand. This chapter briefly discusses the common disorders such as stenosing tenosynovitis, trigger finger, de Quervain's tenosynovitis, Bowler's thumb, Dupuytren's contracture, and rheumatoid deformities of the hand.

■ STENOSING TENOSYNOVITIS (TRIGGER FINGER)

Stenosing tenosynovitis is also called a *trigger finger*. In this disorder, there is the catching of the flexor tendons as they pass through the orifice of the A1 pulley. The patient commonly presents with inability or difficulty to actively extend the flexed finger. Initially, the patient has to put in many efforts, then suddenly the tendon slips out, and the finger extends, mimicking a pistol trigger, and hence it is also called trigger finger. This phenomenon of triggering is the clinical hallmark of the condition. A1 Pulley and the corresponding surface of flexor develop fibrocartilaginous dysplasia, which results in degenerative tendinopathy over time. Most commonly, it affects the ring finger, and other fingers are also affected. Elderly males are commonly affected, but it may also be secondary to hypothyroidism, Cushing's disease, rheumatoid arthritis, osteoarthritis, gout, diabetes, and pregnancy. In Inflammatory disorders, fingers locked in flexion more in morning hours. In severe cases, the finger is locked in flexion and is very painful.

The patients commonly complain of inability or difficulty to actively extend the affected finger. It is also called triggering. On examination, triggering can be elicited. In some cases, there will be tenderness over the A1 pulley. X-ray of the hand may be helpful to rule out any other pathology, and additional examination such as ultrasound, magnetic resonance imaging (MRI) scan of the hand can confirm the diagnosis.

Conservative treatment of early stages includes simple splinting with nonsteroidal anti-inflammatory drugs (NSAIDs), stretching exercises also have been shown to give results in the early stages. Conservative treatment of more severe cases are trials of wax bath, ultrasound therapy, laser, and shock waves. Injection of a depot preparation of corticosteroid into the flexor tendon sheath is effective. The injection is administered using a 25-gauge needle and 1 cc of 2% xylocaine, and local preparation of methylprednisolone acetate or triamcinolone solution is injected at the level of the A1 pulley into the flexor sheath. Care is to be taken that the drug is not injected into the tendon itself, leading to late secondary tendon rupture.

In more resistant cases where nonoperative management fails, trigger finger release is indicated. Trigger finger release is done at the level of the A1 pulley. The percutaneous flexor tendon sheath release can be done by a 20-gauge needle placed percutaneously. Complications of this technique are tendon rupture, scaring of the tendon, incomplete release, and infection.

■ DE QUERVAIN'S TENOSYNOVITIS

De Quervain's tenosynovitis was first identified in 1995 by Swiss surgeon Fritz de Quervain. It is also called texting thumb, gamer's thumb, BlackBerry thumb, radial styloid tenosynovitis, de Quervain's disease, de Quervain's tenosynovitis, designer's thumb, washerwoman's sprain, tenosynovitis, Mommy thumb, mother's wrist. The first dorsal compartment, including abductor pollicis longus (APL) and extensor pollicis brevis (EPB), is involved. A stenosing tenosynovial inflammation of these tendons, thickening, and swelling of the common tendon sheath or extensor retinaculum causes increased tendon friction. Most commonly found in women in the age group of 30–50 years with right-side predominance. Other risk factors are rheumatoid arthritis, other immunoinflammatory diseases, overuse, golfers and racquet sports, post-traumatic, pregnancy, Cushing's disease, and hypothyroidism.

Patients present with radial site wrist pain, exacerbated while lifting the objects with the wrist in the neutral position and sometimes griping. On examination, there will be tenderness around the radial styloid at the level of the first dorsal compartment; the wrist range of movements is normal.

Clinical Provocative Test
- *Finkelstein maneuver*: On abducting the wrist ulnarward, with patient clenches thumb in a fist, the patient complaints of pain around the styloid tip.
- *Eichhoff maneuver*: On abducting the wrist ulnarward, with thumb in a fist, the patient complained of pain around the styloid tip, followed by relief of pain as the patient extends the thumb with the wrist in ulnar deviated position.

Investigations
- X-ray of the forearm and wrist AP are usually normal.
- Ultrasonography and an MRI scan show inflammatory changes in T2-weighted images in the tendon sheath involved.

Treatment
Conservative treatment includes rest, NSAIDs, contrast bath, thumb spica splint. If the patient is not responding to these modalities, then local steroid injection in some refractory cases and injections of platelet rich plasma have shown promising results. Many patients respond well to conservative treatment, but the rate of recurrence is significant.

Operative
In refractory cases, those not responding to a conservative line of treatment and patient having severe pain with limitations of activities of daily living, surgical release of the first dorsal compartment can be done.

The incision is given on the radial side just proximal to the wrist, at the level of radial styloid, the first dorsal compartment is exposed. Care to be taken to protect the superficial radial nerve, and then the common sheath is opened to make the first compartment roomy.

DEFORMITIES AND CONTRACTURES IN RHEUMATOID ARTHRITIS

Rheumatoid arthritis patients with rheumatoid hand presents with a subacute or insidious onset of synovitis of both hands and wrist, distal interphalangeal joints are not involved, with constitutional symptoms such as malaise, weight loss, fatigue, and myalgias. Women are more commonly affected than males. There are involvement and deformities of the metacarpophalangeal joint and proximal interphalangeal joints. The damage to ligamentous and intra-articular structures and the forces acting along the intrinsic and extrinsic muscles may result in deformity. Swelling of proximal interphalangeal and metacarpophalangeal joints, ulnar head, and wrist are tender and boggy presents as an early sign. Limitation of the movements of wrist and finger is common. There is tenosynovitis of both the flexor and extensor tendons. Interosseous muscle atrophy is very common. There is a protrusion of the ulnar head, instability of the distal radioulnar joint with ulnar deviation of fingers, and volar subluxation of the metacarpophalangeal joint. Prominent ulnar head with the inability to extend the little finger due to the rupture of the extensor digit mini tendon with the distal radioulnar joint subluxation is also called Vaughan-Jackson deformity.

Finger deformities are caused by the normal forces applied to damaged joints by the extrinsic flexors and extensors, displacement of the lateral bands of the extensor hood, tightness of the intrinsic muscles, central slip rupture, or rupture of the long extensor or long flexor tendons with loss of active movements. The common deformities include a swan-neck deformity, Boutonniere deformity, and an intrinsic plus deformity.

Swan-neck Deformity
In swan-neck deformity, there is flexion of the distal interphalangeal joint and hyperextension of the proximal interphalangeal joint, sometimes flexing the metacarpophalangeal joint (**Fig. 1**). This deformity may develop in patients with volar plate laxity or patients with conditions such as Ehlers-Danlos syndrome. The mallet deformity patients may later develop the swan-neck deformity due to extensor tendon disruption at the distal joint with secondary overpull of the central slip, causing secondary proximal interphalangeal joint hyperextension. There may be synovitis of the proximal interphalangeal joint because leading to capsular disruption, tightening of the lateral bands and central tendon, and the lateral bands in a fixed dorsal position, leading to proximal interphalangeal flexion. Nalebuff et al. divided swan-neck deformities into four types:
1. *Type I*: Deformities are flexible and can be treated surgically by flexor tenodesis of the proximal interphalangeal joint, the fusion of the distal interphalangeal joint, and reconstruction of the retinacular ligament.
2. *Type II*: Deformities are caused by intrinsic muscle tightness, and hence require intrinsic release in addition to that required for Type I.
3. *Type III*: Deformities are stiff and these deformities require joint manipulation, mobilization of the lateral bands, and dorsal skin release.
4. *Type IV*: Deformities are stiff and have significant destruction of the joint surface and stiff proximal interphalangeal joints, and are managed with arthrodesis of the proximal interphalangeal joints or proximal interphalangeal joint arthroplasty if the metacarpophalangeal joints are well preserved.

Boutonniere Deformity
Boutonniere deformity is described as a flexed proximal interphalangeal joint, with a hyperextended distal interphalangeal joint.

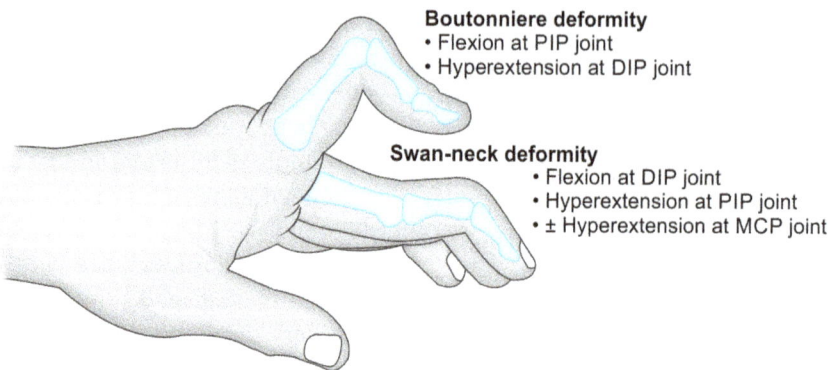

Fig. 1: Deformities in rheumatoid hand. (DIP: distal interphalangeal; PIP: proximal interphalangeal; MCP: metacarpophalangeal)

Chronology of Progression

The synovitis of the proximal interphalangeal joint causes attenuation of the central slip, causing the lateral bands to subluxate volarly. As the deformity progresses, the lateral bands are forced farther over the proximal interphalangeal joint condyles and become locked at their new course. Gradually, they become adhered in this subluxated position and cause flexion of the proximal interphalangeal joint due to an altered line of pull, volar to the joint's axis. The tightening of the lateral bands also hyperextends the distal interphalangeal joint through their insertion at the base of the distal phalanx. The metacarpophalangeal joints assume an extension attitude to compensate for the fixed flexion deformity of the proximal interphalangeal joints. However, this extended attitude does not become a fixed deformity.

Classification

Nalebuff et al. classified Boutonniere deformity based on the radiographic appearance of the joint surface and the amount of active and passive motion as mild, moderate, and severe.

Mild deformity: The proximal interphalangeal joint is in an attitude of flexion which can be passively extended to neutral. The distal interphalangeal joint is in an attitude of extension, with some ability to flex the joint. The proximal and distal interphalangeal joints are normal on radiographs. The passively correctable flexion deformity at the proximal interphalangeal joint is managed by repositioning the lateral bands of the dorsal extensor apparatus, the synovectomy of the proximal interphalangeal joint, and the Dolphin–Fowler procedure, in which an extensor tendon tenotomy is done at the level of the middle phalanx.

Moderate deformity: The proximal interphalangeal joint is an attitude of flexion which can be passively extended. The flexor tendon function is normal, and radiographs of the hand show normal interphalangeal joint space. The distal interphalangeal joint is hyperextended, and the metacarpophalangeal joint is correctable to full flexion passively. A central slip reconstruction is done by mobilizing the lateral bands dorsally and suturing them to each other, to the central tendon insertion, and the posterior capsule of the proximal interphalangeal joint. A tendon graft may also be used for this reconstruction.

Severe deformity: It is characterized by stiff joints. The radiographs show joint destruction. The middle and ring fingers are treated with extensor tendon reconstruction and silastic joint arthroplasty using silicone prosthesis. In the index finger, a fusion of the proximal interphalangeal joint is a suitable option.

Intrinsic Plus Deformity

The intrinsic plus deformity occurs as a result of contracture of the hand's intrinsic mechanism, causing flexion of the metacarpophalangeal joints and extension of interphalangeal joints. The deformity develops simultaneously with the Z-deformity of a rheumatoid hand which consists of ulnar deviation of the digits, volar subluxation of the proximal phalanges metacarpophalangeal joints, and radial deviation of the wrist. The clinical diagnostic test for this condition, described by Sterling Bunnell, evaluates intrinsic tightness, where a greater force is required to flex the proximal interphalangeal joint when the metacarpophalangeal joint is in passive extension as compared to its flexion. In a rheumatoid hand, maintaining the axial alignment of the finger with the metacarpal while checking for intrinsic tightness is essential to ensure the accuracy of this test, as the contracture of intrinsic muscles tends to be more in the medial side of the hand due to ulnar deviation of the fingers.

The treatment of this condition consists of a proximal or distal release of the hand intrinsic muscles. The presence or absence of flexion contracture in the metacarpophalangeal joint guides to the choice of type of intrinsic release required. A distal intrinsic release suffices in the absence of metacarpophalangeal joint flexion contracture, in which resection of the intrinsic tendon is done distal to the transverse fibers. The presence of a metacarpophalangeal joint flexion contracture necessitates a proximal intrinsic release, in which a release of the transverse and oblique fibers of the contracted intrinsic muscles is done proximal to the metacarpophalangeal joint.

DUPUYTREN'S CONTRACTURE

Dupuytren's contracture is a pathology affecting the hand that replaces normal digital and palmar fascia (bands and sheaths) with abnormal, hyperplastic fibrous tissue (nodules and cords), resulting in progressive and irreversible contractures of metacarpophalangeal and interphalangeal joints. Its first description was given by Henry Cline and Astley Cooper.

Applied Anatomy

The palmer fascial complex consists of aponeurosis and fascia. Aponeurosis in the hand, can be subclassified into radial, ulnar and central aponeurosis (**Fig. 2**). The radial aponeurosis consists of the thenar fascia, the pretentious band to the thumb tendon, and the proximal and distal commissural ligaments. The ulnar aponeurosis consists of the hypothenar fascia and the pretentious band to the small finger. The central aponeurosis consists of fibers in longitudinal, transverse, and vertical orientations. The longitudinal fibers give pretendinous bands to the central three digits. Each band bifurcates into three layers, a superficial layer to the dermis, a middle layer to the digit, the "spiral band," and a deep layer to the dorsal side. The transverse fibers constitute the transverse ligament of the palmer aponeurosis proximally and the natatory ligament distally. The vertical fibers consist of the bands of Grapow and the septa of League, which are the first structures to be affected in Dupuytren's disease.

The fasciae of the palmar fascial complex consist of the digital fascia, the palmar fascia, and the fascia around neurovascular structures. The fascia around the neurovascular structures consists of volar, dorsal, medial, and lateral parts named the Grayson ligament, the Cleland ligament, the Thomine fascia the Gosset fascia, respectively. The Cleland ligament is the last structure to be involved in Dupuytren's disease.

Etiology and Risk Factors

It occurs in adults in their 40s to 60s. It is 10 times more common and occurs earlier in men as compared to women. It is most common in white northern European individuals. Other risk factors are diabetes mellitus, epilepsy, alcoholism, smoking, hypercholesterolemia, and the HIV-positive population. An autosomal dominant pattern has been suggested, and the lesions occur earlier and are more frequent in these families.

Associated Conditions

Ledderhose disease, Peyronie disease, and Garrod nodules are the conditions associated with Dupuytren's contracture. Ledderhose disease is characterized by developing well-circumscribed, firm nodules in the medial plantar fascia of one or both feet. Peyronie disease is characterized by plastic penile induration. Garrod nodules or "knuckle pads" are thickenings over the extensor surfaces of the proximal interphalangeal joints. Patients with these associated findings are considered to have a Dupuytren's diathesis. The disease progression and rate of recurrence following surgery are higher in these individuals.

Histology

Histologically, the Dupuytren's contracture begins with proliferative fibroblastic lesions forming nodules of type 3 collagen that gradually blend with the surrounding fascia. An increase in the matrix metalloproteinase activity and abundant mitoses is seen in these lesions' myofibroblasts. Hemosiderin granules can be observed in the most immature areas of cellular proliferation.

Histological Stages

The primary pathology behind joint deformities in hand is transforming the normal fascial bands into cords, which occurs through three histological stages, viz. proliferative, involutional, and residual (**Fig. 3**).

The proliferative stage is characterized by the formation and growth of nodules, composed predominantly of type 3 collagen derived from immature myofibroblasts and fibroblasts arranged in a whorled pattern. These nodules proliferate and adhere to the overlying skin. They appear over the metacarpophalangeal joints and the proximal interphalangeal joints in the palmar aspect of the hand.

In the involutional stage, the nodules stop growing and begin to contract. The fibroblasts get aligned in the longitudinal axis of the hand along the lines of tension. Myofibroblasts later become the predominant cell type and produce type III collagen and resulting in contracture. A progressive contracture tenses the normal fascia, leading to its hypertrophy and nodule-cord units.

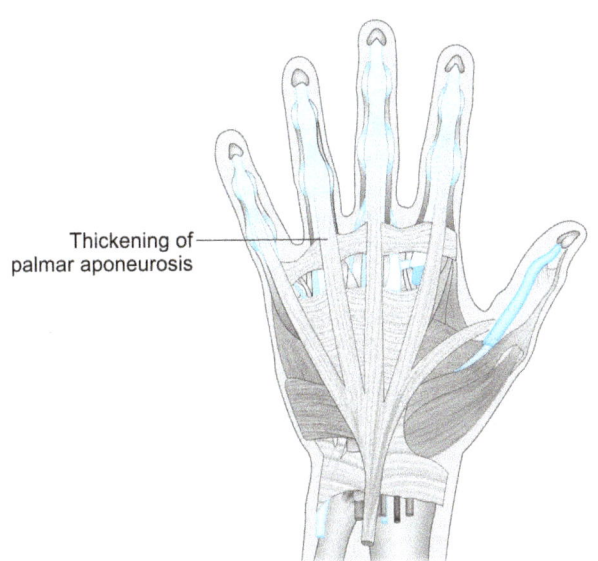

Fig. 2: Thickening of palmar aponeurosis in Dupuytren's disease.

In the residual stage, the nodules become smaller, and the collagen-rich cords remain. The pretentious band, the spiral band, the lateral digital sheet, and the Grayson ligament undergo fibrous thickening to form a spiral cord that runs along with the neurovascular bundle. Contraction of the spinal cord causes the neurovascular structures to migrate toward the midline of the finger. The Cleland ligament is spared in this pathological process.

Bilateral involvement is seen in around 45% of cases and is rarely symmetric. Ring and little fingers are the most commonly affected. The pathology begins on the medial aspect of the hand at the level of metacarpophalangeal joints. Contractures of the metacarpophalangeal and interphalangeal joints become more severe as the fibroplasia matures. These contractures are usually painless. However, nodules have been shown histologically to have neural entrapment and may produce pain in some individuals.

Treatment (Flowchart 1)

Nonoperative

Observation and treatment of underlying medical comorbidities in static disease with minimal contracture may lead to spontaneous subsidence of the lesions. Other nonoperative treatments are external beam radiation and intralesional injections of steroids or purified collagenase derived from *Clostridium histolyticum*. The contractures of the MCP and PIP joints are manually ruptured approximately 18 hours following collagenase injection.

Operative

The surgeries in increasing order of dissection can be as follows:
- *Subcutaneous fasciotomy*: The fascia is divided through a stab incision, and no tissues are excised.
- Fasciectomies, partial or complete
- *Fasciectomies—subtotal or total with skin grafting*: Chronic contractures warrant a release of the flexor tendon sheath, oblique strands, Grayson, Cleland, Checkrein and accessory collateral ligaments, and an arthrotomy of metacarpophalangeal and interphalangeal joints. Open wound resulting from a radical release is addressed with skin grafting.
- Staged external fixation
- Arthrodesis

■ BOWLER'S THUMB

Definition

It is a chronic neuropathy affecting the ulnar digital nerve of the thumb due to long-standing repetitive irritation of this

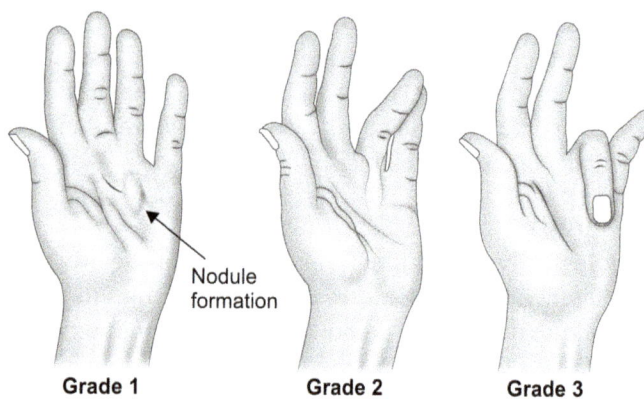

Fig. 3: Stages of Dupuytren's contracture.

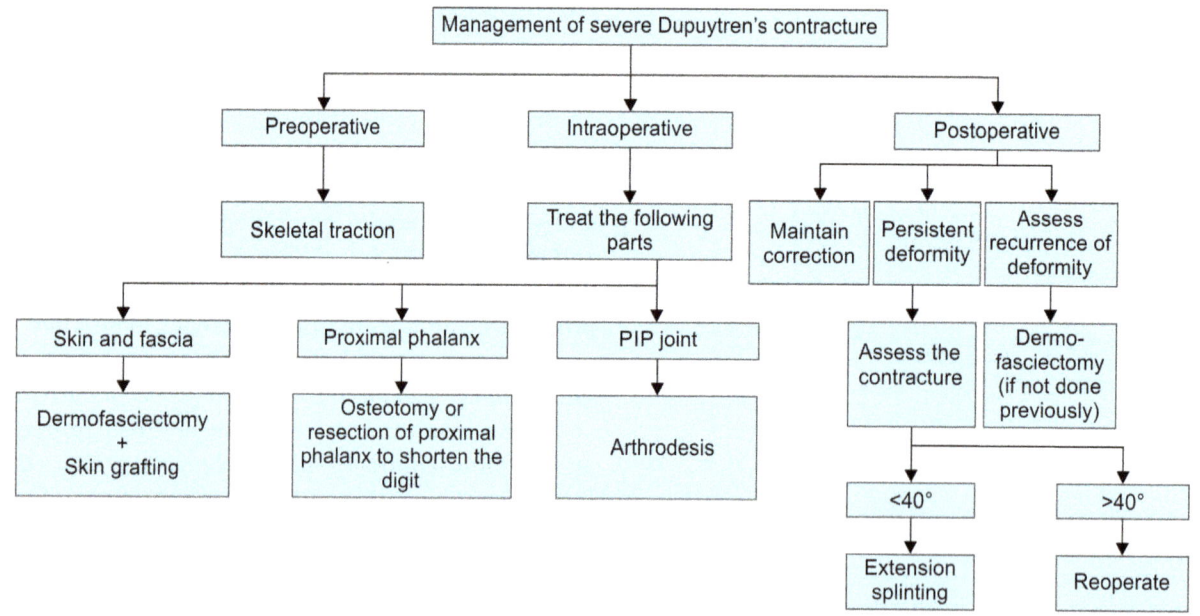

Flowchart 1: Outline for management of severe Dupuytren's contracture.

(PIP: proximal interphalangeal)

nerve in eager or professional bowlers who tend to engage their thumb in the thumb-hole of the bowling ball for a longer duration during ball release to ensure a better spin.

Etiology
Sportspersons or occupations that chronically exert tension on the ulnar digital nerve of the thumb, such as bowlers, baseball players, masseurs, and cherry pitters, are prone to suffer from this condition.

Pathophysiology
Chronic tension or compression on the ulnar digital nerve leads to its inflammation. The resulting long-term neuritis, followed by a healing response in the form of scarring around the nerve, with or without neuroma formation, is responsible for its conspicuous clinical features.

This disorder can occur in two forms, viz. acute neuritis following a single episode of bowling and chronic irritation of the nerve, classically described as "the Bowler's thumb" **(Fig. 4)**. Acute neuritis is a type 1 nerve injury or neurapraxia which resolves spontaneously.

Histology
Persistent irritation around the inflamed nerve leads to scar formation around its epineurium.

The nerve fascicles atrophy with time, and the interfascicular region shows evidence of fibrosis.

Clinical Features
Early symptoms are numbness or abnormal sensations in the first webspace. Gradually the patient starts experiencing pain localized to the medial aspect of the base of the thumb and a weak grip. Chronic cases present with a palpable mass in the volar aspect of the thumb along with the above symptoms.

The diagnostic signs include tenderness along the medial border of the thumb and in the palpable mass. The Tinel's sign is positive. The sensation in the first webspace is diminished, and the two-point discrimination test is altered.

Differential Diagnosis
Carpal tunnel syndrome and cervical radiculopathy have to be ruled out as the differential diagnoses of this condition.

Investigations
Nerve conduction velocity studies show the diminished amplitude of action potentials in the ulnar digital nerve of the thumb.

Treatment (Flowchart 2)
Conservative line of management in abstinence from bowling or other inciting factors, use of a thumb spica splint for immobilization is necessary to curtail the repetitive irritation and tension on the nerve. Conservative treatment is successful in recreational bowlers who comply well with abstinence from bowling and in cases of acute neuropathy.

Surgical management is preferred for professional bowlers who cannot comply with a trial of conservative management. The various surgical modalities available are:
- Neurolysis
- Resection of the neuroma with or without nerve grafting
- Transposition of the ulnar digital nerve

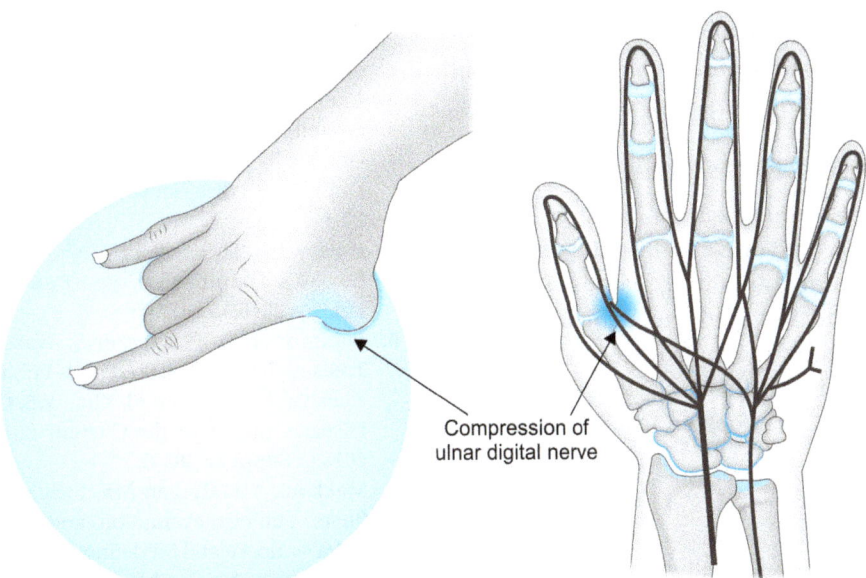

Fig. 4: Compression of ulnar digital nerve in bowlers.

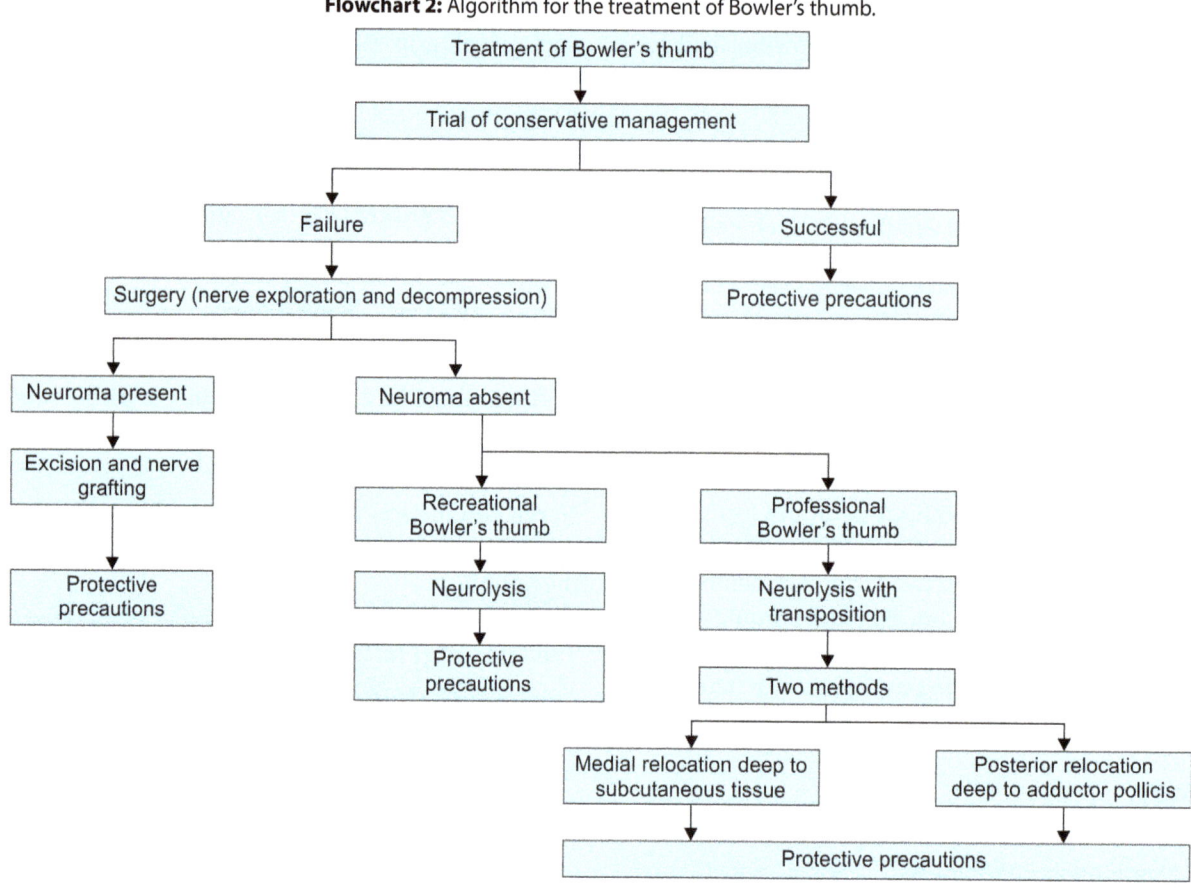

Flowchart 2: Algorithm for the treatment of Bowler's thumb.

Neurolysis

The nerve is dissected along its entire course through a Bruner incision made in the medial side of the thumb. The fibrosis around the nerve is excised, the nerve is freed from adhesion, and is wrapped in a nerve protector to provide a roomy encasement.

Neuroma Resection and Nerve Grafting

In severe nerve, atrophy or a neuroma formation, resection of the neuroma or affected nerve segment and reconstruction with a nerve graft is the preferred treatment.

Transposition of the Ulnar Digital Nerve

Professional bowlers are the ideal candidates for this surgery. Transposition of the nerve can be subcutaneous or submuscular. In subcutaneous transposition, the decompressed nerve is relocated to a medial course, and the epineurium is tagged to the subcutaneous tissue. In submuscular transposition, which is a more preferred method, the nerve is relocated posterior to the adductor pollicis muscle.

Protective Precautions

These include using a protective thumb-guard while bowling, using a light ball, modifications in ball-grip, and alteration in size/slope of the thumb-hole in the ball.

Postoperative Assessment

The subsidence of pain and paraesthesia, return of sensations and grip strength, and improvement in the two-point discrimination test are assessed.

FURTHER READING

1. Apfelberg DB, Maser MR, Lash H, Kaye RL, Britton MC, Bobrove A. Rheumatoid hand deformities: pathophysiology and treatment. Western J Med. 1978;129(4):267-72.
2. Chung KC, Pushman AG. Current concepts in the management of the rheumatoid hand. J Hand Surg. 2011;36(4):736-47.
3. Goel R, Abzug JM. de Quervain's tenosynovitis: a review of the rehabilitative options. Hand (NY). 2015;10(1):1-5.
4. Grazina R, Teixeira S, Ramos R, Sousa H, Ferreira A, Lemos R. Dupuytren's disease: where do we stand? EFORT Open Rev. 2019;4(2):63-9.
5. Halsey JN, Therattil PJ, Viviano SL, Fleegler EJ, Lee ES. Bowler's Thumb: case report and review of the literature. Eplasty. 2015;15:e47.
6. Jeanmonod R, Harberger S, Waseem M. Trigger Finger. Treasure Island (FL): StatPearls Publishing; 2021.
7. Khashan M, Smitham PJ, Khan WS, Goddard NJ. Dupuytren's Disease: review of the Current Literature. Open Orthop J. 2011;(5 Suppl 2): 283-8.
8. Makkouk AH, Oetgen ME, Swigart CR, Dodds SD. Trigger finger: etiology, evaluation, and treatment. Current Reviews in Musculoskeletal Medicine. 2008;1(2):92-6.
9. Swanson S, Macias LH, Smith AA. Treatment of Bowler's neuroma with digital nerve translocation. Hand (NY). 2009; 4(3):323-6.

Foot and Ankle Involvement in Orthopedic Rheumatology

- **Rheumatoid and Neuropathic Foot**
  Alok Chandra Agrawal, Ankit Kumar Garg, Shilp Verma
- **Diabetic Foot**
  RC Meena, Jitesh K Jain, Arun Kumar Sharma
- **Ankle Osteoarthritis**
  J Mangwani, N Nanavati, V Adukia
- **Hallux Valgus**
  Raja TV, Ajay SS, Madhan Jeyaraman

31 Rheumatoid and Neuropathic Foot

Alok Chandra Agrawal, Ankit Kumar Garg, Shilp Verma

FOOT AND ANKLE IN RHEUMATOID DISEASE

INTRODUCTION

Rheumatoid arthritis (RA) is a chronic inflammatory disease that primarily affects the synovial joints. It causes periarticular erosion, cartilage destruction, ligamentous laxity, and deformity at a later stage. In about 10–20% of patients, extra-articular manifestations such as tendonitis, fasciitis, bursitis, neuritis, and vasculitis are common. These extra-articular manifestations highly correlate with high titers of rheumatoid factor.

In patients with rheumatoid arthritis, foot pain is relatively common as per existing literature, but it often gets overlooked in routine clinical examinations. The Disease Activity Scoring (DAS28), which measures disease activity and establishes clinical remission, does not include foot and ankle assessment in its list.

The etiology of peripheral neuropathy in patients with rheumatoid arthritis is not clearly understood. Peripheral neuropathy such as pure sensory, entrapment neuropathy, mono-neuritis multiplex, and distal axonal sensory-motor neuropathy commonly presents in patients with rheumatoid arthritis. The signs and symptoms of peripheral neuropathy such as pain, muscle weakness, numbness, pins, and needle sensation often mimic arthritis and confusion. Some studies suggest drug toxicity, amyloidosis, vasculitis, nerve entrapment, and autoimmune phenomenon as underlying causes. When they coexist, it often leads to poor quality-of-life and a shorter life span.

ETIOLOGY

The continuum of foot and ankle pain encompasses a wide range of differentials from the disorder of ligaments, tendons, muscle, bone, and joint pathologies, disorders of nerve entrapment, and presence of referred pain as shown in **Table 1**.

Osteoarthritis is one of the most frequent causes of ankle and foot pain. It commonly occurs in the hallux (big toe), joints of midfoot, and ankle joint. It results from the destruction of articular cartilage and joints margins leading to pain, inflammation, swelling, stiffness, limitation of function, and deformity. The formation of new osteophytes can lead to secondary mechanical impingement. In the

TABLE 1: Etiology of foot and ankle pain.

Tendon, ligament and muscle:
- Ankle or foot ligament tear or attenuation
- Chronic joint instability secondary to ligament compromise
- Joint impingement caused by ligamentous tear and/or hypertrophy
- Sinus tarsi pathology
- Achilles tendon pathology
- Achilles tendon rupture
- Plantar fasciitis
- Posterior tibial tendon dysfunction (usually with adult acquired flatfoot)
- Flexor hallucis longus tenosynovitis and stenosis
- Tibialis anterior tendon ear
- Peroneus tendon pathology

Bone:
- Acute fractures of the ankle or foot
- Stress fractures
- Freiberg's infraction (osteonecrosis of the second metatarsal head)
- Osteonecrosis of talus and navicular
- Sesamoid bone pathology
- Metatarsal overload (metatarsalgia)

Joint:
- Osteoarthritis
- Gout
- Rheumatoid arthritis
- Other inflammatory arthritis
- Charcot neuroarthropathy
- Osteochondral lesion of the talus
- Joint impingement (bone, synovitis, or ligamentous hypertrophy)
- Hammer toe, claw toe, and mallet toe deformities
- Hallux rigidus

Nerve compression:
- Tarsal tunnel syndrome
- Anterior tarsal tunnel syndrome (involvement of deep peroneal nerve under the superficial fascia of the ankle)
- Morton's neuroma
- Vessels
- Vasculitis
- Atherosclerosis
- Compartment syndrome
- Neuropathic and referred pain
- Neuropathy
- Spinal pathology
- Complex regional pain syndrome

initial stages, the patient typically complains of pain at the initiation and toward the termination of the movements but can later present with rest pain when the disease becomes severe.

The ankle joint is a weight-bearing joint and is subjected to numerous forces during walking, running, and sports. It is also more commonly prone to injuries such as sprains, ligament tear, chondral injuries, and fractures. The risk of degenerative arthritis in the ankle joint is relatively low compared to the hip and knee. The incidence of foot and ankle pain is about 15–20% in newly diagnosed cases, while in chronic patients, the incidence may be as high as 90% or more.

Therefore, it is essential that after a detailed history and physical examination, the patients should be evaluated with any foot and ankle disorders. Using radiographs and advanced imaging techniques such as computed tomography (CT) scan, magnetic resonance imaging (MRI) can help us in the diagnosis and appropriate treatment.

FUNCTIONAL ANATOMY AND BIOMECHANICS

The ankle joint is a hinge joint between the distal end of the tibia and the fibula, and talus. Due to the complex anatomy, it offers dorsiflexion and plantarflexion in the sagittal plane. Furthermore, in the axial plane, some internal and external rotation can occur.

The foot is broadly divided into three anatomic regions: (1) the forefoot, (2) the midfoot, and (3) the hindfoot. Dorsiflexion and plantarflexion movements primarily occur at the forefoot and midfoot with secondary supination and pronation and abduction/adduction in coronal and axial planes. In the hindfoot, the primary movements occur in the coronal plane (inversion/eversion) with secondary movements dorsiflexion/plantarflexion, internal/external rotation in the sagittal and axial plane, respectively. It is essential for a clinician to know and understand the local anatomy due to the polyarticular involvement of the disease.

DIAGNOSTIC EVALUATION

Physical Examination

The physical examination always begins with the gait analysis. The physician should observe the patient as he enters the examination room. A patient with ankle and foot pain will avoid ground contact with the painful part of the foot. Some patients will have shortened stance phase on the affected limb, suggestive of an "antalgic" gait pattern. In the foot-flat and toe-off phase, some patients will have dynamic collapse of the medial longitudinal arch.

After gait analysis, it is essential to inspect the foot and ankle with the patient in both standing and sitting positions. Any swelling around the joint, callosities, deformities,

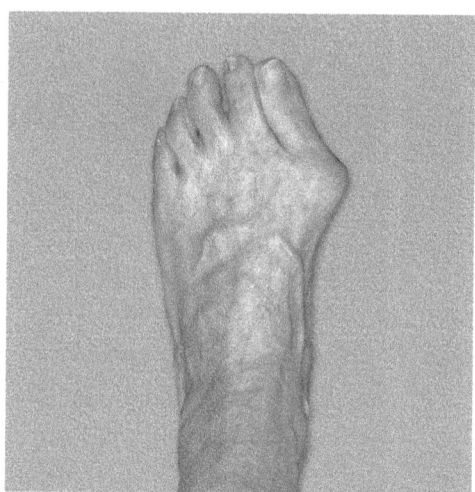

Fig. 1: Hallux valgus.

rheumatoid nodules, and ulcerations should be noted. The callosities form in the area of increased pressure or as a result of constant friction. Hallux valgus **(Fig. 1)**, hammertoes, flatfoot deformity (hindfoot valgus/forefoot abduction) are usually seen in patients with rheumatic arthritis. The wear pattern of soles should always be seen as it gives an idea of pressure zones in the foot.

After inspection, it is important to note any local rise in temperature, bony tenderness, passive correction of deformities. The tenderness must be felt for specific soft tissue, bony landmarks in three anatomical regions (i.e., forefoot, midfoot, and hindfoot). In the forefoot, the first metatarsal head, MTP joint, followed by lateral metatarsal heads and joints can be sequentially palpated. Tenderness, swelling of the bursa, synovitis, instability in second and third metatarsal joints are common findings in RA. In the hindfoot, calcaneum and its parts can be palpated separately. Tenderness over the "sinus tarsi" indicates subtalar joint pathology or sinus tarsi syndrome. Further, pain over Tendo-Achilles insertion may be due to retrocalcaneal bursitis or insertional tendinopathy. Tarsal tunnel syndrome, posterior tibial tendinosis, tenosynovitis may present with posteromedial tenderness.

The possible differential diagnosis with anatomical correlation is shown in **Table 2**.

In movements, the passive range of motion of ankle (normal 20–25° of dorsiflexion to 40–50° of plantar flexion), hindfoot inversion/eversion (normal 20° each), and first metatarsophalangeal joint (normal 70° of extension and 45° of plantarflexion) should be examined.

IMAGING

Weight-bearing radiographs anteroposterior, lateral, and mortise view of the ankle with anteroposterior, oblique, and lateral view of the foot should be part of standard imaging in patients with foot and ankle pain. The joint space narrowing, and deformities often get revealed in weight-bearing films.

TABLE 2: Differential diagnosis with anatomical correlation.

Location	Pathology/Dysfunction
Forefoot	• Arthritis/synovitis • Hallux valgus • Hammertoes, claw toes, and mallet toes • Morton's neuroma • Metatarsophalangeal arthritis/synovitis/instability • Osteonecrosis of the second metatarsal head (Freiberg's)
Midfoot	Arthritis/synovitis, stress fracture, osteonecrosis (navicular)
Hindfoot	• Arthritis/synovitis • Hindfoot valgus deformity • Stress fracture • Plantar fasciitis
Anterior ankle	Arthritis, synovitis, impingement, osteochondral defect
Central ankle	• Osteochondral lesion • Stress fracture
Posterior ankle	• Achilles tendinitis/tendinosis • Retrocalcaneal bursitis • Achilles rupture • Stress fracture
Posterolateral ankle	Peroneal tendinitis, tear, instability
Posteromedial ankle	• Posterior tibial tendinitis dysfunction • Flexor hallucis longus/flexor digitorum longus tendinitis • Tarsal tunnel syndrome

If necessary, the use of advanced imaging techniques such as MRI should be done to search for any early signs of disease activity such as periarticular edema, synovitis, bursal inflammation, and tenosynovitis. It can also evaluate the disease activity, joint destruction, tendinitis/tendinopathy, or for diagnosing tendon rupture in later disease. CT scan can help to study joint morphology and nuclear scintigraphy to evaluate disease activity. Ultrasound, though highly user-dependent, can be used as a bedside tool to assess inflammation and tendon rupture.

DIFFERENTIAL DIAGNOSIS OF FOOT PAIN

Pain and deformity in the forefoot, such as hallux valgus, dorsal dislocation, or subluxation of other toes, are relatively common in patients with rheumatic arthritis. The pathoanatomy can be explained by persistent inflammation and synovitis leading to capsular stretching and attenuation of volar plates. The combination of capsular stretching, tenosynovitis, progressive collateral instability, and destruction of the articular cartilage with bony erosions leads to progressive instability and deformity of the joints. Also, it is commonly associated with metatarsalgia.

The first tarsometatarsal joint is most commonly involved in the midfoot. The complex anatomy and various forces due to deformities in the forefoot and hindfoot cause stress risers across the tarsometatarsal joint. The symptoms are more commonly from altered biomechanics rather than synovitis. This increased tension causes pain in the dorsomedial foot by extension of the first tarsometatarsal (TMT) joint and other TMT joint dorsiflexion and abduction. It can progress to secondary osteoarthritis of the midfoot joints.

In around 21–29% of patients with RA, the hindfoot is involved with talonavicular joint most commonly affected, followed by talocalcaneal joint and calcaneocuboid joint, respectively. Further, the degree of hindfoot affection correlates with the disease duration. In patients with a disease duration of more than 5 years, 25% presents with hindfoot deformity than 8% of patients with a disease duration of fewer than 5 years. The most common hindfoot deformity in patients with RA is an acquired flatfoot deformity (associated with forefoot abduction and heel valgus) which can occur secondary to posterior tibial tendon dysfunction, articular deformity, or hindfoot instability. Clinically, patients presenting with dorsal or medial pain suggest talonavicular joint involvement, while pain on the lateral side of the foot indicates calcaneocuboid or talocalcaneal involvement.

TREATMENT

Nonoperative Treatment

Nonoperative management aims to prevent disease progression and alleviate patient suffering. The three broad pillars of management include footwear modification, medical management, and local steroid injections.

It is equally important to inspect the patient's footwear at the first visit to identify all pressure zones or get a pedobarography. Also, the physician should examine for any associated foot deformity, passive correction of the deformity, and joint suppleness. The patients feel very comfortable with shoes that can accommodate the deformity, provide a soft heel, stiff heel counter with a wide toe box. A separate pair of walking and jogging shoes are recommended. In patients with RA, it is crucial to order softer accommodative orthotics rather than rigid or semirigid, which mainly aims to correct the deformity. Close communication between the orthotist and the treating physician will help properly coordinate the orthotic prescription with diagnosis to make minor modifications as per patients' needs (e.g., use of metatarsals pads will help in relieving pain in patients with metatarsalgia).

The first-line drugs in medical management are disease-modifying anti-rheumatic drugs (DMARDs), followed by nonsteroidal anti-inflammatory drugs (NSAIDs) and biological agents. A team of rheumatologists, orthopedic surgeons, and anesthesiologists can manage the patient better to prevent perioperative problems such as postoperative adrenal insufficiency in patients on chronic steroid therapy.

Finally, to relieve local pain, bursitis, or inflammation, a cocktail injection consisting of local anesthetics and corticosteroids can be judiciously used. It is of utmost importance that such injection should not be placed in and around the tendons, leading to tendon rupture. The injection of a corticosteroid directly into or even near a tendon can adversely affect the biomechanical properties of the tendon and can ultimately lead to rupture. Further, in patients with joint instability (seen on physical examination or stress radiographs), corticosteroids injections are not recommended.

Operative Treatment

The only indication for surgery is the persistence of symptoms, failed medical management, and deformity correction. It is essential to evaluate the status of soft tissue, vascularity of the limb, and patient compliance. Poor limb vascularity may have a negative impact on the outcome. Similarly, the patient needs to adhere to postoperative protocols strictly. Early weight-bearing in fusion surgery may lead to implant failure. The various surgical options include synovectomy, ostectomy, corrective osteotomy, arthroplasty (joint replacement or reconstruction), and arthrodesis (fusion of the joints).

Synovectomy

Synovectomy involves the removal of all inflamed synovial tissue either through open arthrotomy or arthroscopically. It is helpful in patients in the early stage of the disease with preserved joint space and articular surface. It can also slow the progression of the disease activity and provide rapid pain relief for some duration.

Ostectomy

Osteophytes or bony spurs, although less common but can present with a secondary mechanical impingement in some patients with RA. In such isolated cases, a cheilectomy or excision of spurs can provide better results. However, in patients with associated joint destruction, arthroplasty or arthrodesis may be a better option.

Osteotomy

The principle of a corrective osteotomy is not limited to the deformity correction but also to realign the various forces acting on the joint, preventing any undue stress risers. It can prevent the progression of the disease and help in joint preservation. In patients with RA presenting with eccentric ankle arthritis or metatarsalgia, a distal corrective tibial osteotomy to align the axis of metatarsal osteotomies can provide significantly better results as compared to traditional methods such as ankle arthrodesis or metatarsal head excision. Patients with ankle and foot deformities such as pes planovalgus, hallux valgus is common in patients with RA and can be treated with calcaneal osteotomy or metatarsal osteotomies.

Arthrodesis

Arthrodesis or joint fusion surgery is the most promising option for patients with foot and ankle involvement in rheumatoid arthritis. It involves preparing the bony bed to make the opposing surfaces raw, using bone grafts to enhance biology, and compressing them. Once the bony ends become fused, it starts to function as a single unit and, most importantly, alleviates the pain. There may be some functional compromise, change in gait depending on the number of the joints fused.

It can be done via the traditional open, mini-open, arthroscopic approach. The added advantage of the mini-open or arthroscopic approach is minimal soft tissue damage, less periosteal stripping. However, all the patients should refrain from weight-bearing for at least 6–12 weeks irrespective of the approach. Based on the number of joints, degree of destruction, and availability of the bone stock, the surgeon can decide on the need for single, double, triple, or pan-fusion options.

In patients with RA, the first metatarsophalangeal joint is most commonly involved in the forefoot. It is often fused in slight extension to help in the toe-off phase. It is commonly done for severe hallux valgus deformity. In their case series of 47 patients who underwent first MTP joint fusion with a mean follow-up of 6.2 years, Coughlin et al. reported 96% good to excellent results with 100% fusion. As midfoot have less than 10° of movement in the coronal plane, joint fusion has minimal effect on the patient's gait.

In the hindfoot, fusion should be done based on joint involvement. A triple arthrodesis (i.e., fusion of talocalcaneal, calcaneocuboid, talonavicular) maybe preferred in multiple joint involvement with deformities. Since a more significant degree of movement in the coronal plane is from the hindfoot, joint arthrodesis will lead to loss of functional movements, inability to walk on uneven ground or foothills. Ankle arthrodesis with or without triple arthrodesis can also be done in patients depending on the extent of joint damage or deformity. The success rate of ankle arthrodesis was reported to be more than 85%.

Arthroplasty

The most encouraging recent advance in joint reconstruction is total ankle replacement surgery. It can preserve the movements of the ankle. Currently, US Food and Drug Administration (FDA) has approved five different ankle prostheses for elderly individuals or even in middle-aged individuals with low functional needs. However, the technical complexities with surgery, complex revision/fusion in failed cases are significant limitations to its use. It is still not recommended in young individuals who have high functional demands.

Similarly, the first metatarsophalangeal joint replacement is still in the experimental stage. Some studies indicate promising early results, but complications such as implant failure, loosening, synovitis secondary to silastic (polymeric silicone) particle wear are very common. Further, it is not recommended in severe deformity, which occurs in patients with RA.

CHARCOT NEUROPATHIC ARTHROPATHY OF THE FOOT

■ INTRODUCTION

Charcot neuropathic osteoarthropathy is a chronic, progressive degenerative arthropathy of single or multiple joints due to loss of protective sensation. The disease was first described in a patient with tabes dorsalis by Jean-Martin Charcot and later linked with diabetes by Jordan. It is relatively painless and associated with an underlying neurological deficit such as diabetes, tabes dorsalis, leprosy, spinal cord tumor, etc. It commonly affects the joints of the foot and ankle.

■ PATHOPHYSIOLOGY

The cause of Charcot neuropathy is found to be multifactorial. At present, there are two theories—(1) the neurotraumatic, and (2) the neurovascular theory, which explains the pathogenesis.

The neurotraumatic theory described by Volkman and Virchow states that there is a loss of peripheral protective sensation due to peripheral neuropathy. Hence, the bones and joints become susceptible to repeated injuries by trauma, leading to gross destruction, dislocation.

The French hypothesis/neurovascular theory suggests that autonomic neuropathy causes alteration in the blood supply leading to subsequent bony resorption, fracture, and deformity due to increased osteoclast activity.

The current evidence suggests that in patients with peripheral neuropathy, there is upregulation of receptor activator of nuclear factor kappa-B ligand (RANKL) expression due to an unregulated inflammatory process. RANKL stimulates maturation of osteoclast by activating nuclear transcription factor, nuclear factor-κβ (NF-κβ). The nuclear factor-κβ (NF-κβ) also stimulates osteoblasts to produce a glycopeptide, osteoprotegerin (OPG). Repeated trauma results in activation of the proinflammatory cytokines, osteoclasts via RANKL, and NF-κβ, causing bone resorption and severe osteolysis.

■ ASSESSMENT

A typical history suggestive of peripheral neuropathy, and clinical examination supplemented with modern imaging can help in diagnosis. Neuropathy can be assessed using various methods such as Semmes-Weinstein 5.07/10 g monofilament, pinprick test, or neurometer test. Patients with small fiber neuropathy such as autonomic neuropathy may present with additional symptoms such as constipation, gastroparesis, cardiac arrhythmias, and erectile dysfunction.

Clinically, in acute Charcot neuropathy, the patient usually presents with a swollen, erythematous, warm foot, while chronic Charcot neuropathy presents with a structurally deformed foot, undue bony prominence, and deformity. Erythema in the early stage of the disease can raise the suspicion of possible underlying infection or even acute gout.

■ IMAGING STUDIES

Radiographs in the early stage of the disease may suggest degenerative change but, in later stages, will reveal gross obliteration of joint spaces, fragmentation and destruction of the joint, subluxation, and dislocation with surrounding soft tissue edema. It is essential to rule out osteomyelitis, mainly when it is associated with diabetic foot ulcers.

Magnetic resonance imaging can identify the soft tissue lesion, bone marrow edema, joint effusion in the early stage of the disease. A prompt treatment started at this stage can still reverse the progression of the disease. However, the use of MRI is limited as it cannot rule out infection. Advanced nuclear scans such as leukocyte-labeled technetium bone scan (^{99m}Tc-WBC) and indium labeled WBC scan (^{111}In-WBC) are highly sensitive and specific. In indium labeled WBC scan, the neuropathic joint will show cold (negative), and osteomyelitis will show a hot (positive) response.

■ CLASSIFICATION

Eichenholtz in 1966 classified Charcot neuropathy as three-stage as given in **Table 3** and classification of Charcot neuropathy based on MRI is described in **Table 4**.

■ TREATMENT

Conservative Treatment

The nonoperative treatment forms the cornerstone of the therapy. The idea is based on giving adequate joint time to heal by immobilization and delaying weight-bearing. It can be done by total contact casting in which serial casts are changed at weekly intervals and applied for 2–4 months. Alternatively, Charcot Restrained Orthotic Walker (CROW) can be used. The orthosis or contact cast should be used till the inflammation, and local warmth subsides. Once the treatment is completed, an appropriate shoe wear modification should be done to reduce further injury, ulcerations.

Operative Treatment

The various surgical options are resection of the bony prominences (exostectomy), Achilles tendon lengthening,

TABLE 3: Eichenholtz classification of Charcot neuropathy.

Stage	Radiographic finding	Clinical finding
I. Fragmentation	Osteopenia, osseous fragmentation, joint subluxation, or dislocation	Swelling, erythema, warmth, ligamentous laxity
II. Coalescence	Absorption of debris, sclerosis, a fusion of larger fragments	Decreased warmth, decreased swelling, decreased erythema
III. Reconstruction	Consolidation of deformity, fibrous ankylosis, rounding, and smoothing of bone fragments	Absence of warmth, absence of swelling, absence of erythema, fixed deformity

TABLE 4: Classification of Charcot neuropathy based on magnetic resonance imaging.

	Severity grade	
Stage	Low severity: Grade 0 (without cortical fracture)	High severity: Grade 1 (with cortical fracture)
Active arthropathy (acute stage)	Mild inflammation/soft tissue edema	Severe inflammation/soft tissue edema
	No skeletal deformity	Severe skeletal deformity
	X-ray: Normal	X-ray: Abnormal
	MRI: Abnormal (bone marrow edema, microfractures, bone bruise)	MRI: Abnormal (bone marrow edema, fractures, bone bruise)
Inactive arthropathy (becalmed stage)	No inflammation	No inflammation
	No skeletal deformity	Severe skeletal deformity
	X-ray: Normal	X-ray: Abnormal (old healed fractures)
	MRI: No significant bone marrow edema	MRI: No significant bone marrow edema

reconstruction of the foot with the help of deformity correction, arthrodesis. In severe cases, amputation and rehabilitation with prosthesis is recommended.

■ INDICATIONS

The indications of surgical treatment of Charcot neuropathy are given in **Table 5**.

Based on the involvement of joints, Sanders and Frykberg classified Charcot neuropathy on foot as given in **Table 6** and **Figure 2**.

Sanders I

It is also known as the "candy bar" type. The resorptive changes are formed in metatarsal bones, and they can mimic osteomyelitis **(Fig. 3)**. It is managed conservatively.

Sanders II

Once the Lisfranc joints get affected, the metatarsals get translated medially or laterally. This translation is associated with break-in the medial column, secondary development of forefoot abduction, and valgus deformity of the hindfoot. Also, if there is tibialis anterior contracture, it can lead to poor surgical outcomes. It is commonly associated with type III and hence, shares the same treatment strategies.

Sanders III

There occurs a midfoot break leading to rocker bottom deformity with unusual prominence of cuboid insole in this type. The bony prominence leads to skin compromise and nonhealing ulceration.

The surgical management for both type II and type III includes reconstruction and arthrodesis of two columns. In order to correct any associated forefoot deformity, the hindfoot must be placed in a normal position. Hence, in such complex scenarios, triple arthrodesis may be preferred to achieve a stable foot.

TABLE 5: Indications of Charcot neuropathy on foot.

Surgical treatment	Indications
Resection of bony prominences	Focal bony prominences in a stable plantigrade foot
Reconstruction by deformity correction, arthrodesis	• Stable, nonplantigrade foot • Unstable foot
Amputations	• Severe peripheral vascular disease • Recurrent uncontrolled infection • Failed previous surgery

TABLE 6: Sanders and Frykberg classification of Charcot neuropathy.

Type	Localization
I	Metatarsophalangeal and interphalangeal joints
II	Tarsometatarsal articulations (Lisfranc)
III	Midtarsal joint line (Chopart)
IV	Ankle joint and subtalar joint
V	Calcaneus

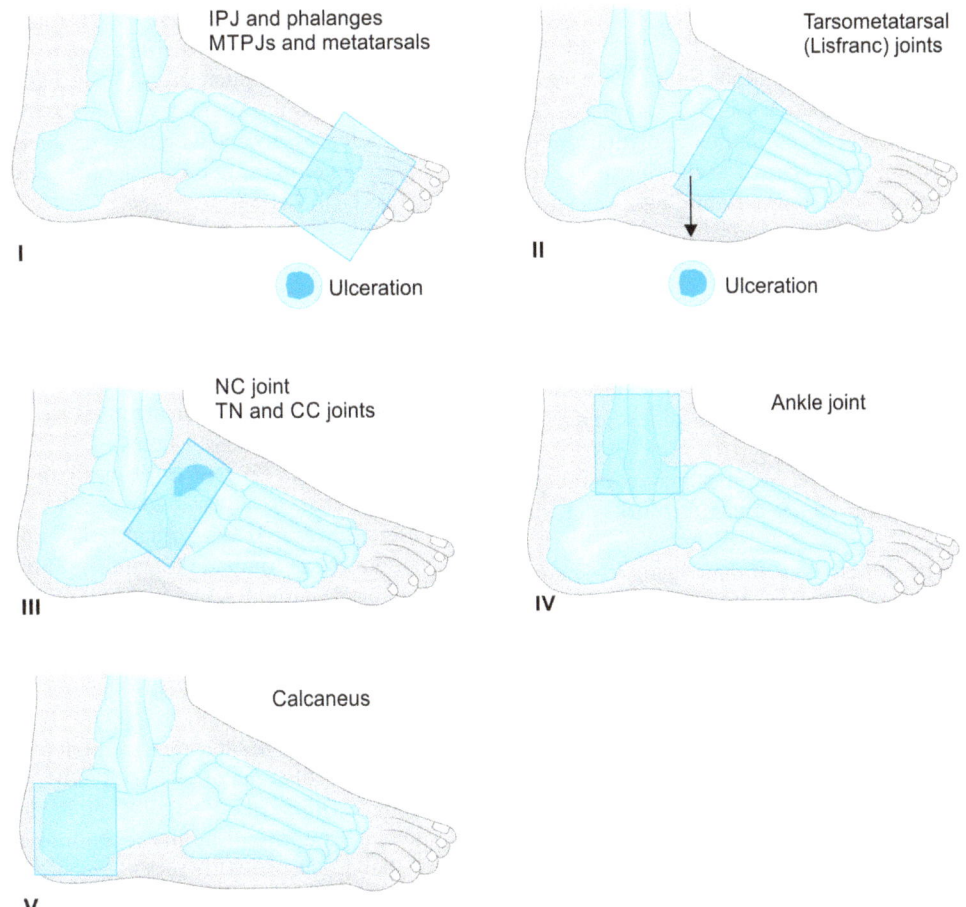

Fig. 2: The Sanders Frykberg patterns of Charcot neuropathy. (IPJ: interphalangeal joint; CC: calcaneocuboid; MTPJs: metatarsophalangeal joints; NC: naviculocuneiform; TMT: tarsometatarsal; TN: talonavicular)

Sanders IV

It involves the ankle and the subtalar joint leading to gross instability and deformity. Ankle and subtalar arthrodesis are the most preferred option. It is essential to assess the soft tissue status, as this area is prone to wound healing complications.

Sanders V

Usually, the involvement of calcaneum is not very common. Due to the high risk of infection, wound healing complications, conservative treatment with an ankle-foot orthosis is the first management line. Care should be taken to prevent ulcerations and provide a stable hindfoot. The role of surgery is limited to the dislocation of fragmentated bone with the action of Tendo-Achilles. A subtalar arthrodesis may be preferred.

CONCLUSION

In the early stages of the disease, Charcot neuropathy of the foot can be effectively managed with offloading joint and total contact casting or CROW. As the disease progresses, arthrodesis can stabilize the joint, and various protective measures can be used. The overall quality-of-life in severe diseases is often lacking.

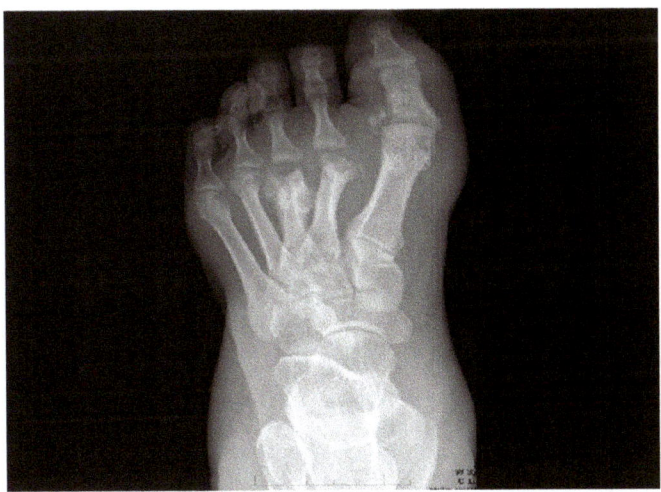

Fig. 3: Sanders I classification.

FURTHER READING

Foot and Ankle in Rheumatoid Disease

1. Action DJ, Deland JT, Otis JC, Kenneally S. Motion of the hindfoot after simulated arthrodesis. J Bone Joint Surg Am. 1997; 79:241-6.
2. Agarwal V, Singh R, Wiclaf, Chauhan S, Tahlan A, Ahuja CK, et al. A clinical, electrophysiological, and pathological study

of neuropathy in rheumatoid arthritis. Clin Rheumatol. 2008;27(7):841-4.
3. Aho H, Halonen P. Synovectomy of the MTP joints in rheumatoid arthritis. Acta Orthop Scand Suppl. 1991;243:1.
4. Bayrak AO, Durmus D, Durmaz Y, Demir I, Canturk F, Onar MK. Electrophysiological assessment of polyneuropathic involvement in rheumatoid arthritis: relationships among demographic, clinical and laboratory findings. Neurol Res. 2010;32:711-4.
5. Bharadwaj A, Haroon N. Interstitial lung disease and neuropathy as predominant extra-articular manifestation in patients with rheumatoid arthritis. Med Sci Monit. 2005;11:CR498-502.
6. Bommireddy R, Singh SK, Sharma P, et al. Long term follow-up of Silastic joint replacement of the first metatarsophalangeal joint. Foot. 2003;12:151-5.
7. Boutry N, Flipo RM, Cotton A. MR imaging appearance of rheumatoid arthritis in the foot. Semin Musculoskelet Radiol. 2005;9:199-209.
8. Bowling A, Grundy E. Activities of daily living: changes in functional ability in three samples of elderly and very elderly people. Age Ageing. 1997;26(2):107-14.
9. Chiodo CP, Martin T, Wilson MG. A technique for isolated arthrodesis for inflammatory arthritis of the talonavicular joint. Foot Ankle Int. 2000;21:307-10.
10. Clark H, Rome K, Plant M, et al. A critical review of foot orthoses in the rheumatoid arthritic foot. Rheumatology. 2006;45:139-45.
11. Coester LM, Saltzman CL, Leupold J, et al. Long-term results following ankle arthrodesis for post-traumatic arthritis. J Bone Joint Surg Am. 2001;83:219-28.
12. Conn DL, Lim SS. New role for an old friend: prednisone is a disease-modifying agent in early rheumatoid arthritis. Curr Opin Rheumatol. 2003;15:192-6.
13. Coughlin M. Rheumatoid forefoot reconstruction. A long term follow-up study. J Bone Joint Surg Am. 2000;82:322-41.
14. Coursin DB, Wood KE. Corticosteroid supplementation for adrenal insufficiency. JAMA. 2002;287:236-40.
15. Daniels TR, Mayich DJ, Penner MJ. Intermediate to long-term outcomes of total ankle replacement with the Scandinavian Total Ankle Replacement (STAR). J Bone Joint Surg Am. 2015;97(11):895-903.
16. Deheer PA. The case against first metatarsal phalangeal joint implant arthroplasty. Clin Podiatr Med Surg. 2006;23:709-23.
17. Golding DN. Rheumatoid neuropathy. Br Med J. 1971;2:169.
18. Groshar D, Gorenberg M, Ben-Haim S, Jerusalmi J, Liberson A. Lower extremity scintigraphy: the foot and ankle. Semin Nucl Med. 1998;28:62-77.
19. Hattrup SJ, Johnson KA. Subjective results of hallux rigidus treatment with cheilectomy. Clin Orthop Relat Res. 1988;226:182-91.
20. Hoppenfeld S. Physical examination of the spine and extremities. Norwalk: Appleton and Lange; 1976.
21. Hugate R, Pennypacker J, Saunders M, Battistella LR, Bértolo MB. The effects of intratendinous and retrocalcaneal intrabursal injections of corticosteroid on the biomechanical properties of rabbit Achilles tendons. J Bone Joint Surg Am. 2004; 86:794-801.
22. Jaakkola JI, Mann RA. A review of rheumatoid arthritis affecting the foot and ankle. Foot Ankle Int. 2004;25:866-74.
23. Kawaguchi Y, Matsuno H, Kanamori M, Ishihara H, Ohmori K, Kimura T. Radiologic findings of the lumbar spine in patients with rheumatoid arthritis, and a review of pathologic mechanisms. J Spinal Disord Tech. 2003;16:38-43.
24. Keysor JJ, Dunn JE, Link CL, Badlissi F, Felson DT. Are foot disorders associated with functional limitation and disability among community-dwelling older adults? J Aging Health. 2005;17(6):734-52.
25. Khoury NK, el Khoury GY, Saltzman CL, Brandser EA. Intraarticular foot and ankle injections to identify source of pain before arthrodesis. Am J Roentgenol. 1996;167: 669-73.
26. Lemming A, Crown JM, Corbett M. Early rheumatoid disease. I. Onset. Ann Rheum Dis. 1976;35:357-60.
27. Magalhaes E, Davitt M, Filho DJ, Battistella LR, Bértolo MB. The effect of foot orthoses in rheumatoid arthritis. Rheumatology. 2006;45:449-53.
28. Matteson EL. Current treatment strategies for rheumatoid arthritis. Mayo Clin Proc. 2000;75:69-74.
29. Menz HB, Morris ME, Lord SR. Foot and ankle characteristics associated with impaired balance and functional ability in older people. J Gerontol A Biol Sci Med Sci. 2005;60(12):1546-52.
30. Menz HB, Morris ME, Lord SR. Foot and ankle risk factors for falls in older people: a prospective study. J Gerontol A Biol Sci Med Sci. 2006;61(8):866-70.
31. Mohan AK, Cote TR, Siegel JN, Braun MM. Infectious complications of biologic treatment of rheumatoid arthritis. Curr Opin Rheumatol. 2003;15:179-84.
32. Peat G, Thomas E, Wilkie R, Croft P. Multiple joint pain and lower extremity disability in middle and old age. Disabil Rehabil. 2006;28(24):1543-9.
33. Pouget J. Vascular neuropathies. Rev Prat. 2000;50:749-52.
34. Riente L, Delle Sedie A, Iagnocco A, Filippucci E, Meenagh G, Valesini G, et al. Ultrasound imaging for the rheumatologist. V. Ultrasonography of the ankle and foot. Clin Exp Rheumatol. 2006;24:493-8.
35. Salih AM, Nixon NB, Gagan RM, Heath P, Hawkins CP, Dawes PT, et al. Anti-ganglioside antibodies in patients with rheumatoid arthritis complicated by peripheral neuropathy. Br J Rheumatol. 1996;35:725-31.
36. Saltzman CL, Mann RA, Ahrens JE, et al. Prospective controlled trial of STAR total ankle replacement versus ankle fusion: initial results. Foot Ankle Int. 2009;30:579-96.
37. Seltzer SE, Weismann BN, Braunstein EM, Adams DF, Thomas WH. Computed tomography of the hindfoot with rheumatoid arthritis. Arthritis Rheum. 1985;28:1234-42.
38. Shankar NS. Silastic single-stem implants in the treatment of hallux rigidus. Foot Ankle Int. 1995;16:487-91.
39. Spiegel TM, Spiegel JS. Rheumatoid arthritis in the foot and ankle diagnosis, pathology and treatment. Foot Ankle. 1982;2:318-24.
40. Thomas R, Daniels TR, Parker K. Gait analysis and functional outcomes following ankle arthrodesis for isolated ankle arthritis. J Bone Joint Surg Am. 2006;88:526-35.
41. Tokunaga D, Hojo T, Takatori R, Kadafi ME, Rajan D, Rowntree M. Posterior tibial tendon tenosynovectomy for rheumatoid arthritis: a report of three cases. Foot Ankle Int. 2000;27:465-8.
42. Vainio E. Rheumatoid foot. Clinical study with pathological and roentgenological comments. Ann Chir Gynaecol Fannie. 1956;45(S):1-107.
43. Vidigal E, Jacoby RK, Dixon AS, Ratliff AH, Kirkup J. The foot in chronic rheumatoid arthritis. Ann Rheum Dis. 1975;34:292-7.

44. Woodburn J, Barker S, Helliwell PS. A randomised controlled trial of foot orthoses in rheumatoid arthritis. J Rheumatol. 2002; 29:1377-83.

Charcot Neuropathic Arthropathy of the Foot

1. Botek G, Anderson MA, Taylor R. Charcot neuroarthropathy: an often overlooked complication of diabetes. Cleveland Clin J Med. 2010;77(9):593-9.
2. Bramham R, Wraight P, May K. Management of Charcot neuroarthropathy. Diab Foot J. 2011;14:163-70.
3. Callaghan BC, Cheng HT, Stables CL, Smith AL, Feldman EL. Diabetic neuropathy: clinical manifestations and current treatments. Lancet Neurol. 2012;11(6): 521-34.
4. Chantelau EA, Grützner G. Is the Eichenholtz classification still valid for the diabetic Charcot foot? Swiss Medl Weekly. 2014; 144:2-9.
5. Gouveri E, Papanas N. Charcot osteoarthropathy in diabetes: a brief review with an emphasis on clinical practice. World J Diab. 2011;2(5):59-65.
6. Low KTA, Peh WCG. Magnetic resonance imaging of diabetic foot complications. Singapore Med J. 2015;56(1): 23-34.
7. Nather A, Lin WK, Aziz Z, Ong CHJ, Feng B, Lin CB. Assessment of sensory neuropathy in patients with diabetic foot problems. Diab Foot Ankle. 2011;2:6367.
8. Sanders LJ, Frykberg RG. Diabetic neuropathic osteo-arthropathy: the Charcot foot. In: Frykberg RG (Ed). The High Risk Foot in Diabetes Mellitus. New York: Churchill Livingstone; 1993. pp. 297-336.
9. Sanverdi SE, Ergen FB, Oznur A. Current challenges in imaging of the diabetic foot. Diab Foot Ankle. 2012;3:9.
10. Wünschel M, Wülker N, Gesicki M. Charcot arthropathy of the first metatarsophalangeal joint. J Am Pediatr Med Assoc. 2012;102(2):161-4.

Diabetic Foot

RC Meena, Jitesh K Jain, Arun Kumar Sharma

INTRODUCTION

Burden of diabetes has increased in the world considerably in recent decades and so has the morbidity and mortality from diabetic foot ulcers (DFU). It is estimated that by 2030 more than 230 million people will have diabetes. Epidemiological studies have estimated prevalence of foot ulcers in diabetic patients ranging from 4 to 27%. DFU is a leading cause of hospital admission and morbidity in diabetic patients. Health care cost due to DFU is huge and estimated to be in billion dollars. One-fifth of total hospital admissions and 20–30% of total expenditure spent on diabetes care is estimated due to foot ulcers and leg problems. Lower limb amputations are 15 times higher in diabetic patients compared to nondiabetic patients.

Five-year survival rate after appearance of a DFU is around 50–60% and 40% of DFU patients develop a new ulcer after healing of one foot ulcer within 1 year. Due to high recurrence rate, it has been suggested that DFU should be considered as in remission and not as cured after healing of the ulcer. In this respect DFU is analogous to cancer. Outcomes of infected diabetic ulcers are universally poor with high rate of mortality and amputation at 1 year after onset of ulcer.

ETIOPATHOGENESIS

Etiology of foot ulceration is multifactorial with many causative and contributing factors **(Table 1)**. In diabetics, with onset and progression of sensory neuropathy, sensation of pain, pressure and proprioception are decreased or lost. This results in loss of protective sensation and increases vulnerability to injuries to foot. Motor neuropathy leads to muscle imbalance in the leg and foot muscles with resultant plantar surface pressure alteration and typical foot deformities, i.e., hammer toe and hallux rigidus. Autonomic neuropathy contributes by causing dry skin, fissures and crusting. All these factors cause multifold increase in the likelihood of physical and thermal foot injuries. High plantar pressure in some contact areas of the foot due to distinguished foot deformities and limited joint mobility at ankle and foot joints further increases the propensity to foot trauma.

Hyperglycemia induced endothelial dysfunction and vasoconstriction in peripheral blood vessels cause hypercoagulability. Atherosclerosis of peripheral leg vessels increases the risk of ischemia and ulcers. Prolonged uncontrolled hyperglycemia also weakens the immune system by cell functions such as phagocytosis, adherence and chemotaxis and subsequent intracellular killing. This disruption of the cellular immunity makes diabetic patients prone to infection.

Hyperglycemia compromises the immune system and diabetic patients are prone for advancement of infection. Infection adversely affects the blood sugar level thus a vicious cycle sets in causing poor control of blood sugar and impairment of immune function with subsequent infection in DFU.

RENAL FUNCTION AND DIABETIC FOOT ULCERS

A considerably high mortality rate has been shown in the diabetics on dialysis after lower limb amputations. Many studies have shown a temporal relationship between simultaneous occurrence of onset of dialysis and foot ulceration in diabetics. Probably inflammation associated with DFU diminishes the renal function.

Foot at Risk of Diabetic Foot Ulcers

Risk factors for DFU are tabulated in **Box 1**. Diabetic patients at greatest risk of ulceration are those having neuropathy, evidence of ischemia, foot deformity, visual impairment, and patients with previous history of foot ulcers.

TABLE 1: Causative and contributing factors to diabetic foot ulcer (DFU).

Causative factors	Contributing factors
Peripheral neuropathy	Peripheral vascular disease
Structural foot deformity leading to high foot plantar pressure	Uncontrolled hyperglycemia
Trauma to foot	

CLASSIFICATION OF DIABETIC FOOT ULCER

Many classifications have been put forward in the literature such as—Wagner classification, University of Texas wound classification system (UT) and PEDIS (Perfusion, Extent, Depth, Infection and Sensation). Wagner's classification is most commonly used and based on the extent of the ulcer. Wagner classification **(Table 2)** does not guide the prognosis and treatment. PEDIS classification **(Table 3)** is more relevant to the prognosis of the ulcer. Higher the grade of PEDIS (2 or >2) poorer is the prognosis. In a study by Ndosi M et al., best predictors of DFU healing were perfusion grade, duration of ulcer and number of ulcers. High grade of perfusion, longer duration of ulcer and multiple ulcers carry the worst prognosis for healing. Based on neurovascular status diabetic foot ulcers can be divided into two types. In neuropathic foot ulcer, foot is warm with palpable pulsation and good perfusion. In neuroischemic foot ulcer, foot is colder with diminished pulses.

EXAMINATION OF DIABETIC FOOT ULCER

Describe the basic ulcer characteristics such as size, depth, margins, location and numbers. Gentle probing with blunt sterile probe determines the base, margins and presence of sinus tract. A direct palpation of the bone with probe increases likelihood of the osteomyelitis. Note is made of any exudate from the ulcer. Surroundings are examined for any erythema, swelling, discoloration, and component of cellulitis **(Fig. 1)**. Further examination should focus on determining the etiopathogenesis. To assess the neuropathy a 10 g monofilament test is currently recommended. A 10 g monofilament exerts 10 g buckling force when it is touched on dorsum and plantar surface of the foot **(Figs. 2A and B)**. With both eyes closed, the monofilament is touched at 90° to the skin and pressed till it buckles to 1 cm, patient is asked to say yes when a touch is felt. A site is visited three times before declaration of neuropathy. Failure to perceive the touch all the three times confirms loss of protective sensation. A graduated tuning fork (128 Hz) is used to screen the vibration perception threshold.

Screen the patient for peripheral vascular disease. History of rest pain and intermittent claudication suggest peripheral arterial disease. Involvement of tibial artery is classical finding in diabetic vasculopathy resulting in absent/diminished pedal pulses and presence of popliteal pulses. Ankle-brachial index is the ratio of the highest systolic blood pressure at the ankle to the systolic blood pressure at the arm, and is measured using a Doppler device. Values between 0.91 and 1.3 are considered normal and below 0.40 are suggestive of critical ischemia.

Culture from a DFU: All ulcers are contaminated so culture from all ulcers is not recommended. When infection is suspected (erythema, purulent discharge) culture is best taken from the purulent drainage or from the ulcer base. In diabetics polymicrobial infection predominates and both aerobic and anaerobic cultures should be asked for. Critical ischemia, osteomyelitis, cellulitis, and abscess increase the likelihood of amputation due to severe infection.

Risk Assessment in Diabetic Foot

- *Low risk foot*: Only callus is present
- *Medium risk foot*: Structural deformity/peripheral neuropathy/peripheral arterial disease
- *High risk foot*: Previous ulceration or amputation along with any of two—structural deformity/peripheral neuropathy/peripheral arterial disease.

Box 1: Risk factors for diabetic foot ulcer (DFU).

- History of prior ulceration
- Poor control of blood sugar
- Long duration of diabetes mellitus
- Chronic renal disease
- Peripheral neuropathy
- Foot deformity and decreased mobility of the foot
- Foot callosity
- Improperly fitted shoes
- Old age
- Visual impairment

TABLE 2: Wagner ulcer classification system.

Grade	Lesion
0	No open lesions; may have deformity or cellulitis
1	Superficial diabetic ulcer (partial or full thickness)
2	Ulcer extension to ligament, tendon, joint capsule, or deep fascia without abscess or osteomyelitis
3	Deep ulcer with abscess, osteomyelitis, or joint sepsis
4	Gangrene localized to portion of forefoot or heel
5	Extensive gangrenous involvement of the entire foot

TABLE 3: The PEDIS classification system and the score system.

Grade	Perfusion	Extent	Depth	Infection	Sensation	Score
1	No PAD	Skin intact	Skin intact	None	No loss	0
2	PAD, No CLI	<1 cm²	Superficial	Surface	Loss	1
3	CLI	1–3 cm²	Fascia, muscle, tendon	Abscess, fasciitis, septic arthritis		2
4		>3 cm²	Bone or joint	SIRS		3

(CLI: critical limb ischemia; PAD: peripheral arterial disease; SIRS: systemic inflammatory response syndrome)

MANAGEMENT

Timely management of diabetic foot can prevent or delay complications such as infection gangrene and amputation. Diabetes is a systemic disease so multidisciplinary approach is required involving vascular surgeon, orthopedician, podiatrist, orthotist, endocrinologist, educator, specialist nurse and dietician for the optimal management of the diabetic foot. Many studies have shown that a team approach as mentioned earlier and self-education can reduce the amputation rate and mortality significantly.

Patient Education

Patients should be taught their responsibility for their own health. Health care givers should teach the patient about importance of controlling blood sugar and regular monitoring of blood glucose level. Written information should be given by educator nurse regarding modifiable cardiovascular risk factor such as diet, BMI, alcohol, smoking and exercise. Patients should be screened at every visit for the risk factors by the clinician for timely involvement of required health care specialist and categorized as having low, medium and high risk for amputation. Structured and repetitive advice on basic foot care along with timely interventions has been emphasized in the literature as an effective measure to prevent foot problems.

Tips for Foot Care involved in Patient Education

- Inspect your foot daily and wash them with water at room temperature.
- Special attention should be given to area between the toes.
- Never walk bare feet. Always wear socks and shoes.
- Trim nails timely and do not try to remove callus at home with knife or chemical agent.
- For dry skin use oil or creams but it should not be applied in between toes.
- Visit your health care giver at earliest whenever you notice a cut, scratch, and changes in the color or texture of the foot or sore/ulcer.

Blood Sugar Control

Hyperglycemia is the main cause of the development of DFU. It delays wound healing by hampering phagocytosis and chemotaxis thus compromising cellular immunity. Early control of blood sugar delays the development of neuropathy in diabetic patients but it has not been shown by any study that glycemic control can revere the established neuropathy. Glycated hemoglobin (HbA1C) level is the best indicator of blood glycemic control of past 3 months. Every 1% increase in HbA1C level increases the relative risk of peripheral vascular

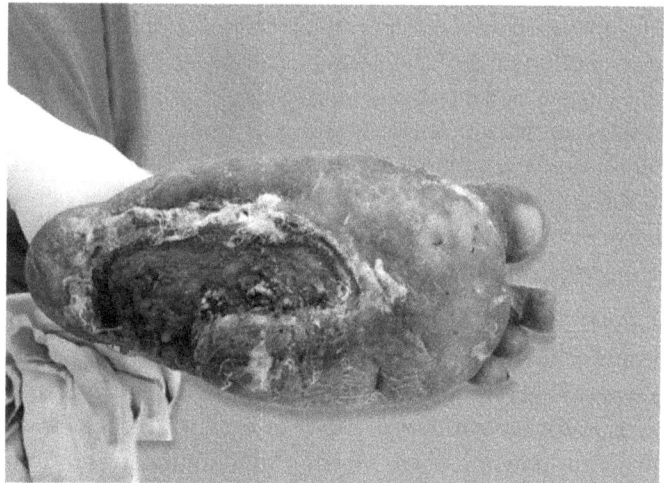

Fig. 1: Infected neuropathic diabetic foot ulcer.

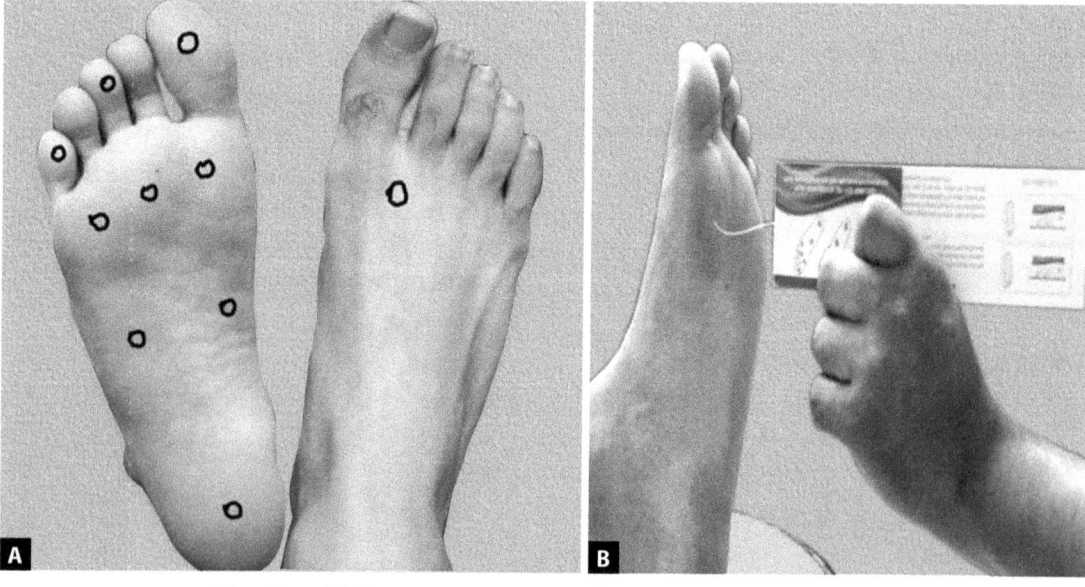

Figs. 2A and B: Sensitivity test with monofilament in a neuropathic foot.

disease by more than 25%. In diabetic people goal should be to keep the HbA1C below 7.0–7.5% (150–170 mg/day).

Surgical and Other Types of Debridement

Sharp surgical debridement is the gold standard for the management of diabetic foot ulcers. Surgical debridement involves removal of all necrotic tissues, debris, and infected tissues and disruption of surface biofilms with scalpel, scissors and curettes. Regular weekly serial debridement should be done if new necrotic tissues form. Serial sharp surgical debridement is associated with improved healing rate of DFU. In severe ischemia aggressive debridement should be avoided and revascularization procedure should be performed before serial debridement if necessary. Other kinds of debridement include enzymatic, autolytic, mechanical, and biological debridement. Enzymatic debridement is useful for ischemic ulcer where aggressive sharp surgical debridement is very painful. Many enzymes such as papain, streptokinase and streptodornase, are used to remove necrotic tissues. In autolytic debridement moist dressings such as hydrocolloids, hydrogels are used to create environment in which body enzymes clear necrotic tissues. Biological debridement utilizes sterile maggots to digest infected necrotic tissues without affecting healthy tissues.

Offloading and Pressure Modulation

Offloading techniques are mainstays of management of neuropathic foot ulcers in diabetic patients. Many offloading techniques are available and their use depends on the patient compliance and location of the ulcer. Commonly used offloading techniques are briefed in **Table 4**.

Foot Wears for Diabetic Patients (Figs. 6A and B)

Ideal foot wear for a diabetic patient should have a wide toe box, soft cushioned soles, and laces/velcro for fitting. Tight fitting shoe may cause sweating and predispose to fungal infection. A tight shoe may also cause shoe bite and neuropathic ulcer in a neuropathic foot. Offloading foot wears are useful in patients with plantar heel/sole ulcers.

Advance Dressings for Diabetic Foot Ulcer

Today, many novel dressings have been introduced for the DFU. Albeit they are commonly used nowadays, but their efficacy is not proven. These are expensive but some studies have shown promising results with these dressing for diabetic foot ulcers. Commonly used dressings are hydrogel, hydrocolloid, alginate dressing, foams, and silver impregnated dressing. Hydrogel and hydrocolloid dressings have a great absorbency and provide moistened environment. They aid in autolysis but better avoided in infected wound due to risk of possible maceration. Alginate and silver impregnated dressings have antibacterial properties and commonly used for infected wound.

SURGERY AND NEWER THERAPIES FOR DIABETIC FOOT

Different types of surgeries which may be required for diabetic foot include vascular surgeries such as bypass graft from femoral to pedal arteries and stenting of lower limb vessels to improve blood flow to ischemic foot, and nonvascular surgeries ranging from debridement to amputation. Newer therapies for management of diabetic foot include hyperbaric oxygen therapy (HBOT), vacuum

TABLE 4: Pressure modulation techniques for neuropathic ulcer.

Technique	Description	Advantage	Disadvantage
Total contact cast (TCC) (**Fig. 3**)	• Plaster of Paris (POP) cast is molded to the shape of the foot with minimal padding • A heel is given for walking. This cast so designed that it allows for equal distribution of the pressure on the sole while offloading the ulcer area	• Most studied and effective for neuropathic ulcer • Faster healing rate compared to other techniques • Gold standard for neuropathic ulcers	• It needs weekly change and expert cast technician • It cannot be applied in case of infection as it does not allow for inspection of the ulcer • If not properly applied, rigid cast can cause irritation or even ulceration to insensate neuropathic foot • It need to be covered during shower • Poor compliance
Removable cast walker (RCW) (**Fig. 4**)	It is a shoe shaped cast-like device that is easily removable	• It allows for self-inspection and topical application of dressing on the ulcer • More compliant for the patient as it can be removed during sleep and shower • It can be used for infected ulcer	Healing rate is slower than TCC
Instant TCC (**Fig. 5**)	It is a combination of TCC and RCW. In this method RCW is worn and elastotape or adhesive bandages are wrapped around it for tight fitting	• Healing rates are comparable to TCC • It can be removed by the patient as and when required	A few studies have shown healing rates comparable to TCC but more RCTs are required to establish it as gold standard for neuropathic ulcer

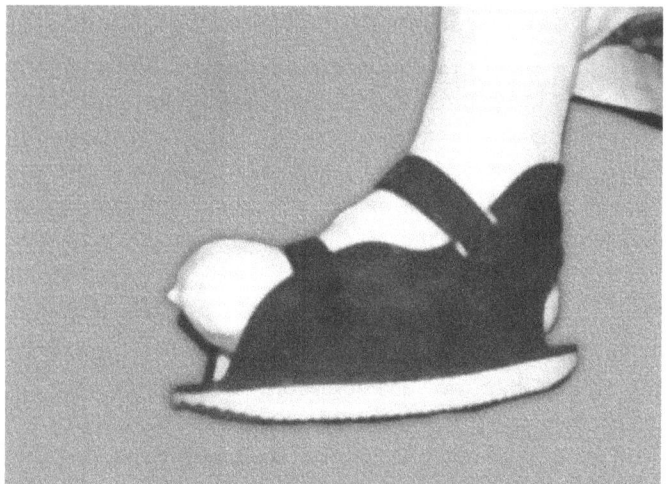

Fig. 3: Total contact cast for patients with diabetic foot ulcer.

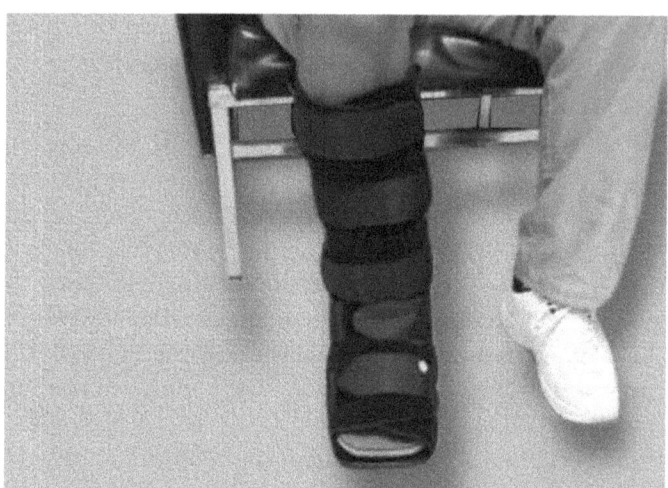

Fig. 4: Removable cast walker (DH Walker) for patients with diabetic foot ulcer.

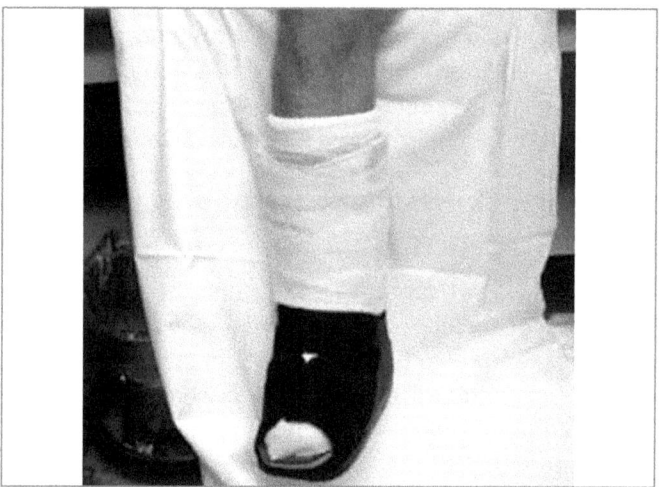

Fig. 5: Instant total contact cast for patients with diabetic foot ulcers.

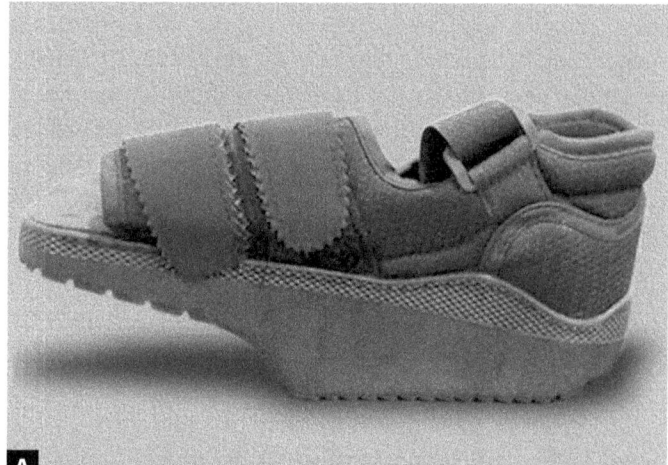

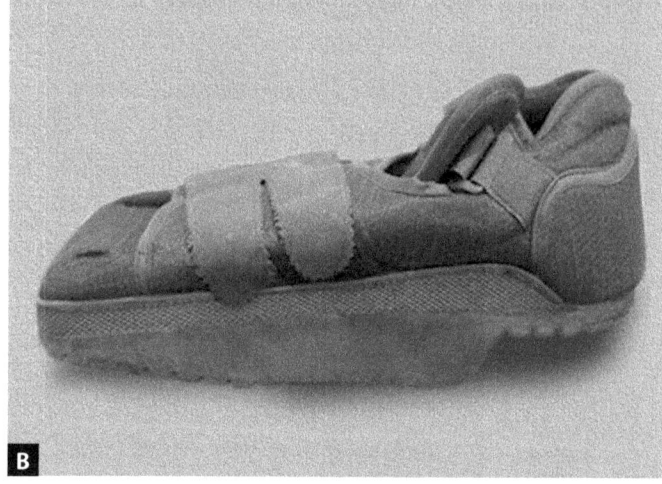

Figs. 6A and B: Offloading shoes for DFU. (A) Forefoot offloader; (B) Heel offloader.

dressing [negative pressure wound therapy (NPWT)], electric stimulation (ES) and bioengineered skin (BES). Many studies have shown significantly high healing rates in DFU after HBOT therapy. Exact mechanism is not known but it has been reported that decreased tissue hypoxia and enhanced tissue perfusion decreases sensitivity to inflammatory cytokines and promotes collagen production and angiogenesis thus improving healing rates. It is mainly used as an adjuvant therapy to debridement and antibiotics. Compared to HBOT, electric stimulation is a safe and inexpensive and many studies have supported their role in chronic ulcer treatment. ES improves blood flow, upregulates cellular responses and decreases infection.

Substantial evidences have been shown in RCTs in favor of NPWT for chronic nonhealing ulcers including DFU. Studies have shown a faster healing rate, faster time for wound closure and less time for healthy granulation tissue in nonhealing ulcers with use of NPWT. A sterile water tight seal is created over the wound with polyurethane or polyvinyl alcohol and adhesive tape. A negative pressure of 80–125 mm Hg is used in pulsed fashion or continuously and suctioned fluid is collected in a container at bed side. By continuously removing wound exudate it reduces bacterial load and promotes cellular proliferation, upregulates cellular function and enhances angiogenesis.

In the last two decades bioengineered skin (BES) has emerged as a new treatment modality for recalcitrant DFU. This method aims at changing the cellular environment to more favorable milieu by replacing the diseased extracellular matrix with a new ground substance matrix with cellular components. Derma graft and Apligraf, are commercially available skin equivalents for use in chronic nonhealing DFU. Oasis is an acellular biomaterial derived from porcine small intestine submucosa. It contains many dermal components including collagen, hyaluronic acid, proteoglycans, fibronectin, and growth factors such as fibroblast growth factor-2, transforming growth factor β1, and VEGF. Numerous RCTs have shown efficacy of these BES products in full thickness nonhealing DFU.

FURTHER READING

1. Al-Waili NS, Butler GJ. Effects of hyperbaric oxygen on inflammatory response to wound and trauma: possible mechanism of action. Scientific World J. 2006;6:425-41.
2. American Diabetes Association. Standards of medical care in diabetes—2017. Abridged for primary care providers. Clin Diabetes. 2017;35:5-26.
3. Ang L, Jaiswal M, Martin C, Pop-Busui R. Glucose control and diabetic neuropathy: lessons from recent large clinical trials. Curr Diab Rep. 2014;14:528.
4. Annersten Gershater M, Pilhammar E, Apelqvist J, Alm-Roijer C. Patient education for the prevention of diabetic foot ulcers: Interim analysis of a randomised controlled trial due to morbidity and mortality of participants. Eur Diab Nurs. 2011;8:102-7.
5. Armstrong DG, Boulton AJM, Bus SA. Diabetic foot ulcers and their recurrence. N Engl J Med. 2017;376:2367-75.
6. Armstrong DG, Lavery LA, Nixon BP, Boulton AJ. It's not what you put on, but what you take off: techniques for debriding and off-loading the diabetic foot wound. Clin Infect Dis. 2004;39(Suppl 2):S92-S99.
7. Armstrong DG, Wrobel J, Robbins JM. Guest Editorial: are diabetes-related wounds and amputations worse than cancer? Int Wound J. 2007;4:286-7.
8. Aydin K, Isildak M, Karakaya J, Gürlek A. Change in amputation predictors in diabetic foot disease: effect of multidisciplinary approach. Endocrine. 2010;38:87-92.
9. Bakri FG, Allan AH, Khader YS, Younes NA, Ajlouni KM. Prevalence of Diabetic Foot Ulcer and its Associated Risk Factors among Diabetic Patients in Jordan. J Med J. 2012;46:118-25.
10. Barnes R, Shahin Y, Gohil R, Chetter I. Electrical stimulation vs. standard care for chronic ulcer healing: a systematic review and meta-analysis of randomised controlled trials. Eur J Clin Invest. 2014;44:429-40.
11. Bello YM, Falabella AF, Eaglstein WH. Tissue-engineered skin. Current status in wound healing. Am J Clin Dermatol. 2001;2:305-13.
12. Boulton AJ, Vileikyte L, Ragnarson-Tennvall G, Apelqvist J. The global burden of diabetic foot disease. Lancet. 2005;366:1719-24.
13. Boulton AJ. Pressure and the diabetic foot: clinical science and offloading techniques. Am J Surg. 2004;187:17S-24S.
14. Cavanagh PR, Bus SA. Off-loading the diabetic foot for ulcer prevention and healing. J Vasc Surg. 2010;52:37S-43S.
15. Diabetes UK. (2015). Putting feet first: Diabetes UK position on preventing amputations and improving foot care for people with diabetes. [online] Available from https://www.diabetes.org.uk/Upload/Shared%20practice/Diabetic%20footcare%20in%20England,%20An%20economic%20case%20study%20(January%202017).pdf. [Last accessed May, 2021].
16. DiPreta JA. Outpatient assessment and management of the diabetic foot. Med Clin North Am. 2014;98:353-73.
17. Dorresteijn JAN, Valk GD. Patient education for preventing diabetic foot ulceration. Diabetes Metab Res Rev. 2012;28(Suppl 1):101-6.
18. Edmonds M. Apligraf in the treatment of neuropathic diabetic foot ulcers. Int J Low Extrem Wounds. 2009;8:11-8.
19. Falanga V. Wound healing and its impairment in the diabetic foot. Lancet. 2005;366:1736-43.
20. Frykberg RG. Diabetic foot ulcerations. In: Frykberg RG (Ed). The high risk foot in diabetes mellitus. New York: Churchill Livingstone; 1991. pp. 151-95.
21. Futrega K, King M, Lott WB, Doran MR. Treating the whole not the hole: necessary coupling of technologies for diabetic foot ulcer treatment. Trends Mol Med. 2014;20:137-42.
22. Game FL, Chipchase SY, Hubbard R, Burden RP, Jeffcoate WJ. Temporal association between the incidence of foot ulceration and the start of dialysis in diabetes mellitus. Nephrol Dial Transplant. 2006;21:3207-321.
23. Game FL, Selby NM, McIntyre CW. Chronic kidney disease and the foot in diabetes--is inflammation the missing link? Nephron Clin Pract. 2013;123:36-40.
24. Hilton JR, Williams DT, Beuker B, Miller DR, Harding KG. Wound dressings in diabetic foot disease. Clin Infect Dis. 2004;39(Suppl 2):S100-3.
25. IDF. International Diabetes Federation, 7th edition. Brussels, Belgium: IDF; 2015.
26. Jude EB, Apelqvist J, Spraul M, Martini J. Prospective randomized controlled study of Hydrofiber dressing containing ionic silver or calcium alginate dressings in non-ischaemic diabetic foot ulcers. Diabet Med. 2007;24:280-8.
27. Kessler L, Bilbault P, Ortéga F, Grasso C, Passemard R, Stephan D, et al. Hyperbaric oxygenation accelerates the healing rate of nonischemic chronic diabetic foot ulcers: a prospective randomized study. Diabetes Care. 2003;26:2378-82.
28. Kirsner RS, Warriner R, Michela M, Stasik L, Freeman K. Advanced biological therapies for diabetic foot ulcers. Arch Dermatol. 2010;146:857-62.
29. Lavery LA, Hunt NA, Lafontaine J, Baxter CL, Ndip A, Boulton AJ. Diabetic foot prevention: a neglected opportunity in high-risk patients. Diabetes Care. 2010;33:1460-2.
30. Lavery LA, Hunt NA, Ndip A, Lavery DC, Van Houtum W, Boulton AJ. Impact of chronic kidney disease on survival after amputation in individuals with diabetes. Diabetes Care. 2010;33:2365-9.
31. Leone S, Pascale R, Vitale M, Esposito S. Epidemiology of diabetic foot. Infez Med. 2012;20(Suppl 1):8-13.
32. Löndahl M, Katzman P, Nilsson A, Hammarlund C. Hyperbaric oxygen therapy facilitates healing of chronic foot ulcers in patients with diabetes. Diabetes Care. 2010;33:998-1003.

Ankle Osteoarthritis

J Mangwani, N Nanavati, V Adukia

EPIDEMIOLOGY

Whilst ankle osteoarthritis (OA) accounts for a significant socioeconomic burden to the society, it is difficult to predict its incidence, due to its low prevalence and lack of correlation between clinical and radiological findings. A cadaveric study by JM Michael et al. has demonstrated a 2% incidence of end-stage ankle arthritis, and suggests that everyone over the age of 66 has a degree of mild wear in the ankle joint. Ankle OA is still not only less prevalent than hip or knee OA, but also has a different pathophysiology. The primary cause of hip or knee OA is idiopathic, whilst post-traumatic arthritis accounts for the majority of patients (78%) with ankle arthritis. Forces going through the ankle joint are over 45% and 64% greater than they are at the hip or knee respectively. Additionally, the ankle has a surface area that is around a third that of the hip or the knee. Despite this, it still has lower rates of idiopathic osteoarthritis, due to unique anatomical and biomechanical factors as discussed below, which protect the ankle from developing primary OA, at the same time predisposing it to developing post-traumatic arthritis, especially following rotational ankle injuries **(Figs. 1A to D)**.

PATHOMECHANICS

The ankle articular cartilage has several properties that help safeguard the joint from degenerative changes. Anatomically, it is a highly thin and uniform layer, with a high tensile strength due to increased cross-linking. It also exhibits a deficiency of interleukin-1 and neutrophil collagenase receptors which protect from cartilage degradation.

Moreover, the ankle joint is unique in that it is a highly congruent joint with a primarily rolling action compared to the knee which involves a combination of movements including rotation and rollback. The congruency results in reduced contact forces transmitted across the joint, and therefore any change in this, as a result of trauma, such as a posterior malleolus fracture, can lead to the development of arthritis. Cadaveric studies have shown that as the size of the posterior malleolus fracture fragment increases, there is a corresponding decrease in the contact area within the tibiotalar articulation resulting in increased contact stresses. Theoretically, it therefore follows that an accurate, anatomical reduction as treatment for an ankle fracture will improve outcomes, however the likelihood of developing

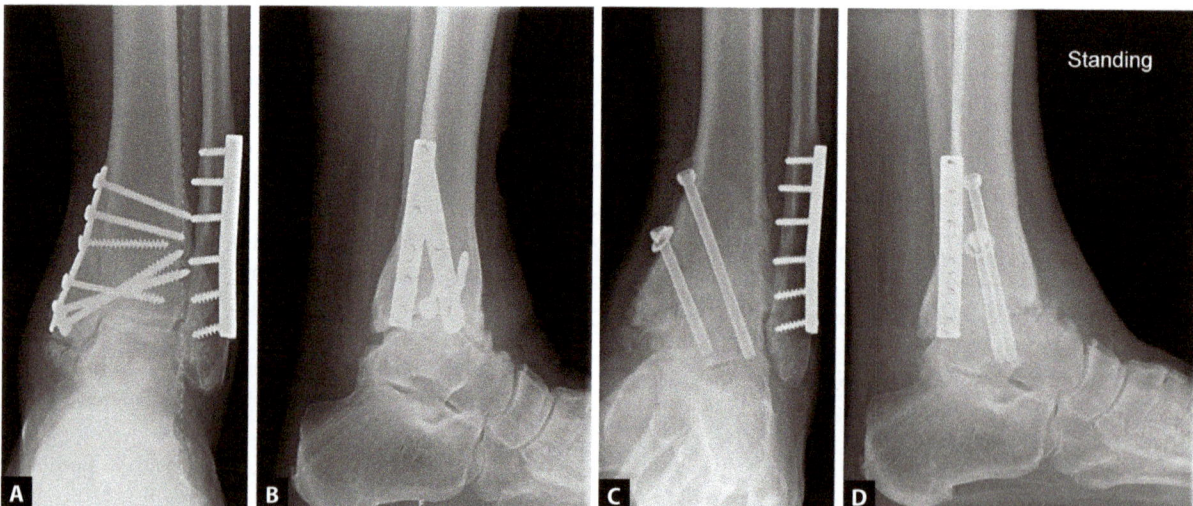

Figs. 1A to D: Weight bearing anteroposterior (AP) and lateral radiographs of a patient with a previous treated bimalleolar ankle fracture, demonstrating significant varus deformity of the ankle joint with development of end-stage ankle osteoarthritis (OA) (A and B). This was subsequently treated with removal of metalwork and an arthroscopic ankle arthrodesis (C and D).

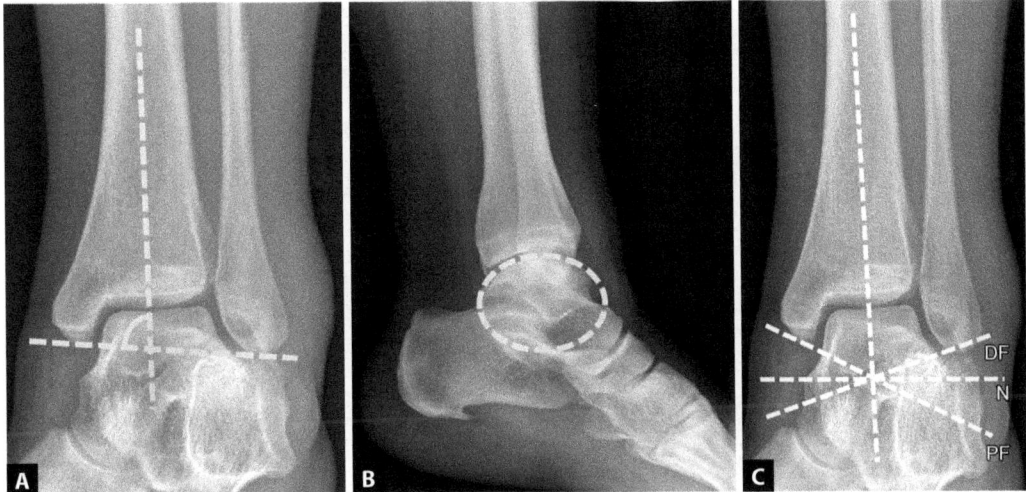

Figs. 2A to C: Normal ankle biomechanics. (A) AP radiograph demonstrating the axis of the ankle joint (normal values between 74 and 94°); (B) Lateral radiograph demonstrating the highly congruent tibiotalar joint and; (C) AP radiograph demonstrating the change in the position of the forefoot and hindfoot on dorsiflexion (abduction and eversion respectively) versus that on plantarflexion (adduction and inversion respectively). (N = neutral foot position; DF = dorsiflexion; PF = plantarflexion)

post-traumatic arthritis may in actuality be dependent more on the severity of trauma than the quality of articular reconstruction **(Figs. 2A to C)**.

DIAGNOSIS

A patient who presents with end-stage arthritis will usually report severe, limiting pain which stops them from performing activities of daily living. They may experience pain at night, on weight bearing or going up or down hill. The pain is usually described as being centered around a 'c' shape configuration anteriorly around the ankle joint margins and this can be evidenced by the patient cupping their ankle between the thumb and index finger when asked to locate the pain.

It is important to establish a history of trauma including fractures or recurrent sprains. A history of recurrent sprains gives clues to the fact that the ankle joint may be unstable and may therefore preclude certain management options. Other less common etiologies to consider include inflammatory or infective arthropathies, gout, hemophilia or neuropathy.

Diffuse ankle pain suggests global disease whereas pain on maximum plantarflexion (such as descending stairs or downhill walking) points towards posterior ankle pathology. Anterior impingement or pain may suggest isolated anterior ankle arthritis with classic anterior osteophytes and talus 'kissing' lesions. Subfibular pain may be indicative of subtalar disease.

EXAMINATION

The ankle examination should always begin with an evaluation of the patient standing and walking. Surgical scars, skin grafts, previous trauma and skin changes may all be visible from this simple inspection. A gait assessment is then performed and the positions of the hindfoot and forefoot noted. A patient with end-stage ankle arthritis will have difficulty with ambulation due to the painful and limited range of motion at the ankle joint. They may compensate by externally rotating the foot whilst walking. Similarly, patients with anterior ankle impingement are likely to suffer with pain during the 2nd rocker of gait due to impingement in maximal dorsiflexion of the ankle.

Following inspection, the ankle and the foot should be palpated to pinpoint areas of tenderness, after which the movements of the joints should be assessed actively and passively. This is done to exclude other common pathologies such as tibialis posterior dysfunction or adult acquired flatfoot. Finally, a neurovascular examination should be performed to complete the assessment.

After physical examination, all patients should have weight bearing anteroposterior (AP), mortise and lateral radiographs of the ankle as well as AP, lateral and oblique radiographs of the ipsilateral foot. In addition, hindfoot alignment views (Saltzmann or Cobey) should be obtained as part of the preoperative planning if there is malalignment of lower limb. Occasionally, it may be prudent to obtain a computed tomography (CT) scan to ascertain the degree of degeneration in different joints to aid in surgical planning **(Figs. 3 to 5)**.

CLASSIFICATION

Tables 1 and 2 show classification of ankle osteoarthritis.

TREATMENT

As with the majority of orthopedic conditions, ankle arthritis can be managed with nonoperative, medical or surgical treatments. Conservative management should be the starting point for all patients. Patients should be appropriately counseled to reduce weight and encouraged

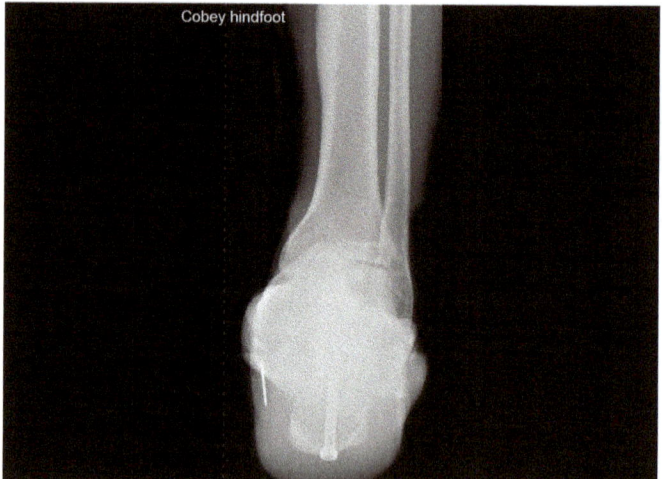

Fig. 3: Cobey view of the right ankle and hindfoot.

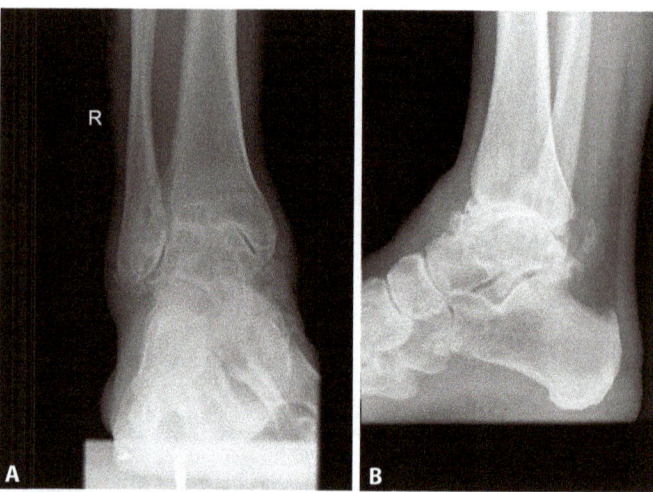

Figs. 4A and B: Weight bearing AP (A) and lateral (B) views of a right ankle demonstrating narrowing of joint space, subchondral sclerosis, and osteophyte formation suggesting osteoarthritis.

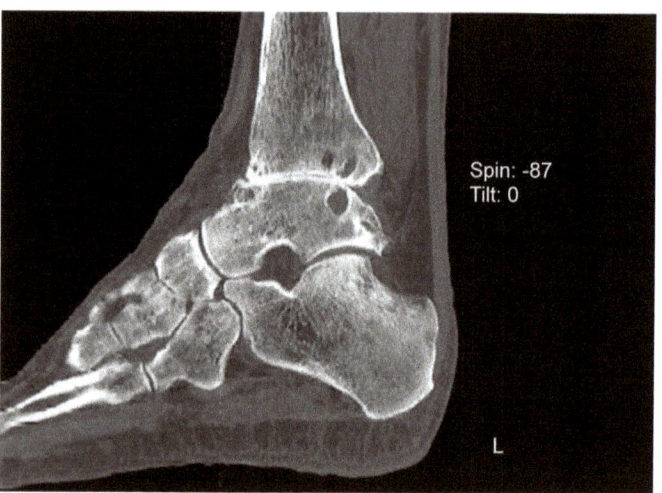

Fig. 5: Sagittal CT scan of a left ankle demonstrating ankle osteoarthritis with bone cyst formation and a relatively normal subtalar joint.

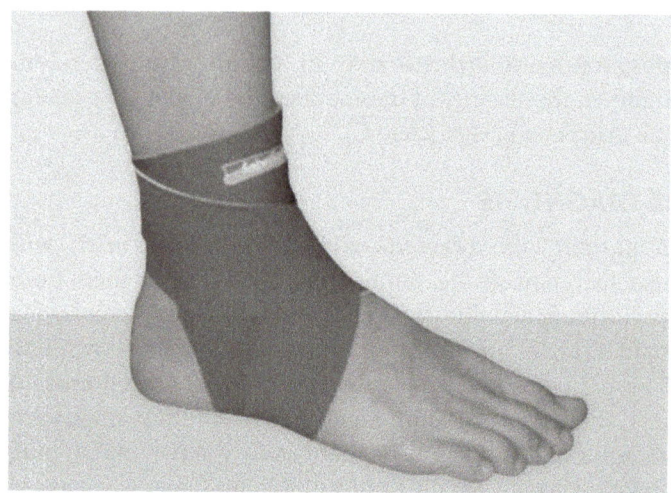

Fig. 6: Off the shelf ankle brace

TABLE 1: Takakura classification of ankle osteoarthritis.

Stage 0	Normal joint or subchondral sclerosis
Stage 1	Presence of osteophytes without joint-space narrowing
Stage 2	Joint-space narrowing with or without osteophytes
Stage 3	Subtotal or total disappearance or deformation of joint space

TABLE 2: Canadian Orthopaedic Foot and Ankle Society (COFAS) classification of ankle osteoarthritis.

Type 1	Isolated ankle arthritis
Type 2	Ankle arthritis with intra-articular varus or valgus deformity or a tight heel cord, or both
Type 3	Ankle arthritis with hindfoot deformity, tibial malunion, midfoot abductus or adductus, supinated midfoot, plantar flexed first ray
Type 4	Types 1, 2, and 3 plus subtalar, calcaneocuboid, or talonavicular arthritis

to participate in nonimpact activities. Nonimpact sports and exercise can reduce the joint reaction forces passing through the ankle, allowing patients to reduce their weight whilst also managing their condition effectively. Adjuncts to conservative management can include offloading braces, walking aids and/or orthotics **(Fig. 6)**.

Medical Management

All patients should be considered for medical treatment prior to any surgical treatment when managing ankle OA. Simple oral analgesics may prove beneficial to patients such that they no longer need or require operative intervention.

Oral supplementation with glucosamine sulfate has been shown to reduce pain in patients with symptomatic knee OA, and its use has therefore been extrapolated to treat patients with ankle arthritis. It is thought to protect cartilage from wear and is safe to use, however more research needs to be carried out in order to determine its efficacy.

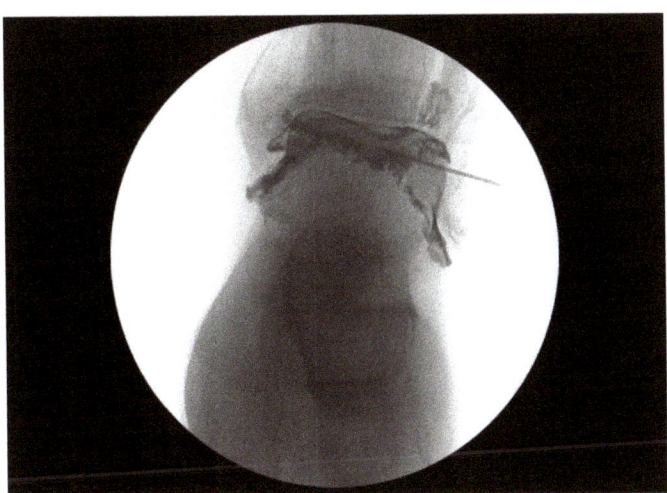

Fig. 7: Fluoroscopy image from X-ray-guided steroid injection to ankle joint.

Intra-articular hyaluronic acid (HA) injections are also used in the treatment of arthritis. It is believed to act as an anti-inflammatory agent as well as help with synovial lubrication by attracting water molecules. Its use however is not recommended by the National Institute for Health and Care Excellence (NICE) as the only studies showing the benefits of HA compared with placebos have been small, poor quality studies with significant bias.

On the other hand, an intra-articular corticosteroid and local anesthetic injection can prove useful as both a diagnostic and therapeutic measure. This is usually performed under image guidance in a sterile environment. A lack of improvement in a patient's symptoms following such an injection usually indicates that ankle OA is unlikely to be the diagnosis or that the injection was not given in the correct joint **(Fig. 7)**.

Patient with inflammatory arthropathies may require disease-modifying drugs or immunologics to reduce and minimize pain, swelling and deformity associated with joint destruction. New biological treatments are proving very useful in suppressing the destructive process induced by autoimmune reactions.

Operative Treatment: Joint Preserving Surgery

Debridement, Chondroplasty and Resection of Osteophytes/Cheilectomy

This procedure involves arthroscopic or open resection of osteophytes, and debridement of torn or fraying edges of the articular cartilage using a shaver or a burr. It is mainly indicated for patients with isolated anterior ankle impingement and is often used in combination with other procedures such as a realignment osteotomy or distraction arthroplasty. It is considered more effective for early arthritis, than for advanced diffuse disease, and requires an ankle which has preserved cartilage space in order to carry out the procedure. A relative contraindication for this procedure is a malaligned ankle, as it will be unable to correct the deformity and restore joint alignment **(Figs. 8 and 9)**.

Distraction Arthroplasty

This technique is usually reserved for young patients with end-stage ankle OA, for whom the only other treatment options would be either a joint arthroplasty or an arthrodesis. It involves using an external fixator which causes distraction at the ankle joint. This in theory helps offload the articular surface, providing pain relief, as well as delaying progression of the disease. It is often used as an adjunct along with bony procedures such as joint debridement and realignment osteotomies, and soft tissue procedures such as chondroplasty and tendoachilles lengthening **(Fig. 10)**.

Realignment Osteotomy

This procedure is generally performed for patients with post-traumatic ankle arthritis who have malunited fractures with localized disease. It can be performed either using internal or external fixation. Internal fixation involves correction of the deformity (usually in the coronal plane) using osteotomies and plate fixation, followed be a period of nonweight bearing to allow the osteotomy to unite. On the other hand, using an external fixator such as a circular frame to hold the osteotomy allows for weight bearing early in the postoperative period with the option to adjust the osteotomy later down the line, but risks complications such as infection, loss of position and/or fracture of the regenerate. Contraindications to this procedure therefore include patients who are noncompliant, smokers (due to the increased risk of infection and nonunion), and patients with peripheral vascular disease or poor tissue quality **(Figs. 11A and B)**.

Uni- or Bipolar Shell Allograft

This involves transplanting osteochondral shell allografts, usually through an open approach to the ankle joint, in order to replace the damaged articular cartilage and preserve joint function. It is reserved for young patients, usually with end-stage ankle OA, and is contraindicated in patients where the blood supply to the tibia or talus is disrupted, e.g., those with peripheral vascular disease, talar avascular necrosis, smokers, as well as in those patients with poor soft tissues who will be susceptible to wound healing problems. It should also be avoided in patients with significant malalignment of the ankle joint as this procedure does not help restore normal joint alignment, which is likely the cause of the OA in the first place.

Operative Treatment: Joint Sacrificing Surgery

Ankle Arthrodesis

Ankle arthrodesis is considered to be the "gold standard" treatment for end-stage arthritis. It provides pain relief,

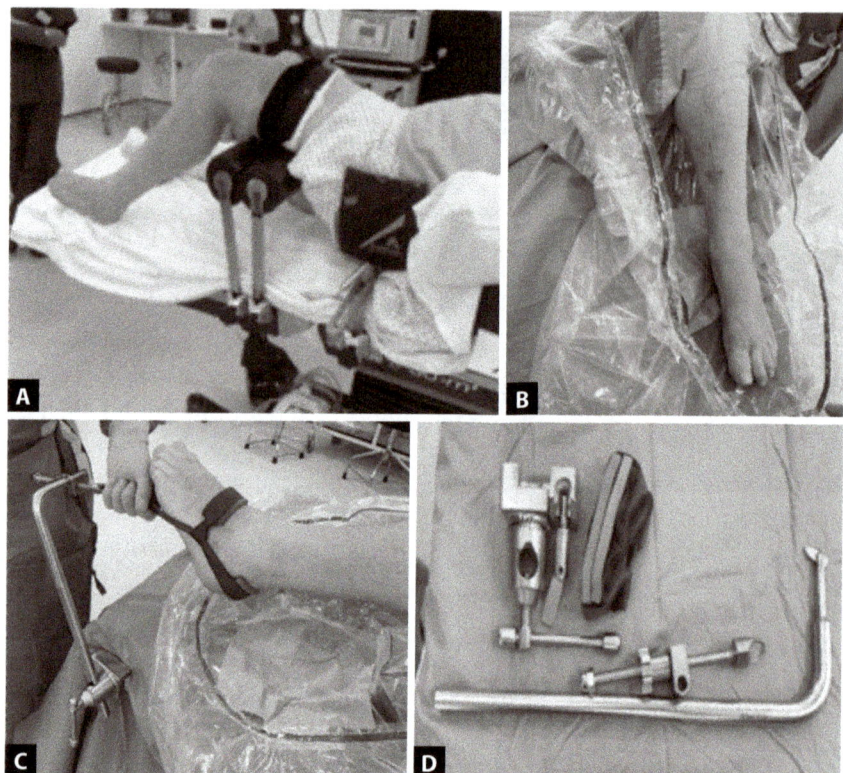

Figs. 8A to D: Clinical photographs displaying the standard set-up for an ankle arthroscopy. A thigh tourniquet is applied and a bolster put under the knee in order to get knee flexion. After prepping the skin, a waterproof sterile drape is used to cover the operative site. In our unit, a noninvasive ankle distractor system (Smith and Nephew) is used with a sterile sling, clamp and support bars, which is applied around the calcaneum. This enables the surgeon to distract the ankle joint by angulating the support bar away from the patient.
Source: Images reproduced from Afifi H et al.

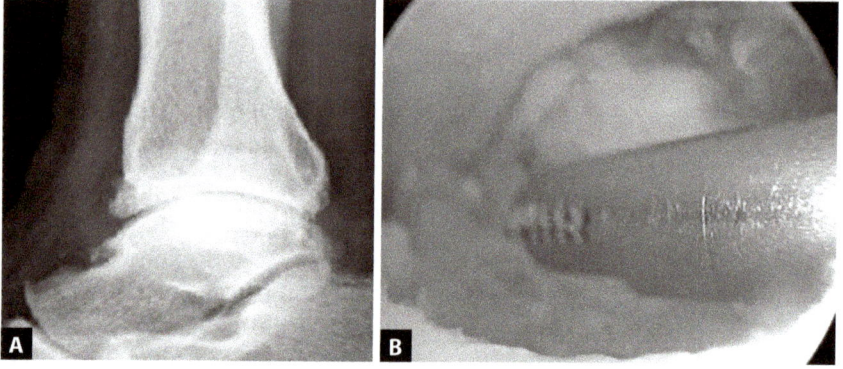

Figs. 9A and B: Anterior ankle osteoarthritis treated with ankle arthroscopy and debridement.

allows for joint deformity correction, and has a wide range of indications including arthritis (post-traumatic, idiopathic, inflammatory), talar osteonecrosis as well as previous joint infection. It can also be used in the revision setting following a failed ankle arthroplasty. Multiple studies have shown ankle arthrodesis to be a reliable procedure with high union rates and good patient reported outcome measures (PROMs).

Traditionally, ankle arthrodesis is carried out as an open procedure, however arthroscopic arthrodesis is rapidly gaining in popularity. An open ankle arthrodesis can be carried out either via an anterior approach, which is used more commonly, or a posterior approach, which tends to be reserved for patients who have a poor soft tissue envelope.

Another less common open approach is the transmalleolar approach which involves excising the lateral malleolus to expose the ankle joint. Arthroscopic ankle arthrodesis involves carrying out the same procedure via percutaneous fusion or a mini-arthrotomy. The ankle joint articular surface is thoroughly debrided till bleeding subchondral bone, and then the joint fused. Arthroscopic ankle arthrodesis has been shown to have fusion rates of over 87%.

Ideally, the ankle is fused in a position that allows for stable, weight bearing. This position tends to be a neutral position in the sagittal plane, 5° of hindfoot valgus and 5–10° of external rotation with the talus posteriorly translated on the tibia.

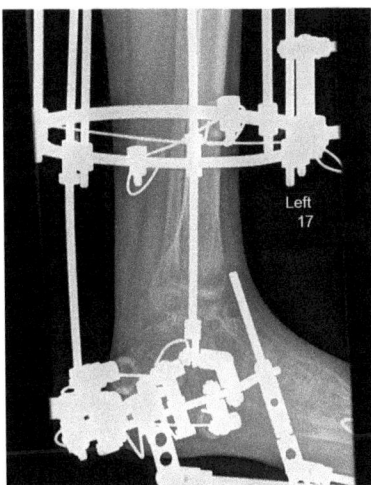

Fig. 10: Lateral radiograph of an Ilizarov frame-assisted distraction arthroplasty.

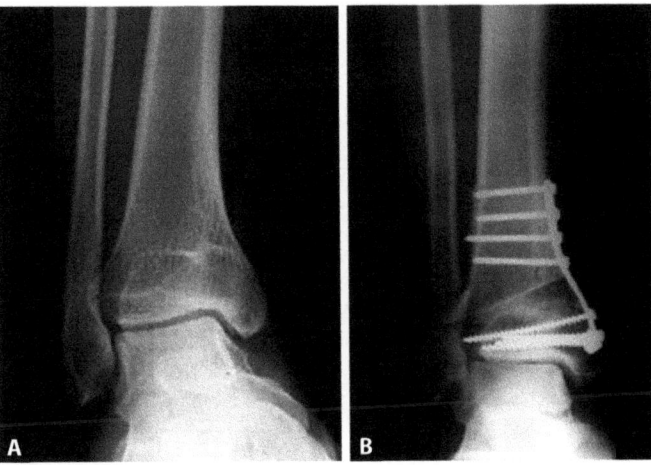

Figs. 11A and B: AP radiographs of an ankle with a significant varus deformity and medial joint OA (A), treated with a supramalleolar osteotomy and restoration of ankle joint alignment (B).
Source: Images reproduced from Bloch B et al.

For fusion of the ankle, internal fixation implants are preferred over external fixators as they are associated with a lower complication rate for infections, wound healing issues and delayed/nonunions. The internal fixation is commonly in the form of 2 crossed, cannulated screws that pass from the medial border of the tibia proximally, through the ankle joint, towards the lateral border of the talus distally.

As expected, range of motion is decreased following a tibiotalar arthrodesis, however studies have shown that the subtalar and midfoot joints of the foot compensate for this loss by allowing a degree of plantar- and dorsiflexion. Overall, the average difference in the range of motion following an ankle fusion is 30.9° when compared with the contralateral, unaffected ankle. Other changes seen postoperatively include a persistent gait asymmetry, with altered biomechanics resulting in hyper-extension of the knee, early heel-lift and reduced hindfoot motion. This results in increased forces going through the other joints of the foot, especially the midfoot, in the stance phase, which can, in theory, lead to the development of OA in those joints, especially the subtalar joint. Despite this, patients still exhibit improvements in their walking speed and distance when comparing preoperative and postoperative measures **(Figs. 12A to D)**.

Ankle Arthroplasty

Total ankle arthroplasty (TAA) has been in development for over 50 years and has come a long way from the early implants which were associated with failure rates of over 70% at the 10-year mark. These implants were generally composed of 2 components, with all the components being cemented, and either constrained or unconstrained. However, these were unable to reproduce the joint kinematics and were therefore prone to failure. More modern implants now are designed to not only restore joint anatomy, but also aim to reproduce normal joint kinematics, ligament stability and mechanical alignment using 2 or 3 components. They are usually metal-backed and have porous surfaces for better integration with bone.

Indications for TAA include patients with end-stage arthritis and a preserved range of motion at the ankle joint, especially the low-demand, elderly patients. However, it has also been used in the revision setting following a painful tibiotalar arthrodesis. Current ankle replacements show a 10% failure rate at 5 years with residual pain being common. It is therefore of paramount importance to select the appropriate patient for a TAA over an ankle arthrodesis to reduce the risks of complications and implant failure. Contraindications for TAA therefore are active local or systemic infection, patients with peripheral vascular disease, osteonecrosis of the talus or neuropathy, and significant joint malalignment. Patients with a poor soft tissue envelope are at a higher risk of developing prosthetic joint infection and/or wound healing problems, and therefore should be counseled appropriately **(Figs. 13 and 14)**.

Outcomes following TAA are improving with newer generation implants, so much so that a prospective cohort study found that TAA demonstrated significant improvements in PROMs when compared with ankle arthrodesis, and no significant differences were found between the 2 groups for complications and revision surgeries when adjusted for patient comorbidities. Currently, a multicenter, randomized trial, titled TARVA, is being carried comparing TAA with ankle arthrodesis in the treatment of patients with end-stage ankle OA. The trial finished recruitment in 2018 and is now undergoing statistical analysis.

SUMMARY

Whilst conservative management options such as analgesics, physiotherapy and joint injections have a place in the treatment of ankle arthritis, often they are only temporary

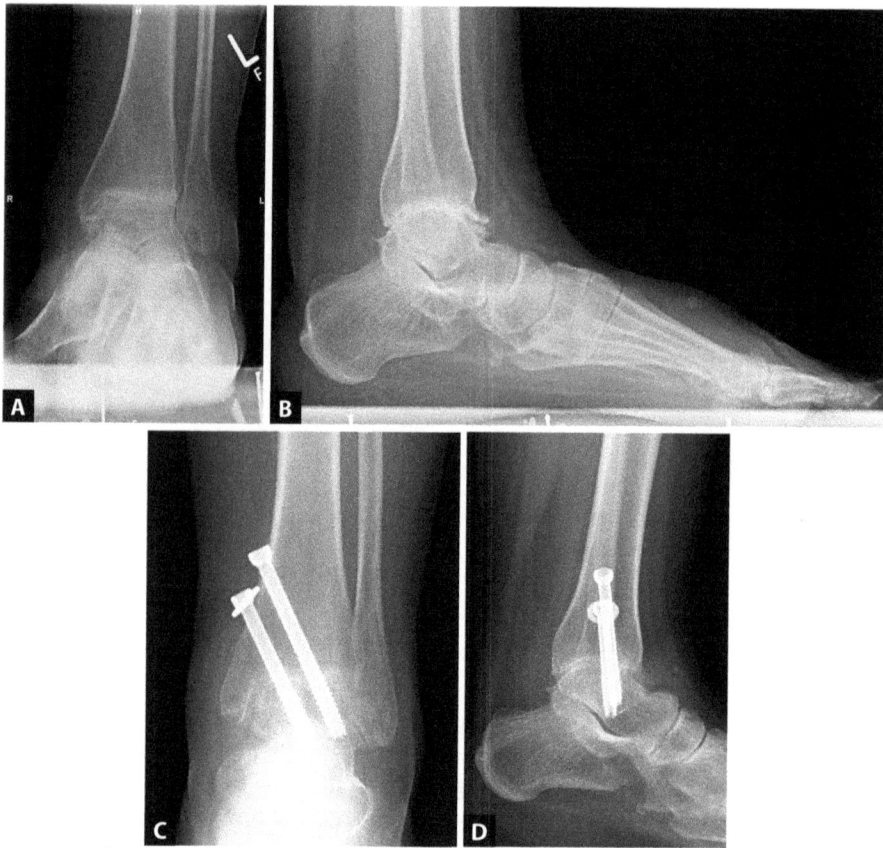

Figs. 12A to D: Anteroposterior (AP) and lateral radiographs of an ankle demonstrating end-stage ankle osteoarthritis (A and B) treated with ankle fusion using 2 cannulated screws (C and D).

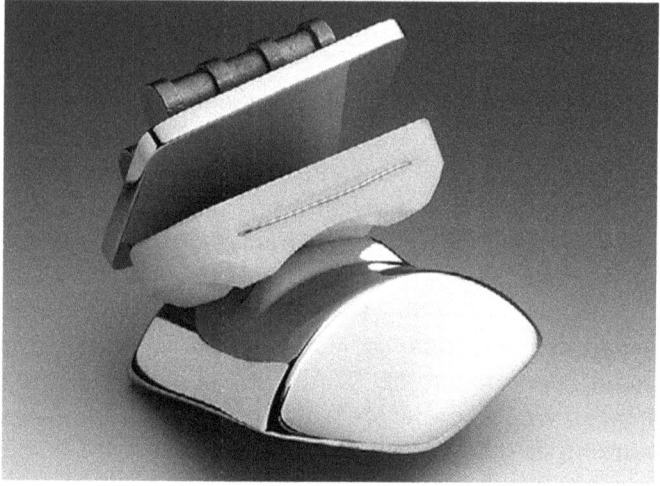

Fig. 13: An example of a STAR ankle replacement prosthesis.
Source: Image provided courtesy of Stryker.

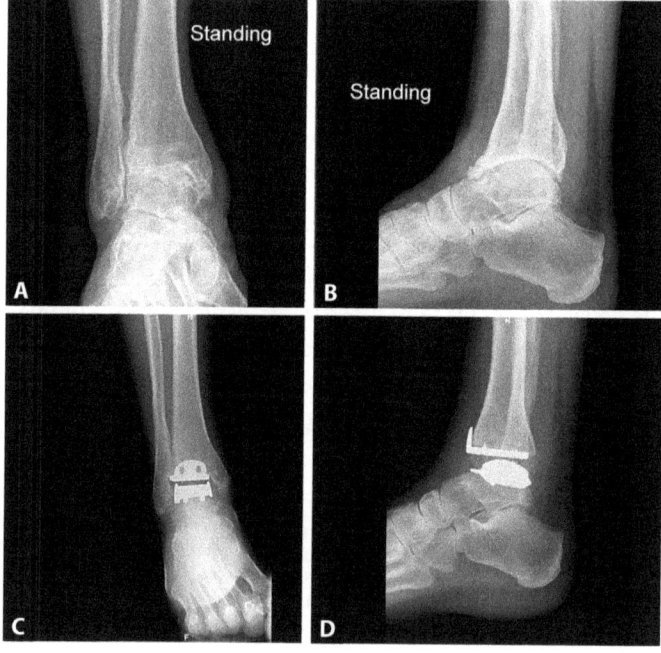

Figs. 14A to D: AP and lateral radiographs of an ankle with end-stage arthritis (A and B), treated with a TAA (C and D).

measures used in order to delay definitive operative management options such as arthrodesis or arthroplasty. However, there is an increasing interest in alternatives such as joint-sparing surgery, which may prove to be a useful next step, especially for the younger, more active patient, before joint fusion or replacement becomes necessary. There have been a number of studies which demonstrate good outcomes following joint preservation techniques, however the studies so far have had small sample sizes, making it difficult to ascertain as to what extent the results can be applied to a more generalized population.

Controversy still exists when discussing ankle arthrodesis versus TAA. Each technique has its pros and cons, and both are

TABLE 3: Summary of management algorithm.

Stage	Age	Ankle joint condition	Surgical procedure
Stage 1	Any age	Impingement only	Arthroscopic debridement
Stage 2	Any age	• Preserved anatomy • Supra-articular malalignment • Heel malalignment	• Arthroscopic debridement • Supramalleolar osteotomy • Calcaneal osteotomy/fusion
Stage 3	Any age Age ≥55	• Nonrestorable ankle anatomy, previous infection, neurological disorders, severe osteoporosis • Normal or restored anatomy with • No adjacent DJD • Adjacent DJD	• Arthrodesis • Arthrodesis/TAA • TAA

developing with the increasing popularity of the minimally invasive arthroscopic technique for ankle arthrodesis, and newer generation implants resulting in better outcomes for the TAA. Results from the ongoing TARVA trial will hopefully help clinicians decide between the two treatment options **(Table 3)**.

FURTHER READING

1. Akra GA, Middleton A, Adedapo AO, Port A, Finn P. Outcome of ankle arthrodesis using a transfibular approach. J Foot Ankle Surg. 2010;49:508-12.
2. Afifi H, Mangwani J, Faroug R. Arthroscopic ankle arthrodesis—surgical technique. J Arthrosc Surg Sports Med. Doi: 10.25259/JASSM_65_2020.
3. Bellamy N, Campbell J, Welch V, Gee TL, Bourne R, Wells GA. Viscosupplementation for the treatment of osteoarthritis of the knee. Cochrane Database Syst Rev. 2006;(2): CD005321.
4. Bloch B, Srinivasan S, Mangwani J. Current concepts in the management of ankle osteoarthritis: a systematic review. J Foot Ankle Surg. 2015;54(5):932-9.
5. Bolton-Maggs BG, Sudlow RA, Freeman MA. Total ankle arthroplasty. A long-term review of the London Hospital experience. J Bone Joint Surg Br. 1985;67:785-90.
6. Buck P, Morrey BF, Chao EY. The optimum position of arthrodesis of the ankle. A gait study of the knee and ankle. J Bone Joint Surg Am. 1987;69:1052-62.
7. Coester LM, Saltzman CL, Leupold J, Pontarelli W. Long-term results following ankle arthrodesis for post-traumatic arthritis. J Bone Joint Surg Am. 2001;83-A:219-28.
8. Collman DR, Kaas MH, Schuberth JM. Arthroscopic ankle arthrodesis: factors influencing union in 39 consecutive patients. Foot Ankle Int. 2006;27:1079-85.
9. Doets HC, Zürcher AW. Salvage arthrodesis for failed total ankle arthroplasty. Acta Orthop. 2010;81:142-7.
10. Florian Nickisch M, Frank R, Avilucea M, Timothy Beals M, Charles Saltzman M. Open posterior approach for tibiotalar arthrodesis. Foot and Ankle Clinics of NA 2011;16:103-14.
11. Gougoulias N, Khanna A, Maffulli N. How successful are current ankle replacements? A systematic review of the literature. Clin Orthop Relat Res. 2010;468(1):199-208.
12. Gougoulias NE, Khanna A, Maffulli N. History and evolution in total ankle arthroplasty. British Medical Bulletin. 2008;89:111-51.
13. Guo C, Yan Z, Barfield WR, Hartsock LA. Ankle arthrodesis using anatomically contoured anterior plate. Foot Ankle Int. 2010;31:492-8.
14. Hassouna H, Kumar S, Bendall S. Arthroscopic ankle debridement: 5-year survival analysis. Acta Orthop Belg. 2007;73:737-40.
15. Helm R. The results of ankle arthrodesis. J Bone Joint Surg Br. 1990;72:141-3.
16. Hendrickx R, Kerkhoffs G, Stufkens S, van Dijk C, Marti R. Ankle fusion using a 2-incision, 3-screw technique. Operative Orthopädie und Traumatologie 2011:1–9.
17. Hintermann B, Barg A, Knupp M, Valderrabano V. Conversion of painful ankle arthrodesis to total ankle arthroplasty. J Bone Joint Surg Am. 2009;91:850-8.
18. Intema F, Thomas TP, Anderson DD, Elkins JM, Brown TD, Amendola A, et al. Subchondral bone remodeling is related to clinical improvement after joint distraction in the treatment of ankle osteoarthritis. Osteoarthritis Cartilage 2011;19:668-75.
19. Kim CW, Jamali A, Tontz W, Convery FR, Brage ME, Bugbee W. Treatment of post-traumatic ankle arthrosis with bipolar tibiotalar osteochondral shell allografts. Foot Ankle Int. 2002;23:1091-102.
20. Krause FG, Windolf M, Bora B, Penner MJ, Wing KJ, Younger ASE. Impact of complications in total ankle replacement and ankle arthrodesis analyzed with a validated outcome measurement. J Bone Joint Surg Am. 2011;93:830-9.
21. Kuettner KE, Cole AA. Cartilage degeneration in different human joints. Osteoarthr Cartil. 2005;13:93-103.
22. Lynch AF, Bourne RB, Rorabeck CH. The long-term results of ankle arthrodesis. J Bone Joint Surg Br. 1988;70:113-6.
23. Macko VW, Matthews LS, Zwirkoski P, Goldstein SA. The joint-contact area of the ankle. The contribution of the posterior malleolus. J Bone Joint Surg Am. 1991;73:347-51.
24. Marsh JL, Buckwalter J, Gelberman R, Dirschl D, Olson S, Brown T, et al. Articular fractures: does an anatomic reduction really change the result? J Bone Joint Surg Am. 2002;84:1259-71.
25. Michael JM, Golshani A, Gargac S, Goswami T. Biomechanics of the ankle joint and clinical outcomes of total ankle replacement. J Mech Behav Biomed Mater. 2008; 1:276-94.
26. Moeckel BH, Patterson BM, Inglis AE, Sculco TP. Ankle arthrodesis. A comparison of internal and external fixation. Clin Orthop Relat Res. 1991;78-83.
27. Muller P, Skene SS, Chowdhury K, Cro S, Goldberg AJ, Dore CJ, et al. A randomised, multi-centre trial of total ankle replacement versus ankle arthrodesis in the treatment of patients with end stage ankle osteoarthritis (TARVA): statistical analysis plan. Trials. 2020; 21(1):197. Doi: 10.1186/s13063-019-3973-4.

28. Norvell DC, Ledoux WR, Shofer JB, Hansen ST, Davitt J, et al. Effectiveness and safety of ankle arthrodesis versus arthroplasty: a prospective multicentre study. J Bone Joint Surg Am. 2019;101(16):1485-94.
29. Ogilvie-Harris DJD, Mahomed NN, Demazière AA. Anterior impingement of the ankle treated by arthroscopic removal of bony spurs. J Bone Joint Surg Br. 1993;75:437-40.
30. Pagenstert GI, Hintermann B, Barg A, Leumann A, Valderrabano V. Realignment surgery as alternative treatment of varus and valgus ankle osteoarthritis. Clin Orthop Relat Res. 2007;462:156-68.
31. Reginster J-Y, Neuprez A, Lecart M-P, Sarlet N, Bruyere O. Role of glucosamine in the treatment for osteoarthritis. Rheumatol Int. 2012;32:2959-67.
32. Rouhani H, Crevoisier X, Favre J, Aminian K. Outcome evaluation of ankle osteoarthritis treatments: Plantar pressure analysis during relatively long-distance walking. JCLB. 2011;26:397-404.
33. Rüedi T. Fractures of the lower end of the tibia into the ankle joint: results 9 years after open reduction and internal fixation. Injury. 1973;5:130-4.
34. Saltzman CL, el-Khoury GY. The hindfoot alignment view. Foot Ankle Int. 1995;16(9): 572-6.
35. Saltzman CL, Hillis SL, Stolley MP, Anderson DD, Amendola A. Motion versus fixed distraction of the joint in the treatment of ankle osteoarthritis: a prospective randomized controlled trial. J Bone Joint Surg Am. 2012;94:961-70.
36. Sealey RJ, Myerson MS, Molloy A, Gamba C, Jeng C, Kalesan B. Sagittal plane motion of the hindfoot following ankle arthrodesis: a prospective analysis. Foot Ankle Int. 2009; 30:187-96.
37. Thomas RH, Daniels TR. Ankle arthritis. J Bone Joint Surg Am. 2003;85-A:923-36.
38. Tulner S, Klinkenbijl M, Albers G. Revision arthrodesis of the ankle. Acta Orthop. 2011;82:250-2.

34. Hallux Valgus

Raja TV, Ajay SS, Madhan Jeyaraman

INTRODUCTION

- It is defined the deformity as an abduction contracture in which the great toe is turned away from the mid-line of the body. This was first defined by Carl Hueterto.
- The adjective valgus implies a static deformity and should not be used interchangeably with abductus which refers to movement caused by muscle function.
- Hallux valgus (lateral deviation of the great toe) is a complicated first-ray deformity that usually includes deformity and symptoms in the smaller toes. It is distinguished by lateral deviation of the great toe and medial deviation of the first metatarsal, as well as static subluxation of the metatarsophalangeal (MTP) joint.
- It is known as a bunion deformity because of the predominant prominence, which is derived from the Latin word "BUNIO," which means "turnip." It is a general term for an enlargement of the MTP joint, such as in cases of hallux valgus, gouty arthropathy, ganglion, or an enlarged bursa overlying the MTP joint.
- Patients often confuse the medial prominence of hallux valgus with the dorsal osteophyte of hallux rigidus and may refer to both disorders as "bunions."
- In most cases, the development of hallux valgus can be directly related to constrictive shoe wear.
- The narrow toe box and raised heel of modern women's shoe wear in particular appear to be the primary culprits in the development of the problem.
- Hallux valgus involves lateral deviation of the hallux at the first MTP joint.
- The toe rotates into pronation along with lateral deviation.
- The nail turns to face toward the instep **(Fig. 1)**.
- As these deformities develop, the lateral structures become contracted and the medial structures become attenuated.
- The first metatarsal deviates to the medial side in the majority of instances, resulting in a deformity known as metatarsus primus varus. During this time, the length of the intermetatarsal ligament connecting the second metatarsal head to the lateral sesamoid stays constant. As a result, the sesamoids maintain their original location in relation to the rest of the foot, and the first metatarsal head subluxate away from them.

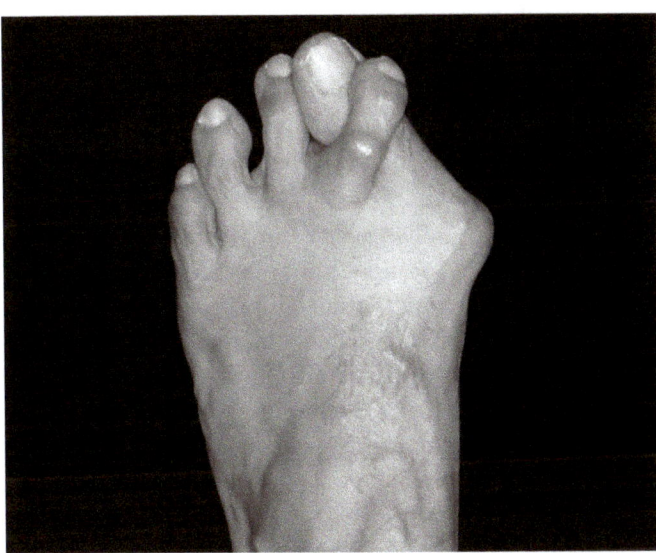

Fig. 1: Hallux valgus with hammer toe deformity.

ETIOLOGY/RISK FACTORS

Extrinsic factors: High-heeled shoes. Narrow toe box and occupational factors.

Intrinsic factors:
- Heredity—60–90%
- Pes planus
- Hypermobility of metatarsocuneiform joint
- Medial slanted metatarsocuneiform joint
- Hyperpronated 1st ray
- Ligamentous laxity
- Pronation of hind foot
- Achilles contracture
- Metatarsus primus varus
- Neuromuscular disorders like cerebrovascular accidents
- Systemic conditions like rheumatoid arthritis
- Female preponderance
- *Age*: 4th-6th decade
- *Miscellaneous factors*: 2nd toe amputation; cystic degeneration of medial capsule.

PATHOANATOMY

- The angle between the first and second metatarsals must be greater than 8-9° to be deemed normal. The valgus angle of the first metatarsophalangeal joint is more than the typical top limits of 15-20°. Pronation of the great toe occurs when the valgus angle of the first metatarsophalangeal joint surpasses 30-35°. The abductor hallucis extends its plantar ward movement **(Fig. 2)**.
- The medial capsular ligament, with its capsule-sesamoid part (inserting to the base of the proximal phalanx) and capsule-phalangeal portion (inserting to the base of the proximal phalanx) is the only restraining medial structure (inserting to the plantar plate). The deep transverse intermetatarsal ligament extends between the plantar plates at the metatarsophalangeal joints, but does not enter into the bone on the metatarsal heads' neighboring sides.
- The great toe is pulled deeper into valgus by the adductor hallucis, which is now unopposed by the abductor hallucis, stretching the medial capsular ligament and weakening it, enabling the metatarsal head to migrate medially from the sesamoids. Furthermore, the flexor hallucis longus, flexor hallucis brevis, adductor hallucis, and extensor hallucis longus enhance the valgus moment at the metatarsophalangeal joint, causing the first ray to bend even further.
- Because of abutment from the tibial sesamoid, the sesamoid ridge on the plantar surface of the first metatarsal head (the crista) flattens. The fibular sesamoid will be displaced entirely or partially into the intermetatarsal area as a result of the bony ridge removal. Because the patient is putting more weight on the lesser metatarsal heads and less on the first ray, secondary diseases such as transfer metatarsalgia, callosities, and stress fractures of a companion metatarsal are more likely.

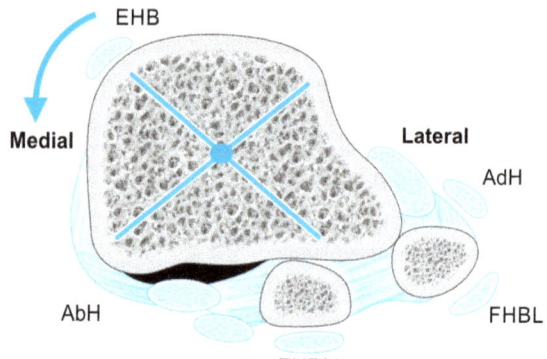

Fig. 2: Pathoanatomy of hallux valgus. (AbH: abductor hallucis; AdH: adductor hallucis; EHB: extensor hallucis brevis; FHBL: flexor hallucis brevis lateral; FHBM: flexor hallucis brevis medial)

- The great toe's valgus posture causes a hammer toe-like deformity in the second toe, which is a severe crossover toe deformity in the second toe coupled with severe hallux valgus of the first ray. The major complaint in this case is discomfort beneath the second metatarsal head, not significant hallux valgus deformity. Splaying of the forefoot causes difficulties wearing shoes with a tight toe box, as well as secondary alterations such corns and bursal hypertrophy on the medial face of the first MTP joint, which can lead to bunion development. Osteoarthritis of the metatarsophalangeal joints is also a result of this.
- Entire spectrum of an established hallux valgus is as follows:
  - Varus deformity of the first metatarsal
  - Valgus of the great toe
  - Bunion formation
  - Arthritis of the first metatarsophalangeal joint
  - Hammer toe of one or more toes
  - Corns, calluses, metatarsalgia.
- Without searching for all of these main and secondary pathological alterations caused by hallux valgus, a foot examination is inadequate, and the patient must be informed about the surgical strategy and prognosis based on these findings.

SIGNS AND SYMPTOMS

- These can range from being asymptomatic to severe
- *Pain*: The primary symptom being PAIN over the medial eminence
- Pressure from footwear is the most frequent cause of this discomfort
- Deformity
- Tenderness
- Aesthetic or cosmetic concerns
- Ligamentous laxity.

DIFFERENTIAL DIAGNOSIS

Gout: Men 40-70 years with acute mono-arthritis of 1st MTP joint, skin may peel over toe and serum uric acid levels elevated in 75% of patient.

Lab findings include monosodium urate crystals in synovial fluid.

Radiographic changes appear after 7-10 years of first episode.

Septic arthritis: Red hot swollen joint with synovial fluid showing leukocytes. Gram stain may be positive, joint fluid/blood culture may be positive.

Osteoarthritis: Affects multiple MTP joints. MTP joints are enlarged but not warm or tender along with painful passive range of motion and exostosis. X-rays show interphalangeal joint space reduction.

Hallux rigidus: Clinically no motion at MTP joint, no acute tenderness and with a dorsal bunion with marked bony overgrowth and ankylosis on X-ray with hallux rigidus.

Hallux valgus with rheumatoid arthritis: Generally symmetrical fibular deviation of all digits may be more severe than isolated hallux valgus, loss of passive range of motion clinically Stage 4 hallux valgus with completely subluxated joint on X-ray, severe deformity with ankylosis demonstrated on X-ray.

Hallux valgus with neuromuscular disease: General presentation of hallux valgus more severe with signs of systemic neuromuscular disease such as spasticity.

■ PHYSICAL EXAMINATION

- With the patient standing and sitting, the foot is examined for:
    - Sites of pain
    - Severity of the hallux valgus deformity
    - Pronation of the great toe
    - *Skin*: For callosity and areas of redness.
- Motion of 1st MTP joint:
    - Range of motion for checking severity of restriction,
    - Pain with or without crepitus.
- *Metatarsocuneiform joint for hypermobility*: Examiner grasps the first metatarsal with the thumb and index finger and pushes it in a plantar lateral to dorsomedial direction and if there is movement >9 mm it represents hypermobility.
- Pes planus deformity, Achilles tendon contractures.
- Deformities of lesser toes.
- *Mobility and structure of foot in general*: Metatarsalgia of other MTP joints.
- Corns, calluses, warts, interdigital neuromas, plantar keratosis.
- Gait analysis.
- Neurovascular status of the limb.

■ MANAGEMENT

Radiographic Assessment

- Radiographs required to evaluate the deformity and help plan the management includes:
    - Weight-bearing radiographs of the foot in anterior-posterior oblique views.
    - Nonweight bearing view of axial or sesamoid view.
- Following information should be checked from the above mentioned radiographs:
    - Evaluate for bone and joint deformity
    - Length and shape of 1st metatarsal
    - The relative lengths of the first and second metatarsals
    - The presence or absence of deformity in the hallux
    - The presence or absence of arthritis at the first MTP or in the midfoot
    - The presence or absence of instability at the first metatarsocuneiform joint
    - Forefoot alignment is evaluated for metatarsus adductus
    - The hallux valgus angle
    - *The intermetatarsal angle*: Formed between the axis of the first and second metatarsals on the AP radiograph.
- The distal metatarsal articular angle: Angle formed between the alignment of the first metatarsal and the margins of the joint surface of the first MTP.
- Joint congruency (congruent vs. incongruent joint).

Hallux Valgus Angle

- Normal <15
- Mild <20
- Moderate 20–40
- Severe >40
- Markers placed in the mid-diaphyseal region of the proximal phalanx and the first metatarsal equidistant from the medial and lateral cortices **(Fig. 3)**
- The longitudinal axis of the proximal phalanx is determined by an axis drawn though points A and B. The longitudinal axis of the first metatarsal is determined by a line drawn through points C and D. Hallux valgus angle is formed by the intersection of these above mentioned lines, AB and CD.

First/Second Intermetatarsal Angle

First-second intermetatarsal angle (IMA) is formed by the intersection of axes of the diaphysis of the first (AB) and the second (CD) metatarsal shafts **(Fig. 4)**.

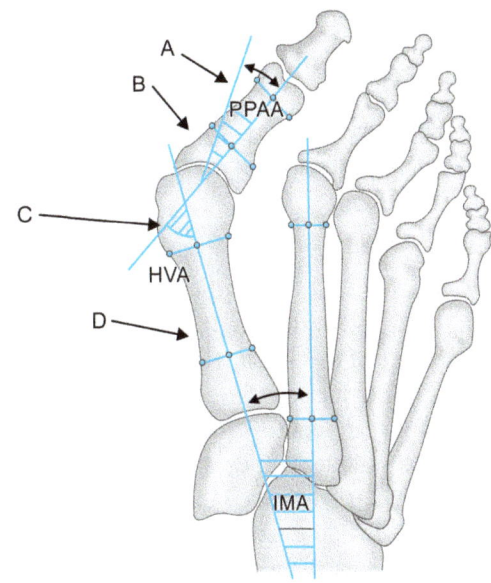

Fig. 3: Hallux valgus angle.

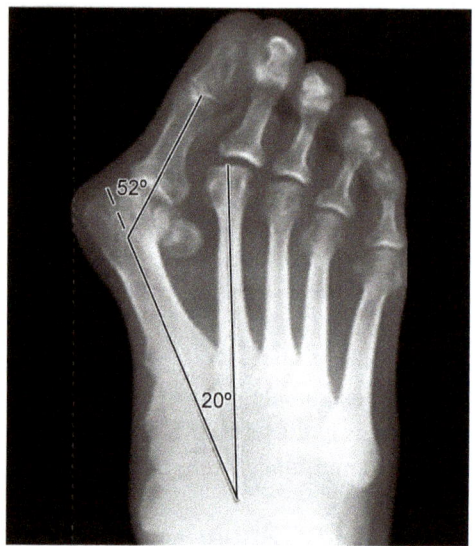
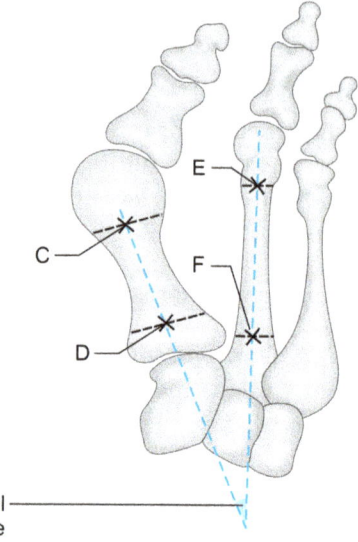

Fig. 4: Intermetatarsal angle.

Distal Metatarsal Articular Angle

- Distal metatarsal articular angle (DMAA) defines the angle formed by the articular surface of the distal first metatarsal with the longitudinal axis of the first metatarsal **(Fig. 5)**.
- Markers for the line are placed on the most medial and lateral extent of the distal metatarsal articular surface (X/Y). Line drawn to connect these two points defines the slope of the articular surface.
- Another line through points W and Z is drawn perpendicular to the first line X'Y'. A third line through points C and D defines the longitudinal axis of the first metatarsal.
- The angle subtended by the perpendicular line (W, Z) and the longitudinal axis of the first metatarsal (C, D) defines the DMAA. The normal limits of this slope subtend an angle which is less than 6°.

Hallux Interphalangeal Angle

This is the angle formed by the long axis of the proximal phalanx and the distal phalanx of the great toe.

Subluxed versus Congruent Joint

- Hallux valgus deformity with subluxation (noncongruent joint) characterized by the in-congruent alignment of the articular surface of the proximal phalanx with respect to the distal articular surface of the distal first metatarsal.
- *Hallux valgus deformity with a nonsubluxated (congruent)*: Characterized by congruent inclination of the distal articular surface of the first metatarsal with normal alignment of the articular surfaces.
- Points X and Y mark the medial and lateral limits of the articular surface of the proximal phalanx.

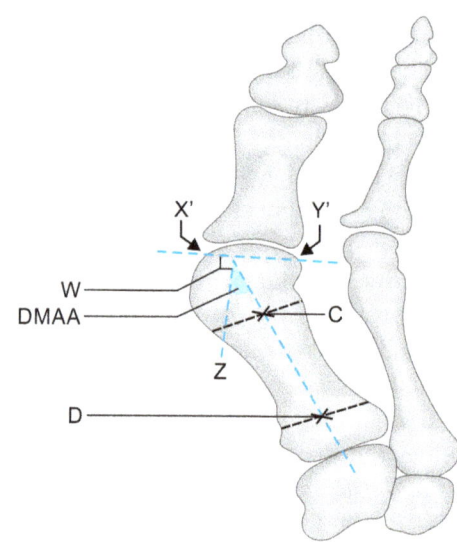

Fig. 5: Distal metatarsal articular angle (DMMA).

Points X' and Y' mark the medial and lateral limits of the metatarsal articular surface. Note the lateral slope of the distal metatarsal articular surface.

Classification

Classification of severity of hallux valgus deformities according to angle measurements are given in **Table 1**.

Treatment

- Conservative management
- Surgical management

Conservative Management (Figs. 6A to F)

- *Foot wear modification*: This is the first line of treatment which includes following modifications and their benefits:

TABLE 1: Classification of severity of hallux valgus.

Classification	Normal	Mild	Moderate	Severe
Hallux valgus angle	<15	<20	20–40	>40
1–2 intermetatarsal angle	<9	<11	12–15	>16
Subluxation of lateral sesamoid	Nil or minimal	<50%	50–75%	>75%

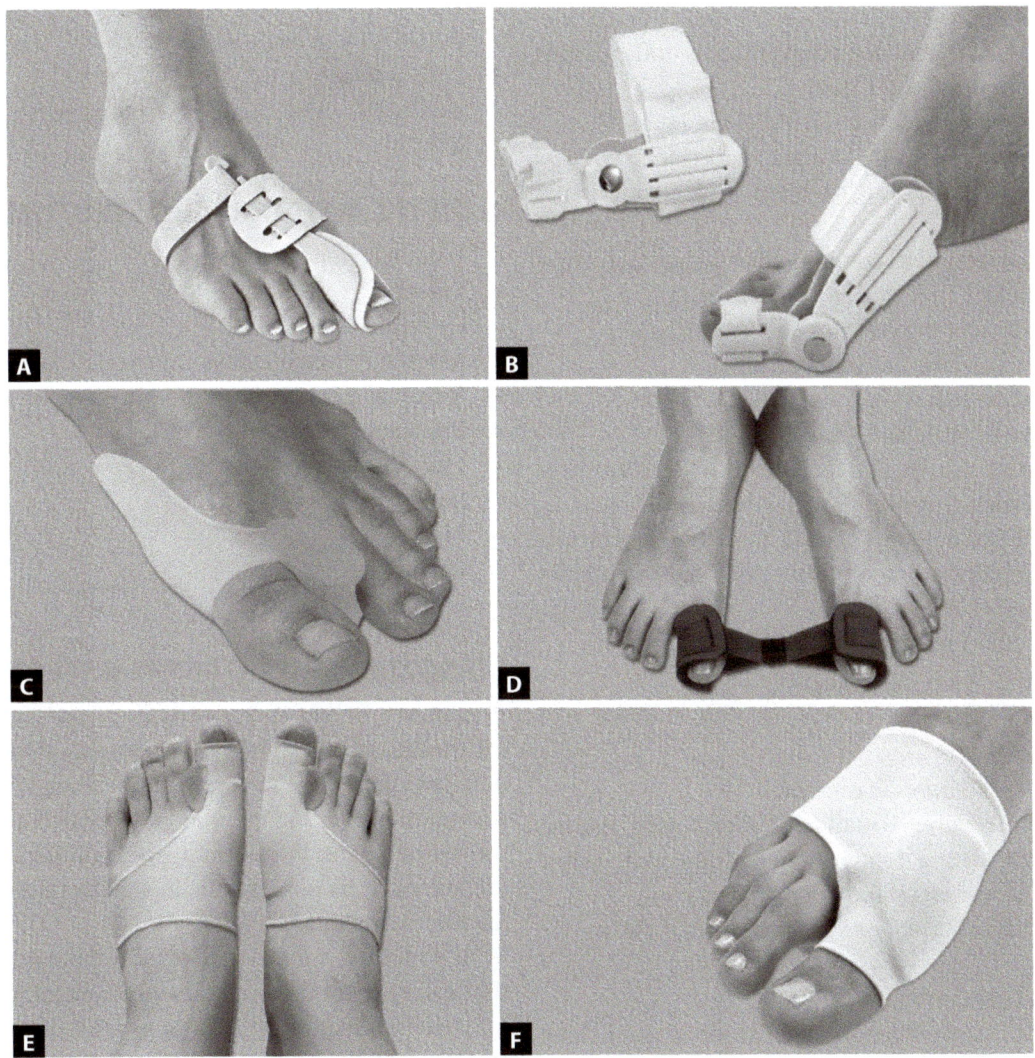

Figs. 6A to F: Hallux valgus: Conservative treatment. (A and B) Night splint Bunion day and night splint; (C) Toe spacer; (D) Toe straightening belt; (E) Toe spacers; (F) Bunion protective pad.

- Widening of toe box decrease lateral deviation of great toe thus decreasing the pressure and inflammation in the joint
- Decreasing the heel height prevents forward sliding of the foot
- Enhanced medial arch support reduces the effects of pes planus.
• TA stretching exercises and TA lengthening.
• Thermoplastic night splints.
• *Bunion aids and strapping*:
  - Bunion pads which are doughnut shapes help to offload the tender inflamed bunion
  - Strapping and night splints have limited positive effects on the bunion.
• Chiropody helps secondary changes such as callosities and skin compromise to reduce.
• Podiatry helps in restructuring the normal foot biomechanics and hence reduces further effects.

Surgical Management

Indications

• Failure of nonoperative modalities:
  - Persistent symptoms for 2 or more years

- Deformity progression
- Should not be done only for cosmetic concerns.

Goals:
- Correction of pathologic elements and yet maintain biomechanically functional forefoot:
  - Correction of the IMT and HV angles.
  - Creation of a congruent 1st MTPJ with sesamoid realignment.
  - Resection of the medial prominence is done parallel and flush with the MT shaft.
  - Retention of function and ROM of the 1st MTPJ.
  - Maintenance of normal weight bearing mechanics.
- To obtain a plantigrade painless and cosmetically acceptable foot.

The following structural components must be taken into consideration before choosing any procedure:
- Valgus deviation of the great toe (hallux valgus)
- Varus deviation of the first metatarsal
- Pronation of the hallux, first metatarsal, or both
- Hallux valgus interphalangeus
- Arthritis and limitation of motion of the first metatarsophalangeal joint
- Length of the first metatarsal relative to lesser metatarsals
- Excessive mobility or obliquity of the first metatarsomedial cuneiform joint
- The medial eminence (bunion)
- The location of the sesamoid apparatus
- Intrinsic and extrinsic muscle-tendon balance and synchrony.

Various surgical procedures in general:
- *Soft tissue procedures:* Usually done for a mild disease especially in young females and along with other procedures, never as a standalone procedure.
- *Distal metatarsal osteotomies:* Procedure of choice for mild disease.
- Proximal MT osteotomies.
- *Combined MT osteotomies:* Done for moderate pathology in MTP joint.
- Phalangeal osteotomies.
- *Fusion procedures/joint arthrodesis:* Indicated in severe disease with progressing degenerative changes.
- *Metatarsophalangeal joint resection arthroplasty:* Indicated in a low functional demand elderly population only.

SOFT TISSUE PROCEDURES
Modified McBride Procedure

Modified procedure includes: Release of transverse metatarsal ligament, adductor hallucis muscle, and the lateral capsule. Bony procedure involves resection of the medial eminence and medially the capsule is plicated. Modification involves retaining the lateral sesamoid which helps in preventing varus deformity common after the original McBride bunionectomy. This procedure is best performed on an incongruent joint as it attempts to realign the MTP joint.

Indications
- History of conservative management initially being failed. 30- to 50-year-old females with clinical symptoms
- HVA — 15–25°
- IMA — less than 13°
- HVI — less than 15°
- No degenerative changes in the 1st metatarsophalangeal joint.

DISTAL METATARSAL OSTEOTOMIES
- Mitchell (step cut osteotomy)
- Wilson
- Chevron
- Modified Chevron **(Figs. 7A to D)**
- Proximal crescentic
- Proximal Chevron
- Opening wedge
- Ludloff
- Mau
- Closing wedge
- Scarf.

PROXIMAL METATARSAL OSTEOTOMIES

If primary or secondary varus of the first metatarsal contributes to the hallux valgus complex, treatment near the deformity's origin is recommended, along with a soft-tissue operation at the first metatarsophalangeal joint to address the hallux valgus. Furthermore, a slight displacement of the metatarsal at its base results in significant improvement at the metatarsal's distal end.

A proximal metatarsal osteotomy and a distal soft-tissue surgery at the metatarsophalangeal joint may assist a patient with substantial degenerative arthritis in the first metatarsophalangeal joint with hallux valgus of more than 35° and an intermetatarsal angle of more than 10°.

A patient with significant degenerative arthritis in the first metatarsophalangeal joint with a hallux valgus of more than 35° and an intermetatarsal angle of more than 10° may benefit from a proximal metatarsal osteotomy and distal soft-tissue surgery at the metatarsophalangeal joint.

An osteotomy at the base of the metatarsal has the following advantages:
- Early stability (3–5 weeks) and union are aided by cancellous bone and large contact surfaces of the fragments (6–8 weeks). Small modifications in position at the osteotomy result in effective treatment of the symptoms at the distal end of the metatarsal.

Unless the surgeon chooses a procedure that purposely shortens the metatarsal, the metatarsal is reduced

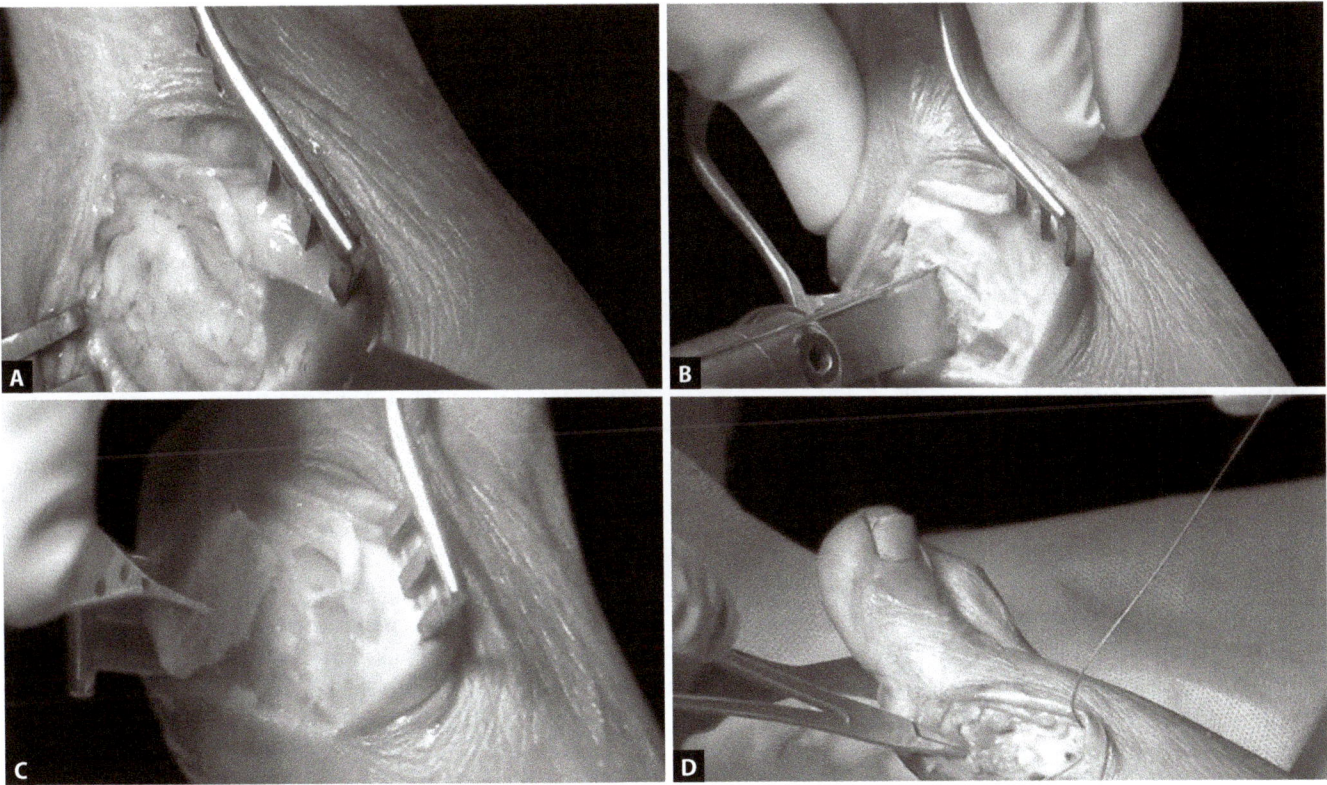

Figs. 7A to D: Steps of modified Chevron osteotomy.

minimally, if at all (the breadth of the osteotomy cut is more than compensated for by the "straightening of the bone").

- It is possible to rectify large angles between the first and second metatarsals. Load bearing by the second metatarsal is reduced by slightly tilting the distal fragment plantarward, lowering the risk of transfer metatarsalgia. Narrowing the forefoot increases the variety of footwear that can be worn and improves the aesthetics.

This type of osteotomy has the following disadvantages:

- It is necessary to dissect a large amount of soft tissue. Unless properly secured internally, the distal fragment tends to move dorsally or migrate medially to its original position. Cast immobilization is frequently needed after this procedure. If the basilar osteotomy is done dorsally, three incisions are required. With regional block anesthesia, the procedure is more difficult to complete.
- The early postosteotomy convalescence is frequently marked by more pain, edema, and immobility than the postosteotomy convalescence. If the fragment displaces or migrates, the second ray may become overloaded.

Currently, the most frequently used proximal metatarsal osteotomies are given in **Table 2**.

Complications

- Roughing of the metatarsal with loss of height resulting in functional malunion with elevation of the first ray (35%)
- Delayed union (5%)

TABLE 2: Most frequently used proximal metatarsal osteotomies.

Type of osteotomy	Approach	Method of IMA correction
Proximal crescentic	Dorsal	Rotation
Proximal Chevron	Medial translational	Rotation
Opening wedge	Medial	Rotation
Ludloff	Medial	Rotation
Mau	Medial	Rotation
Closing wedge	Dorsal	Rotation
Scarf	Medial translational	Rotation

- Rotational malunion (30%)
- Proximal fracture (10%)
- Infection (5%)
- Early recurrence of deformity
- Transfer metatarsalgia
- Osteonecrosis of the first metatarsal head
- Prominent screw causing irritation
- Screw back-out
- Neuralgia.

PROXIMAL PHALANGEAL OSTEOTOMY OR AKIN OSTEOTOMY

The hallux valgus interphalangeus deformity is the most common reason for using this technique. Usually used in conjunction with 1st MT osteotomies for more congruent joint repair. A medial closing-wedge phalangeal osteotomy is performed after medial eminence excision and adductor tenotomy from the base of the proximal phalanx, and the osteotomy is closed and stabilized with the help of two K wires run from distal to proximal through the phalanges and osteotomy site.

The patient profile for the procedure if used alone is as follows:
- Patient older than 55 years
- Excessive hallux valgus interphalangeus (in patient of any age)
- Hallux valgus of no more than 25°
- Intermetatarsal angle of less than 13°
- Good metatarsophalangeal joint motion without localized joint pain.

Contraindications for the procedure are the following:
- Rheumatoid arthritis
- Moderate-to-severe osteoarthritis at the metatarsophalangeal joint
- Intermetatarsal angle more than 13°
- Hallux valgus angle more than 30°
- Subluxation laterally of the tibial sesamoid more than 50% of its width
- Open physis of the proximal phalanx.

COMBINED SOFT-TISSUE AND BONY PROCEDURES

- Keller resection arthroplasty
- Arthrodesis of the first metatarsophalangeal joint
- Arthrodesis with small plate fixation/low-profile contoured dorsal plate and compression screw fixation
- Truncated cone arthrodesis
- Ball and socket arthrodesis (molded arthrodesis)
- Arthrodesis of the first metatarsocuneiform articulation (lapidus procedure).

FURTHER READING

1. Austin DW, Leventen EO. A new osteotomy for hallux valgus: a horizontally directed "V" displacement osteotomy of the metatarsal head for hallux valgus and primus varus. Clin Orthop Relat Res. 1981;157:25-30.
2. Coetzee JC, Wickum D. The Lapidus procedure: a prospective cohort outcome study. Foot Ankle Int. 2004;25:526-31.
3. Coughlin M, Freund E, Roger A. Mann Award: the reliability of angular measurements in hallux valgus deformities. Foot Ankle Int. 2001;22:369-79.
4. Coughlin M, Saltzman C, Anderson R. Mann's Surgery of the Foot and Ankle, 9th edition. Philadelphia: Saunders; 2014.
5. Coughlin MJ, Jones CP. Hallux valgus and first ray mobility. A prospective study. J Bone Joint Surg. 2007;89-A:1887-98.
6. Deenik A, van Mameren H, de Visser E, de Waal Malefijt M, Draijer F, de Bie R. Equivalent correction in Scarf and Chevron osteotomy in moderate and severe hallux valgus: a randomized controlled trial. Foot Ankle Int. 2008;29:1209-15.
7. Durman DC. Metatarsus primus varus and hallux valgus. AMA Arch Surg. 1957; 74:128-35.
8. Easley ME, Trnka HJ. Current concepts review: hallux valgus part 1: pathomechanics, clinical assessment, and nonoperative management. Foot Ankle Int. 2007;28:654-9.
9. Easley ME, Trnka HJ. Current concepts review: hallux valgus part II: operative treatment. Foot Ankle Int. 2007;28:748-58.
10. Fraissler L, Konrads C, Hoberg M, Rudert M, Walcher M. Treatment of hallux valgus deformity. EFORT Open Rev. 2016;1(8):295-302.
11. Grebing BR, Coughlin MJ. The effect of ankle position on the exam for first ray mobility. Foot Ankle Int. 2004;25:467-75.
12. Hardy RH, Clapham JCR. Observations on hallux valgus. J Bone Joint Surg. 1951; 33-B:376-91.
13. Helmy N, Vienne P, Von Campe A, Espinosa N. Treatment of hallux valgus deformity: preliminary results with a modified distal metatarsal osteotomy. Acta Orthop Belg. 2009;75: 661-70.
14. Klaue K. Hallux valgus and hypermobility of the first ray-causal treatment using tarso-metatarsal reorientation arthrodesis. Ther Umsch. 1991;48:817-23.
15. Lee WC, Kim YM. Correction of hallux valgus using lateral soft-tissue release and proximal Chevron osteotomy through a medial incision. J Bone Joint Surg. 2007;89-A(Suppl 3):82-9.
16. Mann RA, Pfeffinger L. Hallux valgus repair. DuVries modified McBride procedure. Clin Orthop Relat Res. 1991;272:213-18.
17. Mann RA. Bunion surgery: decision-making. Orthopedics. 1990;13:951-7.
18. Park YB, Lee KB, Kim SK, Seon JK, Lee JY. Comparison of distal soft-tissue procedures combined with a distal Chevron osteotomy for moderate to severe hallux valgus: first webspace versus transarticular approach. J Bone Joint Surg Am. 2013;95-A:e158.
19. Pfeffinger LL. The modified McBride procedure. Orthopedics. 1990;13:979-84.
20. Richardson EG, Graves SC, McClure JT, Boone RT. First metatarsal head-shaft angle: a method of determination. Foot Ankle Int. 1993;14:181-5.
21. Saltzman CL, Brandser EA, Berbaum KS, DeGnore L, Holmes JR, Katcherian DA, et al. Reliability of standard foot radiographic measurements. Foot Ankle Int. 1994;15:661-5.
22. Stamatis ED, Huber MH, Myerson MS. Transarticular distal soft-tissue release with an arthroscopic blade for hallux valgus correction. Foot Ankle Int. 2004;25:13-8.
23. Steel MW, Johnson KA, DeWitz MA, Ilstrup DM. Radiographic measurements of the normal adult foot. Foot Ankle Int. 1980;1:151-8.
24. Trnka HJ, Hofstaetter S. The Chevron osteotomy for correction of hallux valgus. Interact Surg. 2007;2:52-61.
25. Voellmicke KV, Deland JT. Manual examination technique to assess dorsal instability of the first ray. Foot Ankle Int. 2002;23:1040-1.
26. Wu KPH, Chen CK, Lin SC, Pei YC, Lin RH, Tsai WC, et al. Botulinum toxin type A injections for patients with painful hallux valgus: a double-blind, randomized controlled study. Clin Neurol Neurosurg. 2015;129(Suppl):S58-62.

SECTION 9

Regenerative Science in Orthopedic Rheumatology

- **Introduction to Stem Cells**
  Naveen Jeyaraman, Rashmi Jain, Arunabh Arora

- **Translational Products of Adipose Tissue-derived Mesenchymal Stem Cells: Bench to Bedside Applications**
  Madhan Jeyaraman, Rajni Ranjan, Amrit Kumar Singh

- **Ethical Consideration in Stem Cell Research**
  Manish Khanna, Shashank Tiwari

- **Cellular Therapy in Rheumatoid Arthritis**
  Sathish Muthu, Madhan Jeyaraman, Manish Khanna

- **Cytotherapy in Osteoarthritic Knee**
  Madhan Jeyaraman, Sathish Muthu, Naveen Jeyaraman

- **Promising Role of Regenerative Therapy in AVN and Sports Injuries: An Update**
  Manish Khanna, Madhan Jeyaraman, Arun Gulati

- **Regenerative Medicine in Neurological Disorders: Current Understanding**
  Shilpa Sharma, Prajwal GS, Shivaraj B

- **Ulcers and Regenerative Medicine**
  Sribatsa Kumar Mohapatra, Dushyant Chaudhary, Shivakumar Bingi

35 Introduction to Stem Cells

Naveen Jeyaraman, Rashmi Jain, Arunabh Arora

INTRODUCTION

Stem cells are regarded as unspecialized cells which are capable of turning into specialized ones with each directed to execute specific function. The name "*stem cell*" denotes stemness of multiplication. In simplified manner, stem cells are uncommitted provided these receive any signal of conversion into a specialized cell. Stem cells are earmarked to develop into a variety of cell types wherein enacting as a reservoir of our repair system. These are faceted with the ability to divide unlimited times for the purpose of replenishing the damaged or other cells. On division, each new cell either remains as a stem cell or embraces the caliber of aligning into a new cell type dedicated to render special functions.

The history of stem cell research dates back to mid-1800s period wherein it was discovered that some cells could generate other cells. During early period of 1900s, in fact there was the discovery of the first real stem cells capable of producing blood cells. Since then the platform of stem cell research has opened the doors for medical wonders. The first successful bone marrow transplant discovered in human umbilical cord blood in 1968 has been marked as the revolutionary period in the history of medical sciences. The insight into the serial studies by Martin J Evans and Gail Martin on the embryonic stem cells (ESCs) derived from the inner cell mass (ICM) of mouse blastocysts who coined the term ESC to these cells provided another breakthrough in 1981 in this domain. With advancing years, research work contributed to fit in pieces of stem cell jigsaw. In the year 1997, leukemia was presented as an example of stem cell derived cancer. Later in 1998, James Thomson and coworkers provided the direction for future research in the field of stem cell research through their promising work which included derivation of the first human embryonic stem cell line from the ICM of human blastocysts. Since then the idea of stem cell-based therapies have been subjected to rigorous reformations.

Presently, pioneers are embroiled in a controversy over the use of human ESCs for research. The looming issues involving ethical consideration and technical difficulties in work-up with ESCs have directed the interests of few researchers towards other regenerative avenues. For the same, Japanese researchers Takahashi and Yamanaka published a report of induced pluripotent stem cells (iPSCs) from adult mouse fibroblasts in the year of 2006. In the year of 2012, the Nobel Prize in Physiology or Medicine 2012 was awarded jointly to Sir John B Gurdon and Shinya Yamanaka "for the discovery that mature cells can be reprogrammed to become pluripotent".

Due to recent advances in molecular and tissue engineering and regeneration, the researches on micromolecules have gained the utmost importance in the field of medical sciences. Stem cell offers a greater advantage of biological healing cascade without any significant morbidity to the individuals. The future relies on regenerative medicine called stem cells which has the scientific and ethical controversies.

PROPERTIES

- *Self-renewal*:
  - *Obligatory asymmetric replication*: Renewal of stem cell from a daughter cell.
  - *Stochastic differentiation*: Differentiation of one daughter cell into stem cell and differentiation of one daughter cell to undergo mitosis to form another stem cell.
- *Differentiation*:

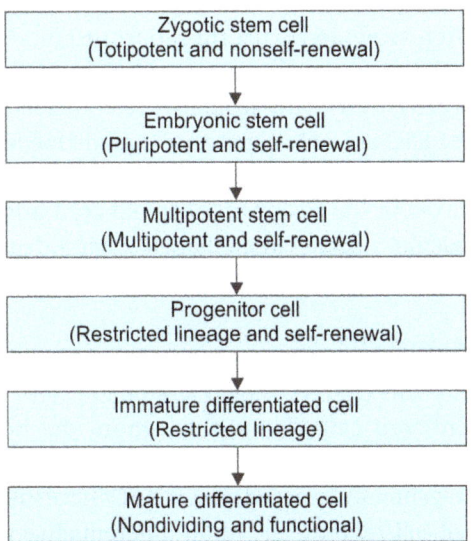

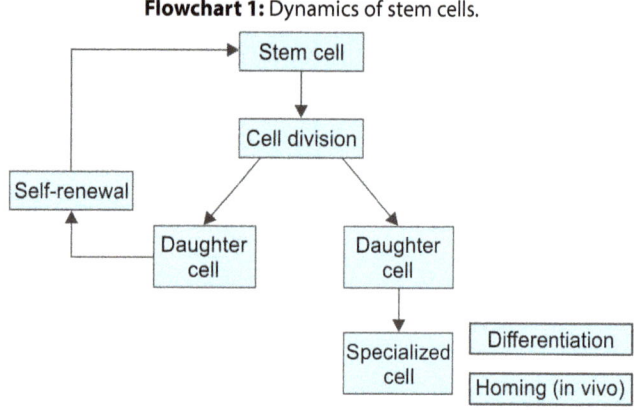

Flowchart 1: Dynamics of stem cells.

- *Homing*: In vivo ability of the stem cells to get along with the tissue or organ in accordance.

DYNAMICS

Dynamics of stem cells are given in **Flowchart 1**.

TYPES

Embryonic Stem Cells

Embryonic stem cells are pluripotent stem cells derived from the ICM of a blastocyst, an early stage preimplantation embryo. Human embryos reach the blastocyst stage 4–5 days postfertilization, at which time they consist of 50-150 cells. Isolating the embryoblast, or ICM results in destruction of the blastocyst, a process which raises ethical issues

Properties

Embryonic stem cells are pluripotent which are able to differentiate to generate primitive ectoderm, which ultimately differentiates during gastrulation into all derivatives of the three primary germ layers: (1) ectoderm, (2) endoderm, and (3) mesoderm. Under defined conditions, ESCs are capable of propagating indefinitely in an undifferentiated state. Conditions must either prevent the cells from clumping, or maintain an environment that supports an unspecialized state. When provided with the appropriate signals, to differentiate (presumably via the initial formation of precursor cells) into nearly all mature cell phenotypes.

Uses of ESC are—(1) regenerative medicine and tissue replacement after injury or disease; and (2) pluripotent stem cells are used in the treatment of spinal cord injuries, age related macular degeneration, diabetes, neurodegenerative disorders (such as Parkinson's disease), AIDS.

Adult Stem Cells

Adult stem cells (ASCs), known as somatic stem cells, are undifferentiated cells, found throughout the body after development, that multiply by cell division to replenish dying cells and regenerate damaged tissues. ASCs have the inherent property of self-renewal and multi-differentiative potential.

The signaling pathways present in ASC are: (1) NOTCH gene pathway for hematopoietic, neural and mammary stem cells, (2) Wnt signaling pathway for proposed stem cell regulators, and (3) TGF-β to regulate the stemness of both normal and cancer stem cells.

Types

- *Hematopoietic stem cell*: Bone marrow and umbilical cord
- *Mammary stem cell*: Luminal and myoepithelial cell types of the gland
- *Intestinal stem cells*: Crypts of Lieberkuhn
- Mesenchymal stem cells (MSCs)
- *Endothelial stem cell*: Cells that line blood vessels
- *Neural stem cell*: Present in the subventricular zone, which lines the lateral ventricles, and the dentate gyrus of the hippocampal formation
- Olfactory ASC
- *Ocular stem cells*: Found in the area of limbus
- *Neural crest stem cells*: Hair follicles which represents a remnant of stem cells of embryonic neural crest. These cells can generate neurons, Schwann cells, myofibroblast, chondrocytes and melanocytes
- *Testicular stem cells*: Spermatogonial progenitor cells found in the testicles of laboratory mice by scientists in Germany and the United States

Induced Pluripotent Stem Cells

Induced pluripotent stem cells are a type of pluripotent stem cell that can be generated directly from adult cells. iPSCs are typically derived by introducing products of specific sets of pluripotency-associated genes, or "reprogramming factors", into a given cell type. iPSC derivation is typically a slow and inefficient process, taking 1–2 weeks for mouse cells and 3–4 weeks for human cells, with efficiencies around 0.01–0.1%. Upon introduction of reprogramming factors, cells begin to form colonies that resemble pluripotent stem cells, which can be isolated based on their morphology, conditions that select for their growth, or through expression of surface markers or reporter genes. The challenges in iPSC are low efficiency, inadequate programming, genomic insertion and tumorigenic potential.

Mesenchymal Stem Cells

- *Location of MSC*: Bone marrow, cord cells, adipose tissue, molar teeth and amniotic fluid.
- *Salient features of MSC*:
  - No expression of HSC markers such as CD 34 and CD 14
  - Expression of matrix markers such as CD 44, CD 29 and CD 71
  - Expression of MSC markers, SH2 and SH105

- *Contains ECM components*: Collagen, proteoglycans and fibronectin
- Growth factors and cytokine receptors for TGFβ
- Antiproliferative activity to inhibit T-cell proliferation into tumorigenic cells
- MSC are multipotent progenitor cells and of stromal origin and may differentiate into a variety of tissues.
- Heterogeneous population of cells that proliferate in vitro as plastic-adherent cells, have fibroblast-like morphology, form colonies in vitro and can differentiate into bone, cartilage and fat cells.
- MSCs have been isolated from placenta, adipose tissue, lung, bone marrow and blood, Wharton's jelly from the umbilical cord and teeth.
- MSCs are attractive for clinical therapy due to their ability to differentiate, provide trophic support, and modulate innate immune response.
- These cells have the ability to differentiate into various cell types such as osteoblasts, chondroblasts, adipocytes, neuroectodermal cells, and hepatocytes.
- Bioactive mediators that favor local cell growth are also secreted by MSCs. Anti-inflammatory effects on the local microenvironment, which promote tissue healing, are also observed.
- The inflammatory response can be modulated by adipose-derived regenerative cells (ADRCs) including MSCs and regulatory T lymphocytes.
- The MSCs thus alter the outcome of the immune response by changing the cytokine secretion of dendritic and T-cell subsets. This results in a shift from a proinflammatory environment to an anti-inflammatory or tolerant cell environment.
- *Properties of MSC*:
  - Well characterized population of ASCs
  - Noncontroversial in terms of ethical issues
  - Diverse differentiation potential
  - Ease of growth in culture
  - Flexible propagation
  - Role in regulatory cells
  - Delivery of gene products
  - Favorable immunoprivilege
  - Allogeneic preparation

Methods of induction of cells:
- Isolate and culture donor cells
- Transduce stem cell-associated genes into the cells by viral vectors. Red cells indicate the cells expressing the exogenous genes
- Harvest and culture the cells according to ES cell culture, using mitotically inactivated feeder cells
- A small subset of the transfected cells become iPS cells and generate ES-like colonies

Immunomodulation of MSCs: The immunomodulatory properties of MSCs enhance their usage in clinical applications. The pathways by which the immunomodulatory mechanisms of MSCs are regulated through.

- *T-lymphocyte system*: MSCs mediate immunoregulation, either produced constitutively by MSCs or released following cross-talk with target cells. Nitric oxide and indoleamine 2,3-dioxygenase (IDO), which are only released by MSCs after triggering by IFNγ produced by target cells. IDO induces the depletion of tryptophan from the local environment, which is an essential amino acid for lymphocyte proliferation. MSC-derived IDO was reported to be required to inhibit the proliferation of IFNγ-producing TH1 cells and, together with prostaglandin E2 (PGE2), to block NK-cell activity.

  Activated CD8+ T lymphocyte by nitric oxide suppresses the proliferation of cytotoxic T cells, inhibits the production of INF-γ and TNF-α, and attenuates the cytotoxic effects. The activated CD4+ T lymphocyte by TGFβ, nitric oxide, hepatocyte growth factor, and PGE2 secreted by MSCs enhances lineage-specific differentiation and cellular proliferation. Upon which the immunomodulatory activities are enhanced via T helper 2 cells through increased IL-4 levels and T regulatory cell through increased TGFβ and suppressed via T helper 1 cell through increased INF-γ levels and T helper 17 cells through increased levels of IL-17A as shown in **Figure 1**.

- *B lymphocyte system*: MSCs enhance antibody production through the activation of B lymphocytes by soluble factors secreted by them.

- *NK cells*: MSCs inhibit cytokine production by NK cells when cultured or co-cultured in the media containing IL-2 or -15. MSCs hamper NK cell cytolytic effects through soluble factors such as HLA-G5, PGE2, IDO system, and also through downregulation of NK receptors like NKp30, NKp44, or NKG2D. Activated NK cells lyse MSCs. Upon exposure with INF-γ increases MHC-I expression on MSCs which conversely decreases the susceptibility to NK cell-mediated lysis as shown in **Figure 2**.

- *HLA-G5 system*: The production of soluble HLA-G5 by MSCs has been shown to suppress T-cell proliferation, as well as NK-cell and T-cell cytotoxicity, and to promote the generation of regulatory T cells.

PRINCIPAL MECHANISM OF ACTION OF STEM CELL

The basis of stem cell action is the formation of new tissues to promote repair and regeneration of damaged tissues thereby restoring normal function. This enables the implication of stem cells in degenerative diseases through remodeling of injured tissues. It was originally hypothesized that upon administration of stem cells it would migrate to sites of injury and will:

- Differentiate into replacement cell types
- Rescue damaged or dying cells through cell fusion

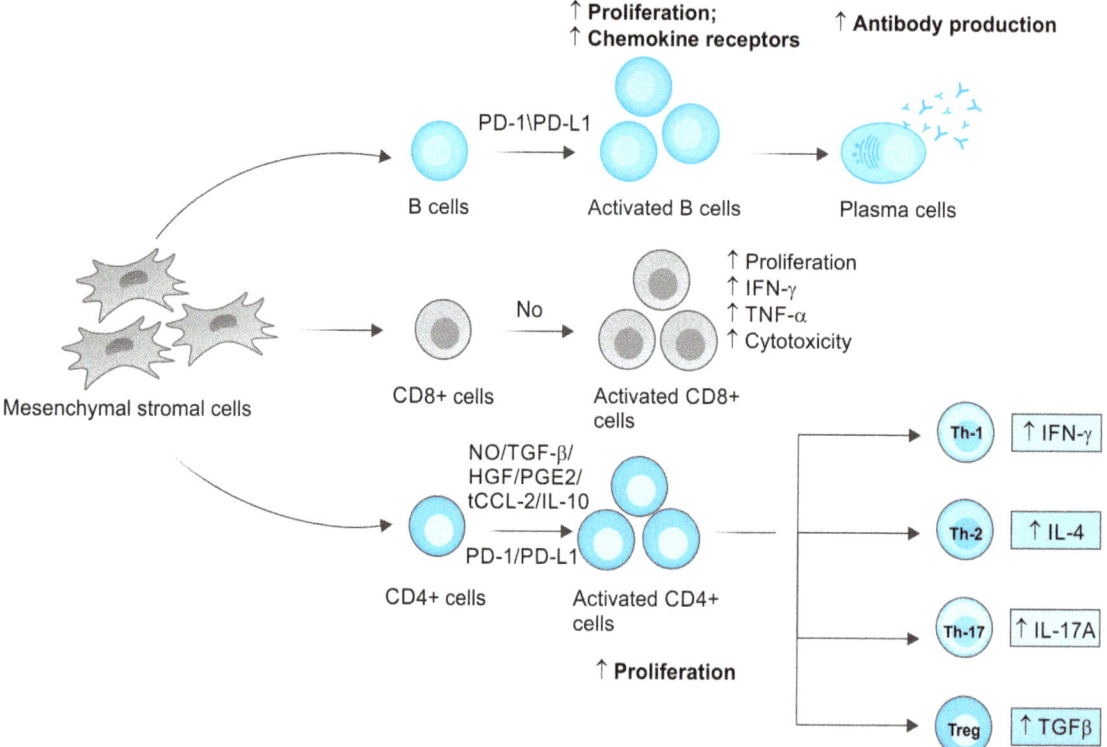

Fig. 1: Immunomodulatory effects of MSCs via T- and B-lymphocyte system. (IFN: interferon; HGF: hepatocyte growth factor; MSCs: mesenchymal stromal cells; PD: program death; PEG2: prostaglandin E2; tCCL: truncated chemokine ligand; TGF: transforming growth factor; TNF: tumor necrosis factor)

- Secrete paracrine factors such as growth factors, cytokines, and hormones
- Transfer of organelles (e.g., mitochondria) and/or molecules through tunneling nanotubes (TNTs)
- Mediate transfer of proteins/peptides, RNA, hormones, and/or chemicals by extracellular vesicles such as exosomes or microvesicles

These functions helps in increase in angiogenesis, plasticity, pluripotency, reduced inflammation, activation of neighboring resident stem cells, beneficial remodeling and this understanding on stem cells function will lead to the development of cell-based therapeutics and regenerative medicine.

▪ TECHNIQUES OF STEM CELL APPLICATION

- *Direct delivery*: The aspirated bone or bone marrow is directly inserted to the injury site. This facilitates direct delivery of stem cells to the injury site and hastens the healing cascade.
- *Cell-based delivery*: Bone marrow is aspirated, and the stem cells are isolated, cultured, and differentiated in laboratory media to increase their numbers before being applied to the injury site.

Application of Stem Cells in Orthopedics

- *Cartilage*: Cartilage is an avascular and aneural structure which has very limited potential for regeneration.

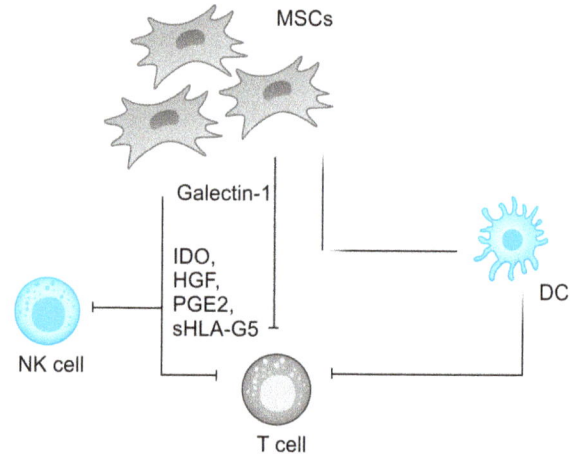

Fig. 2: Immunomodulatory effects of mesenchymal stromal cells (MSCs) via NK cell and HLA-G5 system. (DC: dendritic cell; HGF: hepatocyte growth factor; sHLA: soluble human leukocyte antigen; IDO: indoleamine 2,3-dioxygenase; NK cell: natural killer cell; PGE2: prostaglandin E2)

MSCs are used to provide a scaffold and meshwork to rejuvenate the focal chondral defect by autologous chondrocyte implantation (ACI). ACI is a two-stage procedure, with assessment of the chondral injury and biopsy to harvest 200–300 mg of healthy cartilage, followed by an enzymatic digestion and cell expansion in monolayer culture with cryopreservation of the cells which is further thawed and expanded to the target cell population. During the second stage, a biological reconstruction is performed to repair the articular cartilage defects to hasten the recovery with a successful functional outcome.

For osteoarthritis knee, the delivery of ultrasonicated adipose tissue offers a great advantage in proliferation of chondrocytes along with growth factors leads to better pain relief and functional improvement in quality of life. The dose of adipose tissue to be injected depends upon the grade of osteoarthritis and body mass index (BMI) of the individual.

- *Bone*: Bone morphogenetic proteins (BMPs) receptor 1B is required for mesenchymal stem cell to form osteoblastic lineage in bone defects. MSCs are used to enhance the regeneration of osseous defect in case of segmental bone loss, established nonunion and regeneration of physeal defect in children. The optimal loading of MSC on-to a carrier such as retroviral or adenoviral molecule offers a great advantage in minimally invasive procedure than conventional open surgical techniques. These MSC should possess the properties of osteoinduction, osteoconduction, osteointegration and mechanical stimulation to regenerate osseous defects. In segmental bone loss, calcium carbonate or hydroxyapatite scaffold is inserted upon which MSC are delivered to promote osteogenesis and osteointegration.
- *Tendons*: The chronic and overuse of tendons lead to degenerative conditions such as plantar fasciitis, interscapular fibrofasciitis, tennis elbow, golfer's elbow and tendinopathies. Such degenerated tendon has an inferior potential to regenerate.

  Autologous tenocyte injection is performed by a needle biopsy of healthy tendon which is subjected for isolation of cell of interest called tenocyte. Then tenocyte is amplified in cell cultured media and are injected into the injured or degenerated tendon.

  Tendon bioengineering using mesenchymal stem cells and a silk scaffold, allogenic adipose tissue derived mesenchymal stem cells and injection of microRNA with a loss of miR29 which results in increase in the production of type collagen 3.
- *Ligaments*: Sports injuries will result in concomitant injury to ligaments which have very poor potential to regenerate. MSC along with bone morphogenetic protein 2 and 7 and growth factors enhance neovascularization and regeneration of injured or degenerated ligaments. In anterior cruciate ligament (ACL) and meniscal rupture, intra-articular injection of MSCs with BMP 2 and 7 offers a biological healing of the ruptured ligaments. The scaffold based tissue bioengineering offers a greater advantage in ligamentous healing.
- *Spine*: MSC transplantation into the degenerated disc offers a potential to increase proteoglycans and glycosaminoglycans and induces degenerated spine and disk for regeneration and prevents vertebral collapse. The transported MSC maintain the viability of cells and involve in synthesizing micromolecules responsible for maintenance of disc shape.

  Mesenchymal stem cells have the potent ability to form neural tissue and offer a functional life to patients with traumatic paraplegia. The injection of MSC along with carrier molecule to the injured site allows optimized enhancement of remyelination of the neural tubes and axons thereby restoring the spinal reflex arcs.
- *Miscellaneous disorders*: SC has been tried in osteogenesis imperfecta where the defect lies in type 1 collagen synthesis. MSC are directed to increase the bone strength and integrity and produces type 1 collagen which prevents recurrent fractures with trivial trauma. MSC eliminates the need of immunosuppression in patients with osteogenesis imperfecta.

  In Duchene muscular dystrophy, the defect is due to mutation of *dystrophin gene* leads to the absence of dystrophin protein. MSC administration offers a greater advantage of contractile myotubules differentiation and regeneration of damaged myotubular system.

  In avascular necrosis of bone, the primary pathology is idiopathic. Some theories states avascular necrosis is due to increased intraosseous pressure. The aim of surgery is to decompress the intraosseous pressure by drilling multiple holes in the bone. Delivering of MSCs in the drill holes leads to osteointegration and osteogenesis which helps in remodeling of the bony structures.

DIRECTION FOR FUTURE

Stem cell optimizes the biological healing of diseases. The regenerative capacity of stem cells provides a pavement for clinicians to build up an organ of interest in vitro. Stem cells admixed with micromolecules such as growth factors, cytokines and BMPs provide a three dimensional structure and biomechanically, structurally and functionally compliant to the naïve cells of host origin. Further, research on the dosage and protocols on stem cell for various disorders to be formulated which leads to decreased morbidity and improve the functional quality of life.

FURTHER READING

1. Ahn JI, Terry Canale S, Butler SD, Hasty KA. Stem cell repair of physeal cartilage. J Orthop Res. 2004;22:1215-21.
2. Akiyama Y, Radtke C, Honmou O, Kocsis JD. Remyelination of the spinal cord following intravenous delivery of bone marrow cells. Glia. 2002;39:229-36.
3. Crevensten G, Walsh AJ, Ananthakrishnan D, Page P, Wahba GM, Lotz JC, et al. Intervertebral disc cell therapy for regeneration: mesenchymal stem cell implantation in rat intervertebral discs. Ann Biomed Eng. 2004;32:430-4.
4. Gussoni E, Soneoka Y, Strickland CD, Buzney EA, Khan MK, Flint AF, et al. Dystrophin expression in the MDX mouse restored by stem cell transplantation. Nature. 1999;401:390-4.
5. Horwitz EM, Prockop DJ, Fitzpatrick LA, Koo WW, Gordon PL, Neel M, et al. Transplantability and therapeutic effects of

bone marrow-derived mesenchymal cells in children with osteogenesis imperfecta. Nat Med. 1999;5:309-13.
6. Houdek MT, Wyles CC, Martin JR, Siera RJ. Stem cell treatment for avascular necrosis of the femoral head: current perspectives. Stem Cell Clon. 2014;7:65-70.
7. Hyman J, Rodeo SA. Injury and repair of tendons and ligaments. Phys Med Rehabil Clin N Am. 2000;11:267-88.
8. Jeyaraman M, Muthu S, Jeyaraman N, Ranjan R, Jha SK, Mishra PC. Synovium derived Mesenchymal Stromal Cells (Sy-MSCs) – a promising therapeutic paradigm in the management of Knee Osteoarthritis. Ind J Orthop; 2021. pp. 2-8.
9. Muthu S, Jeyaraman M, Jain R, Gulati A, Jeyaraman N, Prajwal GS, et al. Accentuating the sources of mesenchymal stem cells as cellular therapy for osteoarthritis knees–a panoramic view. Stem Cell Investig. 2021; 8:13.
10. Peretti GM, Caruso EM, Randolph MA, Zaleske DJ. Meniscal repair using engineered tissue. J Orthop Res. 2001;19:278-85.
11. Ramesh R, Jeyaraman M, Chaudhari K, Prajwal GS, Dhamsania HJ. Mesenchymal stem cells–a boon to orthopedics. Open J Regen Med. 2018;7:19-27.
12. Reddi AH. Initiation of fracture repair by bone morphogenetic proteins. Clin Orthop. 1998;355(Suppl):66-72.
13. Rodeo SA, Suzuki K, Deng XH, Wozney J, Warren RF. Use of recombinant human bone morphogenetic protein-2 to enhance tendon healing in a bone tunnel. Am J Sports Med. 1999;27:476-88.
14. Spees JL, Lee RH, Gregory CA. Mechanisms of mesenchymal stem/stromal cell function. Stem Cell Res Ther. 2016;7(1):125.
15. Thomson JA, Itskovitz-Eldor J, Shapiro SS, Waknitz MA, Swiergiel JJ, Marshall VS, et al. Embryonic stem cell lines derived from human blastocysts. Science. 1998; 282(5391):1145-7.
16. Wang AW, Bauer S, Goonatillake M, Breidahl W, Zheng MH. Autologous tenocyte implantation, a novel treatment for partial thickness rotator cuff tear and tendinopathy in an elite athlete. BMJ Case Rep. 2013;2012:7899.
17. Yu J, Vodyanik MA, Smuga-Otto K, Antosiewicz-Bourget J, Frane JL, Tian S, et al. Induced pluripotent stem cell lines derived from human somatic cells. Science. 2007; 318(5858):1917-20.

Translational Products of Adipose Tissue-derived Mesenchymal Stem Cells: Bench to Bedside Applications

Madhan Jeyaraman, Rajni Ranjan, Amrit Kumar Singh

INTRODUCTION

With developments in the field of tissue engineering and regenerative medicine, the usage of biological products for the treatment of various disorders has come into the limelight among researchers and clinicians. Among all the biological products, keen interest has been shown in adipose tissue and its by-products for translation from bench to clinical applications with due consideration to its various unique properties. Due to the heterogeneous population of the cellular mixture in adipose tissue, adipose tissue-derived products possess a greater advantage of regeneration when comparing with bone marrow-derived products.

Traditionally adipose tissue or fat graft transfer was practiced for elective cosmetic procedures and plastic and reconstructive surgeries. Due to the regeneration potential possessed by adipose tissue, the usage has become robust in cosmetic-dermatological procedures, facial rejuvenation, breast and buttocks augmentation, and genital aesthetics. Cellular viability and survival at the transplanted site depends on various factors involving the recipient site, donor site, laboratory processing, and manipulation.

Adipose tissue engineering aims in developing the by-products and their substitutes for regeneration and restoring the function. This further eliminates the need for organ transplants and mechanical device placements. The usage of biodegradable scaffolds along with adipose tissue products plays a major role in cellular growth, proliferation, and differentiation. Once implanted at an appropriate site, scaffolds degrade, progenitor cells proliferate with the help of growth factors, and cytokines to form new tissue. Investigations have been done so far on the ability of biomolecules and biodegradable three-dimensional scaffolds to interact with adipose tissue products in preclinical studies to promote the adipogenesis of stem cells in vitro.

ADIPOSE TISSUE BIOLOGY

An adipocyte is usually 50–150 mm in diameter since it dies from ischemia as the size goes higher and the life expectancy of an adipocyte varies from few months to 10 years in humans. Adipose tissue, a specialized connective tissue with lipid-rich adipocytes, contains a heterogeneous population of cells but adipocyte represents only 20% or less of the cellular mixture. Based on adipocyte morphology, the two types of adipose tissue defined are the white adipose tissue found in adults and the brown adipose tissue found in newborns.

Adipose tissue, apart from being the powerhouse of energy storage, also functions as the largest endocrine organ with the release of various adipokines. Adipose tissue-derived adipokines are leptin, adiponectin, apelin, chemerin, IL-6, 8 and 10, monocyte chemotactic protein-1 (MCP-1), plasminogen activator inhibitor-1 (PAI-1), retinol-binding protein-4 (RBP-4), TNFα, progranulin, CTRP-4, IFN-γ, and inducible protein 10 (IP-10) which are readily available sources to induce stem cells. These adipokines work in a paracrine fashion while transplanted as a cellular therapeutic tool. The components of adipose tissue are lipid-laden adipocytes, fibroblasts, neural and vascular progenitor cells, multipotent progenitor cells, pericytes, extracellular matrices, cytokines, and growth factors as shown in **Figure 1**. The progenitor cells in the adipose tissue are of paramount importance as they ascertain the capacity of regeneration of these tissues. These progenitor cells differentiate into mesodermal, ectodermal, and endodermal lineages. Tissue engineering experts focus on adipose tissue and its products

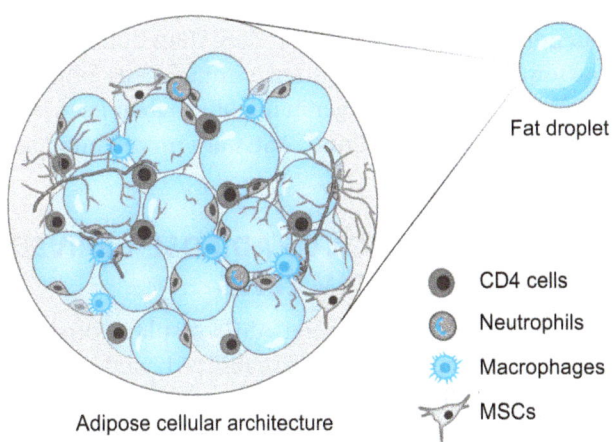

Fig. 1: Organizational structure of adipose tissue.

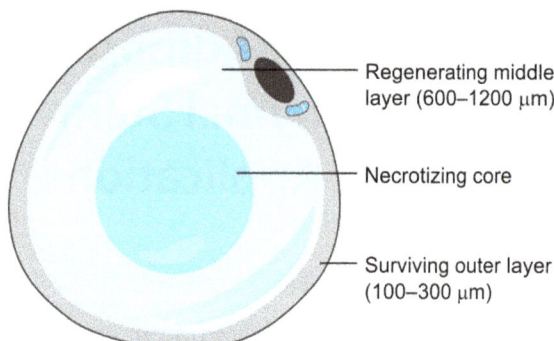

Fig. 2: Zones of an adipocyte.

for their plasticity, relative ease of harvest, and potential autologous usage. The stem cells and progenitor cells from freshly prepared stromal vascular fraction constitute up to 3% which represents 2,500 fold more than the stem cells isolated from bone marrow source (0.002%).

The literature on adipose tissue survival and regeneration depicts "cell survival theory" and "cell replacement theory." Various studies have proven the promising results of adipose-derived stem cell (ASC) assisted fat grafting which provides numerous growth factors and adipokines for improved vasculogenesis, fat graft integration, and survival within the recipient tissue. The adipocyte contains three zones namely (1) outer surviving layer (100–300 μm), (2) middle regenerating layer (600–1200 μm), and (3) inner necrotic layer as shown in **Figure 2**.

Yoshimura et al. demonstrated the sequence of changes that happen after grafting or transplantation of adipose tissue. In preclinical studies, it is shown that all adipocytes undergo apoptosis in the initial few days of grafting. Activation of adipogenesis was due to adipose-derived progenitor cells which were augmented by the adipokines at 3 months postgrafting. By the end of 9 months, lipid droplets get absorbed by macrophages. The final fat graft retention in the recipient site was determined by the rate of successful replacement of the adipocytes.

Adipose-derived stem cell possess various advantages over bone marrow-derived mesenchymal stem cells (BM-MSCs). The harvest action of adipose tissue by liposuction is a less painful procedure than bone marrow aspiration. The number of stem/stromal cells obtained from adipose tissue was larger in quantities than from bone marrow. In long-term culture, ASCs are more genetically stable.

CHARACTERIZATION OF ADIPOSE-DERIVED MESENCHYMAL STEM CELLS

Researchers demonstrated that ASCs display consistent phenotype and reproducing capability based on their cellular yield, cellular viability, adipocyte differentiation, and cell surface markers. During initial culture, ASCs show polygonal-shaped cells which are adhered to the flask surface. They exhibit fibroblastic plastic morphology and expand in-vitro cultures. Around 90% of cells become confluent when subcultured within 2 days of primary culture. The yield and viability of ASCs were 87% and 94% respectively. Luna et al. recovered 1×10^6 adipocytes, 1×10^6 ASCs, 1×10^6 vascular endothelial cells, and 1×10^6 other cells from 1 g of adipose tissue.

During in-vitro cultures, ASCs change the immunophenotype from $CD34^+$, MHC class I and II molecules, $CD80^+$, $CD86^+$, $CD45^+$, $CD11a^+$, $CD14^+$, $CD117^+$, $HLA-DR^+$, NOG^+, $UTF1^+$, $WNT6^+$, and $WNT8A^+$ to increased expression of $CD9^+$, $CD13^+$, $CD29^+$, $CD44^+$, $CD63^+$, $CD73^+$, $CD90^+$, $CD105^+$, $CD166^+$, $BMPR2^+$, $COL6A2^+$, $TGF-\beta R1^+$, and $VEGF-A^+$. The lack of expression of HLA class I and II molecules in the co-culture and serial passages, renders ASCs to possess the property of immunosuppression, and make it suitable for allogenic transplantation.

MSCs from adipose tissue display strong positive expression of $STRO-1^+$, $CD29^+$, $CD73^+$, $CD90^+$, $CD105^+$, $CD166^+$ and $CD44^+$ and weak positive expression for $CD34^+$ and $CD45^+$. MSCs possess enhanced angiogenesis due to the enhanced expression of $CD105^+$ and $CD34^+$ whereas proliferation and differentiation of HSCs were enhanced by $CD9^+$, $CD29^+$, $CD44^+$, $CD49d^+$, and $CD106^+$. Gronthos et al. demonstrated that adipose tissue-derived SVF support hematopoiesis in vitro. Up to about 8 to 12 cellular doubling in culture, AD-MSCs express $CD34^+$. Various theories are available for the attribution of pericytes for stem cell properties. Szoke et al. stated that pericytes present in both MSCs and ADSCs whereas Traktuev et al. and Crisan et al. states that $CD34^+$ and $CD34^-$ pericytes to be the identity of adipose-derived stem cells respectively.

IMMUNOMODULATION OF AD-MSCs

The cellular components of AD-MSC induce and activate quiescent native MSCs to secrete biological micromolecules to the site of injury to establish the local homeostasis through increasing permeability of cells to the injured site, downregulating inflammatory process, and recognition of host tissue progenitor cells for final differentiation into the cell of interest for the injured tissue. Therefore, AD-MSC will activate adaptive cellular response and secretes IL-1Ra, IL-1β, PGE2, IDO, IL-4 and IL-10, and TGF-β which will modulate and prime the native immune cells. These micromolecular interaction leads to a cascade of events responsible for immunotolerance when grafted to a foreign site.

The immunotolerant/immunosuppressive/immuno-modulatory activity of AD-MSC is due to the interplay among regulator T cells, cytotoxic T cells, and B cells as shown in **Figure 3**. Immunomodulatory activity is due to the inhibition of INF-γ and TNF-α production by effector T lymphocytic cells, upregulation of IL-4 and IL-10 by native

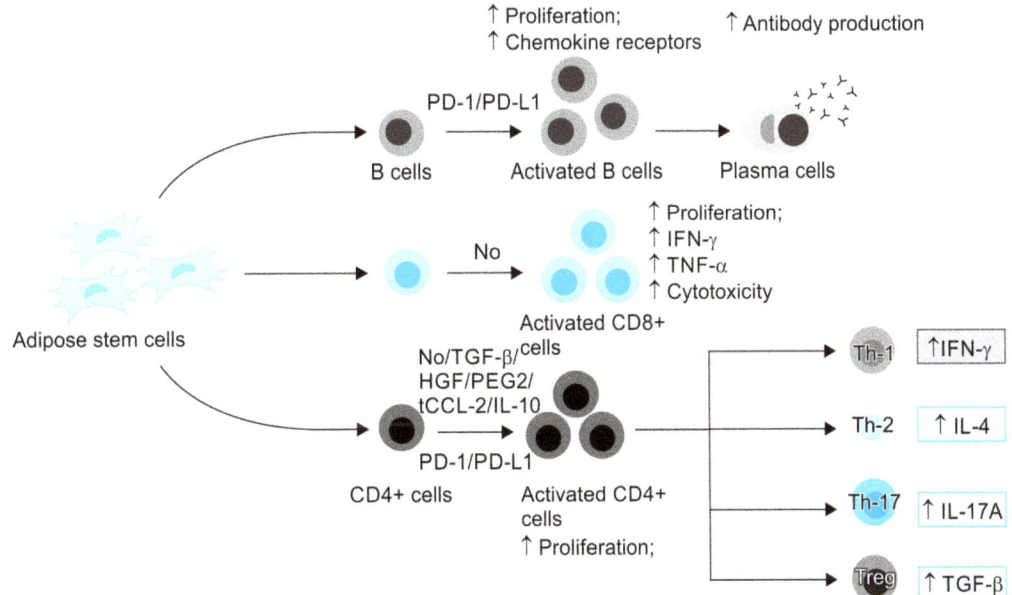

Fig. 3: Immunomodulatory effects of MSCs via T and B lymphocyte system.

immune cells, and inhibition of proliferation, migration, and differentiation of B cells which produce immunoglobulins. Due to the production of indolamine 2,3-dioxygenase by MSC-like cells, the activity of natural killer cells is suppressed. The dendritic cell enhances the expression of IL-4 and IL-10 and suppresses INF-γ and TNFα. This cascade of events directly suppresses the TIMPs and MMPs resulting in the conversion of the proinflammatory environment into an anti-inflammatory environment.

DERIVATIVES AND APPLICATIONS OF ADIPOSE TISSUE

The various derivatives of adipose tissue which are of practical utility with therapeutic potential are given in **Figure 4** and are discussed here:

Adipose Stem Cells

Adipose stem cells are one of the forms of MSC with an inherent property of self-renewal and multipotent differentiation. Due to the advantages of its easy accessibility to the source, abundant availability, and least ethical concern when compared with embryonic stem cells, ASCs render them more suitable in the area of regenerative medicine and tissue engineering. Tissue-engineered 3D scaffolds with ASCs and biomolecules such as growth factors and extracellular matrix materials play a robust role in treating various disorders by the process of cellular proliferation and differentiation. Studies found that ASCs have more grounded immunomodulatory impacts than BM-MSCs.

Adipose tissue contains stem and progenitor cells up to 3% in the uncultured stroma-vascular fraction (SVF) which are 2,500 times more amount of stem cells from bone marrow source. Depending upon the donor and tissue harvesting site, lipoaspirate yields 1 to 10% of stem cells which is approximately 0.5×10^4 to 2×10^5 MSCs per gram of adipose tissue. ASCs act by paracrine fashion by releasing adipocytokines, cytokines, and growth factors that form a secretome.

Following liposuction, the adipose tissue is subjected to phosphate-buffered saline washing along with a 5% antibiotic followed by tissue digestion with the collagenase-1 enzyme. After the disintegration of adipose tissue, the resultant sample was transferred to tubes and subjected for centrifugation at the rate of 2000 rpm for 5 minutes to obtain a stromal vascular fraction that contains ASCs. The resultant cellular pellet is resuspended in 1 mL lysis buffer and recentrifuged at 2000 rpm for 5 minutes. Filter the cellular suspension through a 70 μm cell strainer. Finally plate the cellular mixture in a lysine coated culture plate and incubate at 37°C with 5% CO_2. Inoculate the cellular mixture in well plates for an amount of about 500 mg of adipose tissue to obtain ASCs. According to International Fat Applied Technology Society (IFATS), uncultured ASCs express $CD34^+$, $CD45^-$, $CD235a^-$ and $CD31^-$ whereas cultured ASCs express $CD73^+$, $CD90^+$, $CD105^+$, $CD44^+$, $CD45^-$, and $CD31^-$.

The short- and long-term storage of ASCs were to be investigated. Storage of ASC decreases cellular proliferative capacity in the due course of time. Hence, it has to be supplemented with 10% human sera or PRP in 0.9% saline solution at 4°C for the first 2 hours and not more than 4 hours. For long-term storage, ASCs can be stored at −80°C using liquid nitrogen for up to 6 months.

Microfat

While comparing with nanofat, microfat appears deep yellow, fine granular structure with intact three-dimensional

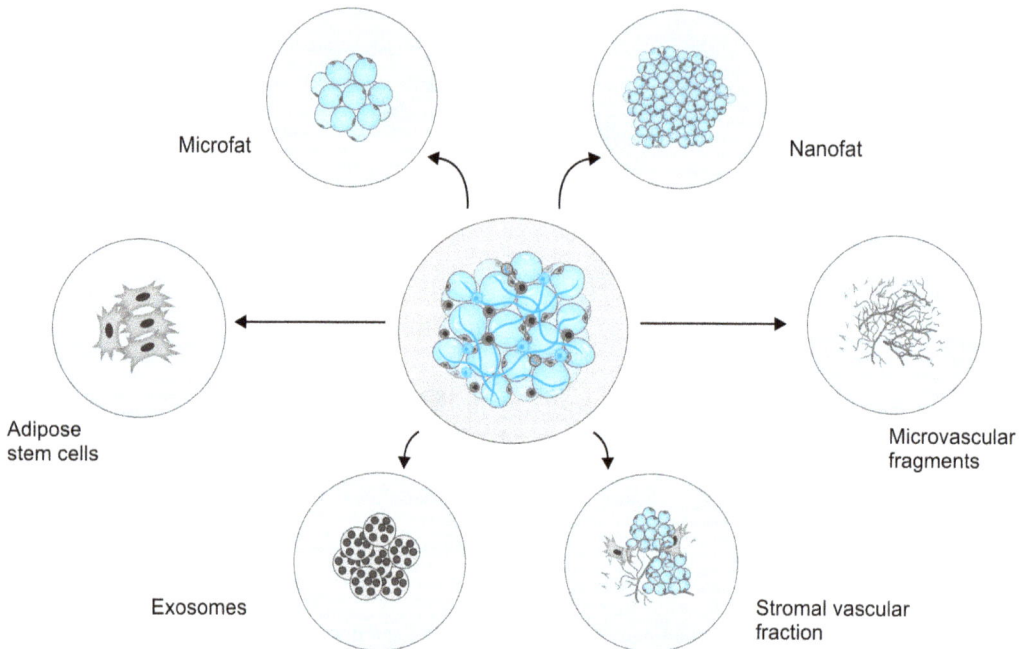

Fig. 4: Derivatives of adipose tissue complex.

adipose tissue architecture. In microfat composition, the mature adipocyte, SVF cells, pericytes, capillary fragments, and fibrous scaffolds were well preserved. Hence, they imbibe with the natural recipient site for survival of graft and provide a niche for SVF cellular mixture for tissue regeneration and rejuvenation.

Yang et al. harvested microfat from adipose tissue through the cannula with side holes of less than 1 mm. Examination of such harvest revealed intact fat lobular structure without any inter-syringing passages and emulsification procedures. The side holes of the cannula with a diameter of 0.8 mm allow the processed microfat to easily pass through the needles without any blockage. Such harvests, used for skin and facial rejuvenation through 27 gauge needles, revealed the preservation of micro functional units of fat tissue to exert the regenerative property of ASCs.

Caggiati et al. demonstrated the higher yield of ASCs from harvested lipoaspirates by barbed cannula than blunt cannula but they found barbed cannula cut the fibrous septum and produce higher quantities of coarse fibers and increases the probability of molecular blockage in the needle. The cellular components in the microfat induce tissue regeneration through the recruitment of monocyte/macrophage differentiation at the recipient site.

The cellular yield in microfat $(2.28 \pm 1.90) \times 10^5$ cells/mL is higher when compared to the yield in nanofat $(4.12 \pm 1.37) \times 10^4$ cells/mL indicating that nanofat involves mechanical emulsification. Microfat components integrate into the local environment due to the intact microintegrity of cellular transplant with inherent resistance to attack by host immune-mediated cells.

Microfat possess various advantages such as (a) no mechanical emulsification or centrifugation involved in preparation other than the shearing forces during harvesting, (b) intact vascular fragments with viable cellular components in the mixture, (c) lessens the ischemic exposure time of adipose tissue harvest while preparing microfat graft and (d) preservation of viable adipocytes restore the degenerated and atrophied skin and subcutaneous tissues.

Nanofat

In 2013, Tonnard et al. developed Nanofat, which is an ultra-purified adipose tissue-derived product that is devoid of mature adipocytes but contains CD34+ ASCs, microvascular fragments, growth factors, biological peptides, and cytokines. It is a liquefied, autologous injectable product with the property of biological integration with adjacent cells and tissues due to its homogenous consistency. The size of nanofat components is approximately 400 to 600 μm. Nanofat behaves on the line of adipose tissue-derived mesenchymal stromal cells. On the site of injury, these stromal cells initiate a site-specific reparative response comprised of remodeling of extracellular matrix (ECM), enhanced and sustained angiogenesis, and immune system modulation.

Due to the multi- and pluripotent nature of cellular components in nanofat, it possesses the ability to differentiate into multiple lineages. Hence nanofat can be extrapolated for preclinical and translational research in tissue engineering. Various preclinical and clinical experiments have proved the antifibrotic, proangiogenesis, neuroregeneration, and enhanced collagen deposition potentials of adipose tissue-derived nanofat.

Sese et al. estimated the total cellular load in the mechanically prepared nanofat to 6.63 million cells/g of lipoaspirate whereas in enzymatically disintegrated SVF it was 0.68 million cells/g of lipoaspirate. The nucleated cellular count in nanofat was 70% and in SVF was 7.3%. The cellular burden in nanofat contains predominantly the stromal cellular population.

Nanofat grafting enhances neoangiogenesis without producing any visible scars and provides a favorable outcome in aesthetic medicine for breast, buttocks, and genital augmentation, facial rejuvenation, and facial volume augmentation. The preclinical and clinical studies with the usage of nanofat have proven the regenerative capacity in various clinical settings.

Microvascular Fragments

Microvascular fragments (MVF), the by-product of adipose tissue ranges between 40 and 180 mm, are composed of arteriolar, capillary, and venular vessel segments. MVF release vascular endothelial growth factor (VEGF) and basic fibroblast growth factor (bFGF) under culture conditions. They are the richest source of proangiogenic factors, which induce vasculogenesis in a paracrine fashion. MVF exhibit positivity for Sca-1/VEGFR-2$^+$, CD44$^+$, CD73$^+$, CD90$^+$, and CD117$^+$. The components of MVF exhibit the morphology of intact lumen, endothelium, and perivascular stabilizing cells. MVF are the building blocks for therapeutic vasculogenesis.

McDaniel et al. illustrated that MVF exhibit higher proliferative potential increased differentiation capabilities and superior ability to form vasculogenesis while comparing with conventionally derived adipose stem cells. Transplanted or injected MVF rapidly integrates with the native tissues to form neoangiogenesis in the physiological environment. The three phases of MVF induced neoangiogenesis are (a) immature vascular segments with higher proliferation capacity, (b) vascular remodeling with high rates of apoptosis, and (c) vascular maturation with microvascular network organization. This complex pattern of neoangiogenesis is associated with the upregulation of angiogenic genes.

Researchers have observed the regenerative potential in cartilage defects and skeletal muscle injury, myocardial infarction, partial or complete thickness skin defects, and diabetes mellitus. MVF loaded scaffolds serve as a tomb for lymphatic network disorders, reducing edema formation, and improvising the vasculogenesis in the area of repair. With the available diverse potentials of MVF, the application of MVF in the clinical setting is plausible with the imperative question over the technical and regulatory compliance from bench to bedside.

Stromal Vascular Fraction

Stromal vascular fraction is an ultra–by-product of adipose tissue through various processing methods. Due to the development of biocellular regenerative medicine and cellular biology, the usage of SVF among regenerative surgeons and researchers has become robust. The components of SVF are MSCs, HSCs, T-reg cells, pericyte endothelial cells, mast-cells, complex microvascular beds (fibroblasts, WBC, dendritic cells, intra-adventitial smooth muscular-like cells, etc.), and extracellular matrix.

Stromal vascular fraction behaves in line with bone marrow-derived MSCs. SVF mixture contains 30% MSCs, 3% endothelial cells and 14% endothelial precursor cells whereas bone marrow-derived MSCs contains 0.001% MSCs, 0.1% endothelial cells, and 2% endothelial precursor cells. About 2% of isolated SVF express hematopoietic markers CD34$^+$ and CD45$^+$ and 7% express MSC markers CD105$^+$ and CD146$^+$. SVF cells express cell surface markers similar to bone marrow-derived MSCs such as CD105$^+$/SH2$^+$, CD90$^+$, CD29$^+$, CD44$^+$, CD71$^+$, and SH3$^+$, along with low expression of CD31$^+$, CD45$^+$, and CD24$^+$.

In literature, various methods of isolation of SVF have been described. SVF isolation needs fat obtained by liposuction and transportation to a cGMP certified laboratory for further processing. The global researchers and clinicians widely use the enzymatic method for isolating and harvesting SVF by collagenase enzymes. After the addition of collagenase enzyme to the lipoaspirate, digestion and disintegration of adipose cells take place and result in the formation of 2 phases in the tubes namely floating adipocyte fraction and settled cellular components as an aqueous mixture. This separation can be enhanced by density gradient centrifugation and filtration. The lower portion of the tube contains a yellowish red pellet which is termed as SVF mixture, which can be intended for in vitro expansion. Due to the ethical issues associated with SVF isolation by the enzymatic method, researchers opted for alternative methods for SVF isolation. Researchers proposed mechanical agitation and disruption of adipose tissue which releases a mixture of cellular components stromal cells. The cellular proportion of SVF by mechanical disruption will be lower when compared with enzymatic degradation but the regenerative potential of those SVF mixture by mechanical disruption remains same as that of enzymatic degradation.

The anti-inflammatory effects of SVF are due to the presence of higher amounts of IL-1 and IL-10 receptor antagonists which are expressed by TNFα and leptin released by monocytes and macrophages in the SVF mixture. SVF mixture provokes adaptive immunity by producing T-reg cells by suppressing the activation of dendritic cells.

Krawiec et al. demonstrated that stromal vascular fraction components being seeded with biodegradable porous scaffolds in vivo for 8 weeks resulted in the generation of tissue-engineered vascular grafts when populated with primary vascular components such as smooth muscle cells, endothelial cells, collagen, and elastin. ASCs or SVF combined with PRP enhances the regenerative potential in the form of neoangiogenesis, cellular proliferation, and differentiation. The combination of SVF with PRP enhances the stemness of MSCs, the growth factors present in PRP induce locally available stem cells and prolong the survival time and rates of cells present in PRP. Such combination treatments have been tried in preclinical and clinical trials for wound healing, osteoarthritis knees, bone and tendon regeneration, periodontal engineering, fat grafting procedures, and vascular diseases. When cocultured with PRP, the viability, motility, proliferation rate, and differentiation of ASCs are increased in the presence of 5% or 20% PRP.

ASC Exosomes

Exosomes form the cell-free regenerative tool in the field of tissue engineering. Exosomes are a part of extracellular vehicles which are formed from endosome-derived lipid bilayered spherical vesicles of 40 to 150 nm in size. Though they are found in all cell types and body fluids, they are comprised of cytokines, proteins, lipids, DNA, and RNA from the parent cell. Exosomes form an integral part of both diagnostic and therapeutic purposes for various diseases. Compared to ASCs, ASC-derived exosomes possess high biosafety profile with low immunogenicity. They protect cargoes from degradation, tissue and target specificity, good tissue permeability, intercellular signaling and communication, immune function, tissue homeostasis, and development of cell fate.

Ogawa et al. observed that mRNAs of adipose tissue-derived exosomes have a significant role in metabolic, immunological, and cellular responses. Various studies demonstrated that adipose tissue-derived exosomes possess the capability of regeneration of muscles and bones, promotion of wound healing, enhancement of cellular proliferation, and neoangiogenesis. There is a future for these exosomes as a diagnostic tool for early identification of pathological processes involved in disease and as a therapeutic tool for a targeted acellular conduit to optimize the pathological milieu at the site of interest.

ETHICAL CONCERNS

An early therapy or a drug development is dependent on the translational phases, the strategy to standardize the process, and regularly acquire data to validate and certify the technologies developed. The safety and efficacy of the developed therapy must be proven from various perspectives including the donor, recipient, product, manufacturing, clinical application, and biovigilance.

The procedure involved in making adipose-derived products involves the collection and preparation of fat tissue. With these procedures, the patient's cells are made available by safer methods without any adverse events. Clinicians who use them in their practice are obliged to abide by the existing laws which control their usage in clinical practice.

The European Medicines Agency (EMA), United States Food and Drug Administration (FDA), and other similar agencies consider adult human cells as biological products of two classes. To take a note, the first one involves cells processed with minimal manipulation (MM) techniques such as filtration, centrifugation, and mechanical disruption done in a single surgical window within a sterile operating environment. The second class of products undergoes a significant manipulation process such as expansion through cell cultures, characterization, cultivation, and other MM techniques when used outside a single surgical window or the operating room.

As per the FDA and EMA regulations, adipose products are considered medicinal products that have to be harvested using validated procedures adhering to stringent regulatory protocols. Clinical Quality Attributes (CQAs) of therapeutic products ensuring safety along with the maintenance of their identity, purity, and potency as per the FDA Guidance for industry. In agreement with the reflection paper EMA/CAT/600280/2010 Rev 1, June 20, 2014, it could be presumed that for autologous use under single therapeutic windows with minimal manipulation in aseptic conditions, adipose-derived products would not require ethical committee underwriting for its clinical use. However, there are no standardized methods or means to isolate ASC with predetermined CQAs making isolation of ASC for targeted therapies difficult. Hence, a modular system configured as a single-use kit that contains all the essential components in exact proportions to follow a specific protocol to establish standardization in isolation of adipose derivatives with targeted action of ASCs with specific CQAs would be ideal and recommended.

CONCLUSION

Of late the interest in the adipose derivatives for regenerative therapies and constructive tissue engineering is on the rise. Having elaborated the biology, characteristics, immunology, and clinical applications of adipose-derived products, it is imperative that evidence to strengthen the clinical applicability of these therapeutic products is needed to warrant an official recommendation from regulatory authorities. Unraveling the utility of various adipose derivatives helps in the improvisation of the existing regenerative therapies and their associated biomedical applications.

FURTHER READING

1. Aronowitz JA, Lockhart RA, Hakakian CS. A method for isolation of stromal vascular fraction cells in a clinically relevant time frame. Methods Mol Biol Clifton NJ. 2018; 1773:11-19.
2. Baer PC. Adipose-derived mesenchymal stromal/stem cells: an update on their phenotype in vivo and in vitro. World J Stem Cells. 2014;6(3):256-65.
3. Bellini E, Grieco MP, Raposio E. The science behind autologous fat grafting. Ann Med Surg. 2017;24:65-73.
4. Bunnell BA, Flaat M, Gagliardi C, Patel B, Ripoll C. Adipose-derived stem cells: isolation, expansion and differentiation. Methods San Diego Calif. 2008;45(2):115-20.

5. Chen F-M, Liu X. Advancing biomaterials of human origin for tissue engineering. Prog Polym Sci. 2016;53:86-168.
6. De Rosa A, De Francesco F, Tirino V, Ferraro GA, Desiderio V, Paino F, et al. A new method for cryopreserving adipose-derived stem cells: an attractive and suitable large-scale and long-term cell banking technology. Tissue Eng Part C Methods. 2009;15(4):659-67.
7. Feinberg AW. Engineered tissue grafts: opportunities and challenges in regenerative medicine. Wiley Interdiscip Rev Syst Biol Med. 2012;4(2):207-20.
8. Flynn L, Woodhouse KA. Adipose tissue engineering with cells in engineered matrices. Organogenesis. 2008;4(4):228-35.
9. Friji MT. Nanofat grafting: basic research and clinical applications. Plast Reconstr Surg. 2014;134(2):333e-334e.
10. Gentile P, Orlandi A, Scioli MG, Di Pasquali C, Bocchini I, Cervelli V. Concise review: adipose-derived stromal vascular fraction cells and platelet-rich plasma: basic and clinical implications for tissue engineering therapies in regenerative surgery. Stem Cells Transl Med. 2012;1(3):230-6.
11. Gentile P, Scioli MG, Bielli A, Orlandi A, Cervelli V. Comparing different nanofat procedures on scars: role of the stromal vascular fraction and its clinical implications. Regen Med. 2017;12(8):939-52.
12. Harrison BL, Malafa M, Davis K, Rohrich RJ. The discordant histology of grafted fat: a systematic review of the literature. Plast Reconstr Surg. 2015;135(3):542e-555e.
13. Hsu VM, Stransky CA, Bucky LP, Percec I. Fat grafting's past, present, and future: why adipose tissue is emerging as a critical link to the advancement of regenerative medicine. Aesthet Surg J. 2012;32(7):892-9.
14. Karina, Samudra MF, Rosadi I, Afini I, Widyastuti T, Sobariah S, et al. Combination of the stromal vascular fraction and platelet-rich plasma accelerates the wound healing process: pre-clinical study in a Sprague-Dawley rat model. Stem Cell Investig. 2019;6.
15. Langer R, Vacanti JP. Tissue engineering. Science. 1993;260(5110):920-6.
16. Mailey B, Hosseini A, Baker J, Young A, Alfonso Z, Hicok K, et al. Adipose-derived stem cells: methods for isolation and applications for clinical use. Methods Mol Biol Clifton NJ. 2014;1210:161-81.
17. Memar O, Nezamabadi A, Milani BY, Milani FY, Djalilian A. Nanofat grafting: basic research and clinical application. Plast Reconstr Surg. 2014;133(5):728e.
18. Ramakrishnan VM, Boyd NL. The adipose stromal vascular fraction as a complex cellular source for tissue engineering applications. Tissue Eng Part B Rev. 2018;24(4):289-99.
19. Simonacci F, Bertozzi N, Grieco MP, Grignaffini E, Raposio E. Procedure, applications, and outcomes of autologous fat grafting. Ann Med Surg 2012. 2017;20:49-60.
20. Tan SS, Ng ZY, Zhan W, Rozen W. Role of adipose-derived stem cells in fat grafting and reconstructive surgery. J Cutan Aesthetic Surg. 2016;9(3):152-6.
21. Tremolada C, Colombo V, Ventura C. Adipose tissue and mesenchymal stem cells: state of the art and Lipogems® technology development. Curr Stem Cell Rep. 2016;2: 304-12.
22. van Dongen JA, Harmsen MC, Stevens HP. Isolation of stromal vascular fraction by fractionation of adipose tissue. Methods Mol Biol Clifton NJ. 2019;1993:91-103.
23. Van Pham P, Hong-Thien Bui K, Quoc Ngo D, Tan Khuat L, Kim Phan N. Transplantation of nonexpanded adipose stromal vascular fraction and platelet-rich plasma for articular cartilage injury treatment in mice model. J Med Eng. 2013;2013.
24. Yang Z, Jin S, He Y, Zhang X, Han X, Li F. Comparison of microfat, nanofat and extracellular matrix/stromal vascular fraction gel for skin rejuvenation: basic research and clinical applications. Aesthet Surg J; 2021.
25. Yoshimura K, Eto H, Kato H, Doi K, Aoi N. In vivo manipulation of stem cells for adipose tissue repair/reconstruction. Regen Med. 2011;6(6 Suppl):33-41.
26. Young DA, Christman KL. Injectable biomaterials for adipose tissue engineering. Biomed Mater Bristol Engl. 2012;7(2): 024104.
27. Zimmerlin L, Donnenberg VS, Pfeifer ME, Meyer EM, Peault B, Rubin JP, et al. Stromal vascular progenitors in adult human adipose tissue. Cytom Part J Int Soc Anal Cytol. 2010; 77(1):22-30.

Ethical Consideration in Stem Cell Research

Manish Khanna, Shashank Tiwari

GENERAL PRINCIPLES

Biomedical and health research involves the four basic ethical principles namely—respect for persons (autonomy), beneficence, non-maleficence and justice have been enunciated for protecting the dignity, rights, safety and well-being of research participants. These four basic principles have been expanded into 12 general principles described here:

1. *Principle of essentiality* whereby after due consideration of all alternatives in the light of existing knowledge, the use of human participants is considered to be essential for the proposed research. This should be duly vetted by an Ethics Committee (EC) independent of the proposed research.
2. *Principle of voluntariness* whereby respect for the right of the participant to agree or not to agree to participate in research, or to withdraw from research at any time, is paramount. The informed consent process ensures that participants' rights are safeguarded.
3. *Principle of nonexploitation* whereby research participants are equitably selected so that the benefits and burdens of the research are distributed fairly and without arbitrariness or discrimination. Sufficient safeguards to protect vulnerable groups should be ensured.
4. *Principle of social responsibility* whereby the research is planned and conducted so as to avoid creation or deepening of social and historic divisions or in any way disturb social harmony in community relationships.
5. *Principle of ensuring privacy and confidentiality* whereby to maintain privacy of the potential participant, her/his identity and records are kept confidential and access is limited to only those authorized. However, under certain circumstances (suicidal ideation, homicidal tendency, HIV positive status, when required by court of law, etc.) privacy of the information can be breached in consultation with the EC for valid scientific or legal reasons as the right to life of an individual supersedes the right to privacy of the research participant.
6. *Principle of risk minimization* whereby due care is taken by all stakeholders (including but not limited to researchers, ECs, sponsors, regulators) at all stages of the research to ensure that the risks are minimized and appropriate care and compensation is given if any harm occurs.
7. *Principle of professional competence* whereby the research is planned, conducted, evaluated and monitored throughout by persons who are competent and have the appropriate and relevant qualification, experience and/or training.
8. *Principle of maximization of benefit* whereby due care is taken to design and conduct the research in such a way as to directly or indirectly maximize the benefits to the research participants and/or to the society.
9. *Principle of institutional arrangements* whereby institutions where the research is being conducted, have policies for appropriate research governance and take the responsibility to facilitate research by providing required infrastructure, manpower, funds and training opportunities.
10. *Principle of transparency and accountability* whereby the research plan and outcomes emanating from the research are brought into the public domain through registries, reports and scientific and other publications while safeguarding the right to privacy of the participants. Stakeholders involved in research should disclose any existing conflict of interest and manage it appropriately. The research should be conducted in a fair, honest, impartial, and transparent manner to guarantee accountability. Related records, data and notes should be retained for the required period for possible external scrutiny/audit.
11. *Principle of totality of responsibility* whereby all stakeholders involved in research are responsible for their actions. The professional, social and moral responsibilities compliant with ethical guidelines and related regulations are binding on all stakeholders directly or indirectly.
12. *Principle of environmental protection* whereby researchers are accountable for ensuring protection of the environment and resources at all stages of the research, in compliance with existing guidelines and regulations.

GENERAL ETHICAL ISSUES

The treating investigator and team are responsible for protecting the rights, safety, dignity, and wellbeing of the patient. The investigator should have the appropriate qualification and shall ensure the team to be adequately qualified, also the whole team shall comply with ethical, medical, legal and social requirements of the research proposal. The important general issues are as mentioned here:

- *Benefit-risk assessment*: Benefit means any favorable outcome of the research which can be used for the welfare of the individual or society. Risk is all potential adverse events faced during the study and which may affect the individuals or the society. The investigator has to assess the benefit and risk of the study depending on the available treatment option and conclude to a final decision.
- *Informed consent*: All the patients shall be adequately consented before start of any procedure. The process involves three components—providing relevant information to potential participants, ensuring the information is comprehended by them and assuring voluntariness of participation. In case the patient is not able to give his/her consent due to any medical condition or age, a legal acceptable representative should consent on the behalf of the patient.
- *Privacy and confidentiality*: Privacy is the right of an individual to control or influence the information that can be collected and stored and by whom and to whom that information may be disclosed or shared. Confidentiality is the obligation of the researcher/research team/ organization to the participant to safeguard the entrusted information. It includes the obligation to protect information from unauthorized access, use, disclosure, modification, loss or theft.
- *Conflict of interest (COI)*: Conflict of interest is a set of situations or conditions where professional judgment concerning a primary interest such as participants welfare or the validity of research tends to be unduly influenced by a secondary interest, financial or non-financial (personal, academic or political). This can be at the level of researchers, EC members, institutions or sponsors. If COI is inherent in the research, it is important to declare this at the outset and establish appropriate mechanisms to manage it.
- *Selection of vulnerable population*: The "vulnerable population", are the disadvantaged subsegment of the community requiring utmost care, specific ancillary considerations and augmented protections in research. Vulnerable population includes but not limited to legal status—children; clinical conditions—cognitive impairment, unconsciousness; or situational conditions including but not limited to being economically or socially disadvantaged, (e.g., certain ethnic or religious groups, individuals/communities which have hierarchical relationships, institutionalized persons, humanitarian emergencies, language barriers and cultural differences).

INFORMED CONSENT

Informed consent is a formal communication between the patient and health care provider that often leads to agreement or permission for care, treatment, or services. The researcher must obtain voluntary written informed consent from the prospective participant for any biomedical and health research involving human participants. This requirement is based on the principle that competent individuals are entitled to choose freely whether or not to participate or continue to participate in the research. Informed consent is a continuous process involving three main components—providing relevant information to potential participants, ensuring competence of the individual, ensuring the information is easily comprehended by the participants and assuring voluntariness of participation.

Requirements of an Informed Consent

- The participant must have the capacity to understand the proposed research, be able to make an informed decision on whether or not to be enrolled and convey her/his decision to the researcher in order to give consent.
- The consent should be given voluntarily and not be obtained under duress or coercion of any sort or by offering any undue inducements.
- In the case of an individual who is not capable of giving voluntary informed consent, the consent of legal acceptable representative must be obtained.
- It is mandatory for a researcher to administer consent before initiating any study related procedures involving the participant.
- It is necessary to maintain privacy and confidentiality of participants at all stages.

ETHICAL CONSIDERATION IN STEM CELL RESEARCH

The basic ethical principle has been already explained in the beginning of the chapter. The specific ethical considerations in relation to stem cell research are health, safety, and rights of the patient.

Prior to any procedure the patient shall be adequately consented through preferably audio video methods. The donation of gametes, embryos, and fetal tissues raise special ethical and moral concerns; hence it is necessary to ensure that the patients are neither exploited nor commoditized. The confidentiality and privacy of the subject shall not be disclosed unless required as per Law of Land.

The patient can be screened by the criteria which are given in **Table 1**.

TABLE 1: Criteria for the screening of the patient.

Inclusion criteria	Exclusion criteria
• Healthy individuals of both sexes in the age group of 18–40 years • Willingness and ability of the patient to comply with the program • The patient should be able to comprehend the Institutional Ethics Committee (IEC) approved information, need for informed consent including audio-video consent, patient rights, voluntary nature of donation and then sign the informed consent form (ICF)	• Refusal or inability to give informed consent • An illness that precludes the use of general anesthesia/local anesthesia (whichever applicable) • Illness such as tuberculosis, malaria or any other infection • Autoimmune disorders (diabetes mellitus), hypertension, heart disease • Past history of any malignancy • Features of any genetic or chromosomal disorders • Family history of any inherited disorders • *Abnormal laboratory investigations:* Hb ≤ 11.0 g%, serum creatinine ≥2.0 mg%, serum total bilirubin ≥1.0 mg% • Pregnant and nursing women • Patients found positive for any of the infectious disease markers • Participation in a similar donation program within the last 6 months

The patient must be informed about the need for screening of transmittable diseases (about which she/he may or may not be aware of) and of any other risk factors including possible genetic disorders as is practiced for blood and other organ/tissue/cells donation.

Further, procedural risks involved during collection of organ/tissue/cells (e.g., ovum, bone marrow, etc.), under local or general anesthesia should be adequately explained. These details must be included in the information sheet and should be understood by the patient in his/her preferred language.

The patient shall also be informed that under exceptional circumstances, cell lines/products may be generated from the donated material and that these may be banked and shared with other scientific groups.

The cell lines/products may also undergo genetic manipulation and have the potential for commercialization. In the latter event, the Intellectual Property Rights (IPR) of the biological material will not vest with the patient. However, if commercialization brings any benefits, say financial, efforts should be made to pass on the same to the patient/community wherever possible.

The patients should be made aware that they may be contacted in future for any specific requirements.

APPROVALS REQUIRED FOR STEM CELL RESEARCH

Stem cell research is associated with unique ethical, legal and social concerns that require additional oversight and expertise for efficient scientific and ethical evaluation (**Flowchart 1**).

A separate mechanism for review and monitoring is essential both at institutional and national levels.

A National Apex Committee for Stem Cell Research and Therapy (NAC-SCRT) has been established. It monitors and oversees research activities at the national level and lays guidelines for basic and clinical research.

It is mandatory for all institutes and entities engaged in stem cell research to establish an IC-SCR and register the same with NAC-SCRT.

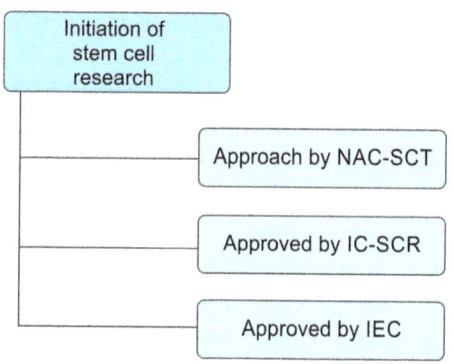

Flowchart 1: Mechanism of approval of stem cell research.

(IEC: Institutional Ethics Committee; IC-SCR: Institutional Committee for Stem Cell Research; NAC-SCT: National Apex Committee for Stem Cell Research and Therapy)

The Institutional Committee for Stem Cell Research (IC-SCR) approves and monitors stem cell research (basic and clinical) at the institutional level. The Institute should also constitute its Institutional Ethics Committee for over view of the clinical studies.

All the clinical studies or research shall be registered with Clinical Trial Registry of India (CTRI) before initiation of the study. The composition, functions and responsibilities of NAC-SCRT and IC-SCR are as per guidelines released by Indian Council for Medical Research.

These oversight committees shall ensure that the review, approval and monitoring processes of all research projects in the field of stem cell research is conducted in compliance with the national guidelines.

In a nut shell all the stem cell research shall be approved by NAC-SCT, IC-SCR, IEC and with Central Drugs Standard Control Organization (CDSCO, in case of drug).

Stem Cell Research Categorization

Largely, it is categorized into three major categories (**Table 2**)—(1) permissible area of research, (2) restrictive areas of research, and (3) prohibited areas of research.

TABLE 2: Three major categories of stem cell research.

Permissible area of research	Restrictive areas of research	Prohibited areas of research

It includes:
• In vitro studies using stem cells isolated from tissues can be done with prior approval of IC-SCR and IEC
• Establishment of new human ESC lines from spare embryos or iPSC lines from fetal/adult somatic cells or SSCs from fetal or adult tissues, with prior approval of the IC-SCR and IEC
• In vitro studies using established cell lines can be carried out with prior approval of the IC-SCR
• In vivo studies in experimental animals with established cell lines from any type of human pluripotent stem cells, viz. ESCs, iPSCs, including their differentiated cells, and human SSCs (fetal, neonatal or adult) from any tissue, are permitted with the prior approval of IC-SCR and Institutional Animal Ethics Committee (IAEC)
	It Includes:
	• Creation of human pre-implantation embryos by in vitro fertilization (IVF), intracytoplasmic sperm injection (ICSI), somatic cell nuclear transfer (SCNT) or any other method with the specific aim of deriving ESC lines for any purpose
	• Clinical trials using stem cells of any type, source, and level of manipulation for homologous/non-homologous transplantation in indications other than listed in National Guidelines
	• Clinical trials sponsored by multinationals, employing cell products developed outside India, should have clearances from the regulatory authorities of the country of the origin, and shall need prior approval from CDSCO following clearance from both IC-SCR and IEC of the trial site
	• All international collaborations require approvals from the respective funding agencies followed by approval from the Health Ministry's Screening Committee (HMSC) as per Government of India guidelines
	• Import of any type of stem cells and/or their products/derivatives requires license from CDSCO as per the established regulations. These should have prior clearances from the regulatory authorities of the country of origin
	• Research involving introduction of human ESC/iPSC/SSCs into animals (including primates), at embryonic or fetal stages of development for studies designed to understand the patterns of differentiation and integration of human cells into non-human animal tissues shall conform to the following:
	  – If the expected outcome of the study is suggestive of a possibility that human stem cells could contribute in a major way to the development of brain or gonads of the recipient animal, the scientific justification for such experiments must first be substantiated with data
	  – Animals derived from such experiments shall not be allowed to breed
	  – Such proposals would need approval of the NAC-SCRT for additional oversight and review after clearance has been granted by the IC-SCR, IEC and IAEC (or CPCSEA)
	• Studies on chimeras where stem cells from two or more species are mixed together at any stage of early development (embryonic or fetal), for understanding patterns of development and differentiation would also require prior approval of NAC-SCRT after clearance has been granted by the IEC and IC-SCR
	• Genome modification including gene editing of stem cells, germ-line stem cells or gamete and human embryos is restricted only to in vitro studies
		It Includes:
		• Research related to human germ-line gene therapy and reproductive cloning
		• In vitro culture of intact human embryos, regardless of the method of their derivation, beyond 14 days of fertilization or formation of primitive streak, whichever is earlier
		• Clinical trials involving xenogeneic cells
		• Any clinical research on Xenogeneic-Human hybrids
		• Use of genome modified human embryos, germ-line stem cells or gametes for developmental propagation
		• Research involving implantation of human embryos (generated by any means) after in vitro manipulation, at any stage of development, into uterus in humans or primates
		• Breeding of animals in which any type of human stem cells have been introduced at any stage of development, and are likely to contribute to chimeric gonadal cells

(CDSCO: Central Drugs Standard Control Organization; IEC: Institutional Ethics Committee; IC-SCR: Institutional Committee for Stem Cell Research; NAC-SCT: National Apex Committee for Stem Cell Research and Therapy)

RESPONSIBILITIES OF SURGEON AND INSTITUTIONS

Indian Council of Medical Research (ICMR) defines responsibilities of the surgeons and Institutions conducting research as follows:

- The investigators and institutions where stem cell research is being conducted bear the ultimate responsibility of ensuring that research activities are in accordance with the national regulations and guidelines.
- The investigator shall endeavor to avoid any activity that leads to hype, or unrealistic expectations in the minds of human participants or general public regarding the status of stem cell research and application.
- Investigators should demonstrate respect for autonomy and privacy of those who donate gametes, blastocysts, embryos or somatic cells for stem cell research, and be sensitive to public concerns about research involving human embryos.
- Investigators should also ensure confidentiality of the human patients to safeguard their rights and dignity.
- Biological material can be procured only from clinics/hospitals that have IEC. The IEC must ensure that the standard operating procedures (SOPs) are in compliance with the guidelines.
- Investigators should treat the biological material with utmost respect and adequate care to avoid misuse.
- Creation of human embryos falls under the restrictive areas of research and shall be resorted to only when all other alternatives have been exhausted.
- Special care should be taken for research involving introduction of human cells in animals, particularly in early developmental stages, since this may lead to development of chimeras or incorporation of stem cells into brain and gonads which can be potentially hazardous.
- Research involving stem cells can be conducted only after approval both from the IC-SCR and NAC-SCRT.

- The proposal should first be reviewed by the IC-SCR which primarily evaluates the scientific and technical aspects of the study followed by the IEC that will review overall work plan with major focus on ethical issues.
- Clinical trials can be permitted only in institutions/hospitals having registered IC-SCR (with NAC-SCRT) and IEC (with CDSCO).
- It is the responsibility of the investigator to generate robust scientific evidence through well designed clinical trials that could yield valuable information for the benefit of patients.
- The study subject and/or legal representative should be provided adequate and unbiased information about the trial protocol, its limitations, and potential adverse effects.
- A clinical trial must have a medical specialist registered with Medical Council of India (MCI) and holding MCI approved postgraduate qualification in the subject domain of the trial. This can only be conducted in a medical institution/hospital with adequate infrastructure and clinical facilities in accordance with Para 2 (1)(ii) of Schedule Y, Drugs and Cosmetic Act, 1940 and rules therein. All medical professionals involved in clinical trials should have a valid Good Clinical Practices (GCP) certification obtained from agencies such as Central Drug Service Agency (CDSA) or online courses conducted by National Institutes of Health (NIH), USA.
- All records pertaining to clinical trials must be maintained for a period of at least 15 years. The head of the institution should facilitate the maintenance of records through investigator and IC-SCR.
- Participants enrolled for clinical trials are not liable to pay any charges toward procedures, investigations and/or hospitalization related to the trial.
- An institution or laboratory developing or processing stem cells for human use should obtain National Accreditation Board for Testing and Calibration (NABL), accreditation for all laboratory procedures required for product development.
- The cells or cell-based products used in the trial should be processed in a CDSCO certified GLP and GMP facility (Schedule L1 and M of Drugs and Cosmetic Act, 1940 and rules therein).
- Those working with human iPSCs should be cautious with the vectors and genes used for induction of stemness against possible malignant transformation.
- Sponsors shall take note of their responsibilities and liabilities under various statutes, regulations, and guidelines governing research and development in this field in the country.
- Government agencies/sponsors facilitating stem cell research must ensure that the projects submitted for financial support has prior approval of IC-SCR in addition to IEC/IAEC/IBSC (whichever applicable).
- For multicentric clinical trials, all participating sites should obtain approvals form their own IC-SCR and IEC.
- Each institution shall have an empanelled roster of investigators conducting stem cell research and ensure that national guidelines, regulations, and best practices are followed.
- Institutions conducting stem cell research shall establish suitable mechanism for creating awareness among the scientific community and the public at large.

IMPORTANT DEFINITIONS

- *Adult stem cell*: It is also known as somatic stem cell. A relatively rare undifferentiated cell found in many organs and differentiated tissues with a limited capacity for both self-renewal (in the laboratory) and differentiation. Such cells vary in their differentiation capacity, but it is usually limited to cell types in the organ of origin. This is an active area of investigation.
- *Conflict of interest*: A situation in which a person is in a position to derive personal benefit from actions or decisions made in their official capacity.
- *Induced pluripotent stem cell (iPSC)*: These are adult differentiated cells that have been genetically reprogrammed to become an embryonic stem cell-like cell by being forced to express genes and factors important for maintaining the properties of pluripotent stem cells.
- *Adverse event*: Any untoward medical occurrence in a patient or participant involved in a study which does not necessarily have a causal relationship with the intervention. The adverse event can therefore be any unfavorable or unintended sign or experience, whether or not related to the product under investigation.
- *Clinical trial registry*: An official platform for registering a clinical trial, such as Clinical Trial Registry of India.
- *Vulnerability*: Vulnerability in research pertains to individuals who are relatively or absolutely incapable of protecting their own interests because of personal disability, environmental burdens or social injustice, lack of power, understanding or ability to communicate or are in a situation that prevents them from doing so.
- *Institutional Ethics Committee*: An independent body (a review board or a committee, institutional, regional, national, or supranational), constituted of medical professionals and nonmedical members, whose responsibility is to ensure the protection of the rights, safety and wellbeing of human subjects involved in a trial and to provide public assurance of that protection, by, among other things, reviewing and approving/providing favorable opinion on, the trial protocol, the suitability of the investigator(s), facilities, and the methods and material to be used in obtaining and documenting informed consent of the trial subjects.

IMPORTANT GUIDELINES

- National Ethical Guidelines for Biomedical and Health Research Involving Human Participants, Indian Council of Medical Research, 2017.
- National Guidelines on Stem Cell Research, Indian Council of Medical Research and Department of Biotechnology, 2017.
- Schedule Y—the Drugs and Cosmetics Act, 1940.
- Indian Good Clinical Practices (GCP) guidelines, CDSCO. Ministry of Health, Government of India.

FURTHER READING

1. Govt. of India. The Drugs and Cosmetics Act, 1940 (Schedule Y). New Delhi.
2. ICMR. National Ethical Guidelines for Biomedical and Health Research Involving Human Participants. New Delhi: Indian Council of Medical Research; 2017.
3. ICMR. National Guidelines on Stem Cell Research. New Delhi: Indian Council of Medical Research/Department of Biotechnology; 2017.

Cellular Therapy in Rheumatoid Arthritis

Sathish Muthu, Madhan Jeyaraman, Manish Khanna

INTRODUCTION

Rheumatoid arthritis (RA) is an autoimmune disorder essentially triggered by the activation of fibroblast-like synoviocytes (FLS) which in turn triggers a series of inflammatory reactions leading to the disease process. The treatment of the disorder has been closely evolving with an understanding of its pathogenesis. Before the middle of the 1980s, the drugs used were nonsteroidal anti-inflammatory drugs (NSAIDs) and steroids. Then the main modality of treatment was through the disease-modifying anti-rheumatoid drugs (DMARDs). Decoding the molecular basis of inflammation in RA opened new arenas in its management with the introduction of the regenerative science.

ROLE OF PLATELETS IN RHEUMATOID ARTHRITIS

Platelets apart from their role in coagulation are immunomodulators. Particularly in RA, their number and activation correlates with the disease activity. The proinflammatory products released in RA and the products of articular cartilage degradation lead to recruitment and dysregulated activation of the platelets. Platelets are known to contribute IL-1 alpha, IL-1 beta, platelet derived growth factor, transforming growth factor-beta, chemokine ligands CXCL4 and CXCL7, platelet-activating factor, thrombin and thromboxane A2 among others which play an important role in various stages of inflammation in RA. The diverse role of platelets in the pathogenesis of RA has attracted trial of drugs-targeting platelets for the management of RA. Another facet of platelet function in RA is the immune crosstalk. There exists a crosstalk between the immune cells and platelets by which platelets modulate both innate and adaptive immunity. This is facilitated by the expression of diverse ligands and receptors. For example, they express receptors of innate immunity, coreceptors, toll-like receptors, complement receptors, and chemokine receptors. The platelet ligand CD40L promotes B- and T-cell responses like isotype switching in B cells and dendritic cell activation and maturation.

Adding to the complexity of the role of platelets in immunomodulation is their ability to exhibit opposite effects. For example, the platelet released chemokine–beta thromboglobulin increases neutrophil recruitment while the proresolving protein annexin A1, lipoxin A4, and marecin 1 hamper it. Platelets release both pro- and antiangiogenic mediators platelet-derived growth factor, vascular endothelial growth factor, basic fibroblast growth factor, and angiopoietin are all pro-angiogenic while the thrombospondin 1 and CXCL4 are anti-angiogenic. They exhibit both pro- and anti-inflammatory properties which probably change according to the microenvironment. There are major knowledge gaps in the complex role of platelets in inflammation and immunomodulation, mainly because of difficulty in reproducing the in vivo microenvironments in vitro.

MOLECULAR BASIS OF PLATELET RICH PLASMA IN RHEUMATOID ARTHRITIS

Apart from the high concentration of growth factors in platelet rich plasma (PRP) with wound and cartilage healing capacity which formed the rationale for their use in many disease conditions, there are some mechanisms to be considered specific to RA. Newer insights into platelet–lymphocyte interactions suggest that they may dampen the disease process in RA. Zamora et al. in their in vitro study noted that the coculture of platelets and T cells reduced the levels of interferon-gamma and TNF-alpha from T cells. They also reduced T-cell proliferation and expression of CD25, PDL1, and SLAM. This immunomodulatory action mainly by interaction through P-selectin and was partly contributed by soluble proteins such as CXCL4, transforming growth factor-beta and soluble CD40L.

When cocultured with synovial fluid cells from RA patients the platelets reduced the inflammatory cytokine production and increased IL-10 production. The effect of platelets on T cells was dose-dependent and donor independent. Activated platelets injected into joints suppress the release necrosis factor kappa B from chondrocytes halting the disease progress in degenerative arthritis. The results have been supportive in knee and hip osteoarthritis. PRP has shown promising effects in other inflammatory conditions. The topical use of PRP in skin ulcers of systemic sclerosis has shown beneficial results. They have been tried in psoriasis with good results.

Effects of PRP on RA: In vitro Studies

Yan et al. evaluated the effects of the PRP on the invasion and migration of RA–FLS cells. They concluded that PRP induces migration and invasion of FLS by increased expression of MMP-1 (matrix metalloproteinase-1) and actin cytoskeletal reorganization. Wang et al. extracted platelet-derived microparticles (PMS) from PRP and evaluated its effects on the RA-FLS. They concluded that PMS promoted ECM adhesion, migration, and invasion of RA-FLSs. The underlying mechanism may be the increased expression of MMP1 by activation of the NF-κB pathway, which is activated by Erk phosphorylation.

Tohidnezhad et al. used the K4IM line of synoviocytes. They used tumor necrosis factor-alpha (TNF alpha) stimulation to induce rheumatoid arthritis-like inflammation in these cells. The platelet-releasing growth factors extracted from the PRP was applied to such cells. These factors reduced the proinflammatory cytokines. Tong et al. tried PRP on RA-FLS MH7A cell lines and Hela, human FLS-like cells in two different experiments. They induced RA-like inflammation using LPS (lipopolysaccharides) stimulation in the first experiment and TNF-alpha stimulation in the second experiment. PRP effectively downregulated the proinflammatory cytokines in both the studies. PRP also inhibited abnormal angiogenesis and decreased the longevity of the diseased cells.

Effects of PRP on RA: Animal Studies

Lippross et al. conducted studies on the effect of PRP in pigs with RA changes. PRP, apart from reducing the level of proinflammatory markers, restored the prearthritic level of chondral proteins and attenuated chondral and synovial changes in arthritis. Tong et al. evaluated the effects of PRP in RA induced mice and concluded that PRP decreases synovial hyperplasia, inflammatory cell infiltration, and cartilage and bone destruction in RA.

Shafiq et al. evaluated the effect of PRP in RA induced rats. They have also compared the effects with that of glycyrrhizin and a combination of glycyrrhizin and PRP. They found that PRP and glycyrrhizin both produced a significant decrease in arthritic index in rats, along with the decrease in the biochemical markers of arthritis with a positive histopathological change.

Effects of PRP on RA: Human Studies

The only study on the effects of PRP on RA in human subjects is a case series by Badsha et al. in 2019. They administered the PRP to four RA patients in seven joints who had inadequate response to intra-articular steroids injection. All the patients were on oral antirheumatoid drugs before and after steroid and PRP injection. They used the Visual Analogue Scale (VAS), Disease Activity Score (DAS), and ultrasonographic evaluation of joints to grade the improvement after PRP injection. Three patients had immediate pain relief with improvement in synovial changes. One patient had only improvement in synovial changes while VAS score remained the same.

Inference from in vitro Studies

Of the four in vitro studies included—only two studies used PRP. Two studies used extracts from the PRP. Wang et al. used PMS from PRP while Tohidnezhad et al. used platelet-releasing growth factor extracts. Based on the studies utilizing specific extracts, the holistic effect of PRP cannot be concluded. However, considering the paucity of literature on the subject it is essential to include all the available evidences in review to arrive at an inference.

Two studies that investigated the effect of PRP and PMS on migration of RA-FLS point out that PRP increased the migration and invasion of RA-FLS. They, however, did not analyze the other effects of PRP on inflammation. Since Tohidnezhad et al. used platelet-releasing growth factor extract in the analysis of effects on inflammation, the two experiments by Tong et al. remain the only studies that evaluated the complete effects of PRP on RA cell lines. Their studies show encouraging results. To conclude, in the in vitro studies while platelets increase the migration and invasion of RA-FLS, they seem to suppress the inflammation on the whole.

In an in vitro study by Anitua et al., the platelet released growth factors increased the hyaluronic acid secretion from the synovial cells derived from knee osteoarthritis patients. Mishra et al. in in vitro studies showed that buffered PRP increased mesenchymal cell proliferation and chondrogenic differentiation. Kruger et al. in their in vitro analysis showed improved migration and chondrogenic differentiation of subchondral progenitor cells with the addition of PRP. Thus, PRP is chondroprotective.

Inference from Animal Studies

Available animal studies on pigs, rats, and mice show encouraging molecular, histologic, and clinical results. There has been no evidence of exacerbation of inflammation in these studies. Pan et al. evaluated the effects of a combination of PRP, black phosphorus nanoparticles, and chitosan thermoresponsive hydrogel with phototherapy in an in vitro environment and mice with collagen-induced arthritis along with controls. This concoction included osteogenic and thermoresponsive black phosphorus delivered through chitosan thermoresponsive hydrogel intra-articularly along with PRP followed by phototherapy. The addition of PRP to the concoction in vitro increased the binding of mesenchymal stem cells to the hydrogel. In vivo, it reduced the synovial hyperplasia and bone destruction even without phototherapy.

Human study, a case series by Badsha et al. has also shown encouraging results in RA not responding to steroids.

Safety Profile of PRP on RA

Platelet rich plasma is an autologous product. Hence there is no or minimal risk for disease transmission, immunogenic reactions, or cancer. Though long-term studies evaluating its safety profile in the musculoskeletal field is lacking, long-term studies from the oromaxillary field show that PRP is relatively safe. Hypersensitivity to the bovine thrombin that was previously used for activation of PRP is now rare because of the switch to modern alternatives. The development of antibodies against clotting factors—V and IX leading to life-threatening coagulopathies has been reported. There is no compelling evidence of any systemic effects to a local PRP injection. Local complications include scar tissue and calcification at the injection site.

EFFECTS OF HEMATOPOIETIC STEM CELL TRANSPLANTATION ON RHEUMATOID ARTHRITIS

Despite the usage of both conventional DMARDs, and newer biologicals, 40% of the patients with RA continue to have frequent relapses with active and progressive disease. Autologous hematopoietic stem cell transplantation (HSCT) has been considered as an alternative modality of management of such resistant candidates. Although HSCs are multipotent stem cells with the potential to give rise to blood, endothelial cells, and immune cells, in the context of their role in autoimmune diseases they are viewed as immune stem cells. The major complication from the HSCT arises not by the HSCs transfer itself but from the immunosuppressive conditioning regimens utilized to inhibit the autoreactive immune cells prior to the transfer. The rationale of using the immunosuppressive conditioning regimens is not to myeloablate the host immune system but to lymphoablate the autoimmune cells so that immune regeneration starts from the transferred HSCs. These nonmyeloablative regimens used in the included studies commonly employed CYC. Special attention is given to the regimen-related side effects particularly from the high dose CYC which forms the backbone of these regimens.

Response to the HSCT was shown by the reduction in the serum autoantibody titers noted in the included studies. This shows a temporal relationship between the immune balance restoration and clinical response outcomes as a precondition to get immune tolerance in RA patients. However, to obtain optimal results from the HSCT patient selection is of key importance. Although recommended for patients who failed conventional spectrum of management, good results from HSCT are obtained from patients presenting with an early aggressive disease with poor prognostic factors who also have enough residual functional capacity to benefit out of the procedure.

Hematopoietic stem cell transplantation also has considerable morbidity and treatment-related mortality (TRM) associated with it. Based on the registry data, 1-year transplant-related mortality due to autologous HSCT for hematological malignancies was 2–5%. However, from the included studies we noted <1% TRM from the HSCT procedure for RA. The most common complication encountered with HSCT from all the included studies is an infection due to the immunosuppression that accompanies the conditioning protocol followed. Owing to the neutropenia, bacterial or fungal infections may occur and lymphopenia may lead to latent viral and opportunistic infections. This has been counteracted by the empirical use of broad-spectrum antibacterial, antiviral and antifungal medication in this high-risk period post-transplantation.

The risk of TRM and toxicity depends not only on the HSCT protocol used but also on the source of the donor cells. Allogeneic HSCT is associated with a higher risk of complications especially due to the GVHD associated with them. Most of the adverse events are associated with the conditioning regimens utilized following allogeneic HSCT. To clear the autoreactive inflammatory cells from causing GVHD an array of conditioning regimens including drugs such as fludarabine, melphalan, alemtuzumab, treosulfan along with CYC have been utilized in the included studies. To optimize the safety of the procedure, the treatment must be offered after preliminary screening for comorbidities and cardiopulmonary ailments and administration of the regimens in dedicated centers with appropriate supportive care to make the procedure successful and safe.

Is Stem Cell Rescue Necessary after High Dose Immune Ablation?

With the studies reporting complete remission of severe cases of RA after a myeloablative dose of CYC without being followed by HSCT, a question arises whether the procedure is needed first hand. Regeneration of the marrow function similar to HSCT was noted but at a slower pace. Introducing the autoimmune lymphocytes into the host following a high dose of CYC may be a reason for noted failure in some of the cases of autologous HSCT. Although the concept appears appealing, whether it could be qualified to be investigated under a clinical trial poses ethical considerations. However, one could plan for a trial with and without immediate stem cell rescue following high dose CYC therapy for RA patients.

Ideal Source of Hematopoietic Stem Cells

There has been a shift in the source of autologous HSCT from bone marrow (BM) to peripheral blood stem cells (PBSC) because of the rapid hematological recovery especially platelet and neutrophil counts following reinfusion when PBSC is used as a source of HSCT. It also makes the procedure more cost-effective. But it is also noted that, when PBSC is used as a source of HSCT, an 11-fold increase in T cells and an 8-fold increase in B cells were noted, thereby making them less likely to provide any sustained benefit compared to BM source which has a less cellular load on reinfusion. It is also not evident whether the peripheral T cell counts have any temporal association to the damage caused by the disease. One other finding in allogeneic HSCT is that patients who undergone HCST with PBSC source did not document any proportional increase in GVHD compared to BM source. Hence, comparative long-term clinical trials to explore the ideal source of HSCs need further exploration.

Depletion of T Cells from the Harvested Hematopoietic Stem Cells

Although Phase I and Phase II clinical studies established the therapeutic potential, clinical safety, and efficacy of HSCT therapy. There is a paucity of literature to provide a consensus whether the lymphocytes from the collected peripheral HSCs should be depleted before reinfusion. Although T-cell depletion (TCD) prevents the re-entry of autoimmune cells in the system, the procedure bears the risk of late opportunistic infections especially cytomegalovirus and Epstein-Barr virus. There is a current understanding that complete lymphoablation may not be needed since the immune reset happens with the development of the immune regulatory networks and immune tolerance. Moreover, Joske et al. in their study did not find any significant difference due to CD34+ selection either. Hence, the need for TCD has to be further explored with randomized controlled trials to arrive at a definite conclusion on this aspect of HSCT.

Ideal Conditioning Regimen for Rheumatoid Arthritis

Most of the included studies utilized CYC based regimen to minimize the effect of residual autoreactive clone in the body. The effect of the conditioning regimen used on the results of the transplant remains unexplored although the intensity of the conditioning might play a role. Most of the included studies utilized CYC at a high dose of 200 mg/kg administered for four days. Such high dose chemotherapy has its side-effects such as hemorrhagic cystitis. Further research to identify alternative conditioning regimens that are immunosuppressive without being myelosuppressive and also prolongs the remission achieved in patients is needed. Other combinations such as regimens containing ATG were also tried in some of the included studies. Administration of G-CSF in the post-transplant state would shorten the recovery period but in some cases, G-CSF has been shown to trigger an exacerbation of arthritis which needs further exploration. Moreover, clinical trials are needed to evaluate the difference between regimens with enhanced immunoablative capacity where the greater toxicity is justified with prolonged remission and conventional regimens with added post-transplant immune suppression to prolong the remission.

Ideal Timing of HSCT for Rheumatoid Arthritis

The major challenge in utilizing HSCT for RA is the timing of initiation of the treatment in the course of the disease. If the patient is considered for HSCT after a trial of response to immunosuppressive therapy with DMARDs, the disease could have evolved beyond the point of maximum benefit from HSCT since they are less effective in patients with advanced organ damage and immune dysregulation. Since there are no specific guidelines to the timing and patient profile selection for enrolling into HSCT, the decision largely lies in the hands of the patients and their treating physicians. Clinicians should help the patients choose the right treatment by weighing their pros and cons together and provide clear information to aid in the decision-making process considering the prognostic factors associated with the disease process in the individual patients. Although the treatment seems promising, the guidelines drafted by the European League against Rheumatism (EULAR) and EMBT for patient selection for optimal response need further improvement on the above-mentioned areas.

The small sample size of the included studies with heterogeneity in their patient selection methods, HSCT protocols utilized, the reported results, and their definition of remission limit their utility in decision making. In the absence of large clinical trials, a Markov clinical decision analysis to compare the conventional therapy with HSCT could be utilized. The model predicted HSCT to be superior to conventional therapy if the TRM could be maintained <3.3% or if the treatment results are sustainable for 5 years. Having done in the early era of biological therapy, these analyses emphasize that a subset of RA patients could also benefit from HSCT. The differences in the Quality Adjusted Life Years (QALY) between the two groups involved in the model reinstate the role of the patients in the decision-making process. With the improvement in the treatment methods, the safety of the procedure has largely been improved. In selected cases, HSCT may remain the only effective method available making these risks acceptable. Yet, the decision lies in the hands of the patient hence it needs careful discussion before making the treatment choice. With the rise in the resistance to traditional therapy for RA, earlier identification of those nonresponders based on clinic-serological profile and prognostic markers remains a key element to reap the maximum benefit out of this modality.

CONCLUSION

With the rising proportion of nonresponders to conventional DMARDs and biologic therapy, PRP and HSCT therapy would find a place in the treatment spectrum of RA provided large clinical trials with longer follow-up are conducted to establish the ideal treatment strategy to get optimal results out of this treatment modality.

FURTHER READING

1. Anitua E, Orive G. Short implants in maxillae and mandibles: a retrospective study with 1 to 8 years of follow-up. J Periodontol. 2010; 81:819-26.
2. Bingham SJ, Snowden J, McGonagle D, Richards S, Isaacs J, Morgan G, et al. Autologous stem cell transplantation for rheumatoid arthritis—interim report of 6 patients. J Rheumatol Suppl. 2001;64:21-4.
3. Bl C, Ja S, Gj M, Re C. Redo cardiac surgery: late bleeding complications from topical thrombin-induced factor V deficiency. J Thorac Cardiovasc Surg. 1993;105:222-7.
4. Bouffi C, Djouad F, Mathieu M, Noël D, Jorgensen C. Multipotent mesenchymal stromal cells and rheumatoid arthritis: risk or benefit? Rheumatol Oxf Engl. 2009;48:1185-9.
5. Brodsky RA, Petri M, Smith BD, Seifter EJ, Spivak JL, Styler M, et al. Immunoablative high-dose cyclophosphamide without stem-cell rescue for refractory, severe autoimmune disease. Ann Intern Med. 1998;129:1031-5.
6. Brown AJ, Sepuru KM, Sawant KV, Rajarathnam K. Platelet-derived chemokine CXCL7 dimer preferentially exists in the glycosaminoglycan-bound form: implications for neutrophil-platelet crosstalk. Front Immunol. 2017;8:1248.
7. Chakravdhanula U, Anbarasu K, Verma VK, Beevi SS. Clinical efficacy of platelet-rich plasma in combination with methotrexate in chronic plaque psoriatic patients. Dermatol Ther. 2016;29:446-50.
8. Chellamuthu G, Muthu S, Khanna M, Khanna V. Platelet-rich plasma holds promise in management of rheumatoid arthritis: systematic review. Rheumatol Int. 2021.
9. Durez P, Toungouz M, Schandené L, Lambermont M, Goldman M. Remission and immune reconstitution after T-cell-depleted stem-cell transplantation for rheumatoid arthritis. Lancet. 1998;352:881.
10. Everts PAM, Knape JTA, Weibrich G, Schönberger JP, Hoffmann J, Overdevest EP, et al. Platelet rich plasma and platelet gel: a review. J Extra Corpor Technol. 2006; 38:174-87.
11. Gabriel SE, Crowson CS, Luthra HS, Wagner JL, O'Fallon WM. Modeling the lifetime costs of rheumatoid arthritis. J Rheumatol. 1999;26:1269-74.
12. Giuggioli D, Colaci M, Manfredi A, Mariano M, Ferri C. Platelet gel in the treatment of severe scleroderma skin ulcers. Rheumatol Int. 2012;32:2929-32.
13. Jenne CN, Urrutia R, Kubes P. Platelets: bridging hemostasis, inflammation, and immunity. Int J Lab Hematol. 2013; 35:254-61.
14. Joske DJ, Ma DT, Langlands DR, Owen ET. Autologous bone-marrow transplantation for rheumatoid arthritis. Lancet Lond Engl. 1997;350:337-8.
15. Lippross S, Moeller B, Haas H, Tohidnezhad M, Steubesand N, Wruck CJ, et al. Intra-articular injection of platelet-rich plasma reduces inflammation in a pig model of rheumatoid arthritis of the knee joint. Arthritis Rheum. 2011;63:3344-53.
16. M F Silva J, Ladomenou F, Carpenter B, Chandra S, Sedlacek P, Formankova R, et al. Allogeneic hematopoietic stem cell transplantation for severe, refractory juvenile idiopathic arthritis. Blood Adv. 2018;2:777-86.
17. Moore J, Brooks P, Milliken S, Biggs J, Ma D, Handel M, et al. A pilot randomized trial comparing CD34-selected versus unmanipulated hemopoietic stem cell transplantation for severe, refractory rheumatoid arthritis. Arthritis Rheum. 2002;46:2301-9.
18. Pavletic SZ, Klassen LW, Pope R, O'Dell JR, Traynor AE, Haire CE, et al. Treatment of relapse after autologous blood stem cell transplantation for severe rheumatoid arthritis. J Rheumatol Suppl. 2001;64:28-31.
19. Sampson S, Gerhardt M, Mandelbaum B. Platelet-rich plasma injection grafts for musculoskeletal injuries: a review. Curr Rev Musculoskelet Med. 2008;1:165-74.
20. Santos-Moreno P, Valencia O. Experience of biological therapy units in rheumatoid arthritis and other autoimmune diseases. Reumatol Clin. 2019;15:61-2.
21. Shafik NM, El-Esawy RO, Mohamed DA, Deghidy EA, El-Deeb OS. Regenerative effects of glycyrrhizin and/or platelet rich plasma on type-II collagen-induced arthritis: targeting autophay machinery markers, inflammation and oxidative stress. Arch Biochem Biophys. 2019;675:108095.
22. Spero JA. Bovine thrombin-induced inhibitor of factor V and bleeding risk in postoperative neurosurgical patients. Report of three cases. J Neurosurg. 1993;78:817-20.
23. Tong S, Zhang C, Liu J. Platelet-rich plasma exhibits beneficial effects for rheumatoid arthritis mice by suppressing inflammatory factors. Mol Med Rep. 2017;16:4082-8.
24. Verburg RJ, Sont JK, van Laar JM. Reduction of joint damage in severe rheumatoid arthritis by high-dose chemotherapy and autologous stem cell transplantation. Arthritis Rheum. 2005;52:421-4.
25. Wang MJ, Huang Y, Huang RY, Chen X, Zhou Y, Yu, W et al. Determination of role of thromboxane A2 in rheumatoid arthritis. Discov Med. 2015;19:23-32.

Cytotherapy in Osteoarthritic Knee

Madhan Jeyaraman, Sathish Muthu, Naveen Jeyaraman

INTRODUCTION

The large economic burden on the global health care systems is due to the increasing number of symptomatic osteoarthritis (OA) knee patients whereby accounting for greater morbidity and impaired functional quality-of-life. The hyaline cartilage provides friction-free joint movements that protect the underlying bone from excessive load and trauma by distributing the forces equally across the joint. Due to the limited intrinsic healing potentiality and avascular nature of cartilage, once it gets injured, it gradually degenerates and results in osteoarthritis. The booming ideology of "Orthobiologics" has brought up the practice of procedures that are less invasive in nature by administering substances with osteoinductive and osteogenic facets; thereby offering the benefit of decreased morbidity over classic techniques.

The recent developments and impulses in molecular and regenerative medicine have paved the way for inducing the biological active cells such as stem cells, bioactive materials, and growth factors toward the healing and tissue regenerative process. In this connotation, mesenchymal stem cells (MSCs) are the ideal cell-based resort for treating disorders under a minimally invasive environment in conjunction with tissue regeneration. The efficacy of such cell therapies in animal models has been widely recognized.

Mesenchymal stem cells act as a minimally invasive procedure that bridges the gap between pharmacological treatment and surgical treatment for osteoarthritis. It provides a strong and positive balance between proapoptotic and antiapoptotic molecules, proinflammatory and anti-inflammatory cytokines and proangiogenic and antiangiogenic factors for rejuvenation of degenerated cartilaginous tissues. MSCs upregulate tissue inhibitors of metalloproteinases such as TIMPs-1, -3, and -4 by downregulating the signaling molecules of matrix metalloproteinases such as MMP-1, -3, -13, and -28 and upregulating ADAMTS-4 and 5 which lead to normal joint homeostasis.

PHYSIOLOGY OF MSC ACTION IN OSTEOARTHRITIS KNEE

Growth factors and BMP 2 and 7 are reported to exercise anabolic and anti-inflammatory effects and noteworthy these are present in higher concentrations in BMAC. There is induced production of interleukin-1 receptor antagonist (IL-1Ra) molecule in significant concentration by the MSCs and these produced molecules execute the bioactivity of inhibiting IL-1 catabolism. This interesting biological approach renders symptomatic relief in pain. MSCs also support neoangiogenesis through VEGF-A, VEGF-D, HGF, IGF-1, PDGF, PIGF, IL-6, EPO, MCP-1 and cellular proliferation through KGF, FGF-2, VEGF, IGF, PDGF, HGF. MSCs exerted enhanced chondroprotection through diminished proinflammatory mediator production and increased anti-inflammatory cytokine production including IDO, PGE2, TGF-β, TSG-6, HGF, NO, HO-1, HLA-G. They mediate their antiapoptotic actions through VEGF, HGF, IGF-1, TGF-β, GM-CSF. A schematic diagram elaborating on the physiological action of MSC in immunomodulation of OA pathogenesis is given in **Figure 1**.

SOURCES OF MESENCHYMAL STEM CELLS

Mesenchymal stem cells are pluripotent cells with the potential to differentiate into the chondrogenic and osteogenic lineage. They can be derived and isolated from various autologous sources such as bone marrow, adipose tissue, synovium, endometrium, peripheral blood, and allogeneic sources such as placenta, umbilical cord, amniotic fluid as shown in **Figure 2**. However, evidence to delineate the ideal source of MSCs for use in osteoarthritis knee remains unclear. In this review, we elaborate on the various types of MSCs available for therapeutic use and their merits and demerits to address the gap in knowledge in literature.

Embryonic Stem Cells

Embryonic stem cells (ESCs) are derived from the inner cell mass of the blastocyst. Preclinical and clinical studies have proved the significant potential for cartilage engineering. ESCs are totipotent cells. ESCs provide numerous numbers of undifferentiated cells which may differentiate into a cell of a particular lineage. The cultured ESCs provide 3D scaffolds for cartilage engineering. Embryonic stem cells are pluripotent, but their use raises ethical concerns, and additionally

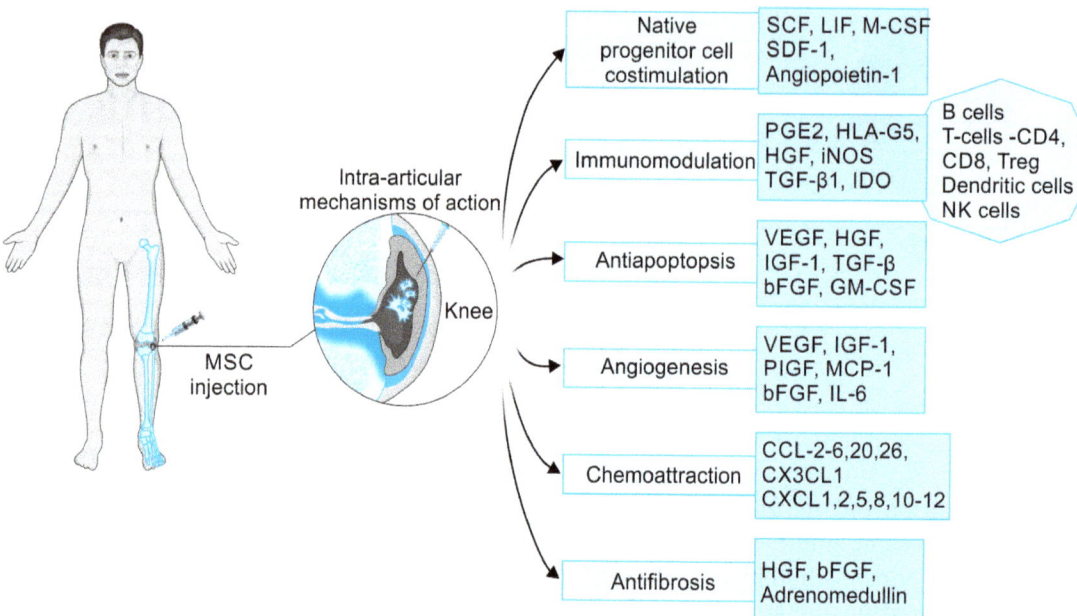

Fig. 1: Schematic diagram elaborating on the physiological action of mesenchymal stem cells (MSCs) in immunomodulation of osteoarthritis (OA) pathogenesis.

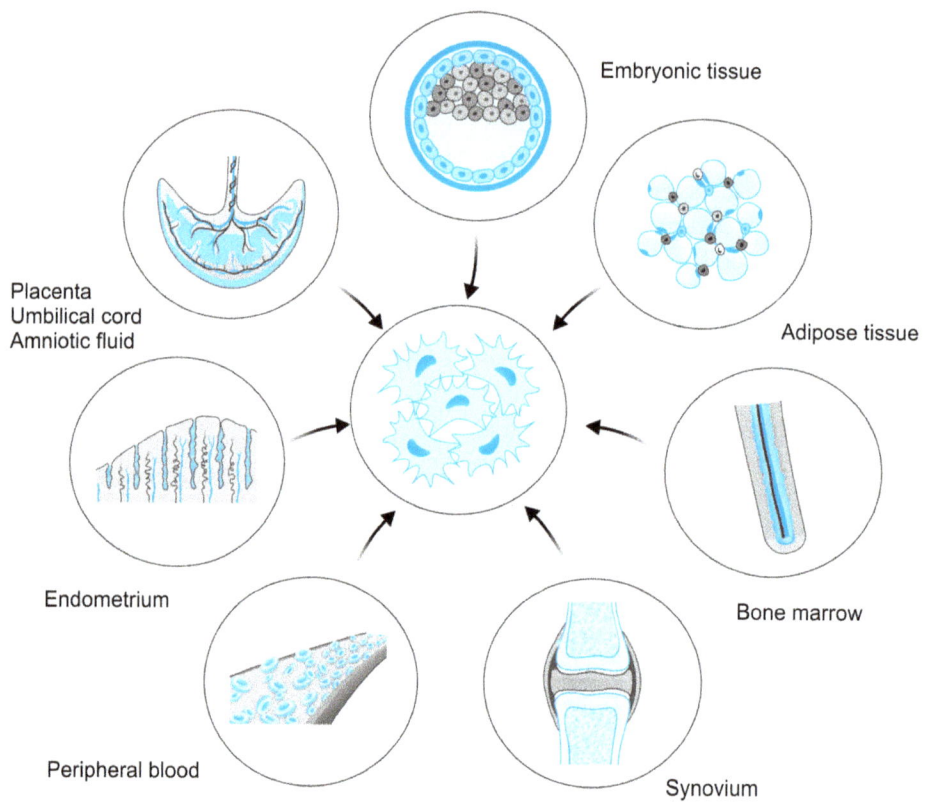

Fig. 2: Sources of mesenchymal stem cells with therapeutic potential.

upon transplantation, they potentially give rise to tumors. Under the controlled growth conditions, ESCs maintained phenotype and genotype along with maintenance of MSC surface markers and exponential proliferation of cellular lineage. Toh et al. demonstrated neochondrogenesis and ECM production under appropriate growth factors, cytokines, and hyaluronic acid-based hydrogels.

Bone Marrow-derived MSCs

In 1970, Alexander Friedenstein demonstrated the definitive regenerating capacity of bone marrow. The major source of bone marrow-derived MSCs (BM-MSCs) is the iliac crest and shafts of long bones. Various researchers have reported that BM-MSCs showed fibroblastoid cells with plastic adhered morphology and nonphagocytic in nature. BM-MSCs showed differentiation toward osteogenic, adipogenic, and chondrogenic responses with the expression of endothelial or hematopoietic specific markers. BM-MSCs express CD146 in humans and CXCL12, Nestin, leptin receptor, and Prx-1 in mice. The osteogenic potential of BM-MSC varies as a few studies prove the greater osteogenic potential and a few prove the equal osteogenic potential when compared with adipose tissue-derived MSCs (AD-MSCs). BM-MSC exhibits an inferior chondrogenic potential when compared with AD-MSC and superior response when compared with Sy-MSCs.

Adipose Tissue-derived MSCs

In recent years, the cells with major regenerative, rejuvenative, and reconstructive potentials were attributed to adipose tissue-derived MSCs due to the possession of characteristics of mesenchymal stem/stromal cells. AD-MSCs are isolated from lipoaspiration as an aqueous fraction from abdominal fat. The components of stromal vascular fraction (SVF) are the combination of adipose-derived stromal cells, endothelial precursor cells, mature endothelial cells, lymphocytes, pericytes, preadipocytes, and mature adipocytes. For bone and cartilage regeneration, the recent advances in the field of molecular and translational medicine have placed SVF at the highest regenerative potential horizon. Since they possess MSC-like properties, SVF renders a better regenerative potential, immunomodulation, anti-inflammation, and neoangiogenesis at the site of action. Despite the better translational potential of SVF in regenerative medicine, the challenges are viewed in the form of isolation and quantification of cellular components in SVF. Due to the presence of various cellular components in the SVF mixture, adipose-derived stem cells share a common cell surface antigen of hematopoietic stem cell CD34 as proposed by the International Society of Cellular Therapy (ISCT). Various researchers stated that SVF has a strong potential for regenerating tissues like MSCs.

An SVF mimics the morphology of fibroblasts and possesses mesenchymal stem cells like properties. Due to the MSC-like property of SVF, it induces the differentiation of different lineage of cells such as osteoblast, chondroblast, myoblast, and adipoblast. The cellular mixture of SVF possesses cell surface antigens of both HSCs (CD-34 and 45) and MSCs (CD-105 and 146). SVF cells share common cell surface antigens of bone marrow-derived mesenchymal stem cells such as CD-24, 29, 31, 44, 45, 71, 90, 105/SH2, and SH3. Since adipose tissue contains various components of a cellular mixture, the concept of allogenicity with adipose tissue-derived stem cells is questionable. AD-MSCs exhibit significant osteogenic potential with the cytokines secreted by the cellular mixture and hence act as a promising therapeutic agent for bone and cartilage engineering in orthopedic disorders. Our recent meta-analysis found AD-MSCs to have an upper hand compared to BM-MSCs in the management of OA knee in terms of their efficacy and safety.

Synovium-derived MSCs

Mesenchymal stem cells in synovial fluid are increased along with degenerated cartilage in osteoarthritis and the gene profile of these cells is more similar to the synovial MSCs indicating their role in OA. In humans, MSCs derived from synovial tissue may have superior chondrogenic potential. In a study, the transplantation of synovial MSC resulted in full defect filling of the cartilage without any adverse clinical events. Animal models have revealed that the joint microenvironment has endogenous populations of synovial MSCs which have chondrogenic differentiating potential and to some extent, contribute to cartilage repair. Mak and colleagues demonstrated that intra-articular injection of autologous or allogeneic synovial MSCs has beneficial effects when infused into a diseased joint. Delgado-Enciso and colleagues recently recommended an inventive approach for cartilage regeneration which is based on the intra-articular injection of bioactive cell-free formulation (BIOF2), a compound that could promote expansion and chondrogenic differentiation of endogenous populations of synovial MSCs. Horie and Mizuno reported that synovium-derived MSCs (Sy-MSCs) injected into rat knees accommodated themselves to the lesion, differentiated into chondrocytes directly, and promoted cartilage regeneration without traveling to distant organs. Repeated injections of Sy-MSCs have shown a chondroprotective effect and promising results in rat OA models. Successful cartilage repair following direct injection of Sy-MSCs may reflect the ability of synovial MSCs to home to chondral lesions.

Endometrium-derived MSCs

Endometrium-derived MSCs (En-MSCs) drew attention from global researchers for their accessibility from the source and non-posting ethical issues. In a reproductive life cycle of a woman, the endometrium undergoes over 400 cycles of regeneration. En-MSCs pose a greater potential for chondrogenesis via TGF-β, FGF-2, -9 and -18 and IGF-1. The isolation of En-MSCs is through the collection of menstrual blood, hysterectomized specimens, or endometrial biopsy. En-MSCs possess OCT-4, SSEA-4, and CD49a but lacks STRO1 expression. En-MSCs exhibited higher colony-forming units and proangiogenic properties than BM-MSCs. Miranda et al. exhibited that En-MSCs produce less cytokine activation and immunosuppressive molecules than BM-MSCs. Wolff EF et al. demonstrated chondrogenic differentiation potential in En-MSCs. Evidence proved the presence of epithelial cell nests in the endometrium which further shown stromal-epithelial interaction for differentiation into cells of bone, cartilage, and adipose tissue. Chen and his colleagues proved the inferior potential of En-MSCs toward chondrogenic and osteogenic nature when compared with BM-MSCs and Pl-MSCs.

Placental-derived MSCs and Umbilical Cord-derived MSCs

The appeal of using umbilical cord-derived stem cells (Um-MSCs) and placenta-derived stem cells (Pl-MSCs) is that they are the youngest stem cells available for osteoarthritis treatment. They are considered "Day Zero Cells". Umbilical cord blood as well as umbilical cord tissues contain cells with good proliferative capacity and chondrogenic potential. Also harvesting these cells is a painless and noninvasive procedure. Recently, clinical outcomes of human UCB-MSCs (hUCB-MSCs) for cartilage regeneration have been reported. In a trial, it was seen that a single intra-articular injection of placental MSC derived allogenically resulted in significant symptomatic improvement as well as improvement in the thickness of cartilage in knee OA. Soltani et al. reported that an allogeneic placental MSC-based product appeared safe and effective for the regeneration of hyaline-like cartilage in OA of the knee after 24 weeks of follow-up, obtained favorable clinical outcome. At the end of 24 weeks follow-up, they observed 10% improvement in cartilage thickness in the intervention group. Wang et al. found that Warton jelly-MSCs secreted more glycosaminoglycans than did BM-MSCs during chondrogenic differentiation. A study showed the repair of articular cartilage in animal models with the help of placenta-derived MSCs grown on silk fibroin material. Human umbilical origin stem cells are found to mitigate OA progression in large animal models too. In the phase I/II trial, a repeated UC-MSC dose strategy led to a favorable safety profile and improved clinical results for the treatment of long-term pain in knee OA patients.

Amniotic Fluid-derived MSCs

The applications of amniotic fluid-derived MSCs (AF-MSCs) have proven and hold a wide range of promising healing effects in sports injuries and pathologies of bone, tendon, and cartilage disorders. AF-MSCs have a higher differentiation potential for osteogenic and chondrogenic lineage than adult stem cells. AF-MSCs confer a low risk of tumor development without catering to the ethical concern and epigenetic memory over embryonic stem cells. In vitro studies suggest that the amniotic membrane proved to be a scaffold for cellular therapy in cartilage tissue repair. Preclinical studies suggested that dehydrated human amnion chorion membrane act as a disease modifier in OA knee. Attenuation of cartilage degeneration has been proved with a minced amniotic membrane in a rat MMT OA model. Willett et al. injected a dehydrated human amniotic membrane for the management of OA knee in the rat model and found lowered cartilage attenuation with enhanced proteoglycan and collagen II content in the regenerated cartilaginous tissue. In the literature, only two clinical trials on amniotic fluid-derived MSCs for management of OA knee were available. Vines et al. and Farr et al. proved the safety, efficacy, and functional outcome of amniotic fluid-derived MSCs on the management of OA knee in various KL grades.

Peripheral Blood-derived MSCs

An increasing number of studies have suggested that peripheral blood (PB) is a potential alternative source of MSCs, which have shown similar chondrogenic differentiation potential with bone marrow-derived MSCs (BM-MSCs) in both in vitro and in vivo studies. In a series of studies performed by Saw et al., a significant amount of articular cartilage regeneration, as well as profound symptomatic relief, was seen with autologous peripheral blood progenitor cells. In a clinical trial published in the year 2017, it was cited that intra-articular injection of allogenically harvested peripheral blood stem cells combined with hG-CSF helped in alleviating pain, disability, and better cartilage regeneration in OA patients and avoided total knee arthroplasty (TKA) in these patients offering a safe and exciting possibility in the treatment of OA. A study by Skowroński showed superior results for cartilage regeneration by PB-MSC as compared to bone marrow-derived cells. Another study demonstrated good evidence of articular cartilage repair, an increase in cartilage thickness as well as enhanced physical function by use of repeated injections of PBSC into the damaged joint. A recent review article established the use of PB-MSCs in cartilage repair and regeneration to be very safe and efficacious. In phase II clinical trial on the use of PBSCs in an arthritic knee, it was found that these cells increase the mean cartilage thickness and improve the quality-of-life.

ETHICAL CONCERNS

With the rapid advances in regenerative medicine using stem cells, ethical concerns for their use on patients have also been more stringent. The ethical issues that all stem cell researchers face begin with the development of a meaningful question before the clinical translation of the technology in hand which might bring about an answer which is both scientific and social value. The risk and benefits of the therapy to society and patients must be balanced at each stage of their research. Sound justification is needed to upgrade the research from animal models to human subjects. Minimizing the risk and harm, appropriate selection and recruitment of the subjects, and making an informed decision through consent forms are the ethical considerations involved in any clinical research, and stem cell therapy is no exception. With the increase in concerns for the use of animals in preclinical research, good animal models are often inadequate to equate the effects in humans. Hence, an uncertainty continues in the first human trials using stem cells even with increased safety protocols are in place.

Comparative characteristics of the individual sources and the level of ethical consideration with the sources and significance are elaborated in **Table 1**.

ONGOING RESEARCH AND FUTURE DIRECTIVES

Several preclinical studies and clinical trials have revealed that mesenchymal cells can be used to treat OA knees because of their self-renewal property and capacity for differentiation into the functional chondrocytes to form cartilage tissues, release various cytokines and chemokines, and provide an appropriate conducive microenvironment to promote cartilage repair.

Although the reliability of such treatment methodology for OA knee is being tested in human subjects by a few clinical trials, they provide us with conflicting results and thereby clouding this only ray of hope for OA knee patients. To date, 87 trials have been registered in the clinical trials registry, with 57 ongoing trials and 29 completed trials with their protocols given in **Table 2**.

TABLE 1: Comparative characteristics of the varied sources of mesenchymal stem cell (MSC) therapy for osteoarthritis (OA) knee.

Sources of MSCs	Ethical consideration	Sources	Significance	Invasiveness
ESCs	+++	Inner cell mass	Totipotent in nature; Allogenicity	+
BM-MSCs	+	Iliac crest	↑ potential to regenerate bone and cartilage; Easy to isolate stem cells; Auto and allogenicity ++; No culture required	–
AD-MSCs	+	Abdomen, medial aspect of thigh	↑ potential to regenerate cartilage and soft tissues; Complex natured to isolate stem cells; Autologous ++; Allogenicity	–
Sy-MSCs	+	Synovium around knee joint	↑ potential to regenerate bone and cartilage; Auto and allogenicity ++; Culture required for exponentiation	+
En-MSCs	+	Endometrial shedding	Potent to regenerate bone and cartilaginous tissues; Allogenicity ++; Culture required	+
Pl-MSCs	+	Amniotic membrane, chorionic plate, chorionic villi, decidua	Pluripotent in nature; Difficult to isolate cell mass; ↑ potential to regenerate bone, cartilage and soft tissues; Auto and allogenicity ++	–
Um-MSCs		Umbilical cord, Wharton's jelly	Pluripotent in nature; Auto and allogenicity ++; Culture required	–
AF-MSCs	+	Cytotrophoblast, syncytiotrophoblast	Pluripotent in nature; Auto and allogenicity ++; Culture required	–
PB-MSCs	+	Circulating mononuclear cells	Enhanced osteogenic and adipogenic potential	–

(ESCs: embryonic stem cells; BM-MSCs: bone marrow derived MSCs; AD-MSCs: adipose tissue derived MSCs; Sy-MSCs: synovium derived MSCs; En-MSCs: endometrium derived MSCs; Pl-MSCs: placental derived MSCs; Um-MSCs: umbilical derived MSCs; AF-MSCs: amniotic fluid derived MSCs; PB-MSCs: peripheral blood derived MSCs)

TABLE 2: Completed clinical trials evaluating the role of mesenchymal stem cells (MSC) in the management of osteoarthritis knee with published results.

Sl. No.	Author	NCT No.	Year	Country	MSC source	Cell density	Total patients	Follow-up	Clinical trial phase
1.	de Girolamo et al.	NCT01485198	2010	Mexico	Autologous hematopoietic stem cells from bone marrow	10 mL BMAC	61	6 months	I
2.	Taghiyar et al.	NCT00850187	2012	Iran	Autologous cultured BM-MSCs	-	6	12 months	I

Contd...

Contd...

Sl. No.	Author	NCT No.	Year	Country	MSC source	Cell density	Total patients	Follow-up	Clinical trial phase
3.	Emadedin et al.	NCT01207661	2012	Iran	Autologous cultured BM-MSCs	5×10^5 cells/kg/body weight	6	12 months	I
4.	Shadmanfar et al.	NCT01873625	2013	Iran	Autologous BM-MSCs	-	60	6 months	II and III
5.	Sheinko et al.	NCT01601951	2014	USA	Autologous BMAC	-	12	12 months	I
6.	Pers YM et al.	NCT01585857	2014	France	Autologous AD-MSCs	$2/10/50 \times 10^6$ AD-MSCs	18		I
7.	Vives et al.	NCT01227694	2015	Spain	Autologous cultured BM-MSCs	40×10^6 MSCs	15	12 months	I and II
8.	Orozco et al.	NCT01183728	2015	Spain	Autologous BM-MSCs	40×10^6 MSCs	12	24 months	I and II
9.	Orozco et al.	NCT01586312	2015	Spain	Allogenic ex vivo cultured BM-MSCs	40×10^6 MSCs	30	12 months	I and II
10.	Al-Najar et al.	NCT02118519	2016	Jordan	Allogeneic in vitro cultured BM-MSCs	$61 \times 10^6 \pm 0.6 \times 10^6$ MSCs	13	12 months	II
11.	Pham et al.	NCT02142842	2016	Vietnam	Autologous SVF and PRP	SVF – 1.0 to 5.0×10^7 cells	30	18 months	I and II
12.	Ghani et al.	NCT01448434	2016	Malaysia	Ex vivo cultured adult allogenic MSCs	-	72	12 months	II
13.	Agarwal et al.	NCT01453738	2016	India	Ex vivo cultured allogeneic BM-MSCs	$25/50/75/150 \times 10^6$ cells	60	12 months	II
14.	Royan Institute	NCT01504464	2016	Iran	MSCs		40	3 months	II
15.	Chen PJ	NCT02291926	2017	China	Human UC-MSCs	2×10^7 hUC-MSCs	20	12 months	I
16.	Camilleri et al. and Shapiro et al.	NCT01931007	2017	USA	Autologous BMAC	5 mL of treated cells + 10 mL platelet-poor bone marrow plasma	25	12 months	I
17.	Lamo-Espinosa et al.	NCT02123368	2017	Spain	Autologous ex vivo cultured BM-MSCs	10×10^6 cells	30	12 months	I and II
18.	Song et al.	NCT01809769	2017	China	Autologous AD-MSCs	$1/2/5 \times 10^7$ cells / 3 mL	18	24 months	I and II
19.	Bao and Zhang	NCT02162693	2017	China	Autologous in vitro extended AD-MSCs	-	53	12 months	II
20.	Lim et al.	NCT01041001	2017	Korea	CARTISTEM allogeneic UC-MSCs	Single dose of 500 µL/cm² containing 2.5×10^6 cells	102	60 months	III
21.	Lim et al.	NCT01626677	2017	Korea	CARTISTEM allogeneic UC-MSCs	Single dose of 500 µL/cm² containing 2.5×10^6 cells	103	48 months	III
22.	Matas and Espinoza	NCT02580695	2018	Chile	Allogeneic UC-MSCs	20×10^6 and 3 mL hyaluronic acid	30	12 months	I and II
23.	Ruane	NCT02958267	2018	USA	Autologous BMAC	5–6 mL BMAC	30	12 months	II
24.	Cellular Biomedicine group	NCT02641860	2018	China	Autologous in vitro extended AD-MSCs	-	22	48 months	I
25.	Jas Chahal	NCT02351011	2019	Canada	Autologous MSCs	$1/10/50 \times 10^6$ MSCs	12	60 months	I and II

Contd...

Contd...

Sl. No.	Author	NCT No.	Year	Country	MSC source	Cell density	Total patients	Follow-up	Clinical trial phase
26.	Lee WS et al.	NCT02658344	2019	Korea	Autologous AD-MSCs	1×10^8 cells per 3 mL	24	6 months	II
27.	Ho Ki Wai	NCT04326985	2020	Hong Kong	Autologous MSCs	-	20	12 months	I
28.	Gary Hieronimus	NCT03337243	2020	USA	Human amniotic membrane and human umbilical cord and Wharton's jelly injections	-	60	3 months	I
29.	Nature Cell Company	NCT02674399	2020	USA	Autologous AD-MSCs	-	28	24 months	II

(BMAC: bone marrow aspirate concentrate; BM-MSCs: bone marrow-derived MSCs; AD-MSCs: adipose tissue-derived MSCs; UC-MSCs: umbilical cord derived MSCs; PRP: platelet rich plasma; SVF: stromal vascular fraction)

Future Directives

Globally, regenerative science in orthopedics holds the future to treat certain conditions where clinicians face stagnation and challenges in the available treatment modalities for certain diseases such as the moderate stage of progressive osteoarthritis, uncontrolled rheumatoid arthritis, avascular necrosis of the head of the femur, tendinopathies, delayed and nonunion of fractures, etc. Stem cells and regenerative medicine hold positive health outcomes in various orthopedic disorders, which have a wide range of osteogenic and osteoinductive potentiality. Various researchers have worked on the next generation of platelet-rich plasma-like allogeneic platelet lysate, platelet-rich fibrin, and various types of mesenchymal stem cells.

The scope for further research in platelet-rich plasma and mesenchymal stem cells in osteoarthritis relies on standardization of dosage and frequency of the injection, universal protocol on preparation methods and injection techniques, quantification of growth factors injected, the role of autologous or allogeneic preparation, radiological documentation on cartilage growth, preparation and standardization for allogeneic formulation and conduction of randomized controlled trials to compare the efficacy and safety of various sources of MSCs and between other methods of cellular therapy in osteoarthritis knees.

CONCLUSION

Currently, various qualitative clinical measurements used to assess the outcomes of various sources of MSCs used in OA knee does not give an objective assessment of their efficacy. The development of appropriate surrogate systems of comparative design with more sensitive quantitative methods of outcome assessment to establish a comparative efficacy of various sources is the need of the hour. The available literature is limited to qualify a source to be ideal for clinical use in humans in OA knee. A consistent methodology to objectively evaluate the efficacy and safety of various sources of MSCs has to be utilized in all clinical trials to conclude their comparative effectiveness and safety.

FURTHER READING

1. Bourin P, Bunnell BA, Casteilla L. Stromal cells from the adipose tissue-derived stromal vascular fraction and culture expanded adipose tissue-derived stromal/stem cells: a joint statement of the International Federation for Adipose Therapeutics and Science (IFATS) and the International Society for Cellular Therapy (ISCT). Cytotherapy. 2013;15(6):641-8.
2. Caplan AI. MSCs: the sentinel and safe-guards of injury. J Cell Physiol. 2016;231(7):1413-6.
3. Chen JY, Mou XZ, Du XC, Xiang C. Comparative analysis of biological characteristics of adult mesenchymal stem cells with different tissue origins. Asian Pac J Trop Med. 2015;8(9):739-46.
4. Chen YR, Yan X, Yuan FZ, Ye J, Xu BB, Zhou ZX, et al. The use of peripheral blood-derived stem cells for cartilage repair and regeneration in vivo: a review. Front Pharmacol. 2020;11:404.
5. Crisan M, Yap S, Casteilla L, Chen CW, Corselli M, Park TS, et al. A perivascular origin for mesenchymal stem cells in multiple human organs. Cell Stem Cell. 2008;3(3):301-13.
6. Darzi S, Zarnani AH, Jeddi-Tehrani M, Entezami K, Mirzadegan E, Akhondi MM, et al. Osteogenic differentiation of stem cells derived from menstrual blood versus bone marrow in the presence of human platelet releasate. Tissue Eng Part A. 2012;18(15-16):1720-8.
7. Delgado-Enciso I, Paz-Garcia J, Valtierra-Alvarez J. A phase I-II controlled randomized trial using a promising novel cell-free formulation for articular cartilage regeneration as treatment of severe osteoarthritis of the knee. Eur J Med Res. 2018;23(1):52.
8. Delorme B, Ringe J, Pontikoglou C. Specific lineage-priming of bone marrow mesenchymal stem cells provides the molecular framework for their plasticity. Stem Cells. 2009;27(5):1142-51.
9. De Ugarte DA, Morizono K, Elbarbary A, et al. Comparison of multi-lineage cells from human adipose tissue and bone marrow. Cells Tissues Organs. 2003;174(3):101-9.

10. Dresser R. Stem cell research as innovation: expanding the ethical and policy conversation. J Law Med Ethics. 2010;38:332-41.
11. Dubey NK, Mishra VK, Dubey R, Syed-Abdul S, Wang JR, Wang PD, et al. Combating osteoarthritis through stem cell therapies by rejuvenating cartilage: a review. Stem Cells Int. 2018;2018:5421019.
12. Espinoza F. A Phase I/II, Randomized, Double-blind, Controlled Study to Assess Safety and Efficacy of Umbilical Cord-derived Mesenchymal Stromal Cells (UC-MSCs) in Patients with Knee Osteoarthritis [Internet]. Clin Trial. 2018:NCT02580695.
13. Farr J, Gomoll AH, Yanke AB, Strauss EJ, Mowry KC; ASA Study Group. A randomized controlled single-blind study demonstrating superiority of amniotic suspension allograft injection over hyaluronic acid and saline control for modification of knee osteoarthritis symptoms. J Knee Surg. 2019;32(11):1143-54.
14. Fu WL, Ao YF, Ke XY, Zheng ZZ, Gong X, Jiang D, et al. Repair of large full-thickness cartilage defect by activating endogenous peripheral blood stem cells and autologous periosteum flap transplantation combined with patellofemoral realignment. Knee. 2014;21(2):609-12.
15. Gale AL, Linardi RL, McClung G, Mammone RM, Ortved KF. Comparison of the chondrogenic differentiation potential of equine synovial membrane-derived and bone marrow-derived mesenchymal stem cells. Front Vet Sci. 2019;6:178.
16. Goldberg A, Mitchell K, Soans J, Kim L, Zaidi R. The use of mesenchymal stem cells for cartilage repair and regeneration: a systematic review. J Orthop Surg Res. 2017;12(1):39.
17. Imam MA, Mahmoud SSS, Holton J, Negida AS, Grubhofer F, Gupta R, et al. A systematic review of the concept and clinical applications of bone marrow aspirate concentrate in orthopaedics. SICOT J. 2017;3:17.
18. Jeyaraman M, Muthu S, Ganie PA. Does the source of mesenchymal stem cell have an effect in the management of osteoarthritis of the knee? Meta-analysis of Randomized Controlled Trials. Cartilage. 2020:1947603520951623.
19. Jin CZ, Park SR, Choi BH, Lee KY, Kang CK, Min BH. Human amniotic membrane as a delivery matrix for articular cartilage repair. Tissue Eng. 2007;13(4):693-702.
20. Kazemnejad S, Zarnani AH, Khanmohammadi M, Mobini S. Chondrogenic differentiation of menstrual blood-derived stem cells on nanofibrous scaffolds. Methods Mol Biol. 2013; 1058:149-69.
21. Li X, Bai J, Ji X, Xuan Y, Wang Y. Comprehensive characterization of four different populations of human mesenchymal stem cells as regards their immune properties, proliferation and differentiation. Int J Mol Med. 2014;34(3):695-704.
22. Lopa S, Colombini A, Moretti M, de Girolamo L. Injective mesenchymal stem cell-based treatments for knee osteoarthritis: from mechanisms of action to current clinical evidences. Knee Surg Sports Traumatol Arthrosc. 2019;27(6):2003-20.
23. Miranda-Sayago JM, Fernández-Arcas N, Benito C, Reyes-Engel A, Carrera J, Alonso A. Lifespan of human amniotic fluid-derived multipotent mesenchymal stromal cells. Cytotherapy. 2011;13(5):572-81.
24. Roberts S, Genever P, McCaskie A, De Bari C. Prospects of stem cell therapy in osteoarthritis. Regen Med. 2011;6(3):351-66.
25. Ronzière MC, Perrier E, Mallein-Gerin F, Freyria AM. Chondrogenic potential of bone marrow- and adipose tissue-derived adult human mesenchymal stem cells. Biomed Mater Eng. 2010;20(3):145-58.
26. Sekiya I, Ojima M, Suzuki S. Human mesenchymal stem cells in synovial fluid increase in the knee with degenerated cartilage and osteoarthritis. J Orthop Res. 2012;30(6):943-9.
27. Shariatzadeh M, Song J, Wilson SL. The efficacy of different sources of mesenchymal stem cells for the treatment of knee osteoarthritis. Cell Tissue Res. 2019;378(3):399-410.
28. Toh WS, Lee EH, Cao T. Potential of human embryonic stem cells in cartilage tissue engineering and regenerative medicine. Stem Cell Rev Rep. 2011;7(3):544-59.
29. Tong W, Zhang X, Zhang Q, Fang J, Liu Y, Shao Z, Yang S, et al. Multiple umbilical cord-derived MSCs administrations attenuate rat osteoarthritis progression via preserving articular cartilage superficial layer cells and inhibiting synovitis. J Orthop Translat. 2020;23:21-8.
30. Wang L, Tran I, Seshareddy K. A comparison of human bone marrow-derived mesenchymal stem cells and human umbilical cord-derived mesenchymal stromal cells for cartilage tissue engineering. Tissue Eng Part A. 2009;15(8):2259-66.
31. Wu W, Le AV, Mendez JJ, Niklason LE, Steinbacher DM. Osteogenic performance of donor-matched human adipose and bone marrow mesenchymal cells under dynamic culture. Tissue Eng Part A. 2015;21(9-10):1621-32.
32. Xu L, Liu Y, Sun Y. Tissue source determines the differentiation potentials of mesenchymal stem cells: a comparative study of human mesenchymal stem cells from bone marrow and adipose tissue. Stem Cell Res Ther. 2017;8(1):275.

40. Promising Role of Regenerative Therapy in AVN and Sports Injuries: An Update

Manish Khanna, Madhan Jeyaraman, Arun Gulati

INTRODUCTION

Cell-based therapies in orthopedics holds a positive future in treating conditions, which face a lot of clinical challenges in presently available treatment modalities such as avascular necrosis (AVN) of femoral head, various sports injuries especially internal derangement of knee. Cell therapy is the most important strategy in the management of such clinical conditions. Autologous minimally manipulated mononuclear cells are an ideal option to be used. As minimal manipulation is being done so there should not be any issues regarding safety concern. Various clinical trials should be planned, not only from clinical perspective but also to generate sufficient evidences for the cellular therapy as a treatment option. Ultimately, angiogenesis and chondrogenesis are desired outcomes of cell-based therapies, which help such patients coming back to the normal life. The most important thing to remember is the proper, justifiable case selection protocol while managing such cases.

As we know that stem cells repair tissues without much scarring, so regenerative science is bound to have lot of scientific interests especially in dealing with various challenging orthopedic conditions.

It is now very much evident that mesenchymal stem cells (MSCs) derived from bone marrow can be used in vitro for the production of cartilage, meniscal tissues, ligament, bone, tendons, etc. Lot of clinical research/trials are being carried out using autologous bone marrow-derived MSCs (BMMSCs). MSCs are also richly present in the adipose tissue (which is easily available in all individuals) and this makes it very useful for the research work.

Although MSCs derived from fat are easy to collect and are actually more in number as compared to BMMSCs (so is the preferred source for procurement as well) but still the demarcating line of advantages-disadvantage of MSCs derived from bone marrow or adipose tissue is not clear. These are important points to ponder upon while selecting stem cells from bone marrow/adipose tissue as the source but for sure there is better capacity and efficiency of fat-derived MSCs to further differentiate into various mesenchymal tissues. Few direct comparison have been published in the literature in the past as well, but for all practical purposes, MSCS are being continuously derived from bone marrow as well as adipose tissue in the clinical research work, so a definitive answer is still lacking on which is better one. Usually, in aspirated bone marrow there are 40 million nucleated cells and out of which stem cells are around 2,000 per milliliter. Collectively, in other words one stem cell is present per 20,000 cells in bone marrow but prevalence of stem cells in fat is described to be much higher (one stem cell per 4,000 cells). Only issue is that the adipose tissue is far less cellular (about 6 million cells per cubic centimeter of the tissue as compared to 40 million in the bone marrow aspirates).

OSTEONECROSIS OR AVASCULAR NECROSIS HEAD OF FEMUR

Hip AVN results from interruption of normal blood flow to the femoral head which if diagnosed at an earlier stage, have the relative option of halting this progression with cell-based therapy. Along with autologous bone marrow concentrate (BMC) (mononuclear cell cocktail), the autologous MSCs with or without platelet-rich plasma (PRP) can also be used in treatment of osteonecrosis. MRI changes after using autologous MNC cocktail or MSCs must be clinically correlated.

Avascular necrosis of the femoral head is usually a devastating progressive orthopedic condition most commonly affecting patients younger than 40 years of age. The exact pathophysiology of AVN is still not clear but the disease is characterized by a gross vascular insult to the femoral head blood supply thus leading to collapse of the head (Osteocytes and bone lining cells in the necrotic lesion and the proximal femur undergo apoptosis thus making it prone for the collapse) and thus subsequent degenerative changes. Typically, many patients present with deep typical groin pain with as such no history of trauma. Usual risk factors are the amount and duration of corticosteroids, history of smoking, history of a long standing alcohol intake, various autoimmune diseases, and sickle cell anemia. These

TABLE 1: Risk factors for avascular necrosis of the femoral head.

Nontraumatic	Trauma induced
• Idiopathic • Long-standing corticosteroid abuse • Alcohol abuse • Autoimmune conditions as SLE • Prolong history of smoking • Sickle cell anemia • Postorgan transplantation • Pregnancy • Cushing's disease • Chronic pancreatitis • In various coagulopathies • Chronic renal failure • Caisson disease • Lipid disorders	• Dislocation of hip • Fracture neck femur • Slipped capital femoral epiphysis

risk factors have to be worked up properly while planning management of the osteonecrosis **(Table 1)**. One of the most common risk factor is steroid exposure. It has been usually observed that about 10–30% of patients who receive steroid for the reasons such as in autoimmune diseases or for immunosuppression therapy for the transplanted organs, develop AVN within 12 months of the exposure.

More recently, human immunodeficiency virus infection and organ transplantation, specifically heart, liver, and kidney transplants, have been found to be associated with osteonecrosis. One more condition is trauma, particularly fracture of the femoral neck and dislocation of the hip where osteonecrosis is very commonly encountered. Still in about 20% of the patients, the cause cannot be detected and these cases are referred to as idiopathic osteonecrosis.

If AVN is diagnosed in the early stage then still in some cases it is be possible to attempt certain surgical procedures, which can preserve the hip joint such as decompression of the femoral head along with placing concentrated bone marrow. The use of autologous stem cells has been shown sometime to halt the progression of AVN of the femoral head, and thus there after preventing the young patients from undergoing total hip replacement (THR) (but this depend upon the stage of disease).

Core decompression (CD) remains one of the most commonly used procedures in early AVN as its description by Ficat and Arlet in 1964. Probably one of most useful procedure for treating early AVN (in precollapse stage) is CD along with placing autologous BMC (but very careful patient selection protocol should be followed). For this, after bone marrow aspiration from posterior iliac crest, cold centrifugation process is being done so that an autologous augmented hematopoietic BMC is obtained which can be further then placed inside the core decompressed site. The bone marrow cocktail also contains very few MSCs and various other cells of stromal as well hematopoietic lineages. These various stromal and hematopoietic lineage cells are critical to the therapeutic effect because they provide an optimal physiological as well as cellular environment for the osteogenesis and the angiogenesis.

Many studies show that 70–90% of osteonecrosed femoral head will collapse within next 5 years period, and thus consequently undergo arthroplasty suggesting that conservative treatment procedures should be instituted early. However, it has been seen that till date, no prophylactic management has been completely successful. Because of the young age of many patients, hip replacement cannot be expected to last the patient's lifetime and therefore attempts should be made to save the femoral head prior to collapse with the use of less invasive procedures. Thus, so far, the results of joint preserving surgeries like CD along with placing mononuclear cell cocktail for the early stage osteonecrosis have been variable and are still controversial.

No matter what so ever etiology may be, but the pathophysiology mostly shows decreased number of MSC pool in the proximal aspect of femur, thus resulting in presence of insufficient osteoblasts for the purpose of bone remodeling, which is very much required in the early stage of disease. Further the presence of insufficient osteogenic cells make the repair mechanism inadequate thus making femoral head prone to collapse. The effectiveness of bone marrow mononuclear cell cocktail placed in the CD site also depends upon the availability of stem cells in the proximal femur with osteogenic potential. In the very early stage of AVN, the osteogenic cells placed in CD site may make the lesion reversible by producing sufficient repair, which must be documented by MRI.

The reason for therapeutic effectiveness in case of injected marrow stromal cells is probably due to secretion of angiogenic cytokines (growth factors), which result in angiogenesis and thus improving osteogenesis as well. It has already been shown in one study that the presence of endothelial progenitor cells in the CD34 fraction implanted in the CD site contribute to positive outcome. Not only this, multiple angiogenic factors such as vascular endothelial growth factor (VEGF), basic fibroblast growth factor (bFGF), etc., released from these CD34+ fractions contribute to the repair significantly. The size of the lesion in the head, the stage of the osteonecrosis, the time from the diagnosis when procedure is being done and various other etiological factors decide the outcome of the implantation procedure.

REGENERATIVE THERAPY FOR AVASCULAR NECROSIS

The use of biologic therapy, PRP, tissue engineering, and stem cell therapy, all are forms of regenerative therapy.

Regardless of the specific initiating event, failure of perfusion occur leading to dead bone tissue. The area surrounding the loss of vasculature, or necrotic region of AVN, may degenerate or collapse. If joint architecture is disrupted then progressive degeneration may occur as a result. However, frequently the AVN region is stable, and in these cases it may degenerate under a slow curve just as any injured joint would. This is exactly where the field of Regenerative Medicine is evolving. Recognizing and halting the progression of arthritis development is the key to preventing joint replacement surgery. So, to alter the progressive paradigm the progression of arthritis has to be halted.

Ankle AVN is difficult as ankle replacements are not nearly as successful as knee or hip replacements. Ankle fusion is also less than desirable in many cases, making regenerative therapy an attractive alternative in some cases. Wrist AVN may be associated with the scaphoid bone. As with the ankle, wrist fusion may limit mobility and be undesirable in many cases. Shoulder replacement is still difficult compared to hip and knee procedures. However, a poor outcome with a shoulder replacement may have significant functional limiting effects. Hip and knee replacement are more common procedures, yet they are not without risk.

Athletes and younger adults especially are more interested in avoiding joint replacement and prospects for regenerative therapies such as PRP and stem cell therapy as treatment for AVN are exciting alternatives to preserve future treatment options, and as a means of addressing the progression of secondary osteoarthritis. There is an increasing focus on the development of early interventions for AVN, aimed at preserving the native articulation to avoid or at least delay THR. Core decompression is currently the most widely accepted surgical treatment for early-stage AVN. The rationale of its use is to reduce or decompress the intraosseous pressure in the femoral head, resulting from venous congestion and other pathways, in order to promote vascular invasion and to facilitate regeneration of the necrotic tissue. The overall clinical success rate of CD has been shown to be only 63.5%, and the rate for subsequent THR or hip salvage surgery is about 33%.

With the scope of improving CD results, the use of different regenerative techniques has recently been proposed to address early AVN stages.

Types of Therapy

- *Stem cells applied in the osteonecrotic area*: BMMSCs, mostly as BMC more rarely cultured or simply as bone marrow aspirates, adipose-tissue-derived MSCs (ADMSCs), or allogenic human umbilical cord-derived MSCs (UCMSCs)
- *Intra-arterial injection of stem cells*: The types of stem cells used with this approach are peripheral blood MSC mobilized by G-CSF, allogenic human derived UCMSCs, BMMSCs, or the combination of above.
- *Bioactive molecules*: Recombinant human bone morphogenetic protein: rhBMP-2, rhBMP-7, partially purified human BMP, or rhFGF-2.
- *PRP*: Either used with bone graft, BMC, or ADMSCs and hyaluronic acid.

Bone marrow aspirate concentrate (BMAC) has emerged as a possible alternative for regenerative medicine. It has been spotlighted as a promising biologic tool because of a rich source of pluripotent MSCs and growth factors. Implantation of autologous MSCs into the CD track, particularly when employed at early (pre-collapse) stages of osteonecrosis of femoral head (ONFH), improves the survivorship of femoral head and reduces the need for hip arthroplasty. Although, the most proper number of cells for injection was not determined, based on the current available data, injection of 10^6–10^9 cells may be reasonable.

The application modalities of BMAC such as intra-articular injection or surgical implantation with bioscaffold may also be an issue to be considered in the clinical settings. Intra-articular injection is relatively simple, easy to apply, and does not require hospitalization for the procedure. However, accurate delivery to the lesion site can be difficult. On the contrary, surgical implantation enables precise delivery to the lesion site, and acquires stability when combined with a bioscaffold or membrane.

Bone marrow-derived MSCs are the most commonly used cells, while other types of stem cells, such as ADMSCs, show a more promising prospect, with a robust growth rate and bone differentiation potential, and could be considered as an alternative to BMMSCs. It has been demonstrated that UCMSCs have excellent osteogenic ability and these cells could improve the local blood supply of osteonecrosis of the femoral head and initial effect in the treatment of early osteonecrosis of the femoral head.

Targeted intra-arterial infusion of PBSCs via the medial circumflex femoral artery is capable of enhancing the efficacy of biomechanical support (porous tantalum roads) in the treatment of ONFH. This confirms that the above combination treatment might be a safe and feasible choice for the treatment of early or intermediate stages of ONFH.

Cotransplantation of autologous BMMSCs and allogeneic UC-MSCs has shown therapeutic effect on ANFH without severe adverse effects. Genetic engineering can be used to modify MSCs to produce various factors, such as bone morphogenetic protein-2 (BMP-2), bFGF, hepatocyte growth factor (HGF), VEGF, calcitonin gene-related peptide (CGRP), or their combinations. VEGF alone or combined with BMP-2-modified MSCs have yielded positive results in dog and rabbit experiments. Gene-modified MSCs may be a promising technique for improving treatment efficiency in ONFH patients.

Cells can secrete different types of EVs, such as exosomes and microvesicles (MV), which have been classified according to their subcellular origins. Studies have demonstrated that exosomes from human synovial-derived MSCs could prevent glucocorticoid-induced ONFH in rats by enhancing proliferation and antiapoptotic effects. It has also been reported that exosomes secreted from human-induced pluripotent stem cell-derived MSCs could prevent ONFH by promoting angiogenesis. MSCs are site-regulated and secrete bioactive factors and signals at variable concentrations in response to local microenvironmental cues. Thus, whether MSC-derived vesicles can fully replace MSCs must be further evaluated.

The effectiveness of core decompression combined with implantation of bone marrow–derived cells (BMDC) and rhBMP-2 for ONFH after femoral neck fractures in children and adolescents has been established by clinical work. It relieves hip pain and prevents the progression of osteonecrosis in young patients lasting more than 5 years after surgery. A single local administration of rhFGF-2-impregnated gelatin hydrogel resulting in its sustained release patients with ONFH showed significant improvement of clinical scores at follow up of 1 year.

The beneficial effects and uses of PRP are well known. These can also be put to use in precollapse stages of AVN femur head. The use of PRP has been verified as a useful management strategy for ONFH treatment. Numerous studies have reported that enhancing osteogenesis and angiogenesis to reconstruct the bone structure of necrotic areas is the main mechanism involved in early-stage ONFH treatment. PRP could augment core decompression and bone graft substitutes to treat early-stage ONFH through increasing the levels of various cytokines that initiate and regulate proliferation, differentiation, and angiogenesis. The cytokines identified in PRP include platelet-derived growth factor (PDGF), transforming growth factor beta (TGF-β), basic fibroblast growth factor (bFGF), endothelial growth factor (EGF), insulin-like growth factor (IGF), and VEGF, most of them have been established to be useful in ONFH by many researchers. PRP could create an optimal environment to increase the repair capacity of ONFH by regulating the interactions of numerous growth factors with different systems. A study reported that the mRNA expression levels of VEGF, PDGF, IGF-1, and TGF-β in ONFH mice were upregulated tremendously after PRP treatment compared to those in the control group (PBS-treated). PRP may increase the production of angiogenic factors via upregulation of the angiogenic gene pathway, which may contribute to angiogenesis in femoral head osteonecrosis. The use of PRP with collagen sheet can increase the reparable capacity after drilling of necrotic segment in stage IIb and III ONFH. The cavity left after core decompression can be filled with a composite of bone graft mixed with PRP. When MSCs are combined with PRP to treat ONFH, the necessary growth factors in PRP could promote the potential of MSCs to differentiate into new bone and blood vessels. Thus, PRP enhances the osteoanagenic effect of MSCs to improve the healing of early-stage ONFH.

The use of a minimally invasive decompression augmented with concentrated bone marrow and PRP results in significant pain relief and halts the progression of disease in majority of patients. In addition to BMMSCs, PRP combined with ADMSCs has also been used for ONFH treatment. In fact studies have claimed that the combination of ADMSCs and PRP may produce improved therapeutic effects for ONFH than BMMSC/PRP treatment.

Platelet-rich plasma alone will not work very well to treat ONFH. Because ONFH is characterized by osteocyte apoptosis as a consequence of the interruption of the blood supply, the most important steps for treating ONFH are facilitating osteogenesis and angiogenesis and restoring bone formation to reconstruct the support at the joint surface. PRP must be administered in association with core decompression and other treatments to play its role.

Regenerative therapies offer good clinical results for the treatment of AVN. The combination of CD with regenerative techniques provides a significant improvement in terms of survivorship over time compared with CD alone. The durability of THR is a concern in such young patients, with a considerable risk for revision arthroplasty during their lifetime. Therefore, the success of nonreplacement procedures is of key importance both for patients' quality of life and for the impact on the health care system and society.

CELLULAR THERAPY HAS PROMISING ROLE IN SPORTS INJURIES

Sports injuries and the resultant gradual degenerative joint conditions have a heavy disease burden on society. Once damaged, the knee articular cartilage, anterior or posterior cruciate ligaments, collateral ligaments lacks the ability to properly repair, and regenerate itself.

For restoring joint functions, various surgical procedures like osteochondral transplantation (autologous usually), arthroscopic anterior cruciate ligament (ACL) reconstruction, autologous chondrocyte implantation. However, arthroplasty still remains the treatment of choice today for an extensively damaged joint. Transplantation and implantation procedures described above are useful procedures for treating such chondral defects (but of limited size only). Thus, there is an urgent need for improved cartilage repair modalities. For repairing cartilage tissue it has been seen that adult stem cells are best to be used as these can be easily isolated, have ability to self-renew and can further differentiate well along multiple connective tissue lineage.

Mesenchymal stem cells have special properties to participate in the repair process of damaged cartilage, meniscus, cruciate ligaments after localizing the site of injury. Several in vivo studies have been done previously and it is now being established that MSCs have a positive role in meniscal repair system. In some cases, MSCs are being used as a carrier or even sometime as scaffold. Clinical grade MSCs with or without PRP can be used for managing minor chondral lesions and for partial ACL tear due to sports injury. This is a possible way to avoid further cartilage degeneration leading to secondary osteoarthritic changes. MRI findings postcellular therapy in sports injuries must be clinically correlated. The importance of rehabilitation for achieving expected recovery after the therapy must not be forgotten and regular follow up must be maintained to assess the final outcome.

PROCEDURE

Patient is asked to lie down on table in supine position with knee-flexed 60-degree or even patient can sit with leg hanging side from the table. In cases like partial cruciate injuries, undisplaced meniscal injuries, intra-articular injection of BMC is given by anteromedial or anterolateral approach. The advantage of this path is that the needle faces least obstruction and maximum accessibility to the synovial joint. Sterile needle of 18 gauge preferably is inserted in the joint aseptically. Then the syringe containing autologous concentrated bone marrow aspirate is being attached to the inserted needle and slowly the material is injected (PRP may or may not be injected along with this).

CONCLUSION

There is no doubt that in the management of various orthopedic disorders, cellular therapy has got a very positive role. Medical science could be benefited from various positive advances made in the field of regenerative science such as using mononuclear cell cocktails, mesenchymal (autologous/allogenic) cells. Regenerative science in osteoarthritis knee, in ONFH, in internal derangement of knee is not without any hurdles at this developing stage.

A number of clinical and preclinical studies have already confirmed the positive bone regenerating role of so called osteogenic progenitor cells (bone marrow derived). Thus, Regenerative science definitely holds a very positive future in the management of some of the challenging orthopedic conditions. In coming future, osteogenic, chondrogenic potentials of stem cells along with biomaterials in orthopedics would play a long way in catering various needs of orthopedic surgeons. Research activities would further expand significantly in coming future for sure.

FURTHER READING

1. Agung M, Ochi M, Yanada S, Adachi N, Izuta Y, Yamasaki T, et al. Mobilization of bone marrow-derived mesenchymal stem cells into the injured tissues after intraarticular injection and their contribution to tissue regeneration. Knee Surg Sports Traumatol Arthrosc. 2006;14:1307-14.
2. Arlet J, Ficat P. Mode of onset of primary osteonecrosis of the femoral head. (Stage I. Uncomplicated). Study of 20 cases histologically verified by punch biopsy. Rev Rhum Mal Osteoartic. 1968;35:239-49.
3. Hauzeur JP, Pasteels JL. Pathology of bone marrow distant from the sequestrum in nontraumatic aseptic necrosis of the femoral head. In: Arlet J, Mazières B (Eds.). Bone Circulation and Bone Necrosis. Berlin: Springer; 1990. pp. 73-6.
4. Hernigou P, Beaujean F, Lambotte JC. Decrease in the mesenchymal stemcell pool in the proximal femur in corticosteroid-induced osteonecrosis. J Bone Joint Surg Br. 1999;81:349-55.
5. Hernigou P, Lambotte JC. Bilateral hip osteonecrosis: Influence of hip size on outcome. Ann Rheum Dis. 2000;59:817-21.
6. Inoue A, Ono K. A histological study of idiopathic avascular necrosis of the head of the femur. J Bone Joint Surg Br. 1979;61:138-43.
7. Izuta Y, Ochi M, Adachi N, Deie M, Yamasaki T, Shinomiya R. Meniscal repair using bone marrow-derived mesenchymal stem cells: experimental study using green fluorescent protein transgenic rats. Knee. 2005;12:217-23.
8. Jeyaraman M, Muthu S, Jain R, Khanna M. Autologous bone marrow derived mesenchymal stem cell therapy for osteonecrosis of femoral head: A systematic overview of overlapping meta-analyses. J Clin Orthop Trauma. 2021;13:134-42.
9. Khanna V, Jeyaraman M, Goel S, Khanna M. Functional outcome of autologous bone marrow concentrate implantation in osteonecrosis of femoral head: A two year follow-up study. J Clin Trials. 2019;9:3.
10. Lieberman JR, Berry DJ, Mont MA, Aaron RK, Callaghan JJ, Rajadhyaksha AD, et al. Osteonecrosis of the hip: management in the 21st century. Instr Course Lect. 2003;52:337-55.
11. Mont MA, Jones LC, Hungerford DS. Nontraumatic osteonecrosis of the femoral head: ten years later. J Bone Joint Surg Am. 2006;88:1117-32.
12. Murphy JM, Fink DJ, Hunziker EB, Barry FP. Stem cell therapy in a caprine model of osteoarthritis. Arthritis Rheum. 2003;48:3464-74.
13. Muschler GF, Nakamoto C, Griffith LG. Engineering principles of clinical cell-based tissue engineering. J Bone Joint Surg Am. 2004;86-A:1541-58.
14. Paley D, Young MC, Wiley AM, Fornasier VL, Jackson RW. Percutaneous bone marrow grafting of fractures and bony defects: an experimental study in rabbits. Clin Orthop. 1986;208:300-12.
15. Tateishi-Yuyama E, Matsubara H, Murohara T, Ikeda U, Shintani S, Masaki H, et al. Therapeutic Angiogenesis using Cell Transplantation (TACT) Study Investigators. Therapeutic angiogenesis for patients with limb ischaemia by autologous transplantation of bone-marrow cells: A pilot study and a randomised controlled trial. Lancet. 2002;360:427-35.
16. Tiedeman JJ, Connolly JF, Strates BS, Lippiello L. Treatment of nonunion by percutaneous injection of bone marrow and demineralized bone matrix. An experimental study in dogs. Clin Orthop. 1991;268:294-302.
17. Yamasaki T, Deie M, Shinomiya R, Izuta Y, Yasunaga Y, Yanada S, et al. Meniscal regeneration using tissue engineering with a scaffold derived from a rat meniscus and mesenchymal stromal cells derived from rat bone marrow. J Biomed Mater Res A. 2005;75:23-30.
18. Zuk PA, Zhu M, Mizuno H, Huang J, Futrell JW, Katz AJ, et al. Multilineage cells from human adipose tissue: implications for cell-based therapies. Tissue Eng. 2001;7:211-28.

Regenerative Medicine in Neurological Disorders: Current Understanding

Shilpa Sharma, Prajwal GS, Shivaraj B

INTRODUCTION

Globally, the overall burden on health care professionals is increased due to the epidemiological transmission from communicable to noncommunicable diseases. Among the noncommunicable diseases, neurological diseases pose a major challenge and threat to both the health care workers and the patients. Due to the evolution of molecular biology and biomedical engineering, stem cells and regenerative-translational medicine have become prime importance in the treatment of various degenerative disorders. The concept of medical products of human origin (MPHO) was initiated by WHO in 2004 which provides the platform for procurement and distribution of biological therapeutic products for the treatment of various disorders.

Regenerative medicine uses the principle of permutation and combination of stem cells, growth factors, and extracellular matrix to regenerate the tissue of interest. The concept of "Cellular Therapy" or "Cytotherapy" uses the biological cells along with biomicromolecules to induce or enhance or augment the quiescent or residual stem cells to exerts their action through paracrine effects. Evidences support the usage of cellular therapy to treat diseases of musculoskeletal, dermatological, ocular, otorhinological, endocrinological, gynecological, and neurological disorders both in vitro and in vivo. The usage of medical products of human origin to treat neurological disorders is of the primitive stage. Various combinations of cells and biomicromolecules have to be augmented to explore the regenerative capacity in neurological diseases. In this chapter, we aim to discuss the plausible role of stem cell therapy in Alzheimer's disease, Parkinson's disease, Huntington's disease, stroke, traumatic spinal cord injury, multiple sclerosis, stroke, and amyotrophic lateral sclerosis and to guide the future research on translational medicine principles in neurological disorders.

STEM CELL: SOURCES AND CHARACTERIZATION

The sources of stem cells play a prime role in lineage differentiation in the form of either osteogenesis, chondrogenesis, adipogenesis, or neurogenesis. The therapeutic effects of various sources of stem cells in terms of efficacy, safety, differentiation potential, durability, accessibility, allogeneic preparation, and culture expandability are of paramount importance to decide the optimal source of stem cells for desired therapeutic effects. Out of all available stem cells, mesenchymal stem cells (MSCs) play a major role in multilineage formation and differentiation. The most commonly explored MSCs are of bone marrow and adipose tissue origin. The sources of MSCs which are not explored in various disorders are from the umbilical cord, amniotic fluid, synovium, placenta, dental tissues, and periosteum. Bone marrow and periosteum-derived MSCs are more osteogenic in nature whereas synovial and adipose-derived MSCs are more chondrogenic in nature. MSCs of the placenta, umbilical cord, and amniotic fluid are pluripotent in nature and equivocal in differentiation into all lineages. MSCs harvested from dental tissues show equal osteogenesis and chondrogenesis in both in vitro and in vivo studies. These sources of MSCs enhance neurogenesis when neurotrophic factors or neurogenic signaling molecules are augmented. MSCs along with neural-induced growth factors, cytokines, and intracellular signaling molecules enhance neurogenesis and maintains proliferation and differentiation of neuronal progenitor cells in vitro and in vivo.

Mesenchymal stem cells possess cell markers of MSC lineage [CD-13 (alanyl aminopeptidase), -44, -73 (ecto-5'-nucleotidase), -90, -105 (endoglin), -146, and -166, STRO-1], osteogenic markers (BMP-2, OCN, OPN, osteonectin, and COL-1), adipogenic markers (LPL and PPAR-γ), chondrogenic markers (SOX-9 and COL-2), myogenic markers (myosin, myogenin, and SMA-α), neurogenic markers (nestin, GFAP, MAP-2, and β3 tubulin), and pluripotency markers (OCT-4, SOX-2, Nanog, and IGF-1R). They demonstrate negative staining for hematopoietic markers (CD-14, -19, -34, -45, and HLA-DR). MSCs possess a better immunomodulatory mechanisms which are regulated through lymphocyte system, NK cell system, and HLA-G5 system.

NEUROGENIC SIGNALING OF STEM CELL

Neurogenic signaling for adult stem cells is mediated through various pathways such as Wnt/β-catenin, notch, sonic hedgehog pathways, neurotrophic factors, growth factors, neurotransmitters, bone morphogenetic proteins, transcription factors, and epigenetic regulators as shown in **Figure 1**.

Wnt Pathway

Wnt/β-catenin signaling pathway has a major role in the development of the nervous system whereas its disruption leads to various neurological disorders such as Alzheimer's disease, schizophrenia, and mood disorders. Various researchers have demonstrated that Wnt3 is highly expressed in DG hilar cells and cultured astrocytes. Astrocyte-derived Wnt signaling leads to neuroblast proliferation and differentiation via the β-catenin pathway. Wnt signal participates in axonal and dendrite development, formation of dendritic spine, and synaptogenesis. They control the plasticity of the hippocampus and regulate transmission through synaptic junctions and neurogenesis. Wnt signal stimulates neural stem cell proliferation and self-renewal in the subventricular zone and subgranular zone.

Notch Pathway

Notch signal implicates various neuronal processes in neurogenesis in terms of neuronal proliferation, differentiation, and apoptosis. Notch pathway components are expressed in the subventricular zone and subgranular zone in the adult brain. They control and regulate the maintenance of adult neural stem cell, promote cell cycle exit, and decreases the cellular counts in neural progenitor pool. Hippocampal notch gene helps in amplification and self-renewal of nestin-positive cells in the subgranular zone in vitro and in vivo methods. Aguirre et al. emphasized that the notch gene regulates neural stem cells and controls self-renewal in the subventricular zone and the epidermal growth factor (EGF) receptor maintains the proliferation and migration of neural progenitor cells. Extended EGF receptor signaling results in amplification of neural progenitor pool and hence reducing neural stem cell number and self-renewal capacity.

Sonic Hedgehog Pathway

Sonic hedgehog (SHH) is an extracellular protein found to have a role in cellular differentiation in the nervous system and limbs. Ericson J et al., Hynes M et al., and Wechsler-Reya RJ et al. found the significance of SHH in neuronal differentiation of the forebrain, dopaminergic differentiation of the midbrain, and neural precursor proliferation of cerebellum. Increased SHH expression in the hippocampus

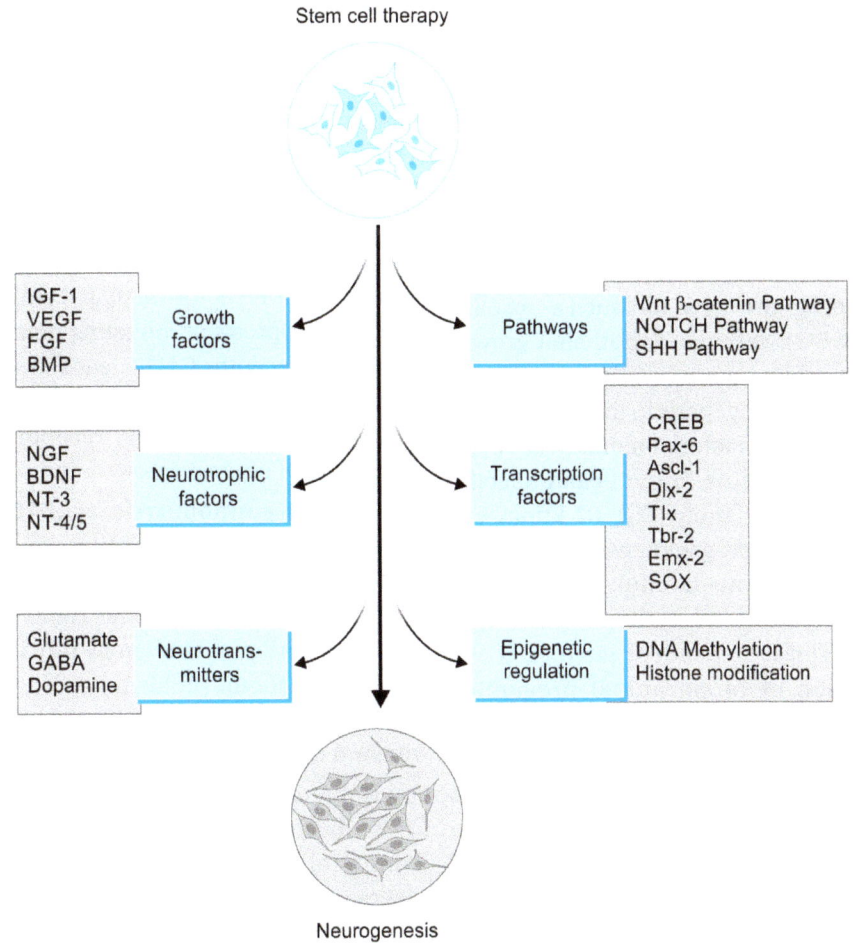

Fig. 1: Factors responsible for neurogenesis.

resulted in in vivo amplification of hippocampal progenitor cell proliferation and maintenance of neuronal progenitor cellular pool in the hippocampus. Angot E et al. insisted that loss of SHH signaling in the subventricular zone results in the failure of migration of type A neuroblasts to the olfactory bulb. Downregulation of SHH signaling leads to cellular senescence and development of age-related disorders, neurodegeneration, type 2 diabetes, and atherosclerosis.

Neurotrophic Factors

A significant role in developing an adult central nervous system is due to the action exerted by neurotrophic factors which are all the extracellular signaling proteins. The major neurotrophic factors involved in mammals are nerve growth factor (NGF), brain-derived neurotrophic factor (BDNF), neurotrophin 3 (NT-3), and neurotrophin 4/5 (NT-4/5). These neurotrophic factors bind to p75NTR on the cellular surface to facilitate the binding to neurotrophic factor-specific tyrosine kinase receptors to exert its therapeutic effects. Brain-derived neurotrophic factor is required for neurogenesis and dendritic path arborization. Intraventricular delivery of BDGF into the lateral ventricle leads to increased neurogenesis from the adult subventricular zone. BDGF-mediated TrkB signaling is of prime importance for neural stem cell proliferation in the hippocampus. Neurotrophin 3 knockout mice resulted in the impaired differentiation of neuronal cells yet there was no evidence of decreased proliferation of neuronal cells in the adult hippocampus. Such mice exhibited deficits in learning and memory processes. Infusion of nerve growth factor into lateral ventricle results in increased neuronal survival capacity in the adult hippocampus.

Growth Factors

Evidences prove that specific growth factors such as insulin-like growth factor 1 (IGF-1), vascular endothelial growth factor (VEGF), and fibroblast growth factor (FGF) are regulating and maintaining neurogenesis in the adult central nervous system. These growth factors mediate via signal transduction processes by binding to the ligand-specific receptor of the tyrosine kinase family. FGF-R1 knock-out mice display impaired neuronal progenitor cell proliferation and amplification of new neurons in adult dental gyrus. IGF-1 maintains neurogenesis of adult hippocampal progenitors in an MAP kinase-dependent manner. IGF-1 stimulates differentiation of hippocampal progenitor into oligodendrocyte in vitro by inhibiting BMP signaling. VEGF supports neurite outgrowth and maturation during evolution, which influences a major impact on the learning and memory process. They exhibit a mitogenic effect via the Flk-1 mechanism on neuronal progenitor cells. Infusion of VEGF in lateral ventricle resulted in enormous production of neuronal progenitor cells and maintains vasculogenesis of newly formed neuronal cells.

Bone Morphogenetic Factors

Bone morphogenetic factors (BMP) belongs to the transforming growth factor-beta (TGF-β) superfamily, which plays a significant role in the process of cellular survival, proliferation, and differentiation. They are inversely regulated by noggin, chordin, and neurogesin-1 which lead to extracellular antagonization of BMPs. In par with neural development, BMP support glial differentiation and inhibit neuronal differentiation of type B and C neural cellular population. In the subgranular zone, noggin mediates proliferation and self-renewal of hippocampal neural stem cells both in vivo and in vitro. Raised noggin levels increase neurogenic activity in the hippocampus by inhibiting BMP signaling. In the early embryo phase, active inhibition of BMP signaling is required for neuroectoderm formation then proceeds with the formation of neural crest and dorsoventral axis. In the postnatal phase, BMP induces astroglial fate commitment of forebrain progenitor cells, while inhibiting neuronal and oligodendral cellular fates. During adulthood, BMP modulate neurogenesis through secretion of BMP ligands and inhibitors, maintain the balance of neurogenesis and differentiation in the subventricular zone and subgranular zone.

Neurotransmitters

Neurotransmitters are the chemical messengers in between neurons which are minute diffusible molecules. These biological molecules help in neuronal progenitor cell proliferation and differentiation, synaptogenesis, and neurogenesis. Increased expression of glutamate, an excitatory neurotransmitter, was demonstrated on neuronal progenitor cells in the subventricular and subgranular zone. NMDA receptor-mediated glutamate knockout model exhibits apoptosis of migrating neuroblasts. The activation of kainate receptor GLU_{K5} leads to a decrease in the speed of migration of neuroblasts. There are increasing evidence of kainic acid and AMPA receptors potentiation in the regulation of neurogenesis.

Gamma-aminobutyric acid (GABA), an inhibitory neurotransmitter, depending on intracellular chloride content, exerts effects on immature new granule cells. In the postnatal subventricular zone, the activation of GABA reduces GFAP proliferation by providing a control feedback mechanism for the proliferation of neuronal progenitor cells. $GABA_A$ receptor knockout model resulted in deprived self-renewal mode of quiescent adult neural stem cells.

Dopamine, a catecholaminergic neurotransmitter, has a significant role in ontogenesis and embryonic germinal zone proliferation in the adult brain. Evidences proved decreased proliferation of subventricular progenitor cells due to dopaminergic denervation of epidermal growth factor receptor-expressing type C cells.

Transcription Factors

Transcriptional factors like cAMP response element-binding protein (CREB), Pax-6, Ascl-1, Dlx-2, Tlx, Sox, Emx-2, and Tbr-2 play an important role in the regulation of growth, development, and sustenance of cells. They mediate via kinase-mediated signaling pathways.

Autophosphorylation of CREB mediated by cAMP enhances neurogenesis by the proliferation of neuronal progenitor cells and regulates neuronal survival and plasticity in the adult hippocampus in vivo. Autonomous CREB signaling enhances neuroblast's survival, plasticity, migration, proliferation, and differentiation in the adult subventricular zone. Pax-6 differentiates neuroblasts to postmitotic dopaminergic periglomerular neurons.

ASCL-1, a member of the basic helix-loop-helix family of transcription factors, is responsible for lineage commitment of neural stem cells during both embryonic and adult neurogenesis. Under physiological conditions, vector-mediated enhanced expression of ASCL-1 factor leads to the production of oligodendrocytic lineages. They maintain the plasticity of neural stem cells and direct the lineage differentiation of neural stem cells in the adult brain.

Along with the Pax-2 factor, Dlx-2, a homeobox transcription factor, promotes neuronal precursor differentiation to dopaminergic periglomerular neurons in the olfactory bulb. Overexpression of Dlx-2 resulted in enhanced neuronal differentiation and migration speed of neuroblasts to the olfactory bulb. Dlx-2 plays an important role in subventricular zone proliferation.

The presence of Tlx factor, an orphan nuclear receptor, leads to glial cell differentiation and regulates adult neurogenesis. Tlx activates the Wnt/β-catenin pathway enhances Tlx-induced proliferation of neural stem cells and self-renewal capacity in the adult brain. Sox genes are abundantly expressed in the brain. Sox-2 is responsible for neural stem cell proliferation and differentiation, neuronal maturation, and the formation of dendrites with decreased adult neurogenesis. Increased expression of Sox-11 resulted in neuronal proliferation and differentiation of neural stem cells. Along with the induction of miR-124, Sox-9 act as a downstream regulator of neuronal differentiation.

Emx-2, a homeobox gene, is responsible for neural system morphogenesis. Evidences state that Emx-2 downregulates subventricular zone progenitor cellular proliferation by promoting the amplification of symmetrical division of neuronal progenitor cells.

Epigenetic Regulators

Epigenetic factors such as DNA methylation and histone modification control gene expression in neural stem cells. Methyl-CpG-binding domain protein 1 (MBD1) knock-out mice model exhibits decreased neurogenesis and resulted in the loss of spatial learning capacity. MBD-1 enhances neuronal differentiation by repressing miR-184. Methyl-CpG-binding protein 2 (MeCP2) exhibits neuronal maturation and formation of the spine along with maintenance of neuronal identity. Along with Sox-2, MeCP-2 suppresses miR-137 expression and thereby promotes differentiation of neural stem cells in adults. Bmi-1 is responsible for self-renewal and differentiation of subventricular zone neural stem cells by repressing p16Ink4a. Mixed-lineage leukemia 1 (Mll1) factor regulates neuronal differentiation.

ROLE IN NEUROLOGICAL DISORDERS

The mechanism of action of stem cells in various neurological disorders is being elaborated in **Figure 2** and they are as follows:

Alzheimer's Disease

Pathologically, Alzheimer's disease (AD) is characterized by loss of neurons and synapses in the cerebral cortex and certain subcortical regions. The pathognomonic feature of AD is the presence of neurofibrillary tangles and senile plaques in the cortex, amygdala, and hippocampus. Loss of neurons leads to atrophy of neural tissue in the temporal, parietal, and a part of the frontal lobe. Till now, no standard curative treatment is available for AD except for symptomatic treatment. CT acts as an augmented therapeutic option for the regeneration of locally available neural stem cells.

Neural stem cell or MSC with neurotrophic factors transplantation results in differentiation into glial cells and neuronal cells. Due to paracrine effects, secretion of neurotrophic factors leads to sustained neurogenesis from the subgranular zone and subventricular zone, which improves memory. Engineered neural stem cells enhance the expression of Aβ degrading enzyme which results in decreased Aβ aggregation and improves the density of synapses. The anti-inflammatory and immunomodulatory capacity of MSCs upregulate neuroprotection and downregulate inflammation. Extracellular vehicles released from MSCs target Aβ deposition through mi-RNAs and si-RNAs.

Neural stem cells transplanted into the lateral ventricle of the rodent AD model resulted in the migration and differentiation of neuronal progenitor cells and glial cells. This regeneration found to reduce Aβ deposition and tau phosphorylation, enhances synaptogenesis and neurogenesis, improved spatial learning and memory in rodents with AD. Fluorescent protein labeled BM-MSCs injection reduces the deposition of Aβ plaques and improves synaptogenesis in the hippocampus in primate models with AD. Restoration of motor, cognitive and memory function is observed in aged rats when human MSCs are transplanted.

Improved neuronal function, enhanced neurogenesis, differentiation into neuron-like and astrocyte-like cells when adipose tissue-derived MSCs (AD-MSCs) were transplanted into rodent AD model. Intravenous administration of

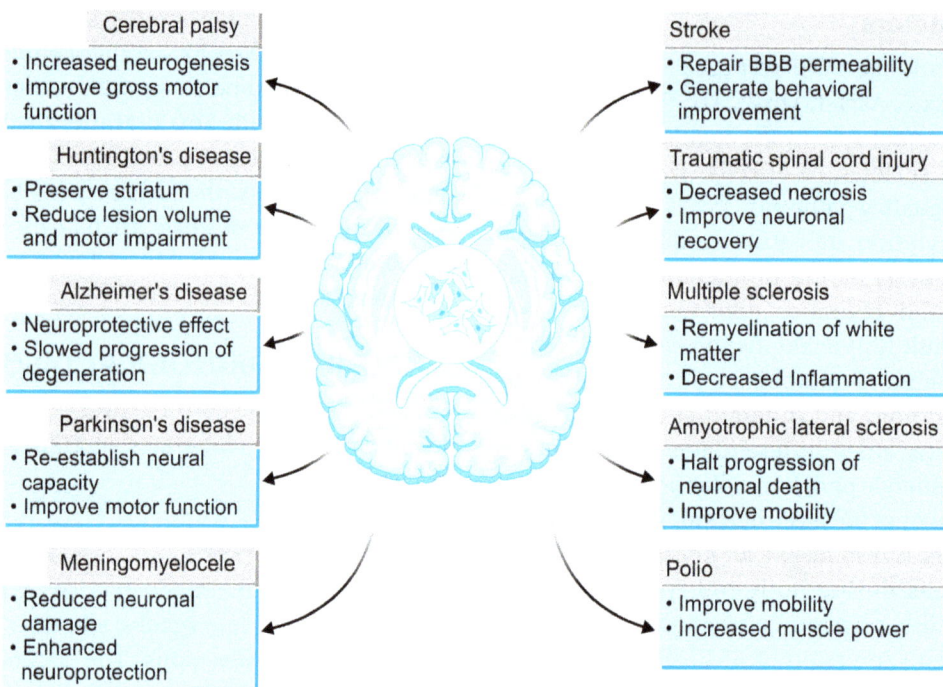

Fig. 2: Therapeutic applications of MSC in various neurological disorders.
(BBB: blood–brain barrier; MSC: mesenchymal stem cell)

AD-MSCs was found in the brain after 12 days of injection in rodents. Transplantation of AD-MSCs into the rodent brain improves cognitive and memory functions with enhanced neurogenesis and reduced Aβ plaque depositions. Neurons and neurospheres can be differentiated from induced pluripotent stem cells. Direct delivery of iPSC into the rodent cortex results in the generation of neuronal progenitors. iPSC treatment of rodent model with AD resulted in the enhanced expression of neprilysin, an Aβ-degrading protease.

Parkinson's Disease

Parkinson's disease (PD) is the most common cortical neurodegenerative disorder, which is characterized by bradykinesia, rigidity, and resting tremor. Evidences are there to support cellular therapy for PD as there are no standard treatment modalities. CT for PD includes autotransplantation (adrenal medullary cells, mesenchymal stromal cells, embryonic stem cells, induced pluripotent neuronal progenitor cells, and carotid body cells), allotransplantation (retinal pigment epithelial cells and human fetal ventral mesencephalon), and xenotransplantation (porcine ventral mesencephalon).

Clinical grade MSC transplantation of 6-hydroxydopamine mouse model exhibits clinical improvement in the natural history of PD. MSC-derived neurotrophic factors stimulate quiescent stem cells and enhance neuroprotection against oxidative stress-induced apoptosis. MSC inhibits microglial activation by increased secretion of immunosuppressive factors such as TGF-β1, PGE2, HGF, IDO, NO, IL-10, and IL-6 or by direct cell-cell contact. Researchers exhibited the generation of more than 80% of PAX-6 and SOX-1 expressing neuroectodermal progenitors with simultaneous inhibition of BMP and SMAD pathways using recombinant noggin and SB431542 factors. Secretion of FGF-8 factor by isthmus enhances the differentiation of SNpc dopaminergic neuronal cells. iPSCs are created by reprogramming of dermal fibroblast with the increased expression of c-myc, klf-4, oct4 and sox2 leads to dopaminergic neuron differentiation which forms the basis of cellular therapy for PD.

Parmar and Jun have formulated the ideal cellular state for PD transplantation used iPSC products. Rodent and monkey models of PD have been transplanted with dopaminergic precursors resulted in enhanced survival of graft and maturation in vivo into dopamine secreting neurons. Those PD models exhibited significant motor improvement without dyskinesia.

In a rat PD model, Rath et al. exhibited improved behavioral and motor symptoms with 650 TH$^+$ dopaminergic neurons. Kikuchi et al. suggested that 16,000 TH$^+$ dopaminergic neurons produce a neurogenic effect and improved behavioral effects in PD models of rodents. In vivo implantation of human embryonic stem cells derived dopamine neurons in PD rats resulted in improved motor and locomotive functions, which forms the basis of PD patients' management.

Huntington's Disease

Huntington's disease (HD) is an inherited genetic disorder with progressive neurodegeneration, which is characterized by dementia, cognitive, affective, and movement disorders.

HD is due to a mutation in the *huntingtin* gene on the short arm of chromosome 4 with trinucleotide (CAG) repeat sequence. No established treatment modalities are available for delaying the onset and progression of HD. Cell-based therapy for HD is in the primitive stage in regenerative medicine.

In the quinolinic acid (QA) rat model of HD, systemic administration of neural stem cells resulted in the migration of neuronal cells into the striate lesion, augments striatal hypertrophy, and long-term functional recovery. Prevention of striatal degeneration in rat HD model by administration of brain-derived neurotrophic factor, which is realized by neural stem cells leads to decreased neuronal damage and enhances neurogenesis. Intrastriatal administration of neural stem cells in rodents with HD resulted in increased migration velocity of neural cells to the striate cortex and provides a long-term functional outcome.

Administration of BM-MSCs in QA rodent model of HD proved improved behavior and the expression of neural phenotype in the regenerate. With the robust release of growth factors from implanted BM-MSCs, enhancement of cell survival and neuronal protection have been visualized in rodents. AD-MSCs transplantation into striatal lesions in HD rodent model reduces the volume of the lesion and improved behavioral and locomotive performances, increased overall survival with HD, and reduction in striatal neuronal loss and mHtt aggregates.

Cerebral Palsy

Cerebral palsy occurs due to perinatal insult, developmental neural abnormalities, infections, trauma, or genetic causes, which result in nonprogressive motor disability. Such a disability poses a major burden in social and financial concern for the family and the affected individual. These cases are the ideal candidate for stem cell therapy to repair and regenerate the lost neural circuit.

Chaitanya et al. reported excellent outcomes with bowel and bladder control, gross motor, sensory, and cognitive functions when five intrathecal injections of bone marrow-derived mononuclear cells were administered in a patient with cerebral palsy. Administration of UC-MSCs along with G-CSF in 2 cases of cerebral palsy resulted in improved functional outcome in the form of independent walking. These MSCs enhance neurovasculogenesis, counterfeit fibrosis, oxidative stress, anti-inflammation, and neuromodulation. To expedite an excellent improvement in gross motor function, the level of motor impairment needs to be considered. A significant motor function is achieved in cerebral palsy if the cellular count is more than 2×10^7.

Chen et al. observed enhanced gross motor functions and language quotient in cases of cerebral palsy when treated with neural stem cell-like cells derived from BM-MSCs. These neural stem cells integrate with host cells and tissues, exhibit plasticity, homing effect, and neuromodulation and synaptogenesis. Li et al. observed increased neurogenesis in the subventricular and subgranular zone when MSCs are transplanted in an animal model with cerebral palsy. They reported the upregulation of IL-10 levels along with decreased apoptosis of neurons in the ischemic zone.

Yasuhara et al. observed enhanced behavioral outcome and neurogenesis when multipotent adult progenitor cells are administered intracerebrally and intravenously in the rodent model of neonatal hypoxic-ischemic injury. Researchers proved that allogeneic or xenogeneic cellular transfer needs no immunosuppression in a rat model of ischemic stroke. Multipotent adult progenitor cell transfer in stroke enhances improvement as long as 6 months following the transfer, where they act by trophicity of growth factors and neurogenic signaling.

Stroke

Stroke poses a serious social stigma in the community and offers a negative impact on the patient's recovery. Among all noncommunicable diseases, stroke remains the most common disease with chronic disability and mortality. The treatment for stroke remains a multidisciplinary approach. The improved neuroperformance, neuroprotection, and neuroregeneration can be offered by cellular engineering and translational medicine.

Though stroke inflicts severe damage to a heterogeneous population of neuronal cells and its vascular circuit, regenerative therapy aims in restoring neural plasticity and its vascular connections. Restoration of behavioral effects, synaptogenesis, neurogenesis, and vasculogenesis has been observed in murine models of ischemia when transplanted with embryonic stem cells. Neural stem cell engraftment in animal models of neural ischemia resulted in synaptogenesis and restoration of electrophysiological properties and neural plasticity. Though immunologically naïve, MSCs restore neurorestorative potential in neuronal disorders through various growth factors and cytokines. UC-MSCs transplantation for stroke models through intravenous or intrathecal route serve as a potent source for cellular regeneration rather than cellular replacement therapy and hence improve neural homeostasis. Menstrual blood-derived MSCs have been explored by various study groups for stroke and emphasized neuroprotection and behavioral changes in animal models when administered through intracerebral or intrathecal route. Meta-analysis on MSC therapy for ischemic stroke concluded that motor improvement has been observed in stroke cases regardless of the dosage of MSCs administered. A few studies have reported fever, headache, and recurrent stroke as side effects of regenerative therapy for stroke.

Engineered stem cells with VEGF and BDGF by vector delivery showed increased paracrine effects with increased survival rate in mice stroke models. Excellent clinical outcomes were seen when engineered BM-MSCs transfected with the Notch-1 gene in stroke models. Advanced therapies with extracellular vehicles released from MSCs of various sources exactly target the pathogenic site and reverse the natural course of the disease and restores the neural homeostasis.

Traumatic Spinal Cord Injury

Traumatic spinal cord injury poses a debilitating course with an increased rate of disability with paraplegia, dysfunctioning of sensorimotor, gastrointestinal, and genitourinary systems. The prognosis and recovery of the neuronal circuit depend on the age, the level of spinal injury, and the time of presentation to the health care facility. To restore the neuronal circuit and plasticity, stem cells and biological peptides offer a greater advantage than classical modalities of treatment. Animal models of SCI treated with various sources of MSCs and engineered and modified cells have been widely accepted.

Induction cocktail with MSCs, biological peptides, and growth factors, embryonic stem cells (ESCs) are used to regenerate neurons and glial cells. In a rat model of SCI, neurons integrate and enhance survival once ESCs are injected. In a demyelinated rat model of SCI, ESCs myelinate the axons deficit with myelin and proven the functional recovery. Cao et al. demonstrated astrocytogenesis when neural progenitors are transplanted in rat model of SCI. Genetically engineered neural precursor along with noggin differentiate into oligodendrocytes which are used to treat SCI, where functional outcomes were excellent.

Olfactory ensheathing cells are harvested from nasal mucosa and are administered as a cellular agent for regenerating axons in the SCI site. These cells enhance the outpouching of neurites, neuroenhancement, neuroprotection, and remyelination of demyelinated neural tissues. Subarachnoid and intra- and extradural administration of UC-MSCs exhibited improved motor function in the extremities in a patient with spinal cord compression. Radiological evidences proved the spinal cord expansion at the injured spinal level. A meta-analysis by Muthu et al. stated that transplantation of MSCs in SCI improves the neurological outcome. They established the safety and efficacy of the source of MSCs being transplanted. They gave an insight into MSC-derived exosomes and secretomes for SCI patients, which hold promise for future treatments.

Intravenous administration of AD-MSCs in SCI individuals showed no adverse effects with a good hindlimb motor function through activation of kinase proteins such as erk1/2 and Akt. AD-MSCs increase the chances of cellular survival at the spinal lesion level. Intrathecal transplantation of AD-MSCs in 14 cases of SCI reported with improved ASIA scores along with the improvement in EMG and MRI.

iPSCs derived neural progenitors exhibit embryonic stem cell-like neuronal differentiation both in vitro and in vivo. In SCI animal models, iPSCs reduce spinal cord inflammation and edema, restores neural circuits, remyelination, and neural pathway regeneration. Further in-depth exploration of the neural regenerative potential of iPSCs with or without vector agents have to be evaluated in terms of safety, efficacy, and long-term functional outcomes in SCI individuals.

Multiple Sclerosis

Multiple sclerosis (MS), an autoimmune neurodegenerative disorder, is characterized by global axonal demyelination which is induced by autoreactive T cells leading to functional neurological disability. Cellular transplantation holds good for the management of multiple sclerosis to produce a better neurological outcome. The rationale of cellular transplantation in MS is immunosuppression which helps to eliminate autoreactive lymphocytes and hence allow installation of a tolerant immune system.

For refractory MS, autologous hematopoietic stem cells (HSCs) along with a high dose of immunosuppression are the treatment of choice to curb the disease. The rationale behind the combination is that chemotherapeutic agents destroy the dysregulated immune system whereas HSC reinstall the new immunotolerant environment. MSCs provide immunomodulatory effect in terms of suppression of T and B cell proliferation, enhancement of Treg cells, and inhibition of NK cells. Therapeutic benefit was observed in 10 patients with advanced MS disease when administered intrathecally with expanded BM-MSCs. Neural stem cells offer therapeutic plasticity through neurotrophic factors and neurotransmitters. Once it reaches the central nervous system, it induces the proliferation of quiescent stem cells present in the subventricular and subgranular zone of the hippocampus. iPSC-derived oligodendrocyte precursor cells in primate model with MS exhibited migration of neuronal progenitor cells to brain and evidence of neurogenesis was observed. Embryonic stem cells when transplanted for MS, the cells differentiated into cells with a myelogenic response. Histological evaluation of transplanted human embryonic stem cells to mice with encephalomyelitis showed migration of neural progenitors to the brain and production of oligodendrocytes.

Amyotrophic Lateral Sclerosis

Amyotrophic lateral sclerosis (ALS), the most common motor neuron disease and a neurodegenerative disorder, is characterized by progressive loss of motor neurons which result in muscular weakness, atrophy, fasciculations, and spasticity. Till now there is no standard treatment for ALS except symptomatic and supportive management with rehabilitation. Stem cell therapy offers plasticity, homing effect, and neuromodulation in neuronal disorders, where stem cells differentiate into multiple neuronal lineages. When stem cells are administered locally or systemically, they migrate to the target site and exert their action through the paracrine effect. Stem cells halt the progression of ALS, modulate host immunity, inhibit inflammation and apoptosis, and regenerate the injured motor neurons.

The transient clinical and functional improvements were observed when human neural stem cells are engrafted in the ALS model and offered neuromodulation and neuroprotection. In the mouse ALS model, when NSCs are administered, the response was observed in the form of prolonged survival of mice and delayed progression of ALS. Mazzini et al. formulated the basis of neural stem cells dosage for ALS to obtain an optimum therapeutic response. UC-MCs, when transplanted intraspinal, improve motor function and attenuate the loss of motor neuron. They increase the survival of G93A-SOD1 mice by 12 days. Genetically engineered retro-orbital injection of UC-MSCs increases the expression of VEGF and FGF in G93A-SOD1 mice and exhibited improvement in motor neuron environment. Retro-orbital injection of UC-MSCs increased the survival rate up to 25% in G93A-SOD1 mice. AD-MSCs transplantation in ALS mice model was performed either intravenously or intracerebroventricularly. Intracerebroventricular injection of AD-MSC exhibited better functional outcomes, delayed the disease progression, and maintained neuroplasticity than intravenous AD-MSCs administration. AD-MSCs were found to secrete robust amounts of VEGF, BDGF, IGF-1, and NGF. These factors enhance the mice survival and offer neuroprotection.

Polio

Postpolio syndrome (PPS) is characterized by delayed onset of neuromuscular symptoms in patients affected with acute polio. The diagnosis is usually clinical and assisted by an electromyogram. No definite treatment modalities are available for PPS. Neurorestoration in PPS poses a great challenge to offer clinical improvement. Due to the rapid development of technologies with stem cells and cellular engineering, the functional improvement in PPS-affected individuals is plausible. There is no evidence available on cellular therapy in PPS except for one case report.

Xi et al. reported a case of 64 years male with a diagnosis of PPS and offered cellular therapy in the form of intrathecal umbilical cord MSCs (UC-MSCs) (1.2×10^7 cells) and neural progenitors with cerebrolysin (2×10^6 cells) around C7-T1 junction followed by intrathecal neural progenitors with cerebrolysin (2×10^6 cells) and schwann cells (5×10^5 cells) around T9-T10 junction. Then intravenous UC-MSCs (1×10^7 cells) were infused followed by implantation of MSC cocktail around T1-T2 junction with intrathecal neural progenitors (2×10^6 cells), olfactory cells (1×10^6 cells), BM-MSCs (3×10^6 cells) along with cerebrolysin. All these MSC implantations were performed in a gap of 4 days each. They observed both clinical and functional improvement in this patient in the form of walking independently and was pain-free in the 4 years follow-up period. The possible mechanisms for this improvement are due to the release of neurotrophic factors, promotion of axonogenesis, remyelination, and conversion of internal neuromuscular environment toward regeneration.

Meningomyelocele

Myelomeningocele (MMC) is the most frequently diagnosed congenital spinal defect by ultrasound where the protrusion of the spinal cord through a vertebral defect is observed. As a result of such pathology, the patient is characterized with paraplegia and bowel and bladder dysfunction. Cellular engineering provided a proper platform to explore the plausibility of treating MMC in a biological way. The therapeutic effects and prognosis of MMC treated with cellular therapy with stem cells remain unclear.

In the fetal rat MMC model, administration of human amniotic fluid MSCs (hAF-MSCs) decreases the intensity of neuronal damage, enhances neuroprotection, and induces astrogliosis in the degenerated neuronal cells. hAF-MSCs migrate to spinal cord defect via CXCL12/CXCR4 signaling and secrete cytokines and growth factors to exert its action. They concluded that hAF-MSCs differentiate into cytokeratin expressing cells and enhances re-epithelialization. In this model, hepatocyte growth factor (HGF) plays an important role in reducing the inflammatory response, promote neuronal outgrowth, neurogenesis, vasculogenesis in cases of neuronal disorders.

A paradigm shift was being observed by researchers in treating MMC with placental-derived MSCs (P-MSCs) and amniotic fluid-derived MSCs (AF-MSCs), who possess low immunogenicity and high pluripotency. Fetal cellular and tissue engineering pace up the neuronal regeneration of spinal cord pathologies when loaded with biosynthetic scaffolds. Due to the regenerative capacity of AF-MSCs, it is preferred to be the alternative treatment for spina bifida. Evidences state that transamniotic stem cell therapy exhibit improvement in motor functions in MMC animal models. Vasculogenesis at the cell-engrafted site is being promoted by VEGF and FGF-2. A wide range of soft tissue coverage in the MMC animal model was demonstrated with intra-amniotic injection with scaffolds like alginate and polylactic-co-glycolic acid molecules.

■ CONCLUSION

Stem cell therapy offers amazing opportunities for the future. With the ability to regenerate human tissues and repair the pathology in various diseases involving brain, and spinal cord, stem cell therapy paves the way for the future in conditions where supportive care was the only available treatment to prevent the situation from becoming worse. The critics of the technology is silenced by the evidences being generated nowadays, however, the ethical challenges are daunting. Well-designed clinical trials are needed to evaluate the clinical efficacy and safety of stem cell therapy for these neurological disorders. On a cautionary note, considering the complexity of the disease complex methods of their management is often necessary and with the public perception of stem cell therapy as a magic bullet, it is unlikely to be used as a monotherapy but rather as a part of the holistic regimen that aims to improve the quality of life of these patients.

FURTHER READING

1. Chen G, Wang Y, Xu Z, Fang F, Xu R, Wang Y, et al. Neural stem cell-like cells derived from autologous bone mesenchymal stem cells for the treatment of patients with cerebral palsy. J Transl Med. 2013;11(1):21.
2. Crigler L, Robey RC, Asawachaicharn A, Gaupp D, Phinney DG. Human mesenchymal stem cell subpopulations express a variety of neuro-regulatory molecules and promote neuronal cell survival and neuritogenesis. Exp Neurol. 2006;198(1):54-64.
3. Faigle R, Song H. Signaling mechanisms regulating adult neural stem cells and neurogenesis. Biochim Biophys Acta. 2013;1830(2):2435-48.
4. Hao L, Zou Z, Tian H, Zhang Y, Zhou H, Liu L. Stem cell-based therapies for ischemic stroke. BioMed Res Int. 2014;2014:e468748.
5. Joyce N, Annett G, Wirthlin L, Olson S, Bauer G, Nolta JA. Mesenchymal stem cells for the treatment of neurodegenerative disease. Regen Med. 2010;5(6):933-46.
6. Katoh H, Yokota K, Fehlings MG. Regeneration of spinal cord connectivity through stem cell transplantation and biomaterial scaffolds. Front Cell Neurosci. 2019;13.
7. Kunisaki SM. Amniotic fluid stem cells for the treatment of surgical disorders in the fetus and neonate. Stem Cells Transl Med. 2018;7(11):767-73.
8. Martin DE. Ethical aspects of medical products of human origin. ISBT Sci Ser. 2017;12(1):281-7.
9. Muthu S, Jeyaraman M, Gulati A, Arora A. Current evidence on mesenchymal stem cell therapy for traumatic spinal cord injury: systematic review and meta-analysis. Cytotherapy. 2021;23(3):186-97.
10. Ottoboni L, von Wunster B, Martino G. Therapeutic plasticity of neural stem cells. Front Neurol. 2020;11.
11. Qu J, Zhang H. Roles of mesenchymal stem cells in spinal cord injury. Stem Cells Int. 2017;2017:e5251313.
12. Therapeutic potential of human adipose-derived stem cells in neurological disorders. J Pharmacol Sci. 2014;126(4):293-301.
13. Weiss ARR, Dahlke MH. Immunomodulation by mesenchymal stem cells (MSCs): mechanisms of action of living, apoptotic, and dead MSCs. Front Immunol. 2019;10:1191.

42. Ulcers and Regenerative Medicine

Sribatsa Kumar Mohapatra, Dushyant Chaudhary, Shivakumar Bingi

INTRODUCTION

Whenever there is a break or disruption in normal skin lining and architecture, repair of the wound is normal response and it requires coordination of a number of cell types as well as cellular signal molecules and is completed in three stages; first is inflammation, next comes proliferation stage and the last being the remodeling. Many secondary factors, which may be local (like ischemia) or systemic (as in diabetes), usually are responsible for dysregulation of this complex physiological homeostasis which leads to formation of a wound which is most of the times chronic in nature. Diabetic ulcers which are chronic and most commonly occur on the foot have an ever increasing incidence and are increasing the healthcare expenses tremendously, as they have a very poor healing potential and keeps on recurring even after multiple treatment therapies, creating a need for newer and advanced treatment strategies. For chronic ulcers or wound, a new potential treatment which is gaining popularity is stem cell therapy. The most common type of stem cells which are now commercially in use are the adult type of stem cells, but the use is limited by several factors such as invasiveness of the procedure to procure them, immunologic complications, and the decreased survival of cells in vivo.

Immediately after a wound occurs, aggregation of platelets accompanied by the coagulation cascade help in achieving homeostasis. A number of chemicals which act as chemotactic signals are released at the wound site; they help in recruitment of neutrophils, fibroblast as well as macrophages which start the repair process. These signals include fibroblast growth factor as well as platelet derived growth factors. Any bacteria or debris is cleared off by the migration of scavenger macrophages at the wound bed which help in clearing of the microdebris, as well as the neutrophils which produce cellular signaling molecules such as tumor necrosis factor α (TNFα), interleukin-1 (IL-1) and vascular endothelial growth factor. These cytokines further help in cellular proliferation and increase the recruitment of cells at the wound site. Initially at wound site, a matrix woven from fibronectin protein along with hyaluronic acid is secreted which acts as a bed for epithelialization. The process of re-epithelialization is aided by the stem cells present around the skin appendages such as the hair follicles. At last, the fibroblasts lay down collagen rich fibers into the previously woven matrix and also angiogenesis takes place at the same time increasing the vascularity of the wound.

For management of a chronic wound, several factors play a major role. These are exact diagnosis and removal of the causative factor, optimizing the blood flow at the wound bed to enhance repair potential and removal of the slough and dead tissue time to time. Also pressure points have to be offloaded and padded well in order to prevent further injury.

An exciting and upcoming potential therapy for wound healing is its treatment by stem cells. When stem cells are transferred into the wound bed, they have a direct as well as paracrine mode of action to stimulate recruitment of cells necessary for repair, remodel the newly formed extracellular matrix, and neovascularization by secretion of cellular signaling molecules and growth factors.

ETIOLOGY

Any disease of vascular supply affecting either veins, arteries or capillaries can lead to a chronic ulcer as it affects the body's ability to heal because of the compromised blood supply. The cause may also be a metabolic one as in diabetes or a neurogenic as in Charcot's disease. One of the main causes for chronicity is the persistence of the underlying etiological factor. These nonhealing wounds are resistant to the usual or conventional methods of treatment.

Some of the common etiologies for chronic ulcers are:
- Diabetes
- Sickle cell disease
- Peripheral vascular disease such as Buerger's disease
- Hansen's disease
- Burn injury leading to formation of an ulcer
- Pressure sores
- Venous ulcers as in varicose veins.

MECHANISM OF ULCER HEALING BY STEM CELLS

The ability of stem cells to point and act on the underlying pathological mechanism and restore a homeostasis as well as bring back the positive balance of the cytokines which promote healing, makes them an encouraging treatment modality for healing of chronic ulcers.

Angiogenesis is a very crucial step for a good wound healing, as it evokes the tissue perfusion and hands over the important micro- and macronutrients and also abates the hypoxic situation present at the wound bed. In patients with long standing uncontrolled diabetes mellitus, the endothelial progenitor cells lose their potential for migrating to site of injury, which further affects the process of angiogenesis which in further leads to poor wound healing.

Stem cells prove beneficial for all the three stages of wound healing. When stem cell therapy is used for wound healing, these stem cells differentiate into a variety of cells which play various roles in different stages of wound healing by their direct as well as paracrine actions. In the first phase or inflammatory phase of wound healing, these cells or their derivatives help in increasing the concentration of growth factors and other cellular signaling molecules at wound site and also increases the cytokines which were previously suppressed and are helpful in wound healing. This results in chemotaxis of wound healing cells such as fibroblasts and epidermal cells such as keratinocytes. These cells are lacking in a chronic wound, so the recruitment of the same leads to enhanced wound healing. Post differentiation of stem cells, they can give rise to fibroblasts, myofibroblast, endothelial cells (for angiogenesis), keratinocytes or even smooth muscle cells. This mainly happens in the proliferative stage.

In the last stage or the remodeling stage, the differentiated myofibroblasts play a major role.

FOOT ULCERS IN DIABETES MELLITUS

Diabetes is a multisystem disease which involves almost everything due to its effect on the small, large blood vessels as well as neuropathy related complications. Even a small thorn prick can lead a big nonhealing ulcer in an uncontrolled diabetic person. An ulcer can go for chronicity, become recurrent or even the whole foot may become gangrenous. Stem cell therapy holds a great promise in aiding the healing of these ulcers which most commonly occur in the foot area in diabetics.

Case 1

This is a case of diabetic ulcer treated with stem cell application (**Figs. 1A to E**).

Case 2

This is a case of chronic ulcer with pus discharging-post amputation (**Figs. 2A to D**).

SICKLE CELL ULCER

In sickle cell disease, which is a congenital disorder; the RBCs formed in the bone marrow have an abnormal hemoglobin (Hb), i.e., HbS. Among all the skin manifestations seen in sickle cell disease, chronic ulcers over the leg are most

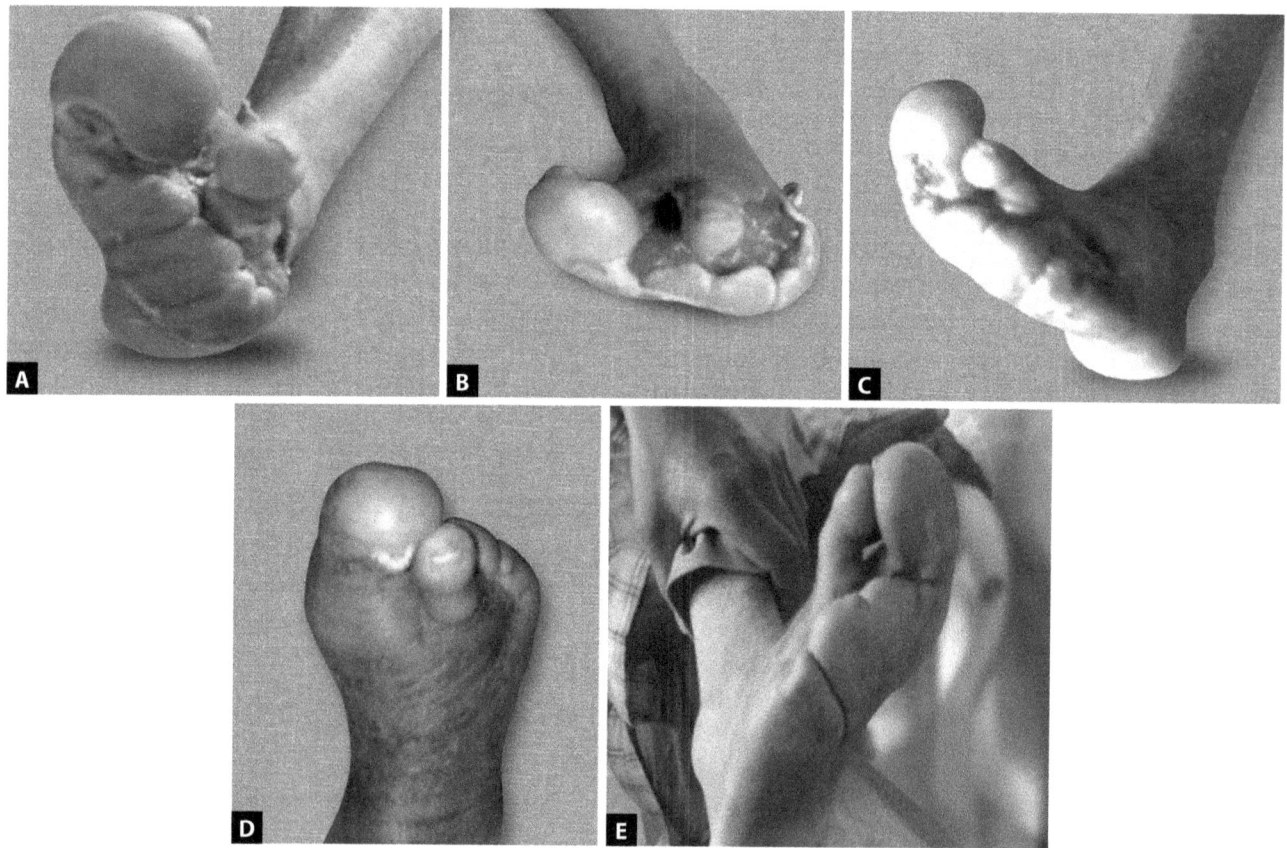

Figs. 1A to E: Case of foot ulcer. (A) At presentation; (B) Single week after application; (C) After 4 weeks; (D and E) 6 weeks post stem cell application.

frequently encountered problem. These are intractable ulcers with a very slow healing potential which is almost sixteen times less than a venous ulcer. They are not just chronic but even recurrent in nature too.

Because of the decreased blood supply at the ulcer site, graft failure is also commonly seen which may lead to more hospitalization time, and this time again increasing the cost of healthcare **(Figs. 3A to E)**.

Case 3

The different stages of bilateral sickle cell leg ulcer are shown in **Figures 4A to E**.

VENOUS ULCERS

The different stages of venous ulcers are shown in **Figures 5A to D**.

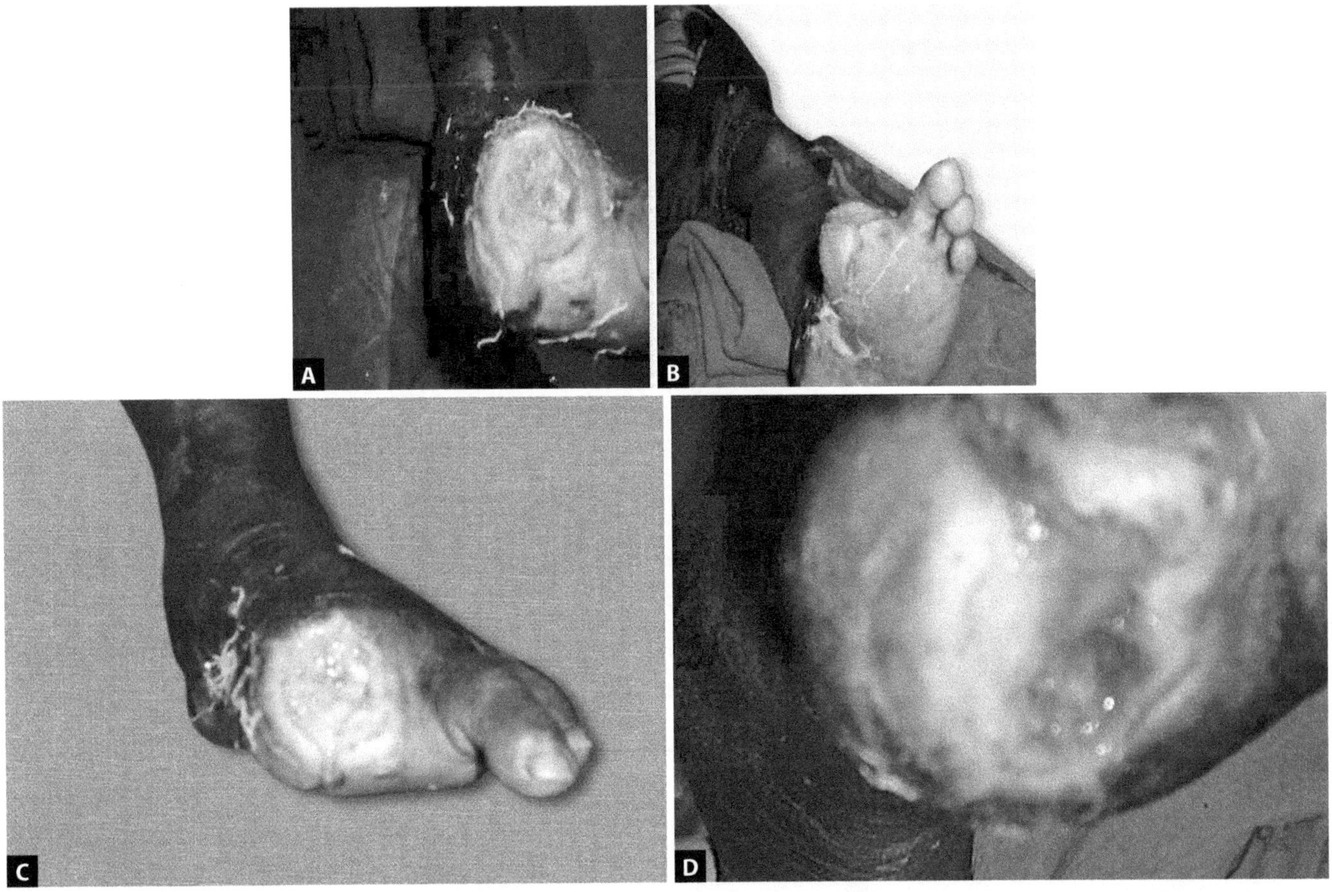

Figs. 2A to D: Case of chronic ulcer. (A and B) At presentation; (C) After thorough debridement; (D) 48 hours postapplication.

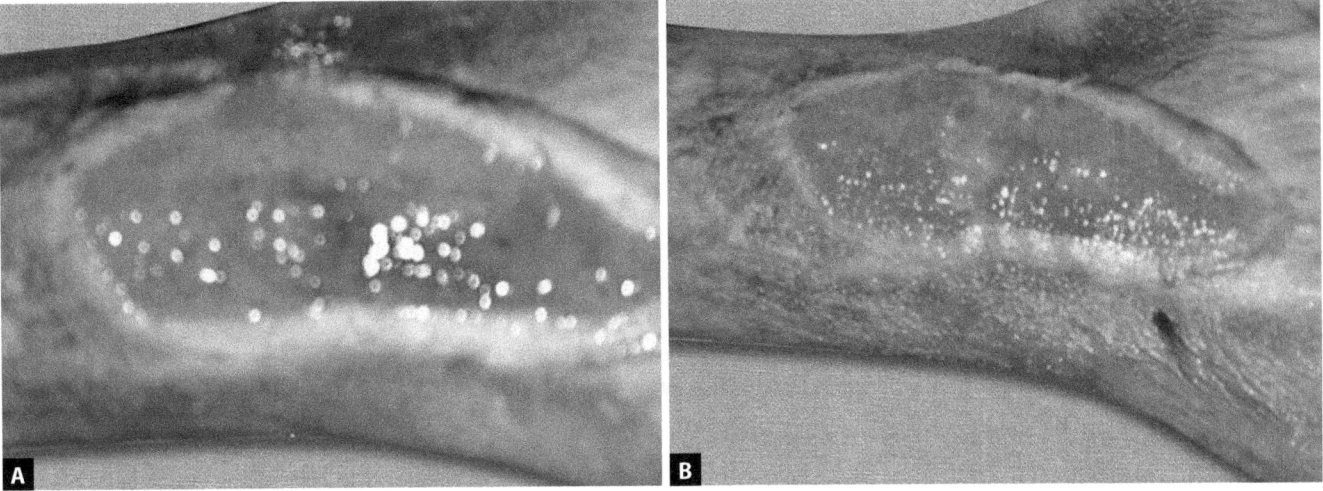

Figs. 3A and B

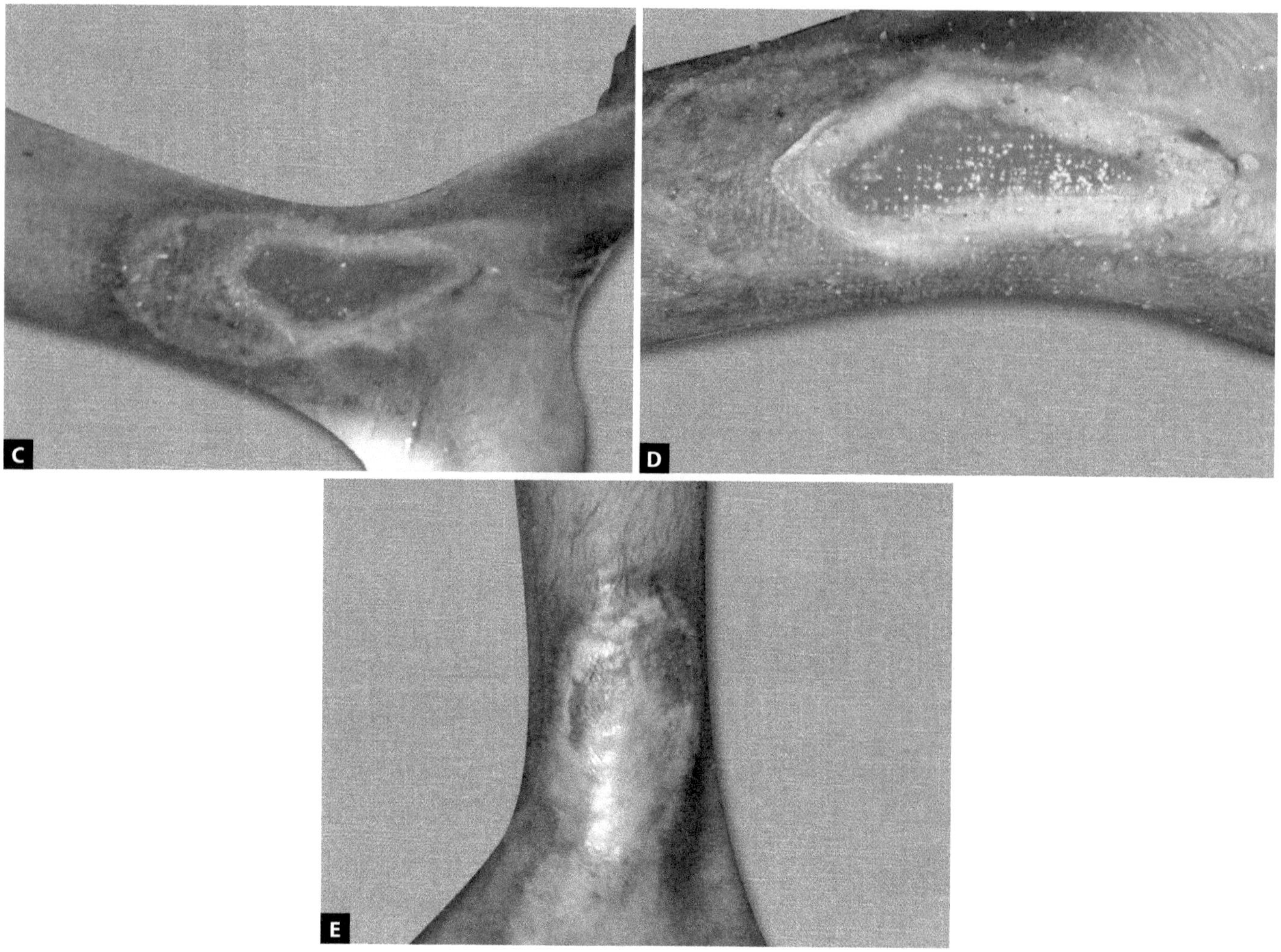

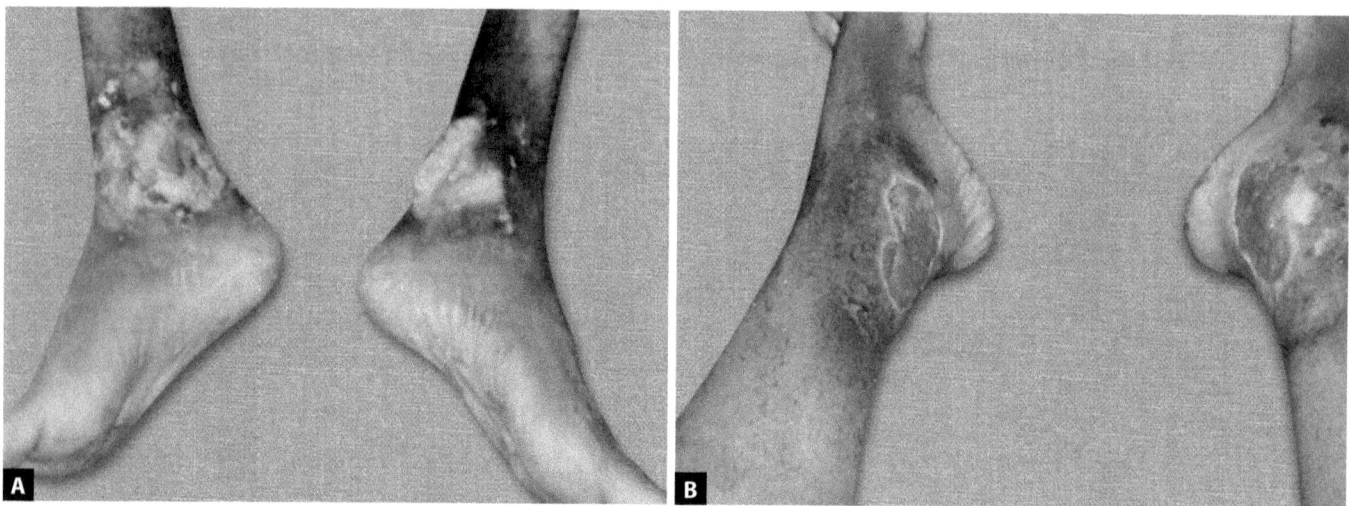

Figs. 3C to E
Figs. 3A to E: Skin manifestations in sickle cell disease. (A) At Presentation; (B) After debridement; (C) 1 week after application; (D) 2 weeks after the treatment; (E) 6 weeks post-treatment.

Figs. 4A and B

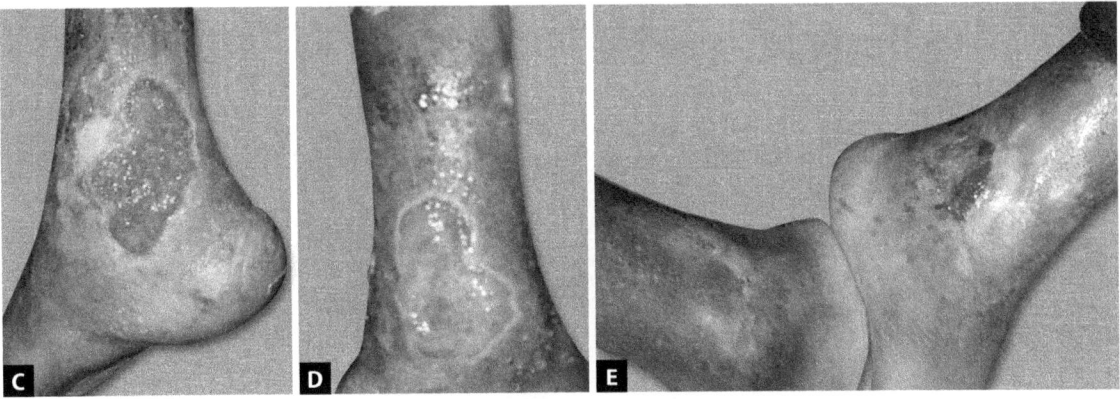

Figs. 4C to E

Figs. 4A to E: Bilateral sickle cell leg ulcer. (A) At presentation; (B) Post debridement; (C and D) After 1 week; (E) After 4 weeks.

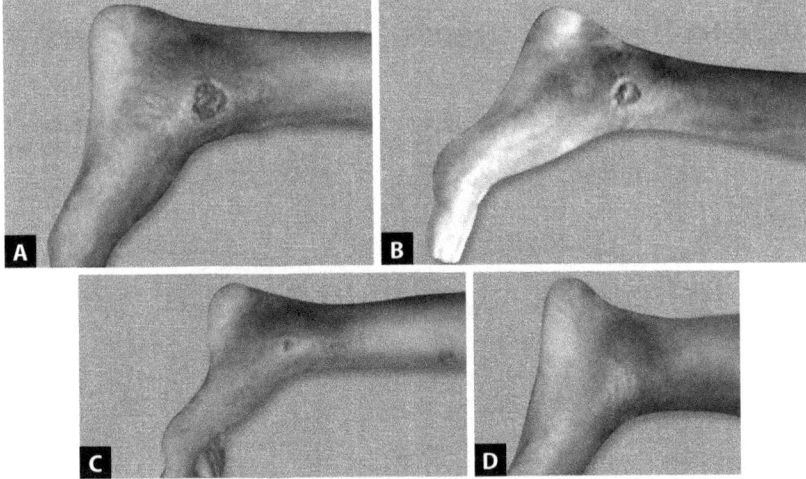

Figs. 5A to D: Case of venous ulcers. (A) At presentation; (B) After debridement; (C) After 2 weeks; (D) After 6 weeks.

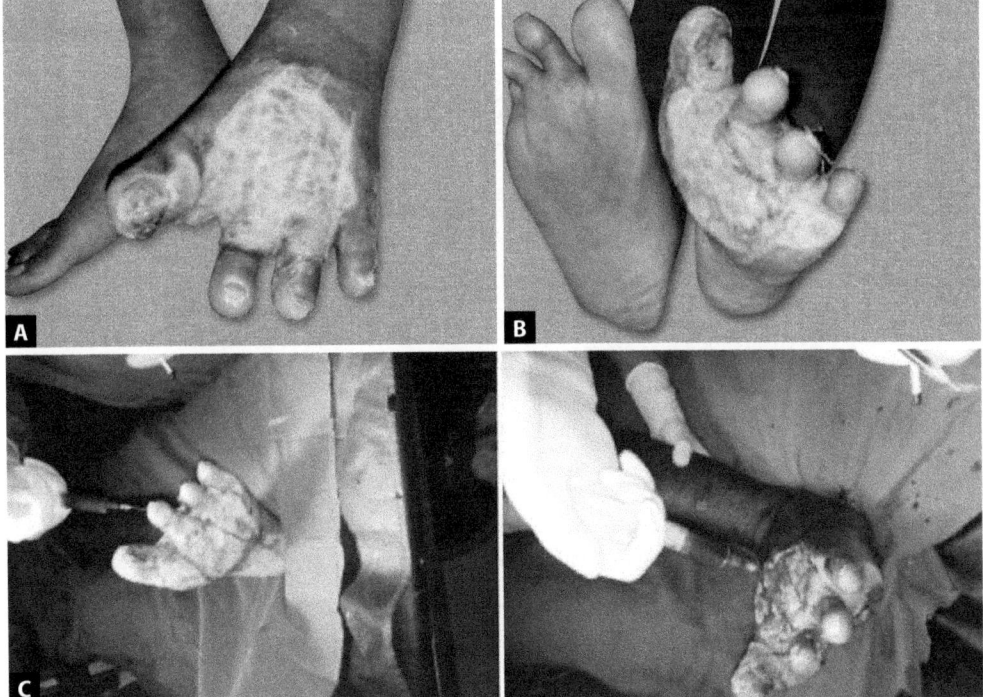

Figs. 6A to C

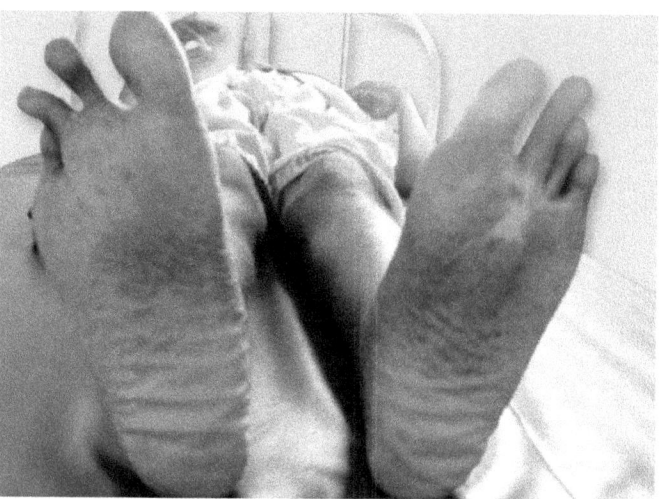

Fig. 6D
Figs. 6A to D: Case of Buerger's disease. (A and B) At presentation; (C) Giving therapy; (D) After full recovery.

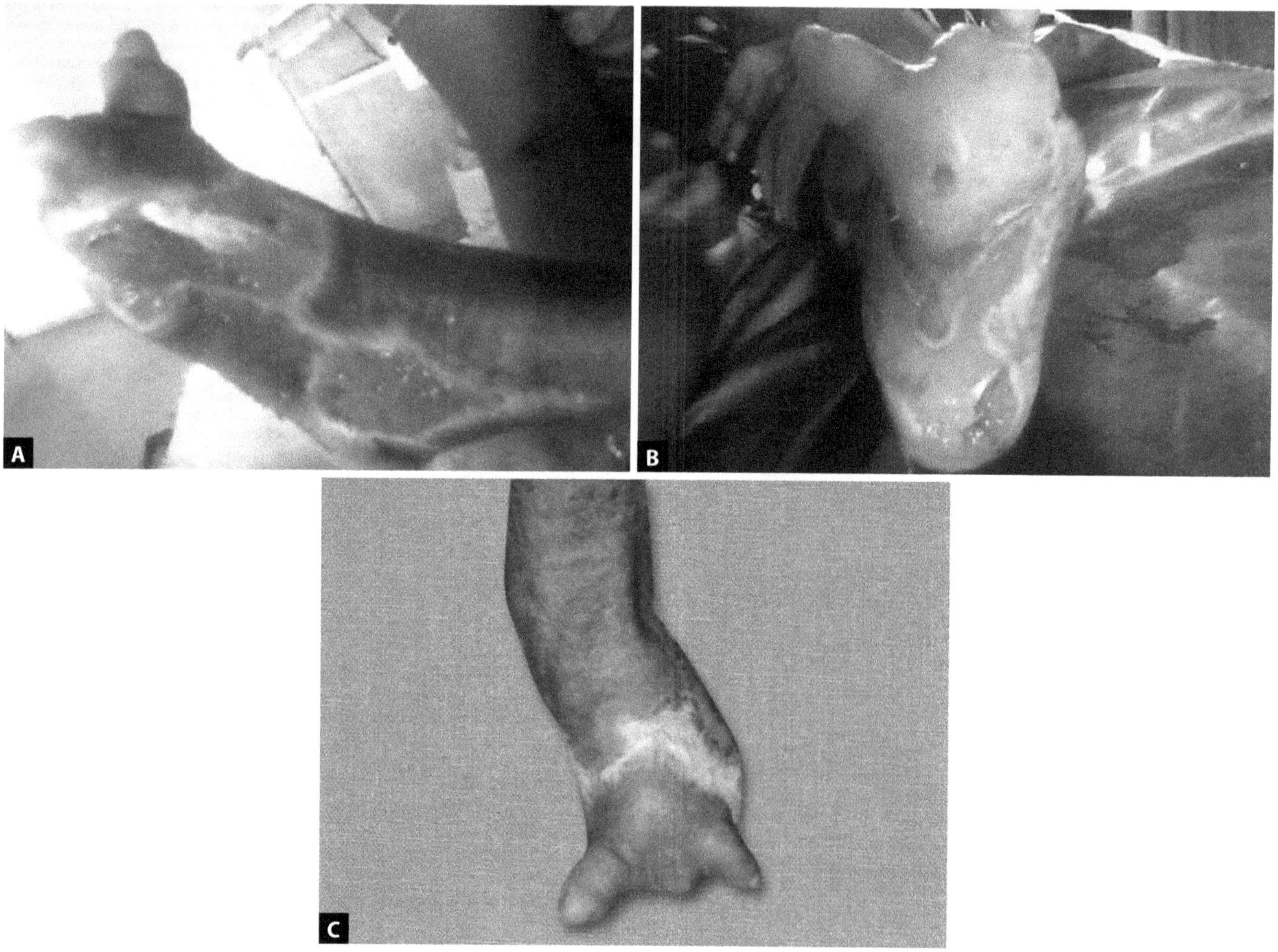

Figs. 7A to C: Case of Hansen's disease. (A) At presentation after debridement; (B) After cell therapy; (C) 6 weeks post-therapy.

BUERGER'S DISEASE

Buerger's disease is an inflammatory disease of arterial wall causing thromboangiitis obliterans of medium and small sized vessels. It may involve the neighboring nerves and veins also **(Figs. 6A to D)**. It affects mostly young individuals and is usually refractory to treatment as bypass or stenting is not possible. In these cases, cell therapy may help in ulcer healing and recovery.

HANSEN'S DISEASE

In this disease, neuropathy involves nerves (N) of both limbs mainly ulnar N, anterior tibial N, posterior tibial N, etc. Repeated trauma due to loss of sensation frequently leads to ulceration. These ulcers are notorious for nonhealing, chronicity and may act as focus of sepsis **(Figs. 7A to C)**. Ulcers are very difficult to treat in leprosy.

FURTHER READING

1. American Diabetes Association. Economic costs of diabetes in the U.S. in 2012. Diabetes Care. 2013;36(4):1033-46.
2. American Diabetes Association. National Diabetes Statistics Report 2014. [online] Available from http://www.diabetes.org/diabetes-basics/statistics/. [Last accessed June, 2021].
3. Blumberg SN, Berger A, Hwang L, Pastar I, Warren SM, Chen W. The role of stem cells in the treatment of diabetic foot ulcers. Diabetes research and clinical practice. 2012;96(1):1-9.
4. Cao Y, Gang X, Sun C, Wang G. Mesenchymal stem cells improve healing of diabetic foot ulcer. J Diabetes Res. 2017;2017:9328347.
5. Eming SA, Martin P, Tomic-Canic M. Wound repair and regeneration: mechanisms, signaling, and translation. Sci Transl Med. 2014;6(265):265-6.
6. Falanga V. Wound healing and its impairment in the diabetic foot. Lancet. 2005;366(9498):1736-43.
7. Galkowska H, Wojewodzka U, Olszewski WL. Chemokines, cytokines, and growth factors in keratinocytes and dermal endothelial cells in the margin of chronic diabetic foot ulcers. Wound Repair Regen. 2006;14(5):558-65.
8. Gallagher KA, Liu ZJ, Xiao M, Chen H, Goldstein LJ, Buerk DG, et al. Diabetic impairments in NO-mediated endothelial progenitor cell mobilization and homing are reversed by hyperoxia and SDF-1 alpha. J Clin Invest. 2007;117(5):1249-59.
9. Gorecka J, Kostiuk V, Fereydooni A, Gonzalez L, Luo J, Dash B, et al. The potential and limitations of induced pluripotent stem cells to achieve wound healing. Stem Cell Res Ther. 2019;10(1):1-10.
10. Isakson M, de Blacam C, Whelan D, McArdle A, Clover AJ. Mesenchymal stem cells and cutaneous wound healing: current evidence and future potential. Stem Cells Int. 2015; 2015:831095.
11. Martin P, Nunan R. Cellular and molecular mechanisms of repair in acute and chronic wound healing. Br J Dermatol. 2015;173(2):370-8.
12. Mizukami H, Yagihashi S. Exploring a new therapy for diabetic polyneuropathy - the application of stem cell transplantation. Front Endocrinol. 2014;5:45.
13. Werner S, Grose R. Regulation of wound healing by growth factors and cytokines. Physiol Rev. 2003;83(3):835-70.
14. Singh VK, Kalsan M, Kumar N, Saini A, Chandra R. Induced pluripotent stem cells: applications in regenerative medicine, disease modeling, and drug discovery. Front Cell Dev Biol. 2015;3:2.
15. Baraniak PR, McDevitt TC. Stem cell paracrine actions and tissue regeneration. Regen Med. 2010;5(1):121-43.
16. Liang X, Ding Y, Zhang Y, Tse HF, Lian Q. Paracrine mechanisms of mesenchymal stem cell-based therapy: current status and perspectives. Cell Transplant. 2014; 23(9):1045-59.
17. Casqueiro J, Casqueiro J, Alves C. Infections in patients with diabetes mellitus: a review of pathogenesis. Indian J Endocrinol Metab. 2012;16(Suppl 1):S27-S36.
18. Clayton ZE, Tan RP, Miravet MM, Lennartsson K, Cooke JP, Bursill CA, et al. Induced pluripotent stem cell-derived endothelial cells promote angiogenesis and accelerate wound closure in a murine excisional wound healing model. Biosci Rep. 2018;38:4.
19. Kim KL, Song SH, Choi KS, Suh W. Cooperation of endothelial and smooth muscle cells derived from human induced pluripotent stem cells enhances neovascularization in dermal wounds. Tissue Eng Part A. 2013;19(21-22):2478-85.
20. Açikgoz G, Devrim İ, Özdamar Ş. Comparison of keratinocyte proliferation in diabetic and non-diabetic inflamed gingiva. J Periodontol. 2004;75(7):989-94.
21. Liu X, Li Q, Niu X, Hu B, Chen S, Song W, et al. Exosomes secreted from human-induced pluripotent stem cell-derived mesenchymal stem cells prevent osteonecrosis of the femoral head by promoting angiogenesis. Int J Biol Sci. 2017;13(2):232-44.
22. Itoh M, Umegaki-Arao N, Guo Z, Liu L, Higgins CA, Christiano AM. Generation of 3D skin equivalents fully reconstituted from human induced pluripotent stem cells (iPSCs) PLoS One. 2013;8(10):e77673.
23. Kuzuya M, Satake S, Esaki T, Yamada K, Hayashi T, Naito M, et al. Induction of angiogenesis by smooth muscle cell-derived factor: possible role in neovascularization in atherosclerotic plaque. J Cell Physiol. 1995;164(3):658-7.

Index

Page numbers followed by *b* refer to box, *f* refer to figure, *fc* refer to flowchart, and *t* refer to table.

A

Abatacept 44, 47, 51
Abdominal pain 105, 111
Abductor halluces 326*f*
Abductor pollicis longus 39*f*, 264, 292
Abscess, cold 180
Achilles guard 208*f*
Achilles insertion 302
Achilles tendinitis 207, 210
    noninsertional 208
Achilles tendinopathy, types of 207
Achilles tendon
    exercises 208
    lengthening 195
Achilles tendonitis, rehabilitation for 209*f*
Acid fast bacilli 69, 171
Acquired flatfoot deformity 303
Acquired syphilis 70
Acrodermatitis chronica atrophicans 69
Acromegaly 191, 191*f*
Active inflammatory disease 76
Acupuncture 254, 257
Adalimumab 32, 48, 51
Addison's disease 21
Adductor halluces 326, 326*f*
Adenosine
    deaminase 98
    triphosphate 239
Adhesive capsulitis 215
Adipocyte
    lipid-rich 341
    zones of 342*f*
Adipose stem cells 343
Adipose tissue 341, 341*f*, 361, 367
    applications of 343
    architecture 344
    biology 341
    complex, derivatives of 344*f*
    literature on 342
    types of 341
Adrenal insufficiency, operative 303
Adrenal medullary cells 376
Adrenocorticotropic hormone 240, 255
Adult human cells 346
Adult stem cell 336, 352
    types 336
Advanced disease 187
Aerobic exercise 252
Aerobic training 252
Affective spectrum disorder 237
Agitation 251
Airway management 89
Akin osteotomy 331
Alcoholic liver disease 65

Alendronate 154
Alkaptonuria 111
Allogeneic
    preparation 365
    transplantation 342
Allopurinol 106, 107
Aluminum toxicity 114
Alzheimer's disease 372, 375
Amikacin C 178
Amino acids, excitatory 238*f*
Amitriptyline 257
Amniotic fluid 362, 372
Amyotrophic lateral sclerosis 378
Anakinra 49, 51, 165
Andersson lesion 84
    clinical features 84
    etiology 85
    management 85
    pathology 85
    radiology 85
Anemia 75, 91, 142, 173
Anesthesia, manipulation under 222
Anesthetic implications 88
Animal studies 355
ANKH gene 109
Ankle 54, 198, 303, 307
    and knee joints 68
    anterior 303
    arthritis 304, 317
    arthrodesis 55, 304, 319, 320
    arthroplasty 321
    articular cartilage 316
    biomechanics, normal 317*f*
    central 303
    fusion 322*f*
    hemophilic arthropathy of 194*f*
    right 318*f*
Ankle joint 302, 316, 319*f*
    alignment, restoration of 321*f*
    left 196*f*
Ankle osteoarthritis 316, 318*t*
    anterior 320*f*
    classification of 317, 318*t*
    diagnosis 317
    end-stage 316*f*, 322*f*
    examination 317
    pathomechanics 316
    treatment 317
Ankle pain 301, 302
    diffuse 317
Ankylosed spine, part of 86
Ankylosing spondylitis 17, 21, 47, 48, 73, 75-78, 81, 86, 91, 92
    index 48

    juvenile 75, 91
    surgical management in 81, 82
    treatment in 77*b*, 91
Ankylosing spondylosis 21
Ankylosis 77
Annulus fibrosis 41, 74
Anorexia 111, 173
Antacids 43
Antagonist 60
Antalgic gait pattern 302
Anti-CD20 agent 50
Anticitrullinated protein antibody 45
Anti-citrulline peptidase antibody 13
Anticyclic citrullinated peptide 30
Anticytokine agents 47
Antidepressants 232
Antigen
    bacterial and viral 15
    presenting cells 13
Antigenicity 49
Anti-inflammatory effects 345
Antinuclear antibody 30, 160
    testing 161
Anti-rheumatic drugs, 44, 45, 75, 91
    disease-modifying 31, 43, 44, 54, 168
Anti-rheumatic therapy 47
Anti-sclerostin antibodies 139
Anti-TNF therapy 54
Anxiety 250
Aortic dissection 88
Aortic pseudoaneurysm 88
Aortic regurgitation 78
Apatite 97
Aplastic anemia 106
Aponeuroses 41
Arnold-Hilgartner staging 193, 193*f*
    modified 194
Arterial disease, peripheral 311
Artery forceps 282*f*
Arthralgia 65, 70
Arthritic hand, treating 270
Arthritic joint disorders 192
Arthritis 21, 58, 69, 70, 93, 97*f*, 159, 160, 187, 267, 320
    active 164, 165
    acute 101, 113
    animal models of 49
    causes of 159
    chronic 97, 113
        destructive 112
    crystal-induced 97, 97*t*
    degenerative 354
    enteropathic 73, 93
    history of 162, 163*t*, 164

idiopathic 49
mutilans 268
post-traumatic 316, 317
progression of 32
reactive 17, 21, 73, 92, 161
seronegative 36
severe 77
tubercular 173
undifferentiated 27, 161
Arthrodesis 54, 56, 58, 167, 195, 198, 275, 276, 304
posterior 180
Arthrofibrosis shoulder 215
Arthrography 270
Arthrokinematic movement 9
Arthropathy 68
chronic 108f
Arthroplasty 54-56, 57f, 124, 277, 304
biomechanics of 10
primary 131
Arthroscopic ankle arthrodesis 320
Arthroscopic capsular release 224, 226f
Arthroscopic management 203
Arthroscopy 114, 124
Arthrotomy 114
Articular cartilage 3, 4, 7, 8t, 40, 58, 100, 109, 117, 120
biomechanics of 118
collapse of 196f
degeneration of 118
normal 117
Articular disease, assessment of 34
Articular neurology 7
Artifacts, crystal-like 114b
Aspirin 102, 107, 167
Asthma 141
Athletes 369
Atrial fibrillation 136
Attack, acute 102, 110
Augmentation techniques 131
Auspitz's sign 68
Autoantibodies production 168
Autoimmune
cells 356
disorders 49, 51
hypothyroidism 21
origin, disorder of 13
Autoimmune disease 17, 18, 20, 21, 128
management of 51
pathogenesis of 13
Autoimmune rheumatic
disease 13, 21
disorders 65
Autologous
blood injection 202
chondrocyte implantation 10, 338
tenocyte injection 212, 212f
Autonomic disturbances 229
Autonomic dysfunctions 242
Autonomic nervous system 240
abnormal 196
Autophosphorylation 375
Autosomal inheritance
dominant 19f
recessive 19f

Avascular necrosis
regenerative therapy for 368
risk factors for 368t
Axial spondylitis 91
Azathioprine 44, 66, 93, 106

B

B cells 14, 43
B lymphocyte system 337
Bacteriology 174
Baker's cyst 35, 41, 64
Balneotherapy 254, 255
Bamboo spine 74, 75, 86
Basic genetics 17f
Bazedoxifene 135
Bedaquiline 182
Behçet's disease 17, 20, 67, 68, 161
Benzbromarone 107
Biceps tendon 219f
Bimalleolar ankle fracture 316f
Bioactive molecules 369
Biochemical parameters, evaluation of 149
Biological therapy 47
use of 368
Bipolar shell allograft 319
Bisphosphonates 77, 135, 154
adverse effects of 136
mechanism of action of 135fc
Blackberry thumb 204
Bladder dysfunction 243
Blood
glucose level 312
peripheral 362
sugar control 312
tests 92
vessels, growth of 14
Blood-brain barrier 376
Blosozumab 139
B-lymphocytes 50
Body mass index 132
Body mechanics 9
Body organ, largest 63
Body planes 6
Body's movement 5
Bone 81, 152, 301, 339, 367
and joints 263
cells 143f
defects 60, 61
deformities 60
density measurements 129
edema 77
effects on 135
formation 143
markers of 129
fractures, long 130
graft 131
substitute 131
lining cells 367
mineral density 125
morphogenetic factors 374
osteopenia 189
porosis 60
production 188
remodeling, mechanism of 127, 128f
resorption marker 129, 142

scan 130
scintigraphy 130
sclerosis 153
trabeculae, resorption of 153
tuberculosis of 171
tumors, benign 161
Bone marrow 87, 341, 350, 360, 369
aspirate concentrate 365, 367, 369
lesions 121
Bony abnormalities 148
Bony destruction 31f
Bony elements 7
Bony osteophytes 188
Bony prominences 305
Borrelia 241
Botulinum toxin 63, 232, 232f
Boutonniere's deformity 27, 58, 66, 268, 293
Bowler's thumb 296, 297
clinical features 297
differential diagnosis 297
etiology 297
investigations 297
pathophysiology 297
treatment of 297, 298fc
Brachioradial pruritus 63
Bradykinesia 376
Breast diseases 35
Brodalimumab 47, 50
Brodalumab 51
Buerger's disease 386, 386f
Bulimia nervosa 237
Bunion deformity 325
Burning micturition 92
Bursa 41, 302
Bursitis 97

C

Cadaveric dissection 282f
Calcaneal stress fracture 210
Calcified zone 118
Calcinosis 66
Calcitonin 134, 154
Calcium 133, 149
channel blockers 66
hydroxyapatite 97
inadequate 129
oxalate 97
role of 129
sulfate 131
Calcium phosphate 97, 131
crystal deposition disease, basic 112
Calcium pyrophosphate
crystals 103
deposition 108, 188
dihydrate 40, 97, 187
calcifications 40
deposition disease 108
Callus formation 149
Campylobacter species 68
Canakinumab 49, 51
Capreomycin C 178
Capsaicin 123, 255
Capsular fibrosis 74
Capsule-phalangeal portion 326
Carbamazepine 63

Carbidopa 116
Cardiac dysfunction 88
Cardiac irregularities 243
Cardiovascular disease 15, 78
Cardiovascular involvement 78
Cardiovascular risk 312
Carpal bone surface, irregular 40
Carpal tunnel
　release, incision for 265f
　syndrome 54, 64, 279
Carpet tack sign 65
Cartilage 4, 13, 117, 338, 367
　and bone, disorders of 95
　changes 39
　degradation of 15
　destruction 104
　injuries 212
　loss 108
　metabolism, biomechanical regulation of 118
Cartilage matrix
　degradation, causes of 119
　protein content 119
　regulation of 120
Cartilage-cartilage interface 4
Cartilaginous tissue 362
Caseous tissue, calcification of 172
Catechol-o-methyltransferase gene 241
Cathepsin 15
　K inhibitors 139
Cauda equina syndrome 78, 84
Celecoxib 105
Cell
　based delivery 338
　death 120
　free formulation 361
　in vivo, survival of 381
　induction of 337
　lining synovium 4
　targeted biologics 47
　types of 3
Cellular biomechanics 5
Cellular component 127
Cellular immunity 14, 172, 310
Cellular therapy 354, 370, 372
Cellulitis 49, 50, 104
Central nervous system 237
　disorders 128
Central sacral line 11
Cerebral palsy 27, 377
Cerebrospinal fluid 239f
Certolizumab 51
　pegol 48
Cervical
　kyphosis, chronic 89
　lordosis 82, 82f
　osteotomy 83
　radiculopathy 281
　spinal disease 63
　spinal involvement 180
　spine 77, 181f
　　fracture 87
Cervicothoracic
　junction 87
　region 11
Charcot's arthropathy 69

Charcot's joints 113
Charcot's neuropathy 306t, 307f
　arthropathy 305
　cause of 305
　classification of 306t
　indications of 306t
　treatment of 306
Charcot's restrained orthotic walker 305
Charcot's triad 197
Charcot-Leyden crystals 114
Cheilectomy 319
Chemical injuries 118
Chemotherapeutic cytotoxics 102
Chemotherapy 172, 178
　before onset of 172
Chest deformity, chin on 90
Chevron osteotomy, modified 331f
Chin-brow vertical angle 82, 82f
Chlamydia 68, 92
　trachomatis 92
Chlorambucil 44
Cholesterol 114
　crystals 114
Chondrocalcinosis 108
　asymptomatic 110
Chondrocyte phenotype, changes in 120
Chondroitin sulfate 117, 118
Chondroplasty 319
Chondrosarcoma 64
Chromosome, structure of 18f
Chronic disease 93
Chronic inflammatory
　arthritis 73
　disease 301
　rheumatic diseases 73
Chronic periarticular syndromes 113
Churg-Strauss syndrome 67
Ciprofloxacin 178
Circinate balanitis 69f
Citalopram 251
Clarithromycin 178
Clodronate 135
Clofazimine C 178
Clofibrate 107
Clostridium histolyticum 296
Clutton's joints 70
Coamoxiclav 178
Coarse pits 68, 68f
Coeliac disease 93
Cognitive behavioral therapy 253
Colchicine 105, 106
　toxicity 105
Collateral ligament
　lateral 119
　medial 119
Colony stimulating factor 15
Combination therapy 32, 140
Common hand disorders 292
Common inflammatory arthritis 40
Comorbid disorders 248
Compartment syndrome 193
Complete blood count 161
Compressive dressings 194
Compromising cellular immunity 312
COMT gene 241
Concavity-compression principle 11

Condyle defects, femoral posterior 62f
Conflict of interest 349, 352
Conjunctivitis 92
Conservative treatment 292
Constipation 251
Contact dermatitis, implant-induced 63
Contracted anterior capsule 226f
Conventional arthrography 217
Core decompression 368
Coronal plane 319
Corticosteroid 43, 60, 106, 107, 168, 270
　injection 113
　　intra-articular 111
Costimulation modulator 50
Costochondral junctions 74
Cranial bone 153
C-reactive protein 61, 163-165, 242, 269
Critical limb ischemia 311
Crohn's disease 73, 267
Crouch gait 11
Cruciate ligament
　anterior 119, 370
　posterior 119
Cryoglobulin crystals 114
Cryoglobulinemia 114
Crystal arthropathies 69
Crystal deposit
　disease 40
　disorders 97, 113
Crystalline foreign bodies 114
Cushing's disease 292
Cutaneous infections, arthritis in 69
Cutaneous rash 63
Cutaneous systemic sclerosis 66
Cyclobenzaprine 250, 257
Cyclooxygenase 43, 167
Cyclophosphamide 44
Cycloserine S 178
Cyclosporine 44, 102
Cyst 108
　ganglion 63
　subcutaneous 64
Cysteine proteinases 15
Cytokine 14, 26, 43, 44, 120
Cytotherapy 372
CZ Hong's technique 233f

D

Dactylitis, signs of 92
Dark skin pigmentation 147
Darrach's procedure 56, 58
de Quervain's tenosynovitis 39f, 204, 205f, 292
Debridement, types of 313
Deformity 112, 153, 268
　correction 11, 82, 84
　　principle of 11
　mild 294
　moderate 294
　pathogenesis of 81
　progression of 180
　severe 294
Degenerative knee, classification of 122
Demyelinating
　disorders 50
　syndromes 49

Dendritic cell 13, 338f
Denosumab 137
Dental caries 29
Dental tissues 372
Depression 111
Dermatofibromas 65
Dermatomyositis 17, 67, 67f, 190
    juvenile 161
Destructive arthropathies 113
D-glucuronic acid 4
Diabetes 283, 381
    mellitus 65, 382
        insulin-dependent 21
Diabetic foot 310
    management of 312
    newer therapies for 313
    risk assessment in 311
Diabetic foot ulcer 305, 310, 310t, 314f, 314f
    advance dressings for 313
    classification of 311
    examination of 311
    risk factors for 311b
    risk of 310
Diabetic patients, foot wears for 313
Diabetic ulcer 310
Diarrhea 105, 106, 251
Diet and activity 167
Dietary factors 13
Dimensional coordinate system 6
Disease
    activity, monitoring of 154
    natural history of 171
Dissection, superficial 282f
Distal metatarsal articular angle 328, 328f
Distal scapula 74
Distal ulna 74
Distal ulnar osteotomy 56
Distraction arthroplasty 319, 321f
Diuretics 102
Diverticulitis 50
Dizygotic twins 20
Dizziness 106, 123, 242, 250, 251
Dopamine 374
    agonists 251
Dorsal extrinsic muscles 264
Double contour sign 40, 41
Drowsiness 251
Drug
    analgesic 231
    anti-inflammatory 44, 75
    antimalarial 44
    antitubercular 177, 177t
    classification of 105fc
    nonsteroidal anti-inflammatory 43, 44, 60, 63, 77, 91, 105, 114, 167, 270, 289, 292, 303, 354
    therapy 134
    toxicity 181
Dry mouth 251
Dual-photon absorptiometry 129
Duloxetine 123, 249, 257
Dupuytren's contracture 65f, 295
    management of severe 296fc
    stages of 296f
Dupuytren's disease 215, 295, 295f
Durkan's test 279

Dynamic compression plate 10
Dystrophic calcification 175

E

Earlier volar plate arthroplasty method 272
Early inflammatory arthritis, ultrasound in 34
Eccentric calf stretching 210
Edema
    neurogenic 243
    trophic 243
Effusion 121
Eichenholtz classification 306t
    modified 197f
Eichhoff maneuver 293
Elbow 54
Electrical nerve stimulation 63
Elimination diet 253
Embryonic stem cells 336, 343, 359, 363, 376
Encephalitis 27
Enchondroma 64
Endocrine disorder 118, 128, 248
Endogenous crystals 97
Endogenous danger signal 99f
Endometrium 361
Endosteal surface 15
Endothelial cells 356
    progenitor 368
Endothelial stem cell 336
Enthesitis 41, 73, 97, 160
    signs of 92
Entrapment syndromes 212
Environmental protection, principle of 348
Enzyme
    angiotensin-converting 161
    hypoxanthine-guanine 115
Enzyme-linked immunosorbent assay 174
Eosinophils, actions of 43
Epicondyle, lateral 74
Epicondylitis
    lateral 201f
    medial 203, 204f
Epigenetic regulators 375
Episcleritis 29
Epithelial barriers 107
Epstein-Barr virus 13, 357
Erosions 40, 103, 188
Erythema marginatum 70
Erythematous border 92
Erythrocyte sedimentation rate 163-165
Esophageal dysmotility 66
Estrogen 129
Etanercept 32, 48, 51
Ethambutol 102, 177
Ethanol 102
Ethical concerns 346, 362
Etidronate 135, 154
Exercise 133, 150, 166, 252
    therapy 122
Exogenous crystals 97
Exosome 213
    therapy 213f
Exostectomy 305
Expansile osteolysis 152
Expansile skeletal hyperphosphatasia 152

Extensor carpi radialis
    brevis 264f
    longus 264f
Extensor digiti minimi 58, 264
Extensor digitorum, left 39f
Extensor hallucis brevis 326f
Extensor indicis proprius 58
Extensor pollicis
    brevis 39f, 264, 292
    longus 264
Extensor tendons 265f
Extracellular component 127
Extracellular matrix, components of 14

F

Facial erythema 67
Familial Mediterranean fever 19
Fasciectomy 296
    subcutaneous 296
Faster healing rate 314
Fatigue 111, 242
Febuxostat 106
    mechanism of action of 106f
Felty's syndrome 17, 22
Femoral fracture
    atypical 136
    condyle split 61f
    management of atypical 137fc
Femoral head 368t
Femur 148, 195
    bone 126f
Fever 75, 91
    high grade 69
    low-grade 173
Fiberglass 114
Fibro fog 242
Fibroblasts 15, 65
Fibrocartilage 7
Fibrocytes 65
Fibromatosis, digital 64
Fibromyalgia 228, 231t, 236, 237, 237f, 239f, 240, 241, 244t, 245f, 252, 253
    assessment of 245f
    criteria 247b
    diagnosing 246f
    pain processing in 238
    pathogenesis 236
    syndrome 248t
    treatment 256
        goals of 249
Fibromyalgianess 245
Fibronectin 315
Fibrous tissue 101
Fibular deviation 28
Fibular osteotomy 124
Filtered urate 97
Finger
    deformities 272, 293
    swelling 39f
Finkelstein maneuver 293
Finkelstein's test 205f
Fissure fractures 153
Fixed flexion deformity 61, 61f
Flat bone fractures 131
Flexor carpi ulnaris 38

Flexor digitorum
    profundus 265*f*
    superficialis 39*f*, 265*f*
Flexor hallucis brevis 326
    lateral 326*f*
    medial 326*f*
Flexor hallucis longus 326
    tendon 58
Flexor tendons 265*f*
    distribution of 265*f*
Fluid collection 37
Foot 197, 305, 306*t*
    care, tips for 312
    deformity 310
    structure of 327
    wear modification 328
Foot and ankle 28, 299
    pain, etiology of 301*t*
    tuberculosis 173
Foot pain 301
    differential diagnosis of 303
Foot ulcer 310, 382, 382*f*
    etiology of 310
Foraminal compression test 281
Forearm and wrist, tunnels in 265*f*
Forefoot 302, 303
    abduction 306
    deformities of 28
    offloader 314*f*
Fracture 153, 193
    first 132
    fixation, biomechanics of 10
    high risk of 144
    transdiscal 86
    transvertebral 86
Frozen shoulder 215, 216
Fusion, partial 276

G

Gabapentin 63, 250
Gait analyses 9, 302
Gamma-aminobutyric acid 374
Ganglion 64
Gastric irritation 106
Gastroenteritis 50
Gastrointestinal bleeding 43
Gastrointestinal disorders 128
Gastrointestinal perforation 50
Gelling phenomenon 159
Gene expression 119
Genetic 115
    factors 26, 128, 152, 241
    studies 20
Genu valgum left knee 61*f*
Giant cells 101
Glenohumeral ligament
    inferior 220*f*
    middle 226*f*
Glomus tumor 64
Glucocorticoids, effects of 143*f*
Glucose-6-phosphatase deficiency 99
Glycated hemoglobin 312
Glycogen storage disease 99
Golfer's elbow 203
    rehabilitation for 204, 205*f*

Golgi tendon reflex 230
Golimumab 48, 51, 76
Gonococcal arthritis 70
Gosset fascia 295
Gottron's papules 67, 67*f*
Gottron's sign 67
Gout 20, 69, 91, 97, 98*f*, 105*fc*, 111*t*, 161, 268, 270, 326
    acute 101*fc*, 102, 105, 110
    arthropathy 189*f*
    chronic 103, 105, 106
        polyarticular 103*f*
    classification for 99*b*, 103
    diagnosis of 100*t*
    differential diagnosis of 104
    drugs in 105
    idiopathic 99
    intercritical 103
    management of 105
    microscopic features of 101
    pathogenesis of 100, 100*f*, 101*f*
    polyarticular 102
    precipitate 102
    primary 99
    secondary 99, 100, 100*f*
Gouty arthritis 98
    acute 102
    painful 97
    pathogenesis of 101*f*
    site of 104*f*
    surgical treatment for 107
Gouty lesions, surgery of 108
Gouty tophi 102*f*, 107, 114
    typical 104*f*
Gradual sublaxation 31*f*
Graft complications 180
Granulocytopenia 106
Granuloma pyogenicum 64
Grattage sign 68
Graves disease 21
Great toe's valgus 326
Gross deformity 188
Growth factors 374
Growth hormone 240, 248, 251, 255
Guanine 99
Guyon's canal 265, 283
    anatomy of 284*f*
    dissection of 282*f*

H

Hallux interphalangeal angle 328
Hallux valgus 28, 29*f*, 302*f*, 325, 325*f*, 329*f*
    angle 327, 327*f*
    classification of severity of 329*t*
    deformity 28*f*, 328
    differential diagnosis 326
    etiology 325
    interphalangeus deformity 331
    management 327
    pathoanatomy of 326, 326*f*
    physical examination 327
    risk factors 325
    signs 326
    symptoms 326
    treatment 328

Hammer toe deformity 325*f*
Hand 267
    and wrist, assessment of 288
    classical deformities in 27
    intrinsic mechanism 294
    pain in 279
    small joints of 275
    surgery, categories of 271*fc*
Hansen's disease 381, 386*f*, 387
Headache 106, 250, 251
    chronic 247
Heartbeats, fast 250
Heel
    cup 211*f*
    offloader 314*f*
    pad 210*f*
    pain 29
    spurs 92
Heliotrope rash 67*f*
Hemarthrosis, post-traumatic 111
Hematoidin crystals 114
Hematologic disorders 128
Hematomas, acute 195
Hematopoietic lineage cells 368
Hematopoietic stem cell 336, 357
    transplantation, effects of 356
Hemochromatic arthritis 189
Hemochromatic arthropathy 189*f*
Hemochromatosis 111
Hemoglobin 114
Hemophagocytic
    lymphohistiocytosis 161
    syndrome, secondary 161
Hemophilia 161, 192
Hemophiliac cyst 193
Hemophilic arthropathy 193*f*
    pathogenesis of 192*fc*
Hemorrhagic gastropathy 105
Henoch-Schönlein purpura 67
Hepatitis
    B 49
    C 49, 237, 248
Hepatocyte growth factor 338*f*
Hereditary 109
Hindfoot 302, 303, 306, 318*f*
    deformities of 29
    instability 303
    motion, reduced 321
Hip 198, 316
    arthroplasty 77
    fracture 128
    pathology 11
Hitchhiker's thumb 268
Hoffmann-Tinel sign 279
Homeobox gene 375
Homozygote 20
Hooked osteophytes 189*f*
Hormone replacement therapy 133
Horn glia, dorsal 238
Hospital admission 166
Human anti-chimeric antibodies 47
Human immune response 172
Human leukocyte antigen 13, 17, 18, 21
Human motion analysis 9
Human origin, medical products of 372
Human skeletal system 3

Humoral immunity 14
Huntingtin gene 377
Huntington's disease 372, 376
Hutchinson's teeth 70
Hyaline cartilage 40, 117f
Hyaluronic acid 7, 117, 121, 315
Hydrodilatation procedure 222
Hydrotherapy 254
Hydroxyapatite 97
   crystal deposition disease 111
   deposition of 147
Hydroxychloroquine 31, 43, 44, 60, 66, 92, 93
Hyperbaric oxygen therapy 313
Hypercalcemia 111
Hypercapnia 142
Hyperemia 175, 281
Hyperesthesia 63
Hyperglycemia 310, 312
   uncontrolled 310
Hyperparathyroidism 111, 189, 190f
Hyperpigmented patch 63f
Hyperuricemia 97, 98, 98f
   asymptomatic 102
   classification of 98t
   sustained 98
Hypnotherapy 254
Hypocalcemia 136, 147
   chronic 148
Hypochromic normocytic anemia 30
Hypoechoic soft tissue 40
Hypogonadal states 128
Hypogonadism 142
Hypophosphatasia 147
Hypophosphatemia 147
Hypopigmented anesthetic patches 69f
Hypotension, neurally-mediated 242
Hypothalamic-pituitary
   adrenal axis 43, 240
   growth hormone 240
   thyroid 240
Hypoxanthine 99
   guanine phosphoribosyltransferase 98
      disorder of 20
Hypoxia 142
   effect of 142f

I

Iatrogenic injuries 90
Ibandronate 154
Idiopathic hypercalciuria 128
Idiopathic hyperphosphatasia 152
Idiopathic osteonecrosis 368
Ilizarov frame 321f
Immune
   ablation, high dose 356
   cells 356
   system 43
      dysregulation of 47
Immunodeficiency virus infection 368
Immunoglobulin 47
Immunomodulators 168
Immunomodulatory adhesion molecule
      integrin 18
Immunomodulatory therapy 93
Indolent tophus ulcers 107

Indomethacin 105, 107
Infection 48, 55, 104, 168
   opportunistic 51
   tubercular 157
Infectious agents 13
Infectious mononucleosis 161
Inflamed granulation tissue 55
Inflamed synovial membrane 100
Inflammasome 109
Inflammation
   chronic 14
   crystal-induced 95
Inflammatory arthritis 267, 269, 272
   etiology of 267
   surgical considerations in 54
Inflammatory bowel disease 21, 93
Inflammatory disorders, acute 110
Infliximab 32, 47, 48, 51
   plus 47
Informed consent 349
Infraspinatus 11
   strengthening 221f
Inherited autosomal disorders 147
Injury
   mechanism of 86
   site of 86
Innate immune system, activation of 13
Inner cell mass 335
Inorganic phosphate 149
Inosine 98
Insomnia 251
Institutional arrangements, principle of 348
Intellectual property rights 350
Interferon
   gamma release assay 49, 174
   signaling 18
Intermetatarsal angle 327, 328f
Interosseous muscle atrophy 293
Interphalangeal joints 54, 57, 58, 264, 307f
   early synovitis of proximal 27f
Interscapular region 63f
Interthenar incision 283
Intervertebral disc 8
Intestinal irregularities 243
Intestinal malabsorption 150
Intestinal stem cells 336
Intra-articular
   fluid 35
   hyaluronic acid 124, 319
   injection 107, 124, 162, 361, 369
   space 175
Intracellular chloride 374
Intracellular signaling pathways 118
Intralesional steroid injection 64
Intramedullary nailing 10, 131
Intrinsic plus deformity 294
Intubating laryngeal mask 90
Ipsilateral foot 317
IRF5 gene 18
Ischemia 310, 381
   critical 311
Ischemic foot 313
Ischial tuberosity 74
Isoniazid 177
Itch, localized 63
Ixekizumab 47, 50

J

Jaccoud arthritis 66
Janus kinase 44, 45
   inhibitors 44
Jaw
   bone 153
   osteonecrosis of 136
Joints 5, 109, 301
   affected 196
      large 110
   alignment 319
   and tendon movements, assessment of 34
   apophyseal 81
   arthrodesis 304
   aspiration 107, 111
   biomaterial attributes, abnormalities in 118
   biomechanics of 5
   calcaneocuboid 303, 307f
   calcification 111
   capsules 74
   classification of 8fc
   compression of 36
   congruent 328
   crepitus in 193
   crystals 113
   deformity 320
   destruction, severe 107, 196f
   disease 97
   distal
      interphalangeal 35, 39f, 58, 91, 66
      radioulnar 55, 271
   dysfunction, permanent 69
   effusion 38
   facet 81
   fewer 162
   fluid, examination of 197
   forces in 118
   function 9
   fusion 304
   gradual deformities of 26
   hip 83
   inflamed 40
   inflammation 114
      signs of 27
   involvement 27, 30, 60, 268
   kinematics 321
   knee 193
   large 36, 112
   lisfranc 306
   lubrication models 7, 8t
   metatarsocuneiform 327
   metatarsophalangeal 104f, 307f, 325, 326, 330
   motion and types 7
   movement 7t
      friction-free 359
   multiple 58
   number of 36
   on palmar aspect 36f
   pain 92
   peripheral small 37
   preserving surgery 319
   proximal interphalangeal 27, 35, 57, 277, 293

radioulnar 189f
replacement 77
sacrificing surgery 319
sacroiliac 27, 73-75, 78, 81
space 187, 305
    loss of 31f
    reduced 189f
spine and sacroiliac 81, 91
sternoclavicular 74
subluxation 188
subluxed 328
surface, irregularity of 100
synovitis in larger 27
talocalcaneal 303
tarsometatarsal 303
tibiotalar 317f
trapeziometacarpal 289
ultrasonography of 31
wrist 55
Jumper's knee 206
Juvenile ankylosing spondylitis, diagnosis of 91
Juvenile idiopathic arthritis 51, 159, 160, 163, 267
    diagnostic considerations 161
    etiopathogenesis 159
    history 159
    investigations 161
    management 162
    medication 167
    physical examination 159
    prognosis 167
    treatment 162

K

K wires 58, 276
Kanamycin C 178
Kawasaki disease 159, 161
Keller resection arthroplasty 332
Kellgren-Lawrence grading 122t
    system 121
Keratan sulfate 117, 118
Keratoconjunctivitis sicca 67
Keratoderma blennorhagicum 68, 69f
Ketoprofen 107
Kidney 102
Kienböck's disease 279, 284, 285, 287
    classification 285
    clinical features 285
    etiological findings 284
    radiological features 285
    systems of 285
    treatment 286
Kissing' lesions 317
Klebsiella 73
Knee 54, 61f, 198, 316
    challenges in 60
    flexion, severe 11
    injuries 212
    osteoarthritis, management for 123fc
    replacement surgery 60
Kyphoplasty 132
Kyphosis, severe 78
Kyphotic deformities 81, 82, 181

L

Lactate dehydrogenase 269
Laminectomy, role of 87
Lapidus procedure 332
Laryngeal mask airway 90
Laser therapy 234
Lead toxicity 102
Leflunomide 31, 32, 43, 44, 60, 164
Leiomyomas 65
Leprosy 69, 69f
Lesch-Nyhan syndrome 99, 101, 115, 115f, 116
    treatment of 115
Lesion
    inflammatory 176
    malignant 176
Leukemia 100
Leukocyte migration test 64
Leukocytosis 75, 91
Leukopenia 106
Lever 5
    classes of 6t
Levodopa 102, 116
Levofloxacin 182
Lifestyle factors 13
Ligament 61, 74, 108, 118, 301, 339, 367
    injuries 212
    intermetatarsal 326
    stability 321
Limb length discrepancy 193
Lipid liquid crystals 114
Lipomas 65
Lipoprotein species, dense low-density 15
Liver
    enzymes 50, 51
    function test 31
Local anesthetic nerve block 63
Local twitch response 229
Locking compression plate 10
Looser's lines 148, 149
Lordotic correction, acute 84
Lubricating substances 4
Lubricin 4
Lumbar lordosis 81
    loss of 81
Lumbar spinal motion 75
Lumbosacral spine 74
Lunate-Capitate joint 188
Luno-Capitate articulation 277
Lupus arthritis 268, 270
Lyme arthritis 69
Lyme disease 69, 161, 228
Lymphoblastic leukemia, acute 161
Lymphocyte
    autoreactive 18
    differentiation 19
    infiltration, diffuse 194f
Lymphoid tyrosine phosphatase 19
Lymphoma 100, 161
Lymphopenia 356
Lysch-Nyhan syndrome 115f
Lytic lesion 189
Löwenstein-Jensen medium 175

M

Macrophage 344
Malar rash 65f
Mallampati grading 89
Malleolus fracture, posterior 316
Mammary stem cell 336
Mannerfelt syndrome 58
Marfan's syndrome 128, 191, 191f
Massage 234, 254
Mast cells 14
    granules of 14
McBride procedure, modified 330
McCarty criteria 40
Measles 152
Mechanical stress 118
Medial epicondyle, biomechanics of 203
Median nerve compression test 279
Medical management 132
Medication 128
    preoperative advice for 60t
MEFV gene 19
Melanotic whitlow 64
Mendelian disease 20
Meningioma 27
Meniscal
    injury 118
    tears 121
    tissues 367
Menkes' steely hair syndrome 128
Menopause, management of 133
Mercaptopurine 106
Mesenchymal stem cells 32, 336, 339, 359, 360f, 361, 363t, 365, 367, 370, 372, 376
    adipose-derived 342
    role of 363t
Mesenchymal stromal cells 338f, 376
Mesenchymal tissue response 14
Metabolic bone disease 130
Metabolic disorders 111
Metabolite allantoin 107f
Metacarpophalangeal joint 27, 35, 55, 56f, 57, 57f, 189, 189f, 263, 271, 275, 293, 294
    digital 57f
    gout affecting first 102f
Metalloproteinase 119
Metatarsal osteotomy 330
Metatarsalgia 304
Methacrylate 114
Methotrexate 31, 43-45, 60, 66, 165
    dose of 47
Methyl methacrylate 97
Microfat 343
Micrognathia 160
Microtrauma 64
Microvascular fragments 345
Midcarpal arthritis 286f
Midfoot 302, 303
Milkman's pseudo fractures 148, 149
Milnacipran 249, 257
Milwaukee shoulder 112
Minocyclines S 178
Misoprostol 43
Modern gait analysis 9
Molecular biomechanics 5

Monoamine oxidase inhibitors 248, 251
Monoarthritis 114
Monoclonal antibody 44
Monocompartmental arthritis 54
Monocyte 344
Mononuclear cell 367
    cocktail 367
    placing 368
Mononuclear phagocyte system 14
Monosodium urate 97, 100
    crystals 99f, 103f
Monozygotic twins 20
Morbidity 78
Mortality 78
    increases, risk of 78
    treatment-related 356
Motion, limited range of 230
Motor disturbances 229
Mouse-human monoclonal antibody 50
Movement, axes of 6
Moxifloxacin 182
Mucin clot test 269
Mucocutaneous lesions 68
Multicomponent therapy 255
Multidrug resistant
    development of 171
    tuberculosis, treatment of 182
Multifocal tuberculosis 173
Multimodal therapy 259
Multiple violaceous papules 67
Multisystem disorder 67
Muscle 15, 81, 264, 301
    activity 9
    atrophy 81
    contraction 5, 65
    flexor 264
    groups, twenty-eight 263
    herniation, tibialis anterior 65
    injuries 212
    intrinsic 264
    microtrauma 240
    palmar 264
    relaxants 232
    stiffness 252
Musculoskeletal
    changes 243
    system 25
    ultrasonography 270
    ultrasound 35
Mushrooming 74
Mycobacteria 26
Mycobacterial infection 171
    diagnosis of 173
Mycobacterium 171
    abscessus 181
    avium complex 181
    chelonae 181
    fortuitum 181
    kansasii 181
    leprae 69
    marinum 181
    metabolism of 171
    tuberculosis 171, 172, 181
Mycophenolate mofetil 66
Mycoplasma 26
Myeloma proteins 114

Myers' cocktail consists 253
Myocardial infarction 102
Myofascial pain 231t
    syndrome 228, 231, 231b
Myofascial trigger point 228, 229b
Myofibroblasts 65
Myopathy 248

N

N-acetyl-d-glucosamine 4
Nanofat 344
    graft 345
Naproxen 107
Natural killer cell 338f
Nausea 105, 106, 111, 123, 251
Neck, movement of 89
Necrotic tissues 313
Negative pressure wound therapy 314
Nephrotoxicity 136
Nerve and blood supply 266
Nerve compression 193, 301
    syndromes 34
Nerve grafting 298
Nerve growth factor 374
Nervousness 250, 251
Neural stem cell 336, 375
Neuroblast's survival 375
Neurocognitive dysfunction 242
Neurodegenerative disorder 376
Neuroendocrine
    dysfunctions 243
    system 240
Neurogenesis, factors responsible for 373f
Neurogenic origin 236
Neuroimmunological interactions 13
Neurologic sequelae 78
Neurological deficit 85, 86
Neurological diseases 372
Neurological disorders 372, 376f
    role in 375
Neurological injury 55
Neurological manifestations 242
Neurological symptoms 87
Neurolysis 298
Neuroma resection 298
Neuromuscular transmission 232
Neuron, apoptosis of 377
Neuronal cells 374
Neuronal disorders 379
Neuronal function 375
Neuropathic arthropathy 195, 197f
    disorders with 196
Neuropathic diabetic foot ulcer, infected 312f
Neuropathic foot 301, 312f
    ulcer 311
Neuropathic pain generators 249
Neuropathic ulcer 313t
Neuropathy 69, 248
Neurotransmitters 374
Neurotraumatic theory 305
Neurotrophic factors 374
Neurovascular theory 196
Neutropenia 50, 356
Neutrophil 105, 110f
    activated 105
    count 51

Newton's laws of motion 9
Nicotinic acid 102
Night splint bunion 329f
Night sweats 173
Nodules, subcutaneous 64
Nonarthritic symptoms 92
Nonbulbar dermal sheath cell 213
    injection 212f
Nonexploitation, principle of 348
Noninfectious arthritis, types of 102
Nonpharmacologic
    therapy 166, 232, 252
    treatment 122
Nonprogressive motor disability 377
Nontuberculous mycobacteria 181
    disease, diagnosis of 174
    infections 171
Notalgia paresthetica 63, 63f
Notch pathway 373
Nucleic acid 100, 100f
    amplification test 176
Numerous techniques 55
Nutrition 133, 253
Nutritional deficiencies 253

O

Obligatory asymmetric replication 335
Oblique retinacular ligament 58
Obstructive pulmonary disease, chronic 141, 144fc
Ochronosis 111
Ocrelizumab 50
Ocular inflammations 136
Ocular stem cells 336
Ocular symptoms 92
Ofatumumab 50
Off shelf ankle brace 318f
Offloading shoes 314f
Offloading techniques 313
Oil drop spots 68
Olfactory ensheathing cells 378
Oligoarthritis, asymmetric 68, 91
Oligoarticular arthritis
    juvenile idiopathic 160
    peripheral 93
Onycholysis 92
Open ankle arthrodesis 320
Open surgical capsular release 224
Opioid 123, 251, 257
    analgesics 123
Oral gabapentin 63
Oral medication 219
Oral steroid, dose of 66
Organ, internal 66
Orthopedic
    conditions 317
    disorders 63, 361
    rheumatology 23, 25, 71, 95, 157, 261, 299, 333
Orthorheumatology, skin manifestations in 63
Orthoscopic resection 64
Orthoses 11
Oscillation, frequencies of 4
Ostectomy 304

Index

Osteoarthritic knee, cytotherapy in 359
Osteoarthritis 10, 61, 97, 110, 111, 117, 118, 120, 153, 187, 188, 268, 288, 301, 318*f*, 326, 359
    calcification in 120
    cartilage, proteinases of 119
    causes of 118, 119*t*
    etiology 117
    inflammation in 120
    management of 117, 121
    pain in 121
    pathogenesis 117
        immunomodulation of 360*f*
    peculiar type of 97
    post-traumatic 119
    risk factors for 118
    secondary 54
    wrist, primary 281
Osteoarthritis knee 359
    management of 363*t*
    therapy for 363*t*
Osteoarthropathy, hypertrophic 190, 190*f*
Osteoarthrosis 279, 287
Osteoarticular tuberculosis, management of 177
Osteoblast 142*f*
Osteoblastic activity 152
Osteocalcin 154
Osteocartilaginous tumor, benign 64
Osteochondral allografts, transplantation of 10
Osteoclastic bone 135
Osteoclasts 77
Osteocytes 367
    cells 143
Osteogenesis imperfecta 125
Osteoid seams 148
Osteokinematic movement 9
Osteolysis, signs of 92
Osteomalacia 147, 149
    causes of 147, 147*t*
    classic 149
    clinical presentation 148
    long-standing 149
    pathogenesis 147
    pseudofracture of 149
    risk factors 147
Osteomalacic syndrome 148, 149
Osteonecrosis 367
Osteophyte 108
    resection of 319
Osteoporosis 60, 61*f*, 77, 104, 125, 129, 141, 141*fc*
    circumscripta 154
    classification of 127*t*
    developement 128
    diagnosis of 125
    management of 143
        steroid-induced 144
    mechanism of steroid-induced 142
    primary 126
    secondary 142
    steroid-induced 142, 143*fc*
    treating 130
Osteoporotic fracture 132*f*, 132*t*, 144
    treatment of 130

Osteoporotic thoracolumbar fractures 132
Osteotomy 54, 124, 167, 179, 304
    angle, determination of 83
    location of 83
    pedicle subtraction 84
    realignment 319
    types of 83, 84*f*, 331
Overlapping disorders, group of 91
Overuse syndromes 212
Ovum 350
Oxalate crystal deposition disease 113
Oxalosis
    primary 113
    secondary 113
Oxcarbamazepine 63
Oxidazes uric acid 107*f*

P

Paget's disease 152
    biochemical 152
Pagetic bones 153
Pain 192, 229, 242, 267
    chronic 248
    medications 251
    perception, mechanism of 238
    referred 229
    relief 319
    signaling, abnormal 239*f*
    subfibular 317
    transmission neuron 238*f*
    visual analog scale for 132
Palmar aponeurosis 295*f*
Palmar fibromatosis 65*f*
Palmoplantar fibromatosis 65
Palpating taut band 229
Pamidronate 154
Papulosquamous lesions 69*f*
Paracetamol 122
Paramyxovirus infection 152
Parathyroid hormone 149
Parathyroidectomy 110
Parent cell 346
Parkinson's disease 215, 216, 372, 376
Parrot' syphilitic osteochondritis 70
Patella 61
Patellar tendinitis 206
Pedis classification system 311*t*
Pelvic
    incidence 82, 83
    tilt 83
Pencil in cup
    appearance 188
    deformity 92
Pendulum exercises 221*f*
Periarthritis 97, 215, 217, 218, 218*f*, 219, 220, 225
    acute 112
    diagnosis of 218
Periarthritis shoulder 215, 223
    causes 216
    diagnosis 217
    etiology 215
    management 219
    pathophysiology 216
    risk factors 216

    signs 216
    symptoms 217
Periostitis, signs of 92
Peripheral arthritis 75
    symptoms 76
    treating 93
Peripheral inflammation 13
Peripheral neuropathy, etiology of 301
Peroneal tendinopathy 208
Phagocytic cells 172
Phalen's sign 279
Pharmacological agents 154
Pharmacology 135
Pharmacotherapy, indications of 154
Phospholipids, surface-active 4
Phosphoribosyl pyrophosphate 98, 115
Physical examination 229, 268
Physical stressors 241
Physiotherapy 77
Piano-Key ulnar head 28
    deformity 28*f*
Piezogenic pedal papules 65
Placenta 372
Plantar fascia
    arthroscopic release of 211*f*
    tear 210
Plantar fasciitis 208, 209*f*
    risk factors for 209
Plasma 98
    cells 26, 101
    proteins 4
Plate fixation 130
Platelet 354
    concentrates, families of 211
    derived growth factor 370
    role of 354
Platelet-rich plasma 354, 367, 370
    injection 202, 211
    intra-articular 124
    molecular basis of 354
    preparation of 211*f*
Pluripotent stem cells 336, 352, 376
Pneumonia 49, 50
Polarizing light microscopy 97
Polio 379
Poliomyelitis 27
Polyangiitis, microscopic 67
Polyarteritis
    asymmetric 268
    inflammatory 111
    nodosa 67, 161
Polyarticular arthritis 248
    types of 111
Polyarticular juvenile idiopathic arthritis 160
Polycythemia 100
Polyethylene 97, 114
Polymerase chain reaction 174, 176
Polymethylmethacrylate 131
Polymorphonuclear cells 269
Polymyositis 17
Polysegmental wedge osteotomy 84
Porcine ventral mesencephalon 376
Porphyria 128
Postpolio syndrome 379
Posture training 234
Pott's spine 63

Prednisone 144
Predominant synovial fluid cell 100
Pregabalin 249, 257
Probenecid 107
Profundus tendons 39f
Progenitor cell 14
    proliferation 374
Proinflammatory cytokines 14, 47, 168, 355
Pronator compression test 281
Pronator Teres syndrome 280
Prophylactic
    procedures 271
        surgeries 55, 57
Prostatitis 92
Prosthesis 11
Prosthetic joint
    flexible 277
    hinged 277
    third generation 277
Protein
    core 117
    crystals 113, 114
Proteoglycans 118, 315
    structure of 117f
Proton pump inhibitors 43
Provocative tests 201
Proximal metatarsal osteotomy 330, 331
Pseudarthrosis 84, 88
Pseudogout 69, 104, 108, 110, 111t
    acute 110
    pathogenesis of 109f, 110f
    pathology of 109
Pseudopodagra 110
Pseudotumor
    cyst 193
    excision 195
Psoriasis 68, 100
    plaques of 68f
    severe 68
Psoriatic arthritis 17, 21, 66, 68, 91, 92, 159, 160, 188, 189f, 268, 270
    hallmark of 92
Psoriatic arthropathy 91, 268
Psoriatic nails 68f
Psoriatic spondylitis 92
Psychological techniques 234
Psychosocial stressors 241
Pubic ramus 148
Pulley exercise 221f
Pulmonary
    changes 29
    diseases 215
    fibrosis 78
    involvement 78
Pure sensory 301
    dysfunction 284
Purine metabolism, disorders of 98
Purine nucleotides 99
Purplish erythema 67
Putative renal urate 100
Pyoderma gangrenosum 67f
    type of 67
Pyogenic infection 173
Pyrazinamide 102, 177
Pyrophosphate arthropathy 108
    chronic 108f, 110

Q

Quality of life 251
Quinolinic acid 377

R

Rabbit femur 119f
Radiation therapy 195
Radio-Lunate joint space 285f
Radionucleotide scans 54
Raloxifene 134
Rasburicase 106
    mechanism of action of 107f
Raynaud's phenomenon 66, 281
Reactants, acute phase 30
Reaction
    hypertrophic 118
    inflammatory 101
    injection site 49
Regenerative medicine 372
Regenerative therapy, promising role of 367
Regional pain syndromes, differential diagnosis of 231
Rehabilitation, biomechanics of 11
Reiter's disease 68, 104, 111
Reiter's syndrome 17, 69f, 73, 92
Remodeling 127
Removable cast walker 313, 314f
Renal dysfunction 97
Renal failure patients 107
Renal function 310
Renal osteodystrophy 149
Residual deformity 172
Respiratory irregularities 243
Restlessness 251
Retrocalcaneal bursitis 210
Rhabdomyolysis 106
Rheumatic disease 17, 18, 22, 47, 243, 248
    childhood 157
    chronic 21
    genetic basis of 17
    management of 47
Rheumatic fever 70
Rheumatoid arthritis 13, 20, 26, 35, 37t, 39f, 43, 47, 54, 56f, 64, 67f, 91, 97, 104, 160, 175, 188, 188f, 189f, 248, 267, 275, 293, 301, 354, 357
    arthroplasty in 60
    clinical features of 26
    contractures in 293
    conventional management of 43
    deformities in 293
    etiopathogenesis 26
    management of 26, 43, 44, 44t
    prevention 48
    treatment of 43f, 44
Rheumatoid disease 35
    classification of 36
    foot and ankle in 301
Rheumatoid factor 13, 26, 45
    negative 160
    positive 160
    test 30
Rheumatoid foot 301
Rheumatoid hand 275
    and wrist, surgery for 55
    deformities in 294f
Rheumatoid knee 55f
Rheumatoid lesions 55
Rheumatoid lung 29
Rheumatoid nodules 29, 29f, 66, 302
Rheumatoid nodulosis, accelerated 66
Rheumatoid tenosynovitis 55
Rheumatoid vasculitis 29
Rheumatoid wrist, arthroplasty of 275, 276
Rheumatologic disease 128
Rheumatologic joint diseases 40
Rickets 161
Rifabutin 178
Rifampicin 174
Rifampin 177
Riley-Day syndrome 128
Rilonacept 49
Risedronate 154
Rituximab 32, 50, 164
Rofecoxib 105
Romberg test 242
Romosozumab 139
Ropes test 269
Rotational ankle injuries 316
Rotator cuff 11
Rotator interval, synovitis of 226f
Rubella 26

S

Sacral slope 83
Sacroiliac arthritis, active 164, 165t
Sacroiliitis 73, 75, 91-93
Saddle nose 70
S-adenosyl methionine 255
Salicylates, coadministration of 107
Salivary glands 34
Salmonella 68, 92
Salpingitis 92
Sanders and Frykberg classification 306t
Sanders classification 307f
Sarcoidosis 191, 191f
    pediatric 161
Sarcopenia 15
Sarilumab 47, 50, 51
Satellite myofascial point 228
Sausage digit appearance 38, 188
Sauvé-Kapandji procedure 56
Scaphoid, fixed deformity of 286f
Scaphotrapezial trapezoid 289
Scapula 149
Schober's test 74, 75
Schwannomas 65
Scleritis 29
Sclerodactyly 66, 66f
Scleroderma 34, 161, 190, 267
Sclerosis, multiple 378
Sclerostin and Dickkopf blocks 140
Sclerostin antibody 140f
Sclerotherapy 64
Scurvy 161
Sea urchin spines 114
Secukinumab 47, 50, 51
Selective estrogen receptor modulators 134
Selective serotonin reuptake inhibitors 250

Sensitivity test 312*f*
Sensory
   disturbances 229
   hyper-responsiveness 247
   neuropathy 310
   symptoms 281
Sepsis, chronic 113
Septic
   arthritis 111, 161, 194, 326
   bursitis 104
Seronegative spondyloarthropathies 91
Serotonin-noradrenalin reuptake inhibitor 251
Serum alkaline phosphatase 150
Sexually transmitted infection 70
Sharpey's fibers 74
Shigella 68
Shock absorber 263
Short wave diathermy 234
Shoulder 54, 198
   biomechanics of 11
   distension 222
   dysfunction 215
   hydrodilatation of 222, 223
   injections, intra-articular 220
   mobilization of 219
   replacement 369
   right 218*f*
Shoulder joint 11, 187, 216
   distension of 224*f*
Sicca syndrome 29, 243
Sickle cell
   disease 382, 384*f*
   leg ulcer, bilateral 385*f*
Silica dust, exposure to 13
Silica exposure 15
Silicone 97
   metacarpophalangeal joint arthroplasty 272, 277
Single gene disorders 19
Single nucleotide polymorphism 241
Single-photon emission computed tomography 129
Sinus 180
   tubercular 173
Sirukumab 44, 47, 50, 51
Sjögren's syndrome 17, 21, 22, 29, 34, 67, 161
   secondary 15
Skeletal effects 136
Skeletal surgery 195
Skeletal tuberculosis, treatment of 176
Skin
   incision 282*f*
   lesions 68, 92
      nonspecific 65
Sleep disturbances 229, 240
Sleep dysfunction 242
Small intestine submucosa 315
Small joint affection 275
Smith-Peterson osteotomy 83, 84
Smoking 13, 15, 128, 141
Smooth muscle cells 382
Social responsibility, principle of 348
Sodium
   fluoride 139
   hyaluronate injection 220
   oxybate 251

Soft tissue 58
   and bony procedures 332
   assessment of 34
   balancing 55*f*
   changes 34
   procedures 330
   reconstruction 272
   rheumatology 35
   severe 278
Soluble human leukocyte antigen 338*f*
Somatic cells 351
Sore throat 247
Spa therapy 254
Spinal ankylosis 73, 78
Spinal column 78
Spinal cord 87
   hematoma 89
   injury, traumatic 378
Spinal disease 77
Spinal flexibility, maintain 75
Spinal fracture 86
   risk of 86
Spinal osteopenia 75
Spinal structure, abnormal 87
Spine 54, 74, 198, 339
   biomechanics of 11
   deformity 54
   enthesopathy in 81
   natural history of 78
   surgery 78
   tubercular 176
Spinopelvic parameters, measurement of 83*f*
Spondylitis 74, 92, 93
Spondyloarthritis 21, 73
Spondyloarthropathy 73, 91
Sports
   equipment, designation of 5
   injuries 367, 370
Spurling's test 281
Staphylococcus 179
Static deformity 325
Stem cell 335, 345, 350, 369, 372, 381, 382
   adipose-derived 342
   application of 338
   dynamics of 336, 336*fc*
   factor 14
   history of 335
   intra-arterial injection of 369
   mechanism of action of 337
   neurogenic signaling of 372
   properties 335
   rescue 356
   research 348-350, 350*fc*, 351
      categories of 351*t*
   therapy 378, 379
   transplantation 356
   types of 336, 369
Stenosing tenosynovitis 205, 292
Stepper exercises 221*f*
Sternal-rib complex 85
Sternomental distance 89
Steroid 143
   exposure, risk factor of 368
   injection 202, 319*f*
      intra-articular 226
   intra-articular 124

Stevens-Johnson syndrome 106
Stiffness 243, 267
Still's disease 267
Strain 10*t*
Streptococci 26
Streptomycin 177
Stressor, preceding 237
Stress-strain curve 199*f*
Stretching 233
Stroke 27, 372, 377
Stromal cells 361
Stromal vascular fraction 343, 345
Strontium ranelate 138
Suave-Kapandji procedures 271
Subarachnoid block 89
Subchondral bone 74, 119, 120
Subchondral sclerosis 318*f*
Subscapular strengthening 221*f*
Substantial evidences 314
Subsynovium 3, 3*f*, 4
Subtalar arthrodesis 307
Subtalar joint, normal 318*f*
Subungual exostosis 64
Subungual hyperkeratosis 68
Subungual verruca 64
Sulfapyridine 44
Sulfasalazine 31, 32, 43, 44, 60, 164
   doses of 48
Sulfinpyrazone 107
Sunlight, exposure to 150
Supracondylar osteotomy 195
Supramalleolar osteotomy 321*f*
Suprascapular nerve block 222
Supraspinatus 11
   tendon 200
Surgeon's lens 271
Surgical carpal tunnel release 283
Surgical release, complications of 283
Swan neck deformities 27, 58, 66, 268, 272, 293
Swelling 192
Symmetric oligoarthritis 68
Symptoms severity scale 245*b*
Syndesmophytes 74, 75
Syndesmotic nonunion 55
Synovectomy 54, 166, 195, 304
Synovial
   biopsy 55, 176, 194
   cell receptors 119
   disease 38
   effusion 36*f*, 37*f*, 39*f*
   hypertrophy 37, 173
   osteochondromatosis 97
   proliferation 36
   tissue 194*f*
Synovial fluid 4, 7, 36*f*, 40, 110, 113
   analysis 31, 122, 269, 269*t*
   composition of 4*f*
   examination 103, 176
   rheology 4
   wet preparations 114*b*
Synovial joints 3, 3*f*, 4, 7, 113
   neural innervation of 9*t*
Synovial membrane 3
   functions 3
Synoviorthesis 195

Synovitis 35-37, 37t, 60, 120, 121, 302
   active 166
   acute 110
   inflammatory 13
Synovium 3, 3f, 4, 372
   hyperplastic 194
Syphilis 70
   type of 70
Syphilitic gumma 70
Syringomyelia 196
Systemic arthritis 164, 165, 187
Systemic biomechanics 5
Systemic consequences 15
Systemic diseases 187
Systemic inflammation 141
   role of 141fc
Systemic inflammatory response syndrome 311
Systemic lupus erythematosus 17, 18, 65, 65f, 97, 161, 267
Systemic sclerosis 17, 66, 66f
Systemic vasculitis 67
   ulcer of 68f

T

T cell 14, 18f, 43
   activated 50
   depletion of 357
Tabes dorsalis 196
Tacrolimus 102
Tai chi and yoga 254
Takakura classification 318t
Talar osteonecrosis 320
Tamoxifen 134
Tarsal tunnel syndrome 210, 302
Technetium bone scan, leukocyte-labeled 305
Telangiectasia 66
Temporomandibular joint, disorders of 236
Tenderness 242
Tendinitis 97, 199
Tendinopathy 199
   epidemiology 199
   etiopathogenesis 200, 201
   molecular mechanism in 200
   pathogenesis of 200f
   treatment for 199
      modalities for 211
Tendinosis 199
Tendo-Achilles sonography 39
Tendon 41, 108, 109, 201, 263, 264, 301, 339, 367
   biomechanical functions of 199f
   disease 37, 213
   disorders 199
      types of 200f
   functional biomechanics of 199
   injury 212
      stages of 201
   metabolism, altered 201
   pathology 34
   rupture 58, 272
   sites of 74
   tears 37
   transfer 58
   xanthomas 37

Tennis elbow 200, 202f, 203f
   rehabilitation for 203, 204f
   splint 202f
Tenosynovial effusion 37, 39f
   sausage finger to 39f
Tenosynovial proliferation 37
Tenosynovitis 36, 38, 39f, 199
Teres minor 11
Teriparatide 139
Tetracycline 113
Thenar atrophy 280
Theophylline 106
Therapeutic effectiveness 368
Thermal injury 201
Thiazides 102
Thiazolidinediones 129
Thomine fascia 295
Thoracic kyphosis 74, 82
Thoracic osteotomy correction 83
Thoracolumbar
   fractures 87
   kyphotic deformity 81
   region 11
Thrombocytopenia 50
Thrombopenia 106
Thumb 27, 58
   deformities 272
   carpometacarpal joint of 279, 287
Thyroid
   acropachy 190, 190f
   dysfunction disorders 215
   hormones 129
Thyromental distance 89
Thyrotropin-releasing hormone 240
Tibial defect 62f
Tibial tendinitis, posterior 210
Tibialis posterior
   primary function of 208
   tendinitis 208
Tibialis tendon dysfunction, classification of posterior 208
Tiludronate 135, 154
Tinel's sign 279
Tinel's test 288
Tissue
   biomechanics 5
   harmonic imaging 35
Tobacco 65
Tocilizumab 47, 50, 51
Toe
   nail dystrophy 92
   off 10
   spacer 329f
   straightening belt 329f
Tophaceous deposits 97
Tophi 97, 103, 104
   large 107
Topical capsaicin 63
Total alkaline phosphatase 154
Total ankle arthroplasty 321
Total contact cast 314f
Total hip
   and knee replacements 167
   replacement 77, 368
Total joint replacement 195, 275
   arthroplasty 107

Total knee
   arthroplasty 362
   replacement 55f
Total wrist
   arthrodesis 276
   arthroplasty 271, 276, 277f
Trabecular bone 142
Tracheal rupture 88
Traditional Chinese medication 124
Tramadol 123, 251, 257
Transcricothyroid instillation 90
Transdiscal fracture 88f
Transverse carpal ligament 282f
Trapezium 58
Trauma 64, 161, 283
Triamcinolone 162
   hexacetonide 168
Triangular fibrocartilaginous complex 263
Tricyclic antidepressants 250
Trigger factors 241
Trigger finger 205, 206f, 292
   fate of 206
   staging of 206
Trigger point
   injection 232, 233f, 257
   types of 228
Tropisetron 232, 251
Tubercular arthritis, X-ray of 175f
Tubercular lesions, types of 173
Tubercular spine, X-rays of 175f
Tubercular spondylitis 175, 181f
Tuberculin skin test 49, 174
Tuberculosis
   diagnosis of 176
   drug-resistant 183
Tuberculous
   arthritis 179
   cavity 175
   dactylitis 191
   spondylitis 179
Tumor necrosis factor 45, 47, 49, 54, 60, 270
   inhibitors 47, 77
Tumor, brown 148
Turner's and Klinefelter's syndromes 128
Twin study 20
Typical deformity 57

U

Ulcer
   and regenerative medicine 381
   healing, mechanism of 381
   nonhealing 314
   venous 385f
Ulcerative colitis 20
   bowel inflammation 93
Ulnar deviation 66
Ulnar digital nerve 297f
   transposition of 298
Ulnar drift 268
Ulnar head arthroplasty 277
Ulnar nerve
   branch of 282f, 283f
   entrapment 279, 283
Umbilical cord 362, 372
Urate crystals, deposition of 101f

Urethral discharge 92
Uric acid 98, 100f, 102f, 107, 115
   crystals 102f
   degradation of 97
   overproduction of 98, 99
   synthesis 106
   under excretion of 98
   urolithiasis 97
Urolithiasis 98
Uveitis
   recurrent 78
   treatment of 167

V

Valgus deformity 306
Valgus knee 61f
Vascular endothelial growth factor 345
Vasculitis 34
Vaughan-Jackson
   deformity 293
   syndrome 58
Venlafaxine 250
Vertebral compression fractures 131
Vertebral fracture, types of 86
Vertebral osteotomy 77
Vertebroplasty bone cement 132
Vertigo 242
Viral diseases 237
Visceral organs, protection of 3

Visceral pain 247
Visual impairment 310
Vitamin
   A 128
   B_{12} deficiency 228
   D 129, 133, 150, 241
      level 150
      metabolism, abnormal 147
   D deficiency 141, 147, 150t, 228
      treatment of 150
Volar tenosynovitis 55
Voluntariness, principle of 348
Vomiting 105, 123
von Willebrand's disease 192
Vulnerable population, selection of 349
Vulvovaginitis 92

W

Wagner ulcer classification system 311t
Walking aids 122, 275, 318
Warfarin 106
Warning signs 269
Weakness 230
   type of 230
Wedge osteotomy 83
Wegener granulomatosis 67
Weight loss 75, 91, 173
Wheel exercises 221f
Widespread pain index 244, 245b

Wilson index 89
Wnt pathway 140f, 373
Wolff's law 5
Wound
   complications 55
   healing problems 321
Wright's stain 113
Wrist 54, 271, 279, 283
   and hand, anatomy of 263
   arthrodesis 56, 275, 276f
   arthroplasty, first 276
   dorsal approach to 56f
   extensor tendons in 264f
   fusion 275
   skeletal articulations of 263f
   volar aspect of 55

Y

Yawning 250
Yersinia 68
   antigen 73
Yoga 254

Z

Z deformity 27, 288
Zig-zag incisions 57
Zoledronic acid 154
Zolendronate 154
Z-thumb deformity 66

EU GSPR Authorised Reprsentative
Logos Europe, 9 rue Nicolas Poussin
1700, La Rochelle, France
Phone: +33 (0) 6 67 93 73 78
E-mail: contact@logoseurope.eu